C0-AWE-458

MAKING WOMEN'S MEDICINE MASCULINE

Making Women's Medicine Masculine

The Rise of Male Authority in Pre-Modern Gynaecology

MONICA H. GREEN

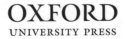
OXFORD
UNIVERSITY PRESS

RG
51
.G74
2008

OXFORD
UNIVERSITY PRESS

Great Clarendon Street, Oxford OX2 6DP

Oxford University Press is a department of the University of Oxford.
It furthers the University's objective of excellence in research, scholarship,
and education by publishing worldwide in

Oxford New York

Auckland Cape Town Dar es Salaam Hong Kong Karachi
Kuala Lumpur Madrid Melbourne Mexico City Nairobi
New Delhi Shanghai Taipei Toronto

With offices in

Argentina Austria Brazil Chile Czech Republic France Greece
Guatemala Hungary Italy Japan Poland Portugal Singapore
South Korea Switzerland Thailand Turkey Ukraine Vietnam

Oxford is a registered trade mark of Oxford University Press
in the UK and in certain other countries

Published in the United States
by Oxford University Press Inc., New York

© Monica H. Green 2008

The moral rights of the author have been asserted
Database right Oxford University Press (maker)

First published 2008

All rights reserved. No part of this publication may be reproduced,
stored in a retrieval system, or transmitted, in any form or by any means,
without the prior permission in writing of Oxford University Press,
or as expressly permitted by law, or under terms agreed with the appropriate
reprographics rights organization. Enquiries concerning reproduction
outside the scope of the above should be sent to the Rights Department,
Oxford University Press, at the address above

You must not circulate this book in any other binding or cover
and you must impose the same condition on any acquirer

British Library Cataloguing in Publication Data
Data available

Library of Congress Cataloging in Publication Data
Data available

Typeset by Laserwords Private Ltd, Chennai, India
Printed in Great Britain
on acid-free paper by
Biddles Ltd, King's Lynn, Norfolk

ISBN 978–0–19–921149–4

1 3 5 7 9 10 8 6 4 2

Contents

University Libraries
Carnegie Mellon University
Pittsburgh, PA 15213-3890

Preface

In 1449, an Italian humanist named Francisco Filelfo wrote excitedly to Filippo Pelliccione, a physician in Milan, asking him, indeed begging him, to be allowed to borrow 'a very ancient book' in Pelliccione's possession. According to Filelfo's letter, the book contained the medical writings of Celsus, Soranus, Apuleius, '. . . and even certain women'.[1] Filelfo didn't mention it, but the 'certain women' were associated with several of the dozen different texts that made up the latter half of the codex, all of which addressed one very specialized medical subject: gynaecology. Nearly a century later, John Leland, an English poet and antiquary, travelled around English religious houses that were now, since the break with Rome, under the authority of King Henry VIII. At the male Augustinian priory of St John the Baptist in Launde (Leicestershire), he found 'The Little Book of Gemissa, for Cleopatra, on the Menses and the Uterus' (*Gemissae libellus ad Cleopatram de menstruis et matrice*). Perhaps reconsidering the potential uses of the text for his reproductively beleaguered king, he crossed out this title and renamed it 'Cleopatra, on Generation' (*Cleopatra de genitura*).[2] For both these Renaissance seekers of 'antiquities', female authorities on women's medicine were an intriguing curiosity. As 'antiquities', however, they were also a thing of the past.

At exactly the same time the non-physicians Filelfo and Leland were engaging in their antiquarian quests, the field of gynaecology was exploding into a fully fledged subdiscipline of medicine. By the end of the sixteenth century, it would be represented not only by dozens of newly published books, including a massive 1097-page oversized compendium, *The Books of Gynaecology* of 1597 (by then in its third edition), but by university lectures, a published list of authorities in the field, and even its own 'insider' controversies. Although there is no evidence that any sixteenth-century physicians or surgeons confined their practice to women's diseases or took on specialist identities as 'gynaecologists', gynaecology had reclaimed from 'the ancients' both its name (*gynaikeia*, from the Greek for 'women's matters') and its rationale for why it should exist as a specialized field. But now, unlike Antiquity, there was no longer any association between the branch of medicine that topically addressed women and female

---

[1] Francisco Filelfo, *Epistolarum familiarum libri VI* (Venice, 1502), f. 43r, as cited in Ann Ellis Hanson, 'The Correspondence between Soranus, Antonius and Cleopatra' (forthcoming); all translations unless otherwise noted are my own. See Chapter 6 below for more on the history of this 'very ancient book'.

[2] T. Webber and A. G. Watson, *The Libraries of the Augustinian Canons* (London: British Library, 1998), p. 104. Leland rarely paid any attention to medical books, which may help explain his difficulty in figuring out that his *Gemissa* was no doubt a corruption of *Genecia* ('Gynaecology').

authority. When at the beginning of the next century the German physician Johannes Georg Schenck compiled a comprehensive list of 'Greek, ancient Latin, Arab, "medieval" and modern Latin and vernacular medical authors who wrote on gynaecology', he could identify some fifty-six individual male authors but only three women—the latter all situated in the long distant past of Antiquity.[3] Neither Schenck nor any sixteenth-century gynaecological writer would acknowledge a medieval or 'modern' woman as his peer.

This sixteenth-century transformation of gynaecology is the end of my story, not its beginning. For I shall argue in this book that the traditions of medical knowledge and practice represented by *The Books of Gynaecology*—a collection of twenty-eight treatises, all of which, with but one exception, were composed (or allegedly composed) by male authors—were in fact a long time in formation. The sixteenth-century gynaecological writers effected a nearly total evisceration of their field, rejecting or simply ignoring the opinions and teachings of medical writers from the previous half millennium. But even if they could not admit it, they had inherited from them something more important: they had inherited the *social structures* as well as the intellectual traditions that allowed men to be authorities in the field of women's medicine. 'Gynaecology' as a specialist field of medical knowledge had indeed been born, but it was a masculine birth—a birth without female involvement, either as maternal principle or assisting midwife.[4]

This transformation in the shifting authorities of women vs. men in the field of women's medicine is all the more remarkable in that what had served as the leading text throughout most of Europe from the late twelfth well into the fourteenth century (and in certain areas, into the sixteenth) was credited to a female author, 'Trotula' of Salerno. Modern researches have shown that 'Trotula' was originally the *title* of a compendium on women's medicine, not its author, though significant parts of the work do indeed derive from a historic twelfth-century female author, Trota (or Trocta) of Salerno. The other parts of the work were male-authored, yet Trota's existence and that of other female practitioners in Salerno made the metamorphosis from the title *Trotula* to the authoress 'Trotula' believable. At least through the fourteenth century many male intellectuals assumed it to be natural that knowledge on women's bodies should

---

[3] Johannes Georg Schenck, *[PINAX] auctorum in re medica, graecorum, latinorum priscorum, Arabum, Latinobarbarum, Latinorum recentiorum, tum et peregrinis linguis cluentium, Exstantium, MS. promissorum vel desideratorum: qui gynaecia, sive muliebria pleno argumento sive ex instituto scriptis excoluerunt et illustrarent* (Strasburg: Lazar Zetzner, 1606). See Chapter 6 below for more on Schenck's *Pinax*.

[4] My use of the term 'masculine birth of gynaecology' throughout this book is a deliberately ironic allusion to the 1603 essay by the English natural philosopher Francis Bacon called *The Masculine Birth of Time*. In that work, Bacon claimed that natural science—reasoned empiricism in all its glory—held the power to restore mankind's rightful dominion over nature that had been lost because of Eve's sin. Quite unsubtly, Bacon added the subtitle 'The Great Instauration of Man's Dominion Over the Universe'.

come from a female authority, and it is therefore unsurprising that 'Trotula' may well have been the most widely read female author in all of high medieval Europe.[5]

Yet both Trota and the author-figure 'Trotula' were anomalies. As this book will show, neither in twelfth-century Salerno nor at any point thereafter did male practitioners, as a group, *not* engage in gynaecological care at some level. Certain individual male practitioners, to be sure, may have refused to treat female patients, either out of a sense of ignorance of women's bodies or a belief that intimate contact with a woman would somehow negatively affect them. And many female practitioners existed who took up that slack; at least one even publicly challenged men to keep out of women's affairs. But there is far too much evidence—textual, iconographic, and anecdotal—to argue that men were completely uninvolved with women's healthcare, including conditions of the reproductive organs. This same evidence also shows that women, however much they continued to attend to the medical concerns of themselves or other women, did not have anything like a *monopoly* over the production of knowledge on or care of the female body. In fact, as this book will demonstrate, male involvement with women's medicine, both medical (control of diet and use of drugs to affect internal conditions) and surgical (the treatment of disorders on or near the surface of the body), increased substantially between the twelfth and sixteenth centuries. Far from being a 'modern' transformation, the masculinization of women's medicine is instead a fundamental feature of western medicine down to its medieval roots.

These are large claims and, to understand them, a crucial distinction must be made, for on this hangs my story. Although obstetrics and gynaecology are not everywhere as tightly linked as they now are in the contemporary United States (and even here they are being uncoupled due to concerns over obstetrical malpractice insurance), modern western medicine has tended to keep them closely associated so that for most observers 'obstetrics and gynaecology' (OB/GYN) are inherently one. And that they are, in so far as both fields necessarily take the organs and physiological functions unique to the female body as their particular concern. This ontological linking of OB/GYN was true of ancient Greek and Roman cultures, and may have been true of other historical societies as well. Yet a linkage of obstetrics and gynaecology based on shared anatomical focus need not

---

[5] Although medieval female authors such as Marie de France, Margery Kempe, Heloise, and others have gotten far more attention from modern scholars, 'Trotula's' work enjoyed a wider *medieval* circulation than any of these. Of the 200 or so Latin and vernacular exemplars of the *Trotula* texts (both extant and attested), over half bear Trota or 'Trotula's' name—a figure all the more remarkable in that two of the three texts that made up the ensemble were anonymous. References to 'Trotula' in such widely circulating texts as Peter of Spain's *Thesaurus pauperum* and Chaucer's *Canterbury Tales* would have also increased her fame. Only the twelfth-century nuns Elizabeth of Schönau and Hildegard of Bingen rivalled her, in the latter case largely because a posthumous collection of her prophecies was so popular; like most other female authors, all Hildegard's other works (including her medical ones) now exist in only a handful of copies.

necessarily dictate that they remained linked in the intellectual frameworks of learned medicine, nor that the social structures of medicine necessarily assigned practice in the two fields to a single group of healers. I will argue here that the gendering of gynaecology took a different path than that of obstetrics, with the result that by the end of the Middle Ages, the two fields were in practice distinct: while care of uncomplicated births remained in the hands of women, gynaecological care (as well as certain aspects of emergency obstetrical care) had passed into the hands of men.

One of the reasons why this very obvious split has not previously been noticed is that modern narratives of the male 'take-over' of women's medicine in Europe (which have themselves overgeneralized from the peculiar English case as if it were true of western cultures generally) are actually narratives about the take-over of midwifery. Female midwives, so the story goes, had a largely unchallenged monopoly up through the eighteenth century, at which point men-midwives began to push them out.[6] Rarely acknowledged is the fact that female midwives really only had a monopoly on normal births; it was already considered normative and acceptable two centuries earlier to call in male surgeons in cases of difficult labour. Yet aside from a 1990 study of the late medieval iconography of Caesarean birth that dated the entry of surgeons into the birthing room to the fifteenth century, little has been made of this fact that early modern obstetrics was 'always already' ambiguously gendered.[7]

Moreover, previous studies, by privileging childbirth as the most important aspect of women's health concerns, have overlooked the fact that long before the eighteenth century male practitioners had also been recognized as competent, and perhaps even inherently more competent, than female practitioners in the treatment of women's gynaecological complaints generally.[8] The present study

[6] A leading textbook on early modern women's history exemplifies the common opinion that the trajectories of obstetrics and gynaecology were similar: 'Women turned to midwives and other women for help with a variety of menstrual ailments, and *by the eighteenth century* they also consulted male physicians' (emphasis added); Merry E. Wiesner, *Women and Gender in Early Modern Europe*, 2nd edn (Cambridge: Cambridge University Press, 2000), p. 56.

[7] Studies of early modern midwifery are now extensive and can readily be identified. Of these, only Adrian Wilson, *The Making of Man-Midwifery: Childbirth in England, 1660–1770* (Cambridge, MA: Harvard University Press, 1995), has examined in detail the extent of male emergency obstetrical care. The 1990 study of Caesarean imagery is Renate Blumenfeld-Kosinski, *Not of Woman Born: Representations of Caesarean Birth in Medieval and Renaissance Culture* (Ithaca, NY: Cornell University Press, 1990).

[8] This point was already made on the basis of a broad survey of evidence more than eighty years ago by Carl Oskar Rosenthal, 'Zur geburtshilflich-gynaekologischen Betätigung des Mannes bis zum Ausgange des 16. Jahrhunderts', *Janus* 27 (1923), 117–48 and 192–212, yet his argument seems to have fallen on deaf ears. In a 1977 essay, 'The Changing Relationship Between Midwives and Physicians During the Renaissance', *Bulletin of the History of Medicine* 51, 550–64, Thomas G. Benedek, who was apparently unaware of Rosenthal's work, spoke of the 'paradox' of learned male physicians having the authority to supervise midwives even though they presumably had no practical experience in routine obstetrics. As I argue in this book, since 'authority' was seen to reside more in book-learning than in hands-on experience, there was no paradox at all. My thanks to

does not contradict the received narrative about female control over normal births, yet by broadening the definition of 'women's medicine' to encompass *all* aspects of the care received by women and by placing questions of the gendering of women's medicine into a longer trajectory, it demonstrates that the ambiguous gendering of early modern obstetrics is but a stage in a longer process that had its roots several centuries earlier.

'Gynaecology', if medievals and early moderns had regularly used the term, would have been understood to encompass almost every aspect of care of a female patient. The medieval physician, in order to develop a particular knowledge of his or her patients' condition, should always calculate their sex along with their age and other contingent factors into a diagnosis. Women's urine was always to be assessed differently than men's when the physician examined it for diagnostic indications, and one of the crucial precepts of the Hippocratic-Galenic model of medicine that dominated western European medicine up through the seventeenth century was that maintenance of women's menstruation (which we now categorize as 'simply' a gynaecological concern) was at the core of what constituted overall health for a woman. Irregular menstruation was not only a sign of some affliction that might impact on fertility, but it could lead to breast cancer, heart disorders, suffocation, and even death.[9] When 'women's health' is defined in this broader way, we can begin to see that any practitioner who treated a female patient was to some extent necessarily a 'gynaecologist'.

As will be discussed in more detail throughout this book, the fact that the organs most specifically involved in women's key physiological function of menstruation were also the sex organs posed no small problem for the cross-sex *practice* of women's medicine. For, in a society that largely assumed heterosexual desire, any male access to the female reproductive/sexual organs could be seen as a sexual encounter. In a few cases, this concern foreclosed male involvement with women's diseases completely. Sometimes male practitioners were willing to address certain conditions but not others. Sometimes, however, and more and more commonly toward the end of the medieval period, concerns over sexual

Kevin Uhalde for sharing with me his observations from the classroom on why there is such general resistance to the idea of male expertise in gynaecology prior to the modern period.

[9] In focusing on the specific field of gynaecology, this book starts from the premise that 'women's diseases' (and therefore, sex differences) were, in fact, recognized to exist. To be sure, there were changing understandings of what these differences were and how they should be understood in formulating therapeutic responses to women's diseases (see, for example, the discussion of surgery in Chapter 2 below). For the purposes of my analysis here, however, it is sufficient to understand that sex differences were seen to lie not only in the *anatomical* differences between men and women, but, more importantly, in differences in their *physiological* processes. For challenges to the thesis that a 'one-sex model' prevailed prior to the eighteenth century, see Monica H. Green, 'Bodies, Gender, Health, Disease: Recent Work on Medieval Women's Medicine', *Studies in Medieval and Renaissance History* 3rd ser., 2 (2005), 1–49; Helen King, 'The Mathematics of Sex: One to Two, or Two to One?', *Studies in Medieval and Renaissance History* 3rd ser. 2 (2005), 47–56; and Michael Stolberg, 'A Woman Down to Her Bones: The Anatomy of Sexual Difference in Early Modern Europe', *Isis* 94 (2003), 274–99.

propriety demanded, not avoidance of female patients, but the deployment of delicate negotiation, verbal interrogation of the patient for her symptoms (sometimes with veiled language), and, most importantly, the employment of female surgeons, midwives, or untrained assistants to do the needed manual observations and operations. By the end of the Middle Ages, the taboo against male sight and touch of the female genitals was no longer absolute, and while midwives were still the normative attendants at uncomplicated births throughout western Europe, emergency obstetrics as well as routine gynaecological care was considered appropriate work for men.

So how did this social and intellectual transformation in the care of women's bodies come about? Indeed, how do we begin to put together a narrative of some of the most private concerns and interactions that medieval women and men faced? It is very rare, as we shall see, to find any detailed evidence of male practitioners' encounters with their female patients of the kind that has fruitfully been used to study women's medicine in more modern periods. We have no bedside charts, no patient diaries, no hospital admission records. Case histories are largely limited to the formulaic genre of the *consilium*, a kind of personalized diagnosis, prognosis, and regimen written for an individual patient that came into use in later medieval northern Italy. Even visual evidence, useful though it may be, demands careful evaluation within the conventions of pictorial representation. We are even more handicapped with respect to evidence for the practices of female healers.

Nevertheless, it is possible to piece together a history of the gendering of women's healthcare in medieval Europe. A surprisingly large body of medical literature that addresses women's health concerns survives from the Middle Ages.[10] The challenge is to explain why it exists and who was using it. In some cases, the 'who' question can be readily answered while the answer to 'why' can at least be inferred. In other cases, however, we come up against the medieval historian's most formidable challenge: the fact that so often we don't have names or other concrete data to attach to much of our evidence. How do we know if the anonymous author, the anonymous reader, or the anonymous practitioner was a woman or a man? I shall argue in Chapter 1 below that although the principal goal of gynaecological knowledge production and delivery was treatment of the sexed female body (meaning that we can assume the sex of the *patient*), for most of the historical actors that surrounded that body we simply cannot know for sure whether they themselves inhabited male or female bodies. Rather than focus on their physical sex, it is more useful for us to assess their social gender: that is, whether they *acted* as a man or a woman in the current definitions of 'masculine' or 'feminine' of their particular social context. It is also this question of *gender*

---

[10] A comprehensive listing of known western medieval gynaecological texts (including separately circulating excerpts) can be found in Monica H. Green, 'Medieval Gynecological Texts: A Handlist', in *Women's Healthcare in the Medieval West: Texts and Contexts* (Aldershot: Ashgate, 2000), Appendix, pp. 1–36.

that I will raise with respect to the creators and users of the main evidence we do have: the physical books that medieval people wrote, read, annotated, bought, sold, bequeathed, and inherited.

My focus on medical books is not a *faute de mieux* choice, occasioned simply by the fact that they survive. A history of medieval women's healthcare could, no doubt, be written entirely from saints' lives or canonization proceedings, culling from these documents written to affirm faith or generate belief tales of difficult birth, incurable diseases, and various attempts to seek out relief.[11] Such sources would, no doubt, probably better capture the world of orally transmitted medical knowledge and belief, a world that, quantitatively, must have far surpassed the culture of literate knowledge that makes up the bulk of my evidence here. While religious sources will be drawn on from time to time in the following pages, rather than showing a world of orality completely distinct from learned traditions such sources tend to confirm that even in the field of women's medicine the growing professionalism of medicine—one that was grounded fundamentally on the valorization of book learning—brought with it a marked masculinization. I argue that the knowledge that came from books began to be seen as *authoritative*: that is, it began to acquire a social power that oral knowledge did not have.[12]

Besides looking at who writes and who reads, of course, I am also looking at who is excluded from these practices. Women, I believe, did not 'lose out' in a struggle for control over gynaecological knowledge production or gynaecological practice because a dominant masculine culture targeted knowledgeable women for suppression. Although the period under discussion here witnessed the inauguration of the first medical licensing regulations, even once women were explicitly restricted to certain ancillary areas of practice there were no effective judicial mechanisms that totally eradicated female practitioners or that could compel or coerce women as patients to accept male practitioners as their caretakers. Rather, the definition of what constituted authoritative knowledge changed and women, because of their general exclusion from cultures of book learning, could not play the game that men did. Or to put it another way, instead of targeting knowledgeable women for suppression, learned masculine culture effectively prevented such women from coming into existence at all. The twelfth-and thirteenth-century literacy revolution in medicine had passed women by, and by the end of the medieval period, when female literacy levels were becoming quite significant, learned medicine—including that part of it that addressed

---

[11] An excellent example of the riches such religious sources can produce is Gabriela Signori, 'Defensivgemeinschten: Kreißende, Hebammen und "Mitweiber" im Spiegel spätmittelalterlicher Geburtswunder', *Das Mittelalter* 1 (1996), 113–34. On how canonization proceedings can be used as a source of medical history, see Joseph Ziegler, 'Practitioners and Saints: Medical Men in Canonization Processes in the Thirteenth to Fifteenth Centuries', *Social History of Medicine* 12 (1999), 191–225.

[12] I am not, of course, claiming that literate knowledge was inherently *better* in the sense of some imagined universal standard of empirical effectiveness. See the Conclusion below on questions of the efficacy of medieval gynaecological practices.

women's internal conditions—had already been defined as a masculine field in which women could claim no authority. Women's limited literacy, therefore, combined with cultural beliefs in women's minimal intellectual capacity and social norms that constrained the public behaviour of women, set clearly *gendered* boundaries to how women could interact with the culture of learned medicine. As will be argued at the end of this book, it was only once that playing field of literacy and advanced education was equalized in the nineteenth and twentieth centuries that women in the western medical tradition would once again achieve stature as learned authorities in women's medicine.

There were, as one would expect, geographical variations in all these trends: northern Europe exhibits less gender polarization than the south, for example, and even these regional categorizations are far too broad to capture many local peculiarities. Nevertheless, this study argues that it is legitimate to make certain claims about a broadly western European culture of women's medicine. Tied together by shared Latin intellectual traditions, among which, importantly, were the *Trotula* texts themselves, western Europe witnessed the creation of a medical culture that valued learned medicine as the best medicine. And men (even many who had never set foot in a university) were the ones who were learned. The norms of propriety that kept men from touching women's genitalia were ultimately trumped by the belief that theoretical understanding about what went on inside the body was more important than practical, manual experience in treating that body or even knowledge gained from the experience of living inside a female body. To be a woman was no longer an automatic qualification for either understanding women or treating the conditions that most commonly afflicted the female sex.

The dozen-plus years spent writing this book have allowed me to learn, in a very personal way, what we historians try to teach our students every day: that the historical moment in which one lives matters greatly in how one can craft a vision of the world and create a life (or, in this case, a historical project) within it. The historical moment in which I have been privileged to live has seen the birth and flourishing of a new era in women's history and its expansion into the truly interdisciplinary field of gender studies; radical developments in the history of the book in general and women's literacy in particular; and, in the field of medical history, the maturation of the study of medieval medicine and especially the phenomenon of vernacularization. I owe debts to scholars in all these fields, most especially to Nadia Margolis and Jocelyn Wogan-Browne, who gave crucial encouragement in tackling the literary aspects of this work, and Margaret Schleissner, for introducing me many years ago to the *Secreta mulierum* tradition; to Michael McVaugh and Linda Voigts, without whose magisterial studies of medieval scientific and medical writings (and their generosity with the same while still in draft!), this project would have been infinitely impoverished; and, most especially, to Montserrat Cabré i Pairet, Helen King, and Katharine

Park, with whom I have had the pleasure of debating 'What is women's medicine?' for many years.

There are countless others who deserve thanks for patiently answering my questions about virtually every topic covered in this book. Most of them are thanked by name in the footnotes, and for those whose name I forgot, know that I have not forgotten your kindness. Three 'group hugs': to the North Carolina Research Group on Medieval and Early Modern Women, which for many years sustained me with great food and even better conversation; to my new colleagues down the hall at the Arizona Center for Medieval and Renaissance Studies, who have truly created an oasis for medieval studies in the desert; and to all my colleagues down that 'virtual hall' of the Internet, the many contributors to the listserv 'medfem-l', who let me knock on their doors and share the best of the spirit of feminist scholarship. Finally, a collective thanks to all my students at the University of North Carolina at Chapel Hill, Duke University, and Arizona State University who over the years have taken my courses on women in medieval society and the history of women in science and medicine. Whether enthusiasts or sceptics of the stories I told them, their questions always helped me keep an eye on 'the big picture' of women's roles in medicine.

While still in utero, this book was tentatively announced as 'forthcoming' under the title *Women and Literate Medicine in Medieval Europe: Trota and the 'Trotula'*. This was planned as a cultural history of the *Trotula* that would include an edition of Trota's *Practica* as an appendix. As the manuscript grew, it became clear that the evidence I had collected for Trota's *oeuvre*, as well as other aspects of women's medical practices in Salerno, was substantial enough to merit publication separately. Readers can look for that material to appear elsewhere.[13]

Portions of several chapters were read before audiences at the Delaware Valley Medievalists Association, the Institute for the History of Medicine at The Johns Hopkins University, the University of Western Ontario, City University of New York, University of Pittsburgh, Medieval Academy of America, New Chaucer Society, Virginia Polytechnic Institute, University of Notre Dame, College of Physicians in Philadelphia, University of Michigan, and the American Association for the History of Medicine. My thanks to all these audiences for their helpful comments. Finally, I must thank the dozens, perhaps hundreds of librarians who over the last decade and a half have facilitated this study by sharing with this modern scholar the 'very ancient books' so many women in the past never would have been able to hold in their hands.

Data on the manuscripts of the *Trotula* were compiled over the course of many years through funding provided by the Josiah Charles Trent Memorial

---

[13] Preliminary results can be found in Monica H. Green, 'Reconstructing the *Oeuvre* of Trota of Salerno', in *La Scuola medica Salernitana: Gli autori e i testi*, ed. Danielle Jacquart and Agostino Paravicini Bagliani, Edizione Nazionale 'La Scuola medica Salernitana', 1 (Florence: SISMEL / Edizioni del Galluzzo, 2007), 183–233.

Foundation (Durham, North Carolina), the National Endowment for the Humanities, the Institute for Advanced Study (Princeton, New Jersey), and the National Humanities Center. A fellowship at the Radcliffe Institute for Advanced Study at Harvard University in 2001–2 allowed me both to dig deeper into the Salernitan context of Trota and to broaden my engagement with women's medicine in other fields, as did a fellowship in 2004 from the John Simon Guggenheim Memorial Foundation. Funds provided by Arizona State University supported the last phases of research.

This book is dedicated to Wesley, Marcia, Charlie, and Peter—because I never had the chance to say goodbye.

M. H. G.

List of Illustrations

List of Tables

List of Abbreviations

BAV	Vatican, Biblioteca Apostolica Vaticana
BLL	London, British Library
BNF	Paris, Bibliothèque Nationale de France
CTC	Cambridge, Trinity College
CUL	Cambridge, University Library
Green, 'Development'	Monica H. Green, 'The Development of the *Trotula*,' *Revue d'Histoire des Textes* 26 (1996), 119–203; repr. in Green, *Women's Healthcare* as Essay V
Green, 'Documenting'	Monica H. Green, 'Documenting Medieval Women's Medical Practice', in *Practical Medicine from Salerno to the Black Death*, ed. Luis García-Ballester, Roger French, Jon Arrizabalaga, and Andrew Cunningham (Cambridge: Cambridge University Press, 1994), pp. 322–52; repr. in Green, *Women's Healthcare* as Essay II
Green, 'Handlist I'	Monica H. Green, 'A Handlist of the Latin and Vernacular Manuscripts of the So-Called *Trotula* Texts. Part I: The Latin Manuscripts', *Scriptorium* 50 (1996), 137–75
Green, 'Handlist II'	Monica H. Green, 'A Handlist of the Latin and Vernacular Manuscripts of the So-Called *Trotula* Texts. Part II: The Vernacular Texts and Latin Re-Writings', *Scriptorium* 51 (1997), 80–104
Green, 'Possibilities'	Monica H. Green, 'The Possibilities of Literacy and the Limits of Reading: Women and the Gendering of Medical Literacy', in Green, *Women's Healthcare*, Essay VII, pp. 1–76
Green, 'Traittié'	Monica H. Green, ' "Traittié tout de mençonges": The *Secrés des dames*, "Trotula", and Attitudes Towards Women's Medicine in 14th- and Early 15th-Century France', in Marilynn Desmond, ed., *Christine de Pizan and the Categories of Difference* (Minneapolis: University of Minnesota Press, 1998), pp. 146–78; repr. in Green, *Women's Healthcare*, as Essay VI
Green, *Trotula*	Monica H. Green, ed. and trans., *The 'Trotula': A Medieval Compendium of Women's Medicine* (Philadelphia: University of Pennsylvania Press, 2001)

Green, *Women's Healthcare*	Monica H. Green, *Women's Healthcare in the Medieval West: Texts and Contexts*, Variorum Collected Studies Series, CS680 (Aldershot: Ashgate, 2000)
LWL	London, Wellcome Library for the History and Understanding of Medicine
OBL	Oxford, Bodleian Library

Introduction: Literacy, Medicine, and Gender

In June of 1410, a female surgeon, Perretta Petone, was brought before the royal tribunal of Paris on charges of unlicensed practice. Perretta never denied that she practised medicine. On the contrary, she proudly claimed that she had been trained by one of her relatives and several other practitioners in a small provincial town and that for the past eight years she had been practising in Paris, evidently with great success. Her patients themselves had demanded her release when she had first been imprisoned more than a year earlier. The intent of the corporation of surgeons that brought the charge, however, was to prove Perretta incompetent. And the key to their arguments was her literacy. According to Perretta's account, at a formal examination of her medical knowledge (which would normally have been performed by only three examiners) some dozen physicians and surgeons all interrogated her together, 'mocking her and eyeing her scornfully'. They took the medical book she had brought with her, a collection of remedies in French, and flipped through the pages in front of her, all the while drilling her with questions about how she prepared her medicines. When asked directly if she could read, Perretta said that she could. Her interrogators, however, concluded that 'she doesn't know an A from a bundle of sticks'.[1]

While Perretta was undergoing her humiliating ordeal in the courts at the Châtelet, there sat on the shelves of the nearby royal library at the Louvre a copy of a Latin medical book on women's medicine bearing the inscription 'Trotula, mistress of women' (*Trotula domina mulierum*). 'Trotula' was, besides the semi-mythical Cumaean Sybil, the only female author represented among the nearly 900 volumes that made up the French king's collection.[2] In fact, the royal library had originally had two copies of 'Trotula's' work: this Latin copy

---

[1] Geneviève Dumas, 'Les femmes et les pratiques de la santé dans le "Registre des plaidoiries du Parlement de Paris, 1364–1427"', *Canadian Bulletin of Medical History/Bulletin canadien d'histoire de la médecine* 13 (1996), 3–27. Dumas provides an analysis and a complete transcript of this case, though see also Laurent Garrigues, 'Les Professions médicales à Paris au début du XVe siècle: Praticiens en procès au parlement', *Bibliothèque de l'École des Chartes* 156 (1998), 317–67, for more on the medical context.

[2] Throughout this book, I shall use *Trotula* as a descriptive label to refer to any or all of the three texts that were eventually subsumed into the *Trotula* ensemble: *Conditions of Women* (*Liber de sinthomatibus mulierum*), *Treatments for Women* (*De curis mulierum*), and *Women's Cosmetics* (*De ornatu mulierum*). When referring to 'Trotula', the purported author of the whole *Trotula* ensemble, I use quotation marks in order to highlight the fact that 'she' is a scribal phantom. See below.

(which was probably rather unimpressive, since it was valued at the modest price of six sous in 1424 when the royal library was dispersed) and a French copy of 'the lesser and the greater *Trotula*' ('le petit et le grant Trotule'). Both copies had been acquired before 1373 by Charles V, who suffered from infertility in the early years of his marriage. Like Charles, a variety of readers in medieval Paris saw great utility in 'Trotula's' work. At least three copies of the Latin texts were owned by the college of the Sorbonne, while individual owners of Latin and vernacular copies ranged from university professors to medical students to surgeons. So renowned was 'Trotula', in fact, that both the Sorbonne and the Abbey of St Victor held works falsely attributed to her. Her name was also cited in non-medical contexts well into the fourteenth century as a premiere authority on women's nature.[3]

The practitioner of questionable literacy, Perretta, and the authoress of enviable fame, 'Trotula, mistress of women', would seem to have little in common. Yet it is the object of this book to show that they represent two extremes of a single spectrum of the ways in which women related to literate medicine in medieval Europe: that is, marginally. It was women's marginality *vis-à-vis* literate medical culture that would make them marginal in the process of creating written knowledge about their own bodies and diseases. By the time the Middle Ages came to a close, neither female practitioners like Perretta nor female textual authorities like 'Trotula' were deemed to have much relevance in the world of medical learning or practice, not even that part of it devoted to women's diseases.

FEMALE AUTHORITY, LICENSING, AND THE POWER OF BOOKS

Perretta's marginality is obvious: a widowed provincial woman, she is jailed, ridiculed, and driven out of practice because she was not able readily to recite the elements of medical theory found in books. 'Trotula's' marginality is more complex, yet it is ultimately akin to Perretta's. The textual figure of 'Trotula' grew up around a core of both lore about and the actual *dicta* of a historic twelfth-century woman, Trota of Salerno, a practitioner who, like Perretta, seems to have been exceptionally skilled in the treatment of men as well as women. Unlike Perretta—and indeed, unlike all but a tiny handful of other medieval women—Trota crossed the threshold into the realm of medical authorship.[4] But

---

[3] On the circulation of the *Trotula* in later medieval France, see Green, 'Traittié'. On the infertility of Charles and his wife, Jeanne de Bourbon, see Chapter 6 below.

[4] On the other documentable female medical writer from the twelfth century, the nun Hildegard of Bingen, see Chapter 1 below. For other written testimonia to women's medical practices, see Monica H. Green, 'Books as a Source of Medical Education for Women in the Middle Ages', *Dynamis: Acta Hispanica ad Medicinae Scientiarumque Historiam Illustrandam* 20 (2000), 331–69, and Chapter 3 below.

only by a few steps. For not only was she disengaged from the theoretical discourse that distinguished the medical writings of her male Salernitan peers, she was ultimately no more accepted as an equal by her fellow twelfth-century medical writers than was Perretta by her fellow surgeons in fifteenth-century Paris.

The figure of 'Trotula', a textually metastasized form of Trota, seems at first glance not to be marginal at all. The *Trotula*, recognized now as a compendium of three different texts of independent twelfth-century authorship, was generally understood in the Middle Ages to be a single text (or perhaps 'a lesser and a greater' pair of texts) by the eponymous author 'Trotula'. 'Trotula's' work was incorporated into handbooks of leading medical writings, and in libraries throughout Europe 'her' work stood side-by-side those of such medical and natural philosophical authorities as Aristotle, Avicenna, and Albertus Magnus. Yet in the very act of granting her a special authority within women's medicine, medieval physicians and natural philosophers also limited 'Trotula's' competence absolutely within those bounds. While it is perhaps ironic, it is not paradoxical that learned Parisian males, both medical practitioners and intellectuals more generally, could (up to a point) accept 'Trotula' as an authority while at the same time dismiss Perretta and indeed all female practitioners in Paris. In fact, 'Trotula' was herself fading into insignificance right around the time Perretta was put on trial. A fifteenth-century French translator of 'Trotula's' work not only simply failed to acknowledge her authorship of the text, he even misinterpreted her name as that of a *disease*.[5] By the following century, nobody any longer assumed that a woman, because she was a woman, would have any greater authority in the field of gynaecology than a man. On the contrary, the opposite was true.

The eclipsing of female practitioners as well as the learned authority 'Trotula' is remarkable, since several centuries earlier there was little to predict this outcome. The Latin *Trotula* texts, composed in southern Italy in the twelfth century, would go on to circulate throughout western Europe, from Spain to Poland, from Sicily to Ireland, and in most of those areas the authoress 'Trotula' would have enjoyed at least a modicum of fame. Likewise, female medical practitioners, marginal though they may have been, can be documented sporadically throughout western Europe and still played a necessary function in the delivery of healthcare to both women and men. But the three centuries separating the historic Trota in twelfth-century Salerno from Perretta in fifteenth-century Paris witnessed extraordinary shifts in the social positioning of medicine within medieval society. The early twelfth century was the last moment in western history when there were no legal restrictions whatsoever on medical practice.[6] Just as in Antiquity, the 'medical marketplace' was open to anyone who wished to lay claim to medical expertise. By the fifteenth century, some form of legal controls or regulation of medical practice had been instituted in what is now Spain, France, Italy, England, and parts of Germany. Although by no means universal, systems of licensing created

---

[5] See Chapter 4 below.   [6] See Chapter 1 below on the origins of medical licensing.

pockets of standardization of what constituted proper medical knowledge and medical skill. Literacy was not a *sine qua non* for licensing; most local licensing panels would conduct oral examinations of prospective licensees to ascertain the extent of their experience and their knowledge of drug lore, surgical technique, etc.[7] Nor were any legal impediments to licensing placed before women prior to the fourteenth century; while such impediments would be enacted thereafter, well into the fifteenth century we have evidence that, at least on an *ad hoc* basis, some women continued to practise medicine without hindrance.[8] Perretta herself would claim as much in 1410, asking why she was being singled out when there were so many other female practitioners in Paris 'of whom nobody demands anything'.

There was, nevertheless, a discernible consensus that licensing was a good thing and that reasonable criteria existed to determine who were the *best* individuals to license. With the rise of the universities out of the cathedral schools in the later twelfth century, medicine took its place as one of the learned disciplines. Precisely because regularized education created a cohort of similarly trained practitioners, authorities looking for some standard against which to assess medical competence began to see university education as the ideal. What university education had to offer was grounding in 'the principles of medical science' and 'verifiable experience'. With the introduction of an Arabic medical corpus into Latinate Europe in the late eleventh century, physicians in Salerno (and later Bologna, Paris, Padua, and Montpellier) could begin to claim to ground their medical beliefs and practices on a real philosophical basis.[9] Whereas empirics might regularly be successful in the cures they performed, they could not explain *why* their cures worked nor explain the causes or predict the outcome of a

---

[7] Danielle Jacquart, *Le milieu médical en France du XIIe au XVe siècle: En annexe 2e supplément au 'Dictionnaire' d'Ernest Wickersheimer* (Geneva: Librairie Droz, 1981), p. 84, notes that there is currently no evidence of university instruction for at least 35% of known Christian French male physicians between the mid 13th and the end of the 15th centuries, at least some of whom may have qualified simply by private study and then submission before an examining body. The most comprehensive collection of published licenses, that of Raffaele Calvanico, *Fonti per la storia della medicina e della chirurgia per il regno di Napoli nel periodo angioino (a. 1273–1410)* (Naples: L'Arte Tipografica, 1962), presents many cases of both men and women who are licensed despite being *ydiota* (illiterate).

[8] Evidence for formally licensed women in the 14th and 15th centuries comes from Spain, the southern Italian Kingdom of Naples, and certain areas of France. In the early 15th century, a 'poor bedeswoman Joan' sought permission from Henry IV of England to practise medicine 'without hindrance or disturbance from all folk'. If her request was granted (we don't know whether it was or not), it would have functioned as a *de facto* licence; see Eileen Power, 'Some Women Practitioners of Medicine in the Middle Ages', *Proceedings of the Royal Society of Medicine* 15, no. 6 (April 1922), 20–3. See also Chapter 3 and the Conclusion below for further evidence of women's medical practices.

[9] Mark D. Jordan, 'The Construction of a Philosophical Medicine: Exegesis and Argument in Salernitan Teaching on the Soul', *Osiris*, 2d ser., 6 (1990): 42–61; and 'Medicine as Science in the Early Commentaries on "Johannitius"', *Traditio* 43 (1987): 121–45; Danielle Jacquart, 'Aristotelian Thought in Salerno', in *A History of Twelfth-Century Philosophy*, ed. P. Dronke (Cambridge: Cambridge University Press, 1988), pp. 407–28.

disease. It was precisely this knowledge of 'hidden causes' that the new learned physicians—who began to style themselves *physicus* ('one learned in the science of nature') as well as *medicus* ('healer')—could claim to offer.[10]

Books were the bearers and transmitters and, indeed, the symbols, of this knowledge. As asserted in a general law passed for the Crown of Aragon in 1359, medical practitioners, just as much as lawyers, were defined by their books:

> we decree that no lawyer in cities, towns, or other significant places may practice law nor exercise the office of judge or assessor *if he does not have all the ordinary books of civil law, or at least the ordinary books of canon law,* or has not studied them for at least five years in a *studium generale*, which he must swear to have done. And we wish the same to be required of physicians in the art of medicine, except that it is enough for them to have studied for only three years in a *studium generale*.[11]

As in the case of Perretta's examination, the physical books themselves might become part of the probative process of competence. For a university-educated practitioner, it was not at all unusual that an examination for licensing involve asking the candidate to read a passage from a book and then offer an *ex tempore* oral commentary on it.[12]

The power of this claim to a 'philosophical' knowledge of medicine can be assessed most clearly among surgeons, who did not gain a firm foothold in the university hierarchy but who nevertheless repeatedly made claims similar to the university physicians to possess a 'science' of healing.[13] Although surgery had been largely passed over as an area of medical writing in twelfth-century Salerno, a written tradition that had begun in Italy *c.*1170 with the pragmatic and descriptive *Surgery* of Roger Frugardi would, by the beginning of the fourteenth century, be represented by fully theorized works by the Italians Bruno of Longobucco, William of Saliceto, Theodoric of Lucca, and Lanfranc of Milan, and the Frenchman Henri de Mondeville. Writing in the mid thirteenth century, Bruno of Longobucco was already identifying Latin literacy as a minimum requirement for practice.[14] Henri de Mondeville, who laid out his

---

[10] Jerome Bylebyl, 'The Medical Meaning of *Physica*', *Osiris*, 2nd ser., 6 (1990), 16–41.

[11] Luís García-Ballester, Michael R. McVaugh, and Agustín Rubio-Vela, *Medical Licensing and Learning in Fourteenth-Century Valencia, Transactions of the American Philosophical Society* 79, pt. 6 (Philadelphia: American Philosophical Society, 1989), p. 8, emphasis added.

[12] See, for example, the record of the examination of Pierre Calberte, bachelor of medicine, at Montpellier in 1307, cited in García-Ballester *et al.*, *Medical Licensing*, pp. 12–13.

[13] University training of surgeons is documented only at Montpellier and certain northern Italian universities, and even then they did not receive a full programme of study. It should be stressed, too, that university-trained physicians were always a numerical minority among the array of medical practitioners. Jacquart, *Milieu*, p. 246, for example, estimates that for Paris (a university town) between the years 1310 and 1329 (which included the year of Jacoba Felicie's trial), there were 84 physicians, 26 (at minimum) surgeons, 97 barbers, and 15 *mires* (empirical healers). It should remembered, too, that practitioners with university associations have a higher likelihood of being identified since their institutional affiliations themselves generate documents chronicling their careers.

[14] Susan P. Hall, 'The *Cyrurgia Magna* of Brunus Longoburgensis: A Critical Edition', DPhil thesis, Oxford University, 1957, p. 4: 'They [ideal surgeons] should be literate men [*uiri litterati*]

own simultaneously empirical and theoretical training as a model for others in the early fourteenth century, stressed that his Latin surgical text was intended for 'intelligent [practitioners], *especially literate ones*, who know at least the common principles of medicine and who understand the terminology of the art'.[15] By 1363, the Frenchman Guy de Chauliac would list literacy as the very first of four qualifications of the good surgeon.[16] While it can be questioned whether literacy alone had the transformative effect on the *practice* of surgery that Mondeville and others had hoped, literacy clearly played a major role in altering the status of surgeons and other practitioners outside the strict confines of the university, what I will call 'peri-university' circles. Some sixty-seven male authors of medical writings in France, for example, have no known university ties and many times that number owned medical books.[17]

This belief in the power of books to confer, not simply collected therapeutic knowledge but also the principles of medical science, was not confined to Latin medical literature. When Ramon Roquer, a surgeon from a small town in Catalonia, was accused, like Perretta, of unlicensed practice in 1338, he asserted that 'he had practised the art of surgery for a long time, and, although he was a layman and unlettered [i.e., not a cleric and not literate in Latin], *he owned good books* and had good cures to his credit'.[18] Ramon's books would probably have been in Catalan, into which at least half a dozen different surgical texts had been translated by the first half of the fourteenth century.[19] To be sure, Latin remained the main language for composition of theoretical medical texts through to the end of the Middle Ages. But just as in Catalonia, many parts of Europe witnessed an efflorescence of vernacular medical writing, often in the form of translations of Latin texts. Thus, in France, we find almost all the major surgical texts—Roger Frugardi, Bruno of Longobucco, Lanfranc, Henri de Mondeville, and Guy de Chauliac—available in French translation by the

---

or at least they should learn the art from someone who knows letters; for I think that hardly anyone who is completely without letters can comprehend this art'. See also Chapter 3 below.

   [15] Henri de Mondeville, *Chirurgia*, in *Die Chirurgie des Heinrich von Mondeville (Hermondaville): nach Berliner, Erfurter und Pariser codices*, ed. Julius Leopold Pagel (Berlin: August Hirschwald, 1892), p. 11.

   [16] Guy de Chauliac, *Inventarium sive Chirurgia magna*, ed. Michael R. McVaugh, with Margaret S. Ogden, Studies in Ancient Medicine, vol. 14, I and II (Leiden: Brill, 1997), vol. I, p. 9. (All citations from this edition will be from vol. 1 unless otherwise indicated.) Chauliac included a full training in medical theory and practice in his definition of literacy. The other qualifications were practical experience (including watching others work), 'ingeniousness' (by which he meant a combination of quick wit, nimble hands, and good eyes), and sound morals (including clinical prudence, chastity, sobriety, and mercy).

   [17] Jacquart, *Milieu*, pp. 199–205.

   [18] Garcia Ballester *et al.*, *Medical Licensing*, p. 9 (my emphasis).

   [19] My thanks to Lluís Cifuentes for sharing with me the results of his many years of research on Catalan scientific and medical texts (personal communication, 5 January 2003). Of course, Ramon may not have been referring specifically to surgical books at all but to remedy books or any number of other medical texts in Catalan; see Lluís Cifuentes i Comamala, *La ciencia en catala a l'edat mitjana* (Barcelona: Universitat de Barcelona, 2001).

fourteenth century, even though authorities in Paris still expected surgeons to have a modicum of Latin.[20] Literacy in at least the local vernacular languages could likewise be expected of apothecaries, who by 1329 in Valencia were assumed to be able to read prescriptions presented to them in the vernacular,[21] and who, in Paris at just about the same time, were being enjoined to have both a corrected copy of the pharmaceutical authority *Antidotary of Nicholas* and at least one literate person in the shop (preferably the master apothecary himself) who could read it.[22] Indeed, the fact that so many later medieval vernacular copies of surgical texts are almost hopelessly corrupt is itself an indication that the value of these books lay more in the symbolic aura of learning they granted to their possessors than any intrinsic knowledge they could have effectively conveyed.[23]

Ramon Roquer, the unlicensed Catalan surgeon, claimed that his prosecution was motivated by other envious surgeons, and there is ample evidence that many cases of prosecution were instigated by fellow practitioners who stood to benefit by removal of their competitors from the medical marketplace. But to cast these developments in licensing and learning as merely the manifestations of self-interest on the part of university-educated practitioners would be to slight evidence that there was a growing *general* belief in the ability of learned medicine to provide desirable medical care. In monasteries and nunneries, which ever since the time of Benedict had been expected to run their own infirmaries to care for their sick, there is widespread evidence for the employment of professional practitioners from outside the community to tend to their more grievously ill. These communities sometimes even signed contracts with licensed practitioners to ensure their attendance when needed.[24] Lay people as well, from the nobility to the middling urban classes, sought out the ministrations of learned

---

[20] On French surgical texts in general, see Helen Valls, 'Studies on Roger Frugardi's *Chirurgia*', PhD dissertation, University of Toronto, 1995; and Claude de Tovar, 'Les versions françaises de la *Chirurgia parva* de Lanfranc de Milan. Étude de la tradition manuscrite', *Revue d'Histoire des Textes* 12–13 (1982–3), 195–262. On Parisian surgeons' Latinity, see the intriguing observations in Geneviève Dumas, 'Les femmes', pp. 13–15. In 1396, the surgeons associated with the Confraternity of Saints Cosmas and Damian ordered that all new apprentices should be able to speak and write good Latin; see Cornelius O'Boyle, 'Surgical Texts and Social Contexts: Physicians and Surgeons in Paris, c.1270 to 1430', in *Practical Medicine*, pp. 156–85, at 183.

[21] García-Ballester, *et al.*, *Medical Licensing*, p. 6.

[22] Henri Denifle (ed.), *Chartularium universitatis Parisiensis* (Paris: Delalain, 1891–9; repr. Brussels: Culture et Civilisation, 1964), 2: 268–9.

[23] For examples of rather astounding levels of textual corruption, see Green, 'Traittié'; Sylvie Bazin-Tacchella, 'Adaptations françaises de la *Chirurgia Magna* de Guy de Chauliac et codification du savoir chirurgical au XVᵉ siècle', in *Bien dire et bien aprandre: Actes du colloque du Centre d'Études Médiévales et Dialectales de Lille III. 'Traduction, transposition, adaptation au Moyen Age'*, Lille, 22–24 septembre 1994, t. 14 (1996), pp. 169–88; and Joris Reynaert, 'Over medische kennis in de late Middeleeuwen: De Middelnederlandse vertaling van Lanfrancs *Chirurgia magna*', *Millenium: tijdschrift voor mimiddeleeuwse Studies* 13, n. 1 (1999), 21–30.

[24] See the evidence collected in Green, 'Books as a Source'.

practitioners and signed contracts with them to ensure their availability.[25] In later medieval Italy, patrician women not simply sought out learned practitioners for cases of infertility and other problems, but even willingly asked to be autopsied by them after their death so that the causes of their disease could be determined for the sake of their children.[26] To be sure, learned practitioners were never numerous enough to attend to the needs of the entire medieval populace, even in densely populated urban areas. Illiterate or only marginally literate practitioners could still be found everywhere and were often used in conjunction with the services of literate healers.[27] But whereas the illiterate empiric might have had the same chance of gaining a local reputation for excellence in healing as a book-learned practitioner at the beginning of the twelfth century, such possibilities for equal competition would have been quite rare by the fifteenth. Literacy is thus a key historical element in the changed landscape of medical licensing and practice in the high and later Middle Ages.

It is also a key element to understanding a broader function that medical literature came to perform in the later medieval period. Even as medicine was becoming more and more professionalized—more concentrated, that is, in the hands of practitioners who took on *identities* as practitioners and perhaps relied on medicine for a major part of their income—it was also developing a broader lay audience for written texts on health. Some readers were simply interested in regimens of health, guides to regulating the six 'non-naturals' (environmental and behavioural factors over which one had some control, such as air, food, sexual activity, and so forth). These interests in health maintenance would often be accompanied by interest in having random recipes or short tracts on the properties of particular herbs, such as betony or rosemary. At this level of reading, we find more or less comparable evidence of male and female interests.[28] Other non-professional readers, however, had more advanced interests, branching into studies of the humours and other elements of physiology, and also allied fields such as alchemy and astrology, which promised even more knowledge with which to control one's relation to the natural world. The genesis of these audiences was likewise a function of the literacy revolution, for we can locate many readers of this type among the mercantile, lawyerly, and notarial classes, those 'pragmatic

---

[25] Katharine Park, *Doctors and Medicine in Early Renaissance Florence* (Princeton: Princeton University Press, 1985), and 'Medicine and Magic: The Healing Arts', in *Gender and Society in Renaissance Italy*, ed. Judith C. Brown and Robert C. Davis (London: Longman, 1998), pp. 129–49; Michael R. McVaugh, *Medicine Before the Plague: Practitioners and Their Patients in the Crown of Aragon, 1285–1345* (Cambridge: Cambridge University Press, 1993); Joseph Shatzmiller, *Médecine et justice en Provence médiévale: Documents de Manosque, 1262–1348* (Aix-en-Provence: Publications de l'Université de Provence, 1989).

[26] Katharine Park, *Secrets of Women: Gender, Generation, and the Origins of Human Dissection* (New York: Zone, 2006).

[27] Park, 'Medicine and Magic'.

[28] Comparable, that is, in type, not in extent. See Chapters 3 and 4 below.

literates' who were increasing in number throughout this period.[29] For example, a grammar teacher and historiographer, Bonvesin de la Riva, estimated in 1288 that there were 1500 notaries in his native Milan, a city that at the time had no university.[30] The rise of such notarial classes was more intense in southern Europe, though by the mid fourteenth century comparable classes of literate, and exclusively masculine, functionaries could be found in urban northern Europe, the majority of whom would have had facility with Latin.[31] Little is known about the training of these bureaucrats, but it is apparent that they could form their own local masculine cultures with shared reading habits (often in the vernacular), such as that in which Geoffrey Chaucer participated at the court of Richard II in England.[32] Medical reading was not necessarily high on the agenda of such socially aspiring male readers, but it figured often enough in the libraries of lawyers, merchants, and gentry to constitute an important element of medical culture.[33] On the island of Majorca, for example, some 660 medical books (most in Latin, but some also in the vernacular) have been found in the possession of eighty-six different individuals between the thirteenth and the mid sixteenth century, at least forty-nine of whom are not professional medical practitioners but rather noblemen, merchants, artisans, and clerics. Aside from one Jewish woman, none of these owners was a woman.[34]

Neither the role of literacy in the processes of medical professionalization nor the rise of lay audiences of medical writings will come as a surprise, of course, when seen in light of the radically changed understanding we have now of the literacy revolution of the high Middle Ages.[35] The work of Michael Clanchy and others has demonstrated that although medieval Europe (at least after its

[29] Richard Britnell (ed.), *Pragmatic Literacy, East and West: 1200–1330* (Woodbridge, Suffolk: Boydell, 1997).

[30] Thomas Behrmann, 'The Development of Pragmatic Literacy in the Lombard City Communes', in Britnell, *Pragmatic Literacy*, pp. 25–42. Ronald G. Witt, *'In the Footsteps of the Ancients': The Origins of Humanism from Lovato to Bruni*, Studies in Medieval and Reformation Thought, 74 (Brill: Leiden, 2000), p. 91, cites modern studies showing only slightly lower numbers of notaries for Bologna and Pisa, nevertheless noting that 'the field [of the notariate] was perennially overcrowded'.

[31] Under Roman-canon law, women could not serve as notaries because they could not legally serve as witnesses to testaments. On the continued use of Latin as the principal language of record throughout Europe, see Britnell, 'Pragmatic Literacy in Latin Christendom', in *idem, Pragmatic Literacy*, pp. 3–24.

[32] Paul Strohm, *Social Chaucer* (Cambridge, MA: Harvard University Press, 1989). See also Witt, *'In the Footsteps'*, for the roles notaries played in the development of humanism and vernacular Italian literature.

[33] I will return to this point in Chapters 4 and 5. For evidence on the circulation among male readers of the French *Régime du corps* (a general regimen of health that had originally been addressed to a female recipient), see Green, 'Possibilities'.

[34] J. N. Hillgarth, *Readers and Books in Majorca, 1229–1550*, 2 vols. (Paris: Éditions du C.N.R.S., 1991), pp. 43–44, 89–96 and 261; Hillgarth in fact suspects that medical volumes are rather underdocumented. On the Jewish woman Alegra, see Chapter 3 below.

[35] The general trends and conclusions of this field of research have been summarized by Charles F. Briggs, 'Literacy, Reading, and Writing in the Medieval West', *Journal of Medieval History* 26 (2001), 397–420, though neither gender nor medicine receive any attention in his analysis.

Christianization) was never completely without letters, it was in the eleventh and twelfth centuries that Europe can be said to have become a truly literate culture. This is not a matter of increasing levels of literacy (though that surely was a by-product of the transition) but of new attitudes about the power of the written word to preserve information in a way that could first compete with and later supersede the powers of individual and communal memory.[36] Clanchy's study centred on the impact of literacy in law and governance; literary scholars have focused on the rise of the vernacular languages and the transition from orality to literacy as it affected composition and performance.[37] Most recently, a variety of researchers have turned to documenting the literacy of medieval women and how medieval gender roles affected women's education and access to different kinds of literature.[38] None of these studies mention medicine, despite its position as one of the archetypal learned professions, next to theology and law among the higher faculties of the medieval universities.

Historians of medicine, for their part, have only begun to pose questions of how literacy or the transition from orality to literacy shaped the content or use of medical knowledge in the premodern period.[39] Studies of medical readers and writers traditionally focused on university physicians whose literacy and Latinity need never be questioned. Prosopographical studies of medical practitioners have occasionally noted their ownership of books or, on the other extreme, instances where practitioners are explicitly called illiterate (*idiota, illiteratus*).[40] Yet thus far there has been no systematic concern to document how literacy or the lack of it may have set up more or less impermeable barriers in the

---

[36] Rosamond McKitterick, *The Carolingians and the Written Word* (Cambridge: Cambridge University Press, 1989); and ead. (ed.), *The Uses of Literacy in Early Mediaeval Europe* (Cambridge: Cambridge University Press, 1990); Michael T. Clanchy, *From Memory to Written Record: England 1066–1307*, 2nd rev. edn (Oxford: Blackwell, 1993). See also his essay 'England in the Thirteenth Century: Power and Knowledge', in *England in the Thirteenth Century: Proceedings of the 1984 Harlaxton Symposium*, ed. W. M. Ormrod (Woodbridge, Suffolk: Boydell Press, 1986), pp. 1–14, which explores some issues of the relation between power and knowledge; and M. B. Parkes, 'The Literacy of the Laity', in *Literature and Western Civilization*, vol. II: *The Mediaeval World*, ed. David Daiches and Anthony Thorlby (London: Aldus, 1973), pp. 555–77.

[37] For example, Franz Bäuml, 'Varieties and Consequences of Medieval Literacy and Illiteracy', *Speculum* 55 (1980), 237–65; Joyce Coleman, *Public Reading and the Reading Public in Late Medieval England and France* (Cambridge: Cambridge University Press, 1996).

[38] I survey this literature in Green, 'Possibilities'. See also Chapter 4 below.

[39] Two early contributions are I. M. Lonie, 'Literacy and the Development of Hippocratic Medicine', in *Formes de pensée dans la collection Hippocratique*, ed. François Lasserre and Philippe Mudry (Geneva: Droz, 1983), pp. 145–61; and Gordon Miller, 'Literacy and the Hippocratic Art: Reading, Writing, and Epistemology in Ancient Greek Medicine', *Journal of the History of Medicine and Allied Sciences* 45 (1990), 11–40. More recently, medievalists have noted the deliberate self-fashioning, both of the individual and of the craft, that the new genre of surgical writing permitted in the late 12th and 13th centuries. There is, moreover, now a growing and very sophisticated literature on issues of audience and uses of medical texts as they crossed from Latin into the vernacular. See Chapter 4 below.

[40] E.g. Shatzmiller, *Médecine et justice*; and McVaugh, *Medicine Before the Plague*. McVaugh has discovered the very intriguing fact that physicians in the Crown of Aragon occasionally functioned as grammar teachers (p. 87), but how they themselves became literate is not known.

transmission of medical knowledge nor how literacy may have played a role in the process of professionalization. Jole Agrimi and Chiara Crisciani, in their several studies of the creation of new medical epistemologies in the high Middle Ages and their effects on medical practice, have come closest to articulating a sense of the importance for medicine of the transition from oral to written forms of communication. As they note, 'The composing of texts can be seen as a fundamental turning point towards more ordered systems of studies which are able to establish a new kind of *societas* [association of master and students], one no longer based on private familiar relationship.'[41] I will argue here that not only did written medical texts enable the formation of these larger *societates* of practitioners, but they also sometimes enabled the formation of larger 'textual communities' (as Brian Stock would call them) of men directly associated neither with the universities nor professional medical practice, yet who had both the literate skills and the intellectual desire to participate in the discourses of medicine.[42]

The present study is also informed by the 'linguistic turn' that has affected so many areas of scholarship in the last twenty years. Like many other historical disciplines, the field of the history of medicine in premodern Europe has broadened considerably to include not only aspects of social history but analyses of the social construction of knowledge. Historians have been faced with the realization that just as medical texts—whether they are works of general medical theory, specialized textbooks on particular diseases, handbooks of regimen, or collections of individualized diagnoses and courses of therapy—cannot be read without an eye to their textual and theoretical affiliations with earlier medical traditions (whether Greek, Arabic or European), so, too, they cannot be read without an eye to aspects of rhetoric, topos, formulicity, and the other discursive traditions in which they participate. Medical texts are not objective records that can provide the historian with transparent witnesses to past realities, but *crafted* documents meant to serve specific, historically contingent purposes. The analytical techniques honed by literary scholars are, in fact, among our most important tools in excavating the shifting meanings and uses of medical texts. As the editors of a recent collection on general uses of the vernacular in England have asserted, medieval texts 'require to be read in quantity, in careful relation to their cultural situation and, above all, with a sense of their strategic function'.[43] Looking at medical texts in quantity is challenge enough (given that the vast

---

[41] Jole Agrimi and Chiara Crisciani, 'The Science and Practice of Medicine in the Thirteenth Century according to Guglielmo da Saliceto, Italian Surgeon', in *Practical Medicine from Salerno to the Black Death*, ed. Luis García-Ballester, Roger French, Jon Arrizabalaga, and Andrew Cunningham (Cambridge: Cambridge University Press, 1994), pp. 60–87.

[42] On this concept of 'textual communities', see below.

[43] Jocelyn Wogan-Browne, Nicholas Watson, Andrew Taylor, and Ruth Evans (eds.), *The Idea of the Vernacular: An Anthology of Middle English Literary Theory, 1280–1520* (University Park, PA: Pennsylvania State University Press, 1999), p. 316.

majority are still unedited), but the payoff from doing so, and from situating them culturally and strategically within their historical contexts, is ample compensation for the effort.

WOMEN AND LITERATE MEDICINE

My primary concern in the present study is to explore the cultural situation and strategic functions of the *Trotula* texts, following them both as they moved through the world of Latin medical literature and as they 'filtered down' (often multiple times) into many of the European vernacular languages. Precisely because they were created prior to the establishment of the universities, and precisely because these texts are gendered feminine in two respects—being both (allegedly) by a female author and addressing women's medicine—the *Trotula* texts offer a unique opportunity to examine how textual communities were formed around treatises on women's medicine, and how and by whom women's medical care was delivered. The history of the *Trotula* was played out on a terrain somewhere between the high learned medicine of the universities and the wholly oral practices of illiterate empirics. I call this terrain 'literate medicine', the realm of medical thought and practice that involves medical knowledge that has been written down, knowledge that has been committed to a textual and not simply oral mode for its transmission. 'Literate medicine' is a much broader category than learned medicine (for example, the formal commentaries and scholastic disputations of the universities), which will demand competence not only with a large technical vocabulary but also with sophisticated philosophical concepts for its interpretation. Literate medicine encompasses learned medicine, of course, but it also includes written material such as recipes jotted down in the back of a notebook or a little handbook of daily regimen. Simply by the fact of its being written down, it involves both its creators and its users in the world of medical books. True, some of these users may not in fact have known how to read, but even if they depended on others to read to them (and so did not have the same intellectual independence as did full literates) these quasi-literates participated all the same in a literate culture.[44] In focusing on literate medicine, therefore, I am by no means ignoring the fact that much, perhaps most medicine in medieval Europe was not literate—that many medical practitioners were probably illiterate, or that many acts of healing and therapy were probably performed without recourse to any texts or textual traditions of knowledge. On the contrary, I take the illiteracy of many practitioners (especially women) very seriously, precisely because it was against this backdrop that literate medicine,

---

[44] I adopt the term 'quasi-literates' from Bäuml, 'Varieties', which he defines as 'those *illiterati* who must and do have access to literacy . . . [and who depend] on the written word for the exercise of their socio-political function' (p. 246).

and especially learned medicine, came increasingly to dominate, and increasingly to disenfranchise, those who could not enter into literate culture.

There are, of course, important distinctions within the realm of literate medicine that must be kept in mind. Already in 1206, the French poet and Cistercian monk Guiot de Provins identified literacy as the key to success for both charlatans and 'good, reliable physicians': 'Any old rascal with the gift of the gab, so long as he's capable of reading, can take in dim-witted folk.'[45] But in fact, literacy plain and simple was never enough. To have basic literacy in the vernacular did not enable one to read Latin; to have some rudimentary knowledge of the properties of herbs did not qualify one to comprehend the subtleties of medical theory that demanded grounding in logic, grammar, and rhetoric; ability to comprehend works of praxis did not necessarily enable one to absorb the highly sophisticated physiological theories of university medical writers. Mastery of as many of these levels of literacy as possible would always give those who struggled for higher status an edge. As the university-trained surgeon/physician Guy de Chauliac warned readers of his Latin surgical text, 'if physicians have not learned geometry, astronomy, dialectics, nor any other liberal discipline, soon leather workers, carpenters, smiths, and others will quit their own crafts and become physicians'.[46]

The higher levels of literate medicine never eclipsed or made obsolete the more humble forms, as is amply attested by continued traditions of more or less random collections of recipes, free of all theoretical trappings, and the continued presence throughout Europe of successful, marginally literate empirical practitioners (of whom Perretta had been one). Nor did Latin always trump the vernacular. As we have already seen, however, there was clearly a sense of hierarchy, a sense that grew as patients themselves came to value more highly the learning of the Latinate, university-trained physician or surgeon who could claim to ground his diagnostic decisions and therapeutic practices in rigorous medical theory. For certain individuals to be excluded from basic literacy, from the grammar schools that taught logic and rhetoric, and from the universities that taught Aristotle, Galen, and Avicenna, meant their exclusion from the small but increasingly powerful circles of literate medical discourse, both as practitioners and as patients who might wish to choose self-treatment or select a practitioner on the basis of informed criteria. It meant, in effect, their exclusion from the mechanisms of power offered by literacy and literate medical culture.

This book is not intended as a definitive exploration of the manifold questions of how literacy and medicine interacted in the Middle Ages, yet in focusing on the question of how literacy, medicine, *and gender* interacted it is in fact able

---

[45] As cited in Tony Hunt, *Anglo-Norman Medicine*, 2 vols. (Cambridge: D. S. Brewer), 2: 15.
[46] Guy de Chauliac, *Inventarium*, p. 9, lines 26–9. Guy was quoting the Greek physician Galen here, making it all the more striking how readily he was able to adopt the rhetoric of ancient medical rivalries to his own day.

to lay bare the central features of that transformation. For it is no coincidence that women—who as a group were excluded from the grammar schools that taught logic and rhetoric, from the universities that taught Aristotle, Galen, and Avicenna, and even from the notarial schools and chanceries that taught bureaucrats their advanced literate skills—were also, as a group, frequently singled out by medical writers and legislators as particularly unsuited for medical practice. Whereas in twelfth-century Salerno male medical writers could refer to the empirical practices of Salernitan women with acknowledgement and even respect, from the mid thirteenth century on denunciation of the practices of women becomes a recurring topos in the writings of theoretical surgery, a field particularly anxious to separate itself from strictly oral and empirical practices. The Italian surgeon Bruno of Longobucco readily adopted the condemnation of medical practice by illiterates from one of his Arabic sources, but it was he who added the particular element of gender: 'What ought to be judged even more indecent and horrible [than medical practice by illiterate men] is that vile and presumptuous women usurp and abuse this art, women who, although they have faith [in what they are doing], have neither art nor understanding.'[47] Lanfranc of Milan, writing some fifty years after Bruno, still relied on the testimony of women, since they 'are without doubt expert in their own diseases', along with his own experience and that of 'revered medical doctors' to confirm the effectiveness of his pharmaceutical recommendations. He nevertheless saw them as a lesser order of practitioner who ought not be delegated responsibilities that properly belonged in the hands of surgeons.[48] His fellow surgical writers Henri de Mondeville and Guy de Chauliac, both writing in the fourteenth century, were even harsher, finding nothing to praise, and much to condemn, in women's medical practices.[49] Early licensing laws either made no explicit mention of women or phrased their stipulations in egalitarian formulae (*medicus vel medica, chirurgicus vel chirurgica*) that assumed that female practitioners not only existed but had the same potential to obtain licenses as did their male counterparts. By the mid fourteenth century, all such egalitarian phrasing had disappeared.[50] In

---

[47] For the full context of this statement, see Chapter 3 below.

[48] Lanfranc, *Chirurgia magna*, in *Cyrurgia Guidonis de Cauliaco. et Cyrurgia Bruni, Teodorici, Rolandi, Lanfranci, Rogerii, Bertapalie* (Venice, 1519), ff. 166va–210vb, Tractatus V (the *Antidotarium*), preface, f. 206va: 'Nullas [medicinas] enim in eo ponemus: nisi illas quibus longo tempore sumus vsi: & quas a reuerendis doctoribus medicis: ac etiam mulieribus habuimus: que omnes sine dubio in casibus suis sunt experte'. In Tractatus I, doctrina 1, on the purpose of surgery, Lanfranc derided his fellow surgeons who, out of arrogance, let such manual tasks as scarifying, cauterizing, and applying leeches fall to the hands of barbers and women (*barberiis & mulieribus relinquantur*, f. 168va).

[49] Henri de Mondeville, *Chirurgia*, p. 65; and Guy de Chauliac, *Inventarium*, p. 1, lines 7–8.

[50] For example, an ordinance from Paris in 1271 reads: 'idcirco firmiter inhibemus ne aliquis cirurgicus seu cyrurgica, apothecarius seu apothecaria, herbarius seu herbaria per juramenta sua limites seu metas sui artificii clam vel palam seu qualitercunque excedere presumat . . .' (Denifle, *Chartularium*, 1:489), while one issued by Philip le Bel in 1311 refers, in French, to 'Chirurgiens et Chirurgiennes' (Edouard Nicaise, *Chirurgie de Maitre Henri de Mondeville: chirugien de Philippe*

1329, the city of Valencia asserted unambiguously that no woman was to practise medicine in the city aside from providing care to other women or children (and even then they were prohibited from prescribing medicinal potions). Similar restrictions specifically on women were put into place (or at least attempted) in England and France by the end of the fifteenth century.[51]

Just seven years before the Valencian ordinance was passed, the well-known trial of Jacoba Felicie was held in Paris. Although Jacoba was accused along with several other women *and men* of unlicensed medical practice, the prosecution of her case took on a particularly gendered focus. A principal argument used by the prosecution against Jacoba was that as it was forbidden for women to practise law, so much the more should they be barred from practising medicine where their ignorance might result in a man's death rather than the simple loss of his case in court. Yet the statute of 1271 which Jacoba allegedly violated said nothing that restricted women more than men from medical practice. On the contrary, the statute was phrased in such a way that put the female surgeon, apothecary, or herbalist under the very same restrictions as her male counterpart—but also outlined the conditions under which *both* men and women could practice legally. Jacoba Felicie claims that she knows medical theory, but nothing in her trial record confirms that she owned books or was literate.[52] Jacoba's trial is also striking because, even as Jacoba tries to separate herself from 'illiterates and empty-headed ignoramuses' (*ydiotas et fatuos ignaros*) to whom, she agrees, medical practice should legitimately be forbidden, and tries to align herself with the theoretical medicine of the university physicians, she also wishes to claim that she, *as a woman*, has a special expertise to treat women that none of her male accusers can claim. And indeed, she has a point: in what ways *could* the learned medicine of university-educated males claim to offer better knowledge or more appropriate treatment to female patients who, according to Jacoba, prefer to 'reveal their secrets' to a female practitioner than to a male? It is notable

---

le Bel, roi de France, composée de 1306 à 1320, Paris: Félix Alcan, 1893, pp. lxiv–v). Ellen E. Kittell and Kurt Gueller, ' "Whether Man or Woman": Gender Inclusivity in the Town Ordinances of Medieval Douai', *Journal of Medieval and Early Modern Studies* 30 (2000), 63–100, find this same use of occupational dyads in mid 13th-century Douai, arguing that there such usages demonstrate the acknowledgement of women's participation in these fields. They also, however, find the same disappearance of such usages by the early 15th century.

[51] García-Ballester, *Medical Licensing*, pp. 29–32; Monica H. Green, 'Women's Medical Practice and Health Care in Medieval Europe', in *Sisters and Workers in the Middle Ages*, ed. J. Bennett, E. Clark, J. O'Barr, B. Vilen, and S. Westphal-Wihl (Chicago: University of Chicago Press, 1989), pp. 39–78, repr. in Green, *Women's Healthcare*, Essay I, at pp. 51–4. This piece originally appeared in *Signs: Journal of Women in Culture and Society* 14 (1989–90), 434–73.

[52] Her accusers, the physicians, likewise tie literacy to proper knowledge of medicine but they throw this back at Jacoba as an accusation: she is, according to them, 'totally ignorant of the art of medicine and illiterate' (*totaliter est ignara artis medicine et non litterata*); Denifle (ed.), *Chartularium*, vol. 2, pp. 255–67. For a recent comprehensive analysis of this case, see Montserrat Cabré i Pairet and Fernando Salmón Muñiz, 'Poder académico *versus* autoridad femenina: La Facultad de Medicina de París contra Jacoba Félicié (1322)'. *Dynamis* 19 (1999), 55–78.

that whereas the Parisian physicians respond point by point to all of Jacoba's other claims (whether the physicians rightly have jurisdiction over the case, the alleged absence of any law forbidding her practice, etc.), on the matter of treating female patients they simply dismiss her arguments as 'worthless' and 'frivolous'.[53] Had the physicians better assessed their own strategic strengths, they might have shifted the debate to who possessed the greater theoretical knowledge of women's diseases. For on this point they, with their medical books, would surely have won.

As the present study will document, university physicians and other male literates would have had within their medical books a not insignificant body of material on female physiology and pathology. Discerning the cultural situation and strategic function of these writings is no easy matter, for it involves exploring how the production and then use of knowledge on the female body was gendered. The rather circuitous path that brought me to this analysis of literacy and the exclusion of women from the production of gynaecological knowledge may help make these connections clear. In my early work, I was concerned to chart the development of ancient theories of female physiology and disease as they were transmitted and transformed in early medieval Latin and Arabic medical traditions.[54] Incidental to that research, I discovered a striking difference in the textual context of early Latin and Arabic material on women's diseases. Whereas the Arabic material was almost entirely subsumed within the genre of the medical encyclopedia—an all-encompassing compendium of diseases usually arranged in head-to-toe order, the diseases peculiar to women being placed among those of the reproductive tract—in the late antique Latin West gynaecological material was more often found in separate, specialized texts. Remarkably, the latter were usually addressed either explicitly or implicitly to women, especially midwives (*obstetrices* or *medicae*).[55] This divergence in genres forced me to think about both the reasons why material on women's diseases might be segregated from other general aspects of medicine, and the possible implications this might have for how we envisaged the actual practice of gynaecology and obstetrics in the period. Not being a historian of medieval Arabic culture, I was unable to explore that aspect of the development. Even limiting myself to the Latin tradition, however, I found the issue becoming increasingly complex. I discovered that, for the most part, gynaecology remained a textually separate field of medicine throughout the early Middle Ages, with new compilations being made up through the twelfth century. But whoever their original intended audiences may have been, the only medieval readers I could document for the late antique treatises were men. My

---

[53] Denifle (ed.), *Chartularium*, vol. 2, p. 267.

[54] Monica H. Green, 'The Transmission of Ancient Theories of Female Physiology and Disease Through the Early Middle Ages', PhD dissertation, Princeton University, 1985.

[55] 'Midwife' was defined much more broadly in antiquity and late antiquity than it would be in the later Middle Ages; in the earlier periods the midwife's responsibilities encompassed the full range of gynaecological as well as obstetrical care. See Chapters 1 and 3 and the Conclusion below.

questions thus kept growing at a pace far exceeding my ability to answer them: Are the original addresses of the late antique Latin texts to midwives evidence for women's literacy in the late antique West? Or is the address to women somehow just a literary conceit, a mechanism to legitimate the publication of material that had all along been intended for men? In either case, what are men doing (a) writing this material and (b) reading it if, as has often been assumed, in the Middle Ages 'women's health was women's business'? All these questions about women's and men's relationship to gynaecological literature were further complicated by the fact that those few studies on medieval literacy that had been done at the time suggested (or assumed) that women's literacy was almost universally minimal throughout the late antique and medieval periods.[56]

My original project surveying the development of early medieval medical theories on the female body had been conceived as a source analysis of the so-called *Trotula* treatises. These twelfth-century works had intrigued me not simply because they were generally reputed to be the most popular medieval texts of their kind, but because they constituted the first attempt to synthesize the very different and in many respects incompatible traditions of Latin and Arabic gynaecological thought. Yet these texts resembled their early medieval predecessors in that they, too, begged questions of their genesis and potential function as practical handbooks of women's medicine. Even if we could postulate literate, Latinate midwives in late antique North Africa, could we plausibly do the same for twelfth-century southern Italy? Or for the rest of medieval western Europe where the texts later came to circulate? If not literate midwives or other female practitioners, were there literate laywomen who would have used such texts privately for their own healthcare? Or were the texts intended not for women at all, but for men? In one respect especially, the *Trotula* made the question of male vs. female involvement with gynaecological literature acute: unique among all later medieval Latin gynaecological texts, they had traditionally been reputed to be the work of a female author, 'Trotula'.[57]

---

[56] In general, in my discussions of literacy I am referring only to the ability to read. It has been widely documented that reading and writing are separate skills, most often learned separately. An inability to write (in terms of the mechanics of putting pen to parchment or paper) need not in itself be an impediment to composition, since dictation to a professional scribe was always a possibility (at least to the upper classes). It was more unusual for a medieval author to write out a text in his/her own hand than to have an amanuensis do it, and this apparently was as true for men as for women. However, because in most instances these amanuenses would have been male (e.g. the cases of Margery Kempe in England or Catherine of Siena), women's dependence on men for access to literate culture would, in this respect, still be a factor.

[57] There is an early medieval Latin gynaecological text associated with the name of the Egyptian queen Cleopatra. The attribution is spurious (the text is almost certainly a late antique composition from earlier Latin sources) but it may derive in some part from the Greek *Cosmetics* traditionally (but equally spuriously) attributed to her. On the late antique Greek text attributed to a woman named Metrodora, see Hélène Congourdeau, ' "Métrodôra" et son oeuvre', in *Maladie et société à Byzance*, ed. Evelyne Patlagean (Spoleto: Centro Italiano di Studi sull'Alto Medioevo, 1993), pp. 57–96; in its Latin translation, however, it was never attributed to a woman. See Monica

The modern history of the *Trotula* has centred around this alleged author 'Trotula', who has been a political pawn in debates about women's capabilities and achievements in medicine ever since the sixteenth century. In 1556, the first formal argument was made that the text (for it was assumed by then to be a single work by a single author) was written not by a woman but by a man. Debates over female authorship are nothing new, of course, and feminist scholars over the last several decades have devoted considerable effort to recovering 'lost' female authors and artists and to exposing the layers of obfuscation and even wilful deceit that have deprived individual women of their historical legacies.[58] Ironically, however, the modern quest for a female author 'Trotula' has obscured several equally pressing questions for a feminist analysis of the *Trotula* texts and for the historical implications of all gynaecological literature. My objective here is to turn the traditional 'Trotula Question' on its head, or rather, to broaden it beyond the simple question 'Did 'Trotula' exist or didn't she? Did she write the text(s) on women's medicine commonly attributed to her?' to an exploration of the historical implications of feminine vs. masculine authorship and readership. I wish to de-centre the question from its traditional emphasis on a presumedly unique author's sex and focus it instead on the broader interface between author and audience, text and social context, and the gender dynamics of the actual practice of women's medicine. In reframing the 'Trotula Question' around the issue of women's participation in the whole culture of literate medicine, several new questions emerge: Did any women *read* these works? Did these texts function to inform women (whether lay or professional) on the causes and cures of women's diseases? Or did they function, instead, as mechanisms by which *men* might learn about and establish authority over the diagnosis and treatment of women's diseases?

WAS WOMEN'S HEALTH WOMEN'S BUSINESS?

The existence of written knowledge on the treatment of women's diseases and conditions raises a conundrum about the social functioning of a system of literate medicine. As mentioned earlier, it has been widely believed that in the Middle Ages 'women's health was women's business': women had exclusive control over gynaecology and obstetrics, meaning that written texts on women's medicine must have been created by women and intended for their use.[59] Although this

---

H. Green, 'Medieval Gynaecological Texts: A Handlist', in Green, *Women's Healthcare*, Appendix, pp. 1–36, at p. 24.

[58] On the authenticity debates surrounding Trota's contemporaries Heloise and Hildegard of Bingen, see most recently Bonnie Wheeler (ed.), *Listening to Heloise: The Voice of a Twelfth-Century Woman* (New York: St Martin's, 2000); and Barbara Newman (ed.), *Voice of the Living Light: Hildegard of Bingen and Her World* (Berkeley: University of California Press, 1998).

[59] See Green, 'Women's Medical Practice'.

belief holds less sway now among medieval historians, the idea that the Middle Ages were some 'golden age' for women's control over their own healthcare is a truism among those working on modern Europe or even doing cross-cultural comparisons.[60] If this scenario of a female monopoly on female medicine were universally true, however, it would beg the question of why knowledge about women's diseases and cosmetics should be written down at all. While women, as a group, might seem to be the most likely generators and users of texts on women's medicine, women, as a group, were also the least likely to have had the kind of access to literate culture that would allow them either to create or to use such texts. In other words, if we are talking about information meant to be kept within a community of women, we need to demonstrate that female literacy was sufficient, or that the author(s) and later copyists of these texts believed it was sufficient, to sustain a written vector of transmission of knowledge among women. An assumption that 'women's health was women's business', at least in so far as it concerns *written* knowledge, therefore demands the positing of a broad community of female readers to explain the existence of the corpus of gynaecological literature that was in fact circulating in medieval Europe.

Unfortunately, the medieval evidence in no way supports such a supposition: most written knowledge about women's bodies is to be found in texts composed *by* male physicians and surgeons, *for* male physicians and surgeons (or if not for them, then for lay male patrons), and incorporated into volumes *owned by* male medical practitioners or other male literates. Despite the wide circulation of the *Trotula* texts throughout Europe and the frequency with which they were copied in Latin and translated into the vernacular, there is only scattered evidence (and that often circumstantial) to suggest that any women owned and used these texts. Women may have had some additional access to the texts through oral readings, but even then it would have often been mediated by men. This, then, raises the question of the relationship between medical writing, medical reading, and medical practice. How is medical knowledge about the female body generated in the first place? Since, so far as I am aware, no medieval author ever explicitly mused on this question, I will have to fill in this lacuna with some speculation.

First of all, I do *not* assume that such knowledge is grounded strictly in biology, that simply because they are born women, women have an innate knowledge of female physiology and pathology. Were medical knowledge of women's bodies innate, there would be no need for its acquisition or transmission, either in written form or orally, since all women would have it from birth. Far

---

[60] In a forthcoming essay, I examine the extraordinary influence that a small 1970 pamphlet, *Witches, Midwives and Nurses*, written by the non-historians Barbara Ehrenreich and Deirdre English, has had not simply in women's history but in anthropological studies of women's health, too.

more important, I believe, is the role of experience, that is, that because they live their lives as women—experiencing not only the biological processes of menstruation, pregnancy, childbirth, lactation, and various disorders consequent to their anatomy and physiology, but also the social expectations of what women should do with their bodies—women individually acquire, to greater or lesser degrees, an experiential knowledge of the workings of the female body. To this individual experience would be added collective knowledge that women gain over many generations and share within their sex-specific communities. This collective knowledge would remain among women, however, only to the extent that there were social pressures to keep it there. If in a society women have a 'separate sphere', if there were a general cultural expectation, inculcated in both men and women, that men should not touch the female genitalia nor should women allow their 'private parts' to be touched or seen by men other than their legitimate sexual partners, *and* if issues surrounding reproductive processes and the organs involved in them are not to be talked about between the sexes, then to that extent women will be the only qualified practitioners of women's healthcare (at least in so far as it involves the genitalia) and the only generators of such knowledge. One of the original *Trotula* texts, *On the Conditions of Women*, explicitly admitted that women, out of shame, do not wish to bare the diseases of their 'private parts' to male practitioners. This would seem to imply that, in medieval southern Italy at least, there were cultural dictates that kept men away from women's bodies at the same time that they fostered an exclusively female context in which experientially acquired knowledge would be used and disseminated.

If, however, gynaecological knowledge can be derived by other means—by, for example, analogical reasoning from the male body or deductive reasoning from certain *a priori* principles—then it is possible that even in a sexually segregated society men could generate a kind of gynaecological knowledge, too. If that knowledge can be added to knowledge gleaned from women (however it is obtained) and to the knowledge found in earlier written texts (the principal source for *Conditions of Women* itself), then even when males are denied immediate access to the female body they can accumulate gynaecological knowledge more or less comparable to women's. If, moreover, males can use female assistants to examine female patients and administer therapeutic measures, then what might have initially appeared to be crucial gender differences—men's lack of personal experience of female bodily functions and their limited access to the female body—might turn out to be immaterial.[61] The only remaining impediment might thus be men's relative freedom to discuss gynaecological matters with their

---

[61] Anatomical dissections of humans do not seem to have occurred prior to the late 13th century, and then only in Italy; prior to that, pigs were used for anatomical training in Salerno. It is possible that certain knowledge was gathered from prostitutes, whose bodies were more accessible to men than those of 'honourable' women. On both these issues, see Chapter 6 below.

patients. In weighing men's ability to acquire gynaecological knowledge against women's, therefore, men are not handicapped in any absolute way. Indeed, if literacy is a tool that men have but women lack, then men might have a real advantage.

It will be the central argument of this book that men's advantage in literacy—and all the intellectual stature and social authority that went with it—was in fact key to the regendering of gynaecological knowledge production and practice between the twelfth and the sixteenth centuries. In short, I am redefining the 'Trotula Question' as an issue about far more than female authorship. It is about women's participation in the whole culture of literate medicine: whether as literate or semi-literate authors, as literate or quasi-literate readers and listeners and practitioners, or, even more distantly, as recipients (as patients) of a form of medicine whose theoretical structures they did not help create and whose precepts they were, perhaps, never expected to understand. To use Brian Stock's term, I am asking who made up the 'textual communities' that surrounded the *Trotula* texts and other medieval gynaecological writings, who viewed the texts as their intellectual property, and who perhaps even found some elements within the texts with which to self-identify.[62] I am therefore of necessity asking whether male as well as female textual communities may have surrounded these texts, how they may have read them, and how, indeed, the very existence of male as well as female readers may have affected not only the practice of but also the discourses surrounding women's medicine.

THE PLAN OF THIS BOOK

The following chapters survey the history of gynaecological literature and the practice of medieval and early Renaissance women's medicine from varying perspectives. I begin with the gender dynamics of medical practice in Salerno and the creation of the *Trotula* texts before the universities and their fixed gendered hierarchies of education came into existence. The so-called 'school' of Salerno was in the late eleventh and twelfth century nothing more than an informal gathering of masters and pupils, not a real physical or legal entity. But having moved beyond the stage of purely empirical (and largely oral) traditions of medical practice,

---

[62] Brian Stock, *The Implications of Literacy: Written Language and Models of Interpretation in the Eleventh and Twelfth Centuries* (Princeton: Princeton University Press, 1983), p. 522, defines 'textual communities' as 'groups of people whose social activities are centred around texts, or, more precisely, around a literate interpreter of them. The text in question need not be written down nor the majority of auditors actually literate. The *interpres* may relate it verbally, as did the medieval preacher . . . [T]he group's members must associate voluntarily; their interaction must take place around an agreed meaning for the text. Above all, they must make the hermeneutic leap from what the text says to what they think it means; the common understanding provides the foundation for changing thought and behavior.'

Salerno's medical school was already engaged in the synthesis of the new, more theoretical medicine coming out of the Arabic world and it was starting to create a style of commentaries on authoritative texts that would characterize formal medical education for the next several centuries. In addition to the group of Latinate male masters who wrote the texts and commentaries for which Salerno is most famous, there was also what seems to have been a significant number of female healers. One of these was Trota who, as John Benton first showed in 1985, was the author of a general treatise on practical medicine, the *Practical Medicine According to Trota* (*Practica secundum Trotam*).[63] She was also, as I will argue here, the source for the most distinctive and novel 'hands-on' text of women's medicine composed in the medieval period, *Treatments for Women* (*De curis mulierum*), which would later form the centrepiece of the *Trotula* ensemble.[64] Within the diverse group of practitioners in twelfth-century Salerno, there was no absolute distinction in the sex of their patients: male practitioners treated female patients, females treated males.[65] There was, however, a clear limit to male access to the female body, with the result that discussions of gynaecological matters by male authors lack certain elements of hands-on knowledge. Conversely, the female practitioners, although they could have intimate contact with both female and male patients, were little engaged in the world of literate medicine being generated by their male peers. Trota was the boundary-crosser: she has an access to the female body unmatched by her male peers, while as a writer she participates in literate medicine. Yet this participation was only marginal; her work evinces little engagement with the high theoretical medical traditions that her learned male contemporaries were actively developing and, with but few exceptions, they were just as oblivious to her. Thus, while at the beginning of the twelfth century, literate medicine was a new enough endeavour not to have been distinctly gendered (thus allowing a skilled female empiricist like Trota to participate), by the end of the century it had become a thoroughly masculine enterprise.

[63] John F. Benton, 'Trotula, Women's Problems, and the Professionalization of Medicine in the Middle Ages', *Bulletin of the History of Medicine* 59 (1985), 30–53.

[64] Benton had dismissed *Treatments for Women* as just another male-authored text that sought, like the male-authored *Conditions of Women* and *Women's Cosmetics*, to control women by controlling their medical care.

[65] Although a range of sexual characteristics was posited by certain medical texts circulating in or around 12th-century Salerno, the *Trotula* texts neither explore sexual ambiguity nor posit 'woman' or 'man' as problematic categories requiring definition or explanation. Sexual ambiguity was not, of course, completely unknown. For example, a text on generation that may have been translated by Constantine the African, called *De spermate* (On the Seed), explained that males were generated on the right side of the uterus, females on the left, and hermaphrodites in the middle. For recognition of the phenomenon of hermaphroditism among surgeons, see Chapter 2 below. The nature of sex differences was also examined at length in a series of natural-philosophical questions that may have originated from Salerno, known as the Salernitan Questions. In the medical texts under discussion here, however, what constituted a 'man' or a 'woman' was not subject to debate.

Chapter 2 turns to the reception of the Latin *Trotula* in thirteenth- and fourteenth-century Europe and to evidence for the gynaecological practice of male physicians and surgeons. Even though the three Salernitan gynaecological texts never established a foothold in university curricula, both individually and as an ensemble the *Trotula* became the most widely circulating specialized texts on women's diseases and cosmetic concerns in medieval Europe. For about a fifth of the documentable copies of the *Trotula*, we know one or more of the owners through whose hands the book passed, and we can therefore be quite specific about the gendered uses of the texts. But for all the rest, the lack of ownership inscriptions raises the need for codicological analysis: that is, examination of how the book, the codex, was put together and what that says about how the volume as a whole might have been used. Thus, for example, I assume that a codex that situates the *Trotula* or other gynaecological texts amid predominantly technical surgical works will likely have been made for a surgeon; one filled with sermons for a preacher. A codex made up entirely of vernacular texts may have been intended for someone who was either ignorant of Latin or felt distinctly more comfortable reading in the local tongue. But a codex that *mixes* Latin and the vernacular cannot be interpreted in the same way. Codicological analysis is, admittedly, inferential in comparison to the more positivist evidence of ownership inscriptions. But precisely because the *Trotula* texts survive in such large numbers (as do other texts on women's medicine), it is possible to reconstruct certain *patterns* of use. And it is these patterns of behaviour, and the meanings attached to them, that make up the societal norms that collectively constitute a gender system.

What all these physical books show, then, together with evidence from other medical writings and illustrations of medical encounters, is that as in Salerno, male practitioners throughout Europe were regularly treating female patients for all kinds of complaints, including gynaecological problems like menstrual irregularities or infertility. Gynaecology (and even what we might call 'advisory obstetrics') had become a fairly normative part of many male physicians' practice, an area in which most healers wished to claim some minimal level of knowledge. Indeed, while the *Trotula* is adopted in the thirteenth century, occasionally even exploited, as the chief authority on women's medicine in large part because it had no effective rival, by the fourteenth century male physicians have developed enough confidence to create a special area of expertise, fertility medicine, which grew from a topic on which a few hasty remedies might be thrown together into an area of specialized thought and writing. Beyond treating disorders of the breasts, surgeons lagged behind the physicians considerably in engaging with gynaecological conditions, yet even they evince developing confidence by the fourteenth century. Both physicians and surgeons are, I argue, clearly inhibited to a significant degree by concerns that cross-sex practice will bring not only shame to the female patient, but dishonour to the male practitioner. Nevertheless, apparently with the consent of female patients, they forge ahead.

Despite occasional denunciations of the dangers of male practice on female patients, a variety of evidence—both textual and iconographic—shows that it was both common and accepted.

Having a better sense of how far the male medical practitioner could and could not go aids us in turning to the question of the extent of women's medical practices. Simply put, the gendered structures of society (including the still unstated prohibition against male sight or touch of the female genitalia) demanded the continued presence of women in medical practice. As I discuss in Chapter 3, female medical practitioners—from specialists in surgery to those engaged in casual practice domestically—can be documented throughout thirteenth- and fourteenth-century Europe; the existence of even more women like them can be inferred precisely because gender segregation would have demanded their existence. Yet there was an important gender differential between these women and their male counterparts. Whereas the medical literacy of male practitioners follows a general upward trajectory in this period, the same was not true of female practitioners. Women's general literacy was clearly rising in the later medieval period, to be sure, but the 'typically feminine' reading habits of women show them turning their reading skills (which only rarely involved full competence with Latin) primarily toward liturgical and devotional reading. Medical books can only rarely be documented in women's hands. While the knowledge encompassed in Latin books may have been conveyed to women through oral readings by literate males, there is scant evidence that the medical book came to function for women as a defining resource for medical learning in the same way it did for men.

Chapter 4 turns from Latin to vernacular texts on women's medicine. The sheer number of translations of the *Trotula* is itself evidence of the existence of new audiences: at least twenty-one different translations were made into Dutch, English, French, German, Hebrew, Irish, and Italian between the late twelfth and fifteenth centuries. A third of the *Trotula* translations are in fact addressed to women and even though we have no woman's signature on any extant medieval copies of these texts, codicological evidence suggests that women probably did own and use some of them. Be that as it may, all the other translations were for either medical practitioners or lay patrons concerned to have knowledge about generation;[66] in neither case was it necessary to specify the gender of the intended audiences since they were assumed to be the same groups that had read the Latin. In both north and south, men not simply continued to read gynaecological literature, they even reappropriated some of the new texts addressed to women: while the enfranchising of female readers was possible, the disenfranchising of

---

[66] I think we mislead ourselves by subsuming all discussions about reproduction under the single rubric 'sexuality', a term unknown and perhaps inconceivable in the medieval period. Although, as I will argue, there was definitely a concern with sexual prurience in some of the warnings that male readers use caution when reading gynaecological literature, the greater motivation for medieval readers really was the desire to understand *and attempt to control* the processes of generation.

male readers was not. Where the vernacular traditions differ from the Latin one, however, is that here we find an explicit contest over who should have access not to the bodies of women but to texts on women's medicine. A peculiar feature of a few of the later medieval vernacular gynaecological texts is that they are prefaced either by warnings to men not to use texts on women's medicine for ill intent, or by apologies to women that such texts are not intended to harm them. These warnings and apologies were not solely concerned with male *practice* of gynaecology. Rather, they reflect an awareness that some male interest in the texts was not therapeutic at all.

Chapter 5 traces the development in the later medieval period of a growing perception that the *Trotula* texts were not repositories of therapies for women's diseases *in toto*, but rather compilations of more specific information on female sexuality and fertility. Chapter 2 has, of course, already shown the activity of male physicians in the field of infertility and Chapter 4 the interests of lay male readers in using gynaecological literature to understand and even control the processes of generation. Chapter 5 takes this story beyond the *Trotula* or even strictly medical writing into a larger genre of 'women's secrets'. Whereas many of the other so-called secrets traditions—in alchemy, astrology, and magic—were inherited or derived from texts of Arabic, Greek, or Hebrew origin, the genre of women's secrets was almost entirely a European creation. Texts circulating under the rubric *The Secrets of Women* took different forms, but most in some way addressed questions of sexuality, foetal development, birth and other issues surrounding generation. The *Trotula* texts came to be allied with this tradition, often being abbreviated or otherwise altered to fit the narrower interests of a new audience interested in generation. The female body was seen not so much as a marvel of generative properties as a site of voracious sexual appetites and mysterious physiological processes that threatened men precisely because they were uncontrollable. The authoress 'Trotula' came to be seen as an authority not on women's diseases, but on 'women's secrets', herself a contributor (according to Chaucer) to the litany of testimonials to the 'wickedness' of women. Here in particular we see the effects of the exclusion of women from literate discussions of their bodies and their conditions, for the university and other all-male institutions provided men with a single sex environment in which to discuss 'the nature of women' without any threat of challenge. Given the larger cultural atmosphere that existed in western Europe in the fourteenth and fifteenth centuries, it is not surprising to find that the 'secrets of women' carried a taint of misogyny, a taint that spread to the *Trotula* as it, too, came to be seen as 'secret'.

'Secrets of women' texts and the larger phenomenon of lay and clerical interest in women's secrets had their own intense afterlife. My focus in Chapter 6, however, returns to the gendering of knowledge production and the practice of women's medicine at the end of the Middle Ages and just beyond. In the fifteenth century, in northern Europe as well as the south, male medical writers began to move beyond their fairly passive levels of involvement in women's medicine to more active, creative roles. In Italy, discussions of women's diseases remained, at least in their original formulation, within the confines of the encyclopedic *Practicae*, where they were perennially linked with conditions of the male genitalia. Yet the size and detail of these sections on reproduction grew to such an extent that several began to circulate independently. More important than the textual form of this material was its content: fifteenth-century Italian writers, both physicians and surgeons, display a new level of engagement with women's medicine; most notably, there is now evidence that the taboo against male sight and even touch of the external female genitalia has finally been breached. Midwives are still the only ones allowed to insert their hands into the female body, but male practitioners were now equipped with a variety of tools that literally opened up the living female body to new levels of inspection. This kind of ocular inspection was not immediately paralleled north of the Alps, but changes in social practice and knowledge occurred there, too. In France, we find male writers confidently adopting the Italian texts, filling the margins of their books with notes on their own gynaecological cures and, in two remarkable cases, composing entirely novel, specialized gynaecological texts, arrogating to the physician the responsibility to supervise the midwife even in the handling of childbirth. We also find extraordinary evidence that male practitioners might contest *among themselves* for the right to treat women's conditions.

By the time the effects of humanism and the printing press spread to medicine, therefore, the field of women's medicine had already been masculinized not only in its theoretical construction but in its clinical application, too. The sixteenth century did witness its own distinct developments, but they built on those of the fifteenth century rather than representing a radical break. First, there was the creation of obstetrics as its own distinct field—the province now of both female midwives and male surgeons, each group having its own texts. Then, there was the creation of gynaecology not simply as a field in which learned practitioners claimed authority, but as a field that now had a rationale for why it should be distinct from 'men's medicine'. The rediscovery of the original Greek Hippocratic corpus of gynaecological texts in the 1520s (and their immediate translation into Latin) contributed not only to this latter development but it gave this new field its own originary masculine source, the Father of Medicine himself, Hippocrates. The medieval inheritance was almost completely wiped from the common consciousness of the field, with the surprising exception of the *Trotula* texts which would be 'cleaned up' by a humanist editor in 1544 and reprinted a total of eleven times over the course of the sixteenth century. They survived, however, not because they were believed to represent a woman's perspective on women's medicine, but because (due to some creative editing) they were believed to be of *classical* origin. The female author 'Trotula' was herself expendable: by 1556, she became a male author Eros, an alteration that could readily be accepted since gynaecology had now been 'birthed' as a field in which female authority played no role whatsoever.

The Conclusion returns to the question of how the creation of a masculine gynaecology affected women, both as practitioners and as patients, and how those effects have extended to the present day. Women were excluded from the institutions and intellectual traditions of western medicine right at the moment that it was establishing its most distinctive features: the grounding of medical science on principles of natural philosophy and the standardization of that knowledge in university curricula. The rise of male authority in gynaecology and emergency obstetrics came at the price of a decline in female authority: a trade-off evidenced both in women's increasingly circumscribed roles as medical practitioners and in the limited ways women's medical competencies were imagined. On several important levels, women had no medical Renaissance: there was a disruption of the late medieval pattern of rendering vernacular gynaecological texts for women and, with but few exceptions, the medical literature available to women in print was narrowed down to a handful of obstetrical texts that spoke to women either as midwives (within a very circumscribed and subordinate role) or to laywomen in their capacity as mothers. While the increasing involvement of at least certain classes of early modern women in literate practices led them to revive a traditional genre of medical writing, the recipe collection, as an arena for feminine expertise, it would not be until the nineteenth and twentieth centuries that the gendering of medical authority that had been established in the Middle Ages would be overturned. Hence the morals of this story of the masculine birth of gynaecology for women's history more generally apply to our own time, including the question of why 'Trotula' has taken on the role she has in modern popular cultural understandings of women's medical history.

The field of gynaecology in medieval and early Renaissance Europe was a territory of interplay, of contest between men and women for access to and control over medical knowledge of the female body. Whatever may have been true of strictly oral traditions of medical practice (where there may indeed have been an all-female world of theorizing and therapy), once we move into the realm of literacy, the gendering of women's medicine instantly becomes complex. I argue that it was probably men who can be credited with many of the layers of authorship and editing of the *Trotula* texts, and that it was certainly men who for the most part claimed the *Trotula* texts as their intellectual property and who formed the principal textual communities surrounding the *Trotula* and other gynaecological literature from the twelfth through the sixteenth centuries. Certain female practitioners, like Trota in the twelfth century and Perretta in the fifteenth, may have recognized the virtues (or, for Perretta, the necessity) of engagement with literate medicine in order to establish their position within the community of medical practitioners, just as certain male translators and the laywomen for whom they wrote recognized the capacity of the vernacular to put gynaecological knowledge back into the hands of women. On the whole, however, women's encounters with literate medicine, whether they were practitioners or patients, were more obstructive than enabling. Only at the point of initial genesis of the *Trotula* texts in twelfth-century Salerno and then again in certain of the late medieval translations is there straightforward acknowledgement and contesting of the paradox of literacy and women's medicine.

1

The Gentle Hand of a Woman? Trota and Women's Medicine at Salerno

[T]here would seem to be no good reason for denying that a book having such decidedly feminine touches as Trotula's was written by a woman. It bears the gentle hand of a woman doctor on every page.

Kate Campbell Hurd-Mead (1930)[1]

Kate Campbell Hurd-Mead, an American obstetrician and ardent proponent of the female medical authority 'Trotula' in the early part of the twentieth century, drew on rhetoric typical of her day when she argued for the feminine authorship of the Salernitan compendium of women's medicine.[2] Women's capacity to practise medicine and especially to treat women and children was 'innate', she and many of her contemporary advocates of female physicians believed, a biologically inherent quality of women. Modern gender theories have rendered such essentialist beliefs in feminine character obsolete and we can no longer assume *a priori* how a woman would have practised medicine or that she would have done so with a 'gentle hand'. Rather, we are accustomed now to see gender roles—the behaviours, occupations, dress, and self-expectations that societies deem appropriate for males or females—as contextually specific and, therefore, historically contingent. What

---

[1] Kate Campbell Hurd-Mead, 'Trotula', *Isis* 14 (1930), 349–67, at p. 364.

[2] Hurd-Mead was, of course, still working on the assumption that the whole *Trotula* ensemble was the work of a single author; ironically, she was particularly persuaded of the author's female identity by what I have identified as the male-authored *Conditions of Women*. For work on Hurd-Mead's late nineteenth and early twentieth-century context, see Regina Markell Morantz-Sanchez, *Sympathy and Science: Women Physicians in American Medicine* (New York: Oxford University Press, 1985); Susan Wells, *Out of the Dead House: Nineteenth-Century Women Physicians and the Writing of Medicine* (Madison: University of Wisconsin Press, 2001); and Montserrat Cabré i Pairet, 'Kate Campbell Hurd-Mead (1867–1941) and the Medical Women's Struggle for History', *Collections. The Newsletter of the Archives and Special Collections on Women in Medicine. The Medical College of Pennsylvania*, Philadelphia, PA, issue 26 (February 1993), pp. 1–4, 8. On 'Trotula's' post-medieval fate, see Monica H. Green, 'In Search of an "Authentic" Women's Medicine: The Strange Fates of Trota of Salerno and Hildegard of Bingen', *Dynamis: Acta Hispanica ad Medicinae Scientiarumque Historiam Illustrandam* 19 (1999), 25–54; and the Conclusion below.

constitutes 'masculine behaviour' in one social context may be deemed 'feminine' in another. For the historian, gender roles must be proven rather than assumed.

This conceptual differentiation between a sexed (physical) body and a gendered (performative) individual actor is, of course, a modern conceit. And in a certain respect it is unhelpful for exploring the history of women's medicine since in reality there never would have been any historical actors (real, living bodies) that were not both sexed and gendered simultaneously. Be that as it may, knowledge of these actors' sex, like their physical bodies, is lost to us. We can, of course, assume universally in the field of gynaecology that the patient's body is female. Yet we have no certain way—barring retrieval of their bones, or even better, their DNA—of knowing whether the authors, readers, and auditors of the Salernitan texts on women's medicine were male or female or even intersexed.[3] I will suggest, however, that it is not really necessary to determine the sex of the attendant circling around the female patient's body, viewing it, touching it, theorizing about its physiological and pathological processes. Rather, for our historical understanding of twelfth-century medicine, it is sufficient to determine the performed gender of the individual authors (or readers or auditors) surrounding our texts, since this will reveal the gendering of medical knowledge and medical practice in medieval Salerno.

Aside from some very fragmentary documentation, the primary evidence we have for any reconstruction of the gendered scenarios of medical practice on women in twelfth-century Salerno are these same medical texts.[4] Analysing any of them individually would no doubt lead to circularity. However, by taking a full survey of the discussions of women's diseases in the Salernitan corpus and by comparing the gendered 'performances' of women's medicine in writings ascribed to known male authors with the comparable 'performances' in the three anonymous, specialized Salernitan texts on women's medicine—the so-called *Trotula* treatises—we can in fact discern the hand of a woman (or women) in

---

[3] This is not meant to imply that female patients were not also *gendered*. In the Salernitan view, a woman is a body with a uterus that can be displaced or become intemperate, with a vagina that can develop lesions or become overstretched, with breasts that can become turgid with milk or eaten away by cancerous lesions. This physical woman shades imperceptibly into the social woman who induces menstruation in order to become fertile, who is concerned to dye her hair and modify the colour of her face or teeth or gums in order to be attractive to men or maintain her social position, the woman who endures painful intercourse or fakes virginity or chooses chastity because of current assumptions about female sexuality. This latter woman is a performer, an active agent choosing to use or manipulate her body in specific ways. See also the Introduction, n. 65, on the question of intersex.

[4] Actually, we should specify that we have their texts as they are embodied in manuscript copies. This latter point is crucial: for none of the 12th-century Salernitan writers is an autograph copy of their work known, and of those copies that have survived into the present day, few even come from southern Italy. While I will concede the possibility of later alterations 'corrupting' the texts that I analyse in this chapter, I have employed all the tools of philological analysis available to me to control for this possibility.

the creation of women's medicine at Salerno. What also becomes clear is where the limits lay both of women's knowledge and of their stature in the social and intellectual hierarchy of Salernitan medicine.

SEXING AUTHORS, GENDERING TEXTS

The idea that gender is 'performed' is in essence the notion that one's identity and actions as a woman or a man do not necessarily arise out of some innate characteristics of having a male or female body, but out of the choices an individual makes about what gender roles they choose to enact within the norms of their historical moment.[5] The gendering of women's medicine did not begin in twelfth-century Salerno, of course, and one of the best examples of the 'performativity' of the practice of women's medicine dates from more than a thousand years before the composition of the Salernitan *Trotula* texts. Right around the beginning of the Christian era, a freedman of the emperor Augustus and friend of Ovid named Hyginus (d. AD 14) composed a series of *Fables*. In a list of *Quis quid invenerit* ('who discovered what'), Hyginus wrote the following account of a midwife named Agnodice:

The ancients did not have midwives [*obstetrices*] and in consequence women often perished because of their shame, for the Athenians had decreed that no slave or woman should learn the art of medicine. A certain young virgin, Agnodice, greatly desired to learn medicine, and out of her desire she presented herself with shorn hair and in male attire to Herophilus as his disciple. When she had learned the art and when she heard of a woman labouring in birth, she came to her. When the woman refused to believe who she [Agnodice] was (thinking her to be a man), Agnodice lifted up her tunic and showed herself to be a woman, and thus she cured her. However, when the male physicians [*medici*] found that they themselves were not admitted to treat women, they began to accuse Agnodice, and they said that he was a 'smooth-faced boy' and a corrupter of women, and that the women were only pretending to be sick. When the Areopagus [the Athenian council] met, they began to bring charges against Agnodice; Agnodice lifted her tunic before them and showed herself to be a woman. But then the physicians began to accuse her even more vigorously, wherefore the leading women [of the city] came before the court and said, 'You are not our husbands but our enemies, because you condemn her who discovered [*invenit*] health for us'. Thus the Athenians changed the law so that free-women might learn the medical art.[6]

---

[5] This theory has been most prominently articulated by Judith Butler, *Gender Trouble: Feminism and the Subversion of Identity* (New York: Routledge, 1990). My analysis here understands gender as a whole concatenation of actions, behaviours, and desires as they relate to the production of medical knowledge and the delivery of medical care. I do not consider gender simply (or even especially) in relation to sexual desire, although the medieval expectation of heterosexual desire clearly underlies the sexual tensions threatening (or imagined to threaten) contact between male healers and female patients.

[6] Hyginus, *Fabulae*, ed. Peter K. Marshall (Stuttgart: Teubner, 1993), Fable CLXXIV, pp. 196–7. For analysis of the meaning of Agnodice's story in its own time, see Helen King, 'Agnodike and

The story of Agnodice is a gender performance *par excellence*. By dressing in drag, Agnodice is able to 'perform' as a man, travelling freely and studying under the great Hellenistic physician Herophilus, who would have been well known in Hyginus's day as one of the most important authorities on anatomy and as the author of a (now lost) treatise on midwifery.[7] Having completed her education, however, and wishing to treat women, Agnodice's masculine identity becomes inconvenient, so she lifts her tunic in front of a reluctant patient and reveals her 'real' identity as a woman. Agnodice's story thus tells a tale about how gender affects medicine from two perspectives. As a 'man', Agnodice's services were refused by the labouring woman; as a woman, they were just as readily accepted. But Agnodice's story also gives us an important model for thinking about the *transfer of knowledge* across gender barriers. Agnodice learns her women's medicine not from other women but from a man, Herophilus. How does Herophilus know so much about women's medicine if women were reluctant to 'bare their ills' to male doctors? Hyginus does not tell us (and I will defer my own answer until we turn to the Salernitan context later). Be that as it may, Herophilus (and apparently the male physicians of Athens) believed that they had some kind of medicine to offer women. Indeed, Agnodice's initial transvestite ruse was motivated precisely because she also believed men had knowledge on women's medicine otherwise unavailable to her.

In what sense, then, did Agnodice 'discover' health for women? Hyginus's story implies that she did so by making the knowledge of men available to female patients in a form they could accept: from a female practitioner who, as a female, did not threaten their sense of sexual shame. The topos of women's shame as an obstacle to adequate gynaecological care did not originate with Hyginus, of course, but stretched back all the way to the first known gynaecological text in the West, the Hippocratic *Diseases of Women*, Book I. Addressing other male physicians like himself, the Hippocratic author noted that problems arise from the patient's unwillingness to communicate with her doctor: '[f]or women are ashamed to tell even if they know, and they suppose that it is a disgrace, because of their inexperience and lack of knowledge'. He also suggested that male physicians err by not thoroughly questioning the woman and instead attempting to treat 'as though they were dealing with men's diseases'.[8] The Hippocratic writer did not, however, suggest that the solution to the 'problem' of women's shame and male physicians' reticence was the institution of female physicians. In fact, close

---

the Profession of Medicine', *Proceedings of the Cambridge Philological Society* 32 (1986), 53–77; and *Hippocrates' Woman: Reading the Female Body in Ancient Greece* (London and New York: Routledge, 1998).

[7] Heinrich von Staden, *Herophilus: The Art of Medicine in Early Alexandria* (Cambridge: Cambridge University Press, 1989). Needless to say, the improbable chronology of Hyginus's story is only one of its many signs of fictionality.

[8] 'Hippocrates', *Diseases of Women* 1.62, as trans. in Ann Ellis Hanson, 'Hippocrates: *Diseases of Women* 1', *Signs: Journal of Women in Culture and Society* 1 (1975), 567–84, p. 582.

analysis of the large body of Hippocratic gynaecological writing shows that men were extensively involved in women's medicine.[9] It is Hyginus, writing in the very different context of early imperial medicine, who rewrites the history of classical medicine: 'the Athenians *changed the law* so that free-women might learn the medical art'. Hyginus's story, therefore, fictively represents a seismic shift in the gendering of medicine from a situation where males were the normative authorities on women's medicine (with no acknowledgement of the problem this created for the *practice* of women's medicine) to a situation allowing women to not simply practise but also to be *trained* to practise on a level comparable with men.[10]

In Hyginus's story, no claim is made that Agnodice's knowledge is, in and of itself, different or better than Herophilus's or the other male physicians of Athens. Agnodice's training may have been simply empirical, an apprenticeship based on observance of the master in action and aural reception of his teachings. Literacy plays no role in the story. About 400 years after Hyginus was writing, however, a North African physician added that next element to the mythography of the gendering of women's medicine. Caelius Aurelianus, in the preface to his Latin translation of the Greek *Gynaecology* of Soranus (late first, early second century CE) offered in essence a summary of Hyginus's tale: 'it was finally decided by the ancients to institute female physicians [*medicas*], so that the diseases of a woman's private parts, when they needed to be examined, would not have to be exposed to male eyes'. 'The ancients', he tells us, 'took care to hand down their secret cures which they called *genecias* ["women's matters"], so that for the sake of women they might be set forth because in women especially, along with other common diseases afflicting them, the shameful parts are affected.'[11] Women's shame, therefore, is not simply the cause for the creation of female physicians, it is also the motivation for *writing down* the traditions of gynaecological and obstetrical knowledge.

Other ancient and late antique gynaecological writings confirm Caelius's implication that written texts on women's medicine were intended principally for a female corps of practitioners. Soranus himself had intended his great *Gynaecology* as an instructional manual for midwives, and the second-century author Galen addressed his sole specialized gynaecological text (a tract on the anatomy of the uterus) to a midwife. The other late antique Latin adaptors of Soranus, Theodorus Priscianus and Muscio, likewise directed their texts to

---

[9] Ann Ellis Hanson, 'A Division of Labor: Roles for Men in Greek and Roman Births', *Thamyris* 1 (1994), 157–202; King, *Hippocrates' Woman*.

[10] Rebecca Flemming, *Medicine and the Making of Roman Women: Gender, Nature, and Authority from Celsus to Galen* (Oxford: Oxford University Press, 2001). There is, of course, no evidence that there ever was a *law* prohibiting women's medical practice in Athens.

[11] Caelius Aurelianus, *Gynaecia*, in Miriam F. Drabkin and Israel E. Drabkin, *Caelius Aurelianus, Gynaecia: Fragments of a Latin version of Soranus' 'Gynaecia' from a thirteenth century manuscript* (Baltimore: Johns Hopkins Press, 1951), p. 1.

midwives. Both of the latter, it is true, 'dumbed down' their writings to make them suitable for what they believed were the lesser intellectual capacities of midwives, but their principal intended audiences nevertheless remained female.[12] In all these cases, it is clear that midwives were never the *only* intended audience: Soranus, for example, was explicit that his book could also be used by those who wished to know how to *choose* 'the best midwife', in other words, the male heads of households who would have been hiring them. Be that as it may, the rendering of gynaecological and obstetrical knowledge directly into the hands of female practitioners was considered normative in this period.

By the time the *Trotula* texts were composed in the twelfth century, in contrast, the social milieu that had generated both literate midwives and texts to put in their hands had long since disappeared. The already diminished intellectual climate of fifth- and sixth-century Roman North Africa would evaporate when the urban environments of the Mediterranean basin were devastated not simply by the influx of migrating tribes from central Asia but also by waves of bubonic plague in the sixth and seventh centuries. The consequent collapse of the political and economic structures in turn brought on the collapse of many elements of the educational structures of ancient Mediterranean society.[13]

This seems to have been particularly disruptive of the networks of education and training that had supported midwifery as an esteemed profession. Whereas midwives (Greek *maiai*, Latin *obstetrices* or simply *medicae*) enjoyed considerable prestige right up through the sixth century, like other specialized medical practitioners who relied on concentrated populations to support their practice, midwives *as medical specialists* seem to have essentially disappeared in the early Middle Ages.[14] Nevertheless, much of the corpus of writings on women's medicine survived. Certain gynaecological texts could be found scattered in isolated libraries across western Europe: the Benedictine monastery of Monte Cassino, just seventy-five kilometres north of Salerno, for example, owned copies of Muscio's text and the late antique pastiche, the *Gynaecology*

---

[12] Theodorus Priscianus, writing in the late fourth century, for example, didn't even attempt to explain obstetrical difficulties, arguing that these needed to be learned through experience rather than reading. Muscio, writing probably in the fifth or sixth century, was not only bemoaning the loss of Greek learning among midwives, but admitted in no uncertain terms that he had had to reduce the expansive text of Soranus's Greek work to a more digestible compendium that sometimes employed a question-and-answer format to make the material more intelligible.

[13] Nicholas Everett, *Literacy in Lombard Italy, c.568–774* (Cambridge: Cambridge University Press, 2003), argues for the continuity of literacy from late Antiquity into the early Middle Ages. But as he himself shows, this is primarily limited to notarial literacy; his evidence for female literacy is negligible.

[14] In the sixth century, the Emperor Justinian ranked *obstetrices* (whom he equated with the male category *medici*) among the most highly valued slaves. See Paul Krüger (ed.), *Corpus iuris civilis*, vol. II: *Codex Iustinianus* (Berlin: Weidmann, 1954), 6.43.3 (anno 531); cf. 7.7.5 (anno 530); I am indebted to Peter Brown for bringing these passages to my attention. For my argument that professional midwives disappeared in the early Middle Ages, see Monica H. Green, 'Bodies, Gender, Health, Disease: Recent Work on Medieval Women's Medicine', *Studies in Medieval and Renaissance History* 3rd ser., 2 (2005), 1–49, at pp. 15–17.

of Cleopatra. The gynaecological chapters of the Hippocratic *Aphorisms* were reworked into a special teaching manual on women's diseases that circulated in France.[15] A gynaecological text attributed in its original Greek form to a female figure, Metrodora, was available in Sicily and it was probably there that it was translated into Latin (anonymously) in the eleventh century. In not a single case is there evidence that a gynaecological manuscript was owned by a woman.

Early medieval Europe thus presents a paradox: the survival of a body of medical writing composed for a specialist audience even after the original target audience ceased to exist. The midwives to whom Theodorus, Caelius, and Muscio had directed their texts were expected to be literate and to have competence in general medical theory. They were expected to be the main caretakers of *all* of women's particular health concerns—that is, gynaecology (which demanded knowledge of the internal workings of the body and the causes of disease) as well as obstetrics. In contrast, none of the newly composed or newly adapted gynaecological texts circulating in eleventh- and twelfth-century Europe (or, as we will see, for several centuries thereafter) make claims to be written specifically for midwives. Two adaptations of Muscio's text, for example, which were probably made in the eleventh century, completely delete Muscio's preface explaining how he expects midwives to make use of his book as well as his clear definition of the midwife as a woman not only literate, but 'learned in all matters pertaining to women, and also experienced in medical practice'.[16] Both texts are distinguished by a systematic suppression of both theory (including anatomy of the female genitalia, the chorion, placenta, etc.) and many instructions on the basic tasks of the midwife such as postpartum procedures, how to wash, swaddle, and cradle the baby. The Latin Metrodora adaptation stresses, unlike its Greek original, the need to 'make what is hidden open' so that women will literally not die of embarrassment because they refuse to discuss their diseases; despite this call for openness, however, there is no expectation that it is *women* who will be the direct reading audience of the text.[17]

[15] Vendôme, Bibliothèque municipale, MS 175, s. xi ex. (S. France), ff. 104r–106v, here entitled *Fisicum medicinalis de iunicia* (The Medical Nature of Women's Diseases).

[16] [Muscio], *Sorani Gynaeciorum vetus translatio latina*, ed. Valentin Rose (Leipzig: Teubner, 1882), pp. 5–6: '3. Quae est aptissima quae obstetrices facere possit? principaliter quae litteras novit et habet ingenium praesens et memoriam, studiosa, munda, in universo iam corpore integra, fortis et laboriosa. 4. Quid est obstetrix? femina omnium muliebrium causarum docta, etiam medicinali exercitatione perita.'

[17] *De passionibus mulierum B*, in BNF, MS lat. 7029, s. xi ex. (Italy), f. 59v: '*De passionibus mulierum.* Utile preuidi uobis scribere superuenientibus plurimis et diuersis passionibus sepius de matrice. ex quibus alique periculose et insanabiles fiunt propter confessionem turpitudinis. alie uero sanabiles ob mediocritatem egritudinis. Qua propter ut ratio pandat quod uerecundia celat. signis uniuscuiusque rei prepositis curationes subiciam.' The Greek text of Metrodora has been edited several times; for a modern French translation, see Hélène Congourdeau, '"Métrodôra" et son oeuvre', in *Maladie et société à Byzance*, ed. Evelyne Patlagean (Spoleto: Centro Italiano di Studi sull'Alto Medioevo, 1993), pp. 57–96.

None of this means, of course, that the *practice* of caring for women's needs in childbirth, or their gynaecological conditions more broadly, necessarily passed out of women's hands. Rather, to the extent that traditions of women's medical knowledge were handed down from generation to generation among women, it must have been through oral means. The ancient texts that had been written to support an educated corps of midwives in Antiquity survived in attenuated form, but the traditions that structured the practice of medicine by women *around written texts* did not. The literate, learned midwife—the kind of broad specialist in women's medicine that Agnodice aspired to be—had disappeared and, as the rest of this book will argue, she never returned with the full array of competence that her ancient predecessor had enjoyed. In this sense, gynaecology in twelfth-century Salerno was already masculine in that the inherited corpus of writings on women's medicine had long since fallen into men's hands.

WOMEN'S MEDICINE AND THE LITERATE MALE PHYSICIAN

If no social power were invested in the written medical text—if, for example, medical texts were seen as a curiosity or as a source for independent learning that carried no inherent prestige—then we could imagine that a book-learned healer had no automatic social advantage over one whose learning was attained through apprenticeship and proven by empirical success. This may well have been the case for the early medieval period, but the twelfth century marks a turning point in the history of western medicine. Medicine in the twelfth century, and specifically at Salerno, was changing from an empirical craft, a manual art, to a field of knowledge that could claim to be based on unifying rational principles. Salerno's reputation as a centre of medical skill extends at least back to the tenth century and, with increasing frequency throughout the latter half of the eleventh century, we find in Salernitan records men taking on the title *medicus* (healer) in the same way they take on specialized occupational epithets like 'judge', 'notary', 'blacksmith', or 'goldsmith'. Some of these practitioners call themselves *medicus et clericus* (healer and cleric), which suggests that the literacy needed for the priesthood could also be used to acquire medical learning. This association was not unique to Salerno, of course, for we find isolated cleric-healers throughout early medieval Europe. What is unique to Salerno, however, from the mid eleventh century on is a growing sense that medical learning was not simply a body of knowledge to be picked up through random reading of whatever medical books were at hand nor was it merely a craft to be transmitted to an apprentice watching and imitating his master or her mistress. Rather, medicine was now being conceived as a body of knowledge that could be taught by sound principles of reasoning that were based on the skills of grammatical, rhetorical, and logical analysis that formed the foundation of a liberal arts education. Medical books should not be read randomly, but in a specific order that moved from basic principles of a scientific understanding of the natural world (what are the four elements? how do elemental properties combine to make up the four humours in the body?) to the more demanding tasks of rational healing like how to derive a diagnosis, prognose the course of a disease, and then prescribe a course of treatment. Medicine was once again becoming *literate*, an endeavour not simply aided by, but defined by the reliance on texts and learned modes of analysis. This was a kind of medicine that no simply oral discourse could achieve.[18]

To the degree that it was becoming literate, medicine was also becoming gendered in a new way. Twelfth-century southern Italian society had, of course, any number of interlocking systems of gender. From practices of inheritance to control of violence, from legal systems to habits of dress and deportment, gender (along with ethnicity, class, religion, and familial identity) structured how all individuals lived their lives. Literacy and access to literate culture were part of this gendered structure. Men, at least those of certain classes, were far more likely to be book-learned than women and more apt to participate in high literate culture. Basic training in literacy, followed by a secondary level of training in the liberal arts, would have been common not simply for boys headed for the priesthood, but also for boys headed for that equally important (and equally masculine) professional class in Italy society: the notariate. Unlike parts of northern Europe where law was only beginning to rely heavily on the written word for contracts, property exchanges, etc., in southern Europe the practices of Roman law and its reliance on written contracts had never disappeared.[19] Women in southern Italy were by no means uniformly illiterate—we can find, for example, a writing case in the possession of one woman, a psalter in the hands of another—but such evidence is rare.[20] Few women would have had more than a rudimentary education in formal grammar, logic, and rhetoric, let alone induction into the world of classical literature. In contrast, male physicians sometimes displayed

[18] I have, of course, had to vastly simplify several centuries of medical developments here. Historians of medicine have still not come to a unitary understanding of how medical literature functioned in the early Middle Ages. Although there was never a period when medical literature was not circulating, how (or how widely) it was being used is difficult to establish beyond the fact that simple recipes for specific ailments and instructions for basic diet or regimen (including periodic phlebotomy) continued to prove popular. On the failure of early medieval medical readers to establish anything like a 'science' of medicine or regularized disciplines of medical teaching, and for the re-emergence of medical teaching in the later 11th century, see Florence Eliza Glaze, 'The Perforated Wall: The Ownership and Circulation of Medical Books in Medieval Europe, *c*.800–1200', PhD dissertation, Duke University, 1999.

[19] Maria Galante, 'Il notaio e il documento notarile a Salerno in epoca longobarda', in *Per una storia del notariato meridionale*, ed. Mario Amelotti, Studi storici sul notariato italiano, VI (Rome: Consiglio Nazionale del Notariato, 1982), 71–94; see also Everett, *Literacy*.

[20] Patricia Skinner, 'Women, Literacy and Invisibility in Southern Italy, 900–1200', in Lesley Smith and Jane H. M. Taylor, eds., *Women, the Book and the Worldly: Selected Proceedings of the St Hilda's Conference, 1993*, vol. 2 (Cambridge: D. S. Brewer, 1995), pp. 1–11. This characterization of women's literacy of course only applies to southern Italy. We have plenty of evidence in other parts of Europe for high levels of learning among upper-class women in the 12th century.

extraordinarily high levels of learning, not simply having exceptional command over Latin style and the writings of classical authors such as Cicero and Boethius, but on occasion even some knowledge of Greek.[21]

Male physicians (or at least those whose practices we can document) are thus characterized as a group by their literacy, their training in the liberal arts and, more and more over the course of the twelfth century, their commitment to establishing medicine as a higher discipline.[22] Male practitioners moved from calling themselves simply 'healers' (*medici*) to 'healers and persons learned in science' (*medici et phisici*), the latter term referring to knowledge of the natural world (and giving birth to the term we still use in English today, 'physician'). Whereas women had been able to achieve considerable success as empirical practitioners in the context of an oral culture of medicine (a visiting Norman monk in the mid eleventh century is said to have found in Salerno no more learned healer than he save for one *sapiens matrona*, a very wise matron),[23] the new commitment to a culture of *literate* medicine radically altered the potential stature of women in medicine since they were so marginal to the culture of literacy itself.

The new learned physicians of twelfth-century Salerno, these 'masters' who within a century would be charged with overseeing the practice of medicine throughout southern Italy,[24] took the whole field of medicine as their province.

---

[21] Paul Oskar Kristeller, 'Fonti per la medicina Salernitana del Sec. XII', *Salerno—Civitas Hippocratica* 1, no. 1–2 (1967), 19–26, at p. 22.

[22] Of some four dozen *medici* who can be documented in Salernitan records between 1050 and 1200, all but two are male. Perhaps two thirds can be inferred to be literate. For example, besides the obvious cases of the known medical writers, many are identified as *clericus et medicus*. None are identified in the documents as *laicus* or *ydiota*.

[23] The Anglo-Norman historian Orderic Vitalis (who died shortly after 1141) recounted the story of Ralph 'the Ill-Tonsured', a member of a powerful Norman family who travelled in the mid 11th century to France and Italy in order to educate himself. As Orderic tells it, Ralph 'was very learned in grammar and dialectic, astronomy and music; and so skilled in medicine that in the city of Salerno, which is the ancient seat of the best medical schools, no one could equal him except one very learned woman' (*sapiens matrona*); Ordericus Vitalis, *The Ecclesiastical History*, ed. Marjorie Chibnall, 6 vols. (Oxford: Clarendon, 1969–80), 2: 28 and 74–6. On the date of Ralph's visit, see John F. Benton, 'Trotula, Women's Problems, and the Professionalization of Medicine in the Middle Ages', *Bulletin of the History of Medicine* 59 (1985), 30–53, at p. 38, n. 22. We learn nothing else of this woman from Orderic's account, though that is what is remarkable: there is no suggestion of surprise that Ralph should have been bested by a woman.

[24] In 1140, the Norman king of Sicily, Roger II, instituted a regulation that 'whoever in the future desires to become a physician should present himself to our officials and judges for an examination according to their judgement'; see the *Assizes* of Roger II, as cited in Leonard C. Chiarelli, 'A Preliminary Study on the Origins of Medical Licensing in the Medieval Mediterranean', *Al-Masaq: Islam and the Medieval Mediterranean* 10 (1998), 1–11, p. 1. Roger may have been emulating Muslim practices of having a royal official supervise the practices of physicians in the same way he supervised merchantile dealings as a whole; in any case, he did not specifically mention the masters of Salerno. Within a century, however, the authority to approve medical practice specifically had passed into the hands of those with the most formal learning, for in 1231 Roger's grandson, Emperor Frederick II, would stipulate that any physician must be 'approved in a convened public examination by the Masters of Salerno' (Frederick II, *Constitutions of Melfi*, as cited in Chiarelli). As we will see in Chapter 3, this transition to licensing pushed neither women nor illiterates out of practice; it did, however, define a clear hierarchy of authority in which the most learned men were in control.

The corpus of writings that came out of twelfth-century Salerno covered theory as well as practice, foundational topics like basic anatomy and clinical issues such as how to choose nourishing foods for one's patients and prepare compound medicines. Old or young, rich or poor, the human body in all its complexity was within these physicians' purview. This universality of perspective encompassed women's medicine, too. Gynaecological recommendations can be found in every single one of the general medical textbooks we have from twelfth-century Salerno (see Table 1.1) and, when several different Salernitan masters composed their commentaries on the Hippocratic *Aphorisms* they did not shy away from commenting on the gynaecological fifth book as well as the rest of the text.[25] From Copho, who was probably writing near the beginning of the century, right up to the cleric John of Saint Paul in the 1170s or 1180s, there is no sense that male practitioners are in any way excluded from this realm of practice.[26] In fact, some of these writers include more on the specific conditions of women than they do on the male genitalia.[27]

The gynaecological chapters in Bartholomeus's *Practica*, for example, which was written prior to 1177, are often quite detailed. He itemizes four distinct causes for menstrual retention and explains the symptoms of each; in his chapter on uterine suffocation he includes a mini-case history of woman who was afflicted by syncope (the fainting that was a principal symptom of this disease) when she went outside to comb her hair while she was still recuperating from another condition. His student, Petrus Musandinus (d. before 1194), begins the gynaecological section of his *Practica* with the assertion that he will write about the cures for each of the many diseases that afflict the generative organs of women 'because I have become expert [in them] through long use'.[28] References to emmenagogues, aids for difficult birth, and uterine pain can regularly be found in works on general pharmaceutics such as the *Circa instans* (an alphabetized textbook on medicinal substances) and the *Antidotary of Nicholus* (a mid twelfth-century textbook of standardized, compound drugs). Indeed, concern to articulate the gynaecological uses of certain substances seems pronounced. A compound medicine that, in an earlier text, had cited its gynaecological properties as just one among many

---

[25] This apparent comfort with incorporating gynaecology into the general definition of 'medicine' is in marked contrast to the one major Salernitan composition of the 11th century, Gariopontus's mid century *Passionarius*, which included no gynaecological conditions at all in an otherwise comprehensive medical compendium.

[26] Even the 11th-century Salernitan archbishop Alfanus (d. 1085) is credited with creating an electuary for aiding conception and preventing miscarriage; CTC, MS R.14.30 (903), s. xiv, f. 221r.

[27] Archimattheus and Petrus Musandinus have no material on diseases of the penis at all. See Table 1.1.

[28] Petrus Musandinus, *Practica*, in Salzburg, Museum Carolino-Augusteum, MS 2166, s. xiii, f. 22rb: 'prout temporis usu expertus sum sufficienter rescribam'. Petrus likewise affirms his personal experience in the chapter on excessive menstruation (f. 22vb: 'credice sola hac medicina multas curaui, et quedam que quatuor mensibus passa fuerat, liberata fuit') and, in the chapter on uterine suffocation, dismisses those who misdiagnose this serious disease as 'inexpert physicians' (f. 23ra: 'imperiti medici').

Table 1.1. Gynaecological and Obstetrical Conditions in the *Practicae* of Male Salernitan Masters

This table summarizes the gynaecological and obstetrical material in the major male writers associated with Salerno. I have also included the *Viaticum* of Ibn al-Jazzār (as translated by Constantine the African) from which several of these writers drew material.[a]

Gyn/Ob Condition	IJ	JA	C	JP	A	B	PM	S	SP
breast disorders[b]	X	—	—	—	—	—	—	—	X
[male genitalia][c]	X	X	X	X	—	X	—	X	[X]
menstrual retention	X	X	X	X	X	X	X	X	X
menstrual excess	X	X	X	X	X	X	X	—[d]	X
uterine suffocation	X	—	X	X	—	X	X	X	X
uterine apostemes	X	—	—	—	—	—	X	X	X
uterine wounds/ulcers	X	—	—	—	—	—	—	X	—
uterine prolapse	X	—	X	X	—	—	X	X	X
pregnancy regimen/ avoidance of miscarriage	X	X	—	—	—	—	X	X	X
infertility	—	X	X	X	X	X	X	X	X[e]
difficult birth	X	X	X	—	—	—	X	X[f]	X
expulsion of the afterbirth[g]	X	[X]	—	—	—	—	—	[X]	X
vaginal problems[h]	—	X	X	—	—	—	X	X	—

 [a] Key
   IJ = Ibn al-Jazzār, *Viaticum*, Book VI (*c*.1080)
   JA = Johannes Afflacius, *Liber aureus* (*c*.1100?)
   C = Copho, *Practica* (*c*.1120?)
   JP = Johannes Platearius, *Practica brevis* (*c*.1150?)
   A = Archimattheus, *Practica* (between *c*.1150 and 1180)
   B = Bartholomeus, *Practica* (before 1177)
   PM = Petrus Musandinus, *Practica* (*c*.1180?)
   S = Salernus, *Catholica* (*c*.1180?)
   SP = Johannes de Sancto Paulo, *Breviarium* (before 1181)

 [b] In the *Viaticum*, this chapter appears in an earlier section of the book along with other conditions of the chest.

 [c] This category will usually include several chapters, ranging from satyriasis to gonorrhea (excessive semen production), swelling of the genitalia, itching, lesions, etc.

 [d] Salernus has only one recipe for menstrual excess, embedded within a general chapter *De matrice*.

 [e] Johannes de Sancto Paulo also includes in his chapter on infertility a section on signs of conception.

 [f] Petrus Musandinus's material on difficult birth is embedded in his chapter on birth in general. He offers brief instructions on how to expel the afterbirth, the lochial flow, and the dead foetus if they don't emerge on their own. All this seems to be adapted from the earlier Salernitan text, *Conditions of Women*.

 [g] In some cases, this topic was included in the chapter on difficult birth, which is signalled by the use of square brackets [].

 [h] I am including under this vague heading conditions such as swelling of the vagina (in Johannes Afflacius, Copho, and Salernus [who is simply quoting JA]), vaginal wounds (Afflacius and Petrus Musandinus), vaginal apostemes (Petrus Musandinus), and methods to constrict the size of the vagina and/or 'restore' virginity (Salernus).

different uses, is transformed in the *Antidotary of Nicholus* into a remedy that is first and foremost defined by its efficacy for women: 'It is called *trifera magna* because it confers great utility to women and makes them fruitful.'[29] While male Salernitan writers were not particularly inventive in theorizing gynaecological disease or recognizing the breadth of disorders that could afflict the female genitalia (a fact which will become more apparent in due course), not a single one of them completely excluded the diseases of women from their purview of the medical art.

What does universally distinguish the work of these male authors, however, is their omission of any direct 'hands-on' recommendations. We know, for example, that Archimattheus, who practised probably from the 1150s to the 1180s, had women among his clientele, for we find them among some two dozen case histories in his brief *Practica*. In the case of a woman with a disorder of her shoulder, Archimattheus readily uses first-person, active verbs to describe how he prepared her medications and applied them. The active first-person ('we') is in fact Archimattheus's most common grammatical construct when he describes his own cures. Yet in the case of a postmenopausal woman in whom he was trying to provoke haemorrhoidal bleeding (the treatment necessarily involving an application to the genital region), the verbal form is passive.[30]

This sort of grammatical 'dance' around women's genitalia can be seen especially clearly in the case of uterine prolapse, a condition that by its very nature demands some kind of hands-on intervention for its treatment.[31] Of the eight general medical compendia we have from male Salernitan writers, uterine prolapse is treated in the *Practicae* of five: Copho, Johannes Platearius, Petrus Musandinus, Salernus, and John of Saint Paul.[32] None of them recommend

---

[29] Cited in Green, *Trotula*, p. 201.

[30] Archimattheus Salernitanus, *Practica Archimathaei*, in *Collectio Salernitana ossia documenti inediti, e trattati di medicina appartenenti alla scuola medica salernitana*, ed. Salvatore De Renzi, 5 vols. (Naples: Filiatre-Sebezio, 1852–59; repr. Bologna: Forni, 1967), 5: 350–76, at p. 358. On the relation between menstrual bleeding (which was generally thought to be salubrious) and haemorrhoids, see Monica H. Green, 'Flowers, Poisons, and Men: Menstruation in Medieval Western Europe', in *Menstruation: A Cultural History,* ed. Andrew Shail and Gillian Howie (New York: Palgrave, 2005), pp. 51–64. When describing treatment of anal prolapse and bleeding haemorrhoids in the 'generic' patient (presumably male), Archimattheus often uses active forms.

[31] The human uterus can prolapse (collapse down into the vagina and, in extreme cases, protrude all the way out to the exterior of the body) when the ligaments that support it are stretched or broken (usually in childbirth) and when the normal muscular and nervous supports of the pelvic floor are compromised (with, again, repeated childbirth and also advanced age being the principal culprits). This condition can also be accompanied by prolapse of the urethra and bladder, by anal prolapse, and by incarceration of portions of the intestines which extrude into the vagina. Although uterine prolapse is not usually a life-threatening condition, incarceration of the intestines can potentially lead to septicemic infection. In modern biomedicine, uterine prolapse is most commonly treated surgically, usually involving hysterectomy and the introduction of structural supports to the pelvic floor.

[32] I omit from this discussion a ninth Salernitan *Practica*, an anonymous text published under the title *Trattato delle cure* (edited in Piero Giacosa, *Magistri Salernitani nondum editi*, Turin: Fratelli Bocca, 1901, pp. 175–279), which also includes a section on prolapse (p. 237). Although there is

any procedures that call for the male physician himself to touch the afflicted woman. Copho, for example, recommends that the woman be given sternutatives (substances that induce sneezing), emetics (medicines to provoke vomiting), or suffumigations of the vagina made with pitch and other ingredients; the one mechanical measure he prescribes is that, with the woman's feet suspended, her womb be filled (his passive) with rain water in which various herbs have been cooked.[33] Petrus Musandinus, who culled much of his gynaecological material from the anonymous *Conditions of Women*, recommends fumigations, applications to the groin, and the use of sweet-smelling substances to the nose; it is the midwife who actually repositions the uterus.[34] John of Saint Paul, a contemporary of Petrus, recommends the use of the same bimodal odoriferous therapy, whereby foul smells are applied to the vagina and sweet smells to the nose; it was believed that the uterus was sensitive to smells and, repelled by the foul odours below while attracted to the pleasant ones above, would return to its proper place.[35] Importantly, aside from Petrus Musandinus, none of these male authors is simply recycling material he has found in other texts. While some textual dependence can at points be discerned, it is clear that they are each giving their own unique opinions on how this rather common condition should be treated. They are, in other words, drawing on their experiences in practice. But in the case of women's gynaecological and obstetrical conditions, their practice is always 'at a distance'.

Again, John of Saint Paul can give us some idea of how a male physician can be said to practise gynaecology or obstetrics even if he does not himself touch, or perhaps even look at, his female patients' genitalia. In his chapter on excessive menstrual flux, John first lists the situations that might cause excessive flux, such as an overabundance of humours, breaks of the veins, or complications during pregnancy or childbirth. It might also be due to haemorrhoids (presumably in the vagina), 'which are recognized by sight and by touch'. John does not specify whose sight or touch is involved here, an omission that continues when he describes how, 'if the mouth of the vagina is opened with a catheter while the pain is increasing, a red humidity will flow out; but when [the pain] subsides a moisture similar to the dregs of wine flows out, sometimes white, sometimes black'. He

good reason to think that this author, too, was male, the evidence of the other texts of undisputed male authorship is sufficient for the purposes of this discussion.

[33] This description comes from the chapter on uterine prolapse attributed to 'M.C'. in the *De egritudinum curatione*, a synthesis of extracts from at least seven different Salernitan authors made late in the 12th century; edited in De Renzi, *Collectio Salernitana*, 2: 340.25–35. In the text of Copho's independently circulating *Practica*, the recommendations are rather different though there is no more 'hands-on' therapy than found here. See below for further discussion of the discrepancies between these two versions of Copho's work.

[34] Petrus Musandinus, *Practica*, in Salzburg, MS 2166, f. 23vb: 'et obstetrix matricem intromittat'.

[35] Johannes de Sancto Paulo, *Breviarium medicine*, in BLL, MS Additional 16385, s. xiii, ff. 4v–78v. For further details on the rationale of this therapy, see Green, *Trotula*, pp. 22–31.

then continues on with some other symptoms that accompany menstrual excess, and then notes that the predominating humour can be known (again, his passive) by the colour of the menses 'and by the colour of the menstrual rag when it is dried out'.[36] In the chapter on impediments to conception, he is the first Salernitan male writer to speak of fleshy obstructions closing off the orifice of the vagina or growing inside the vagina itself. Such obstructions, which not only impede the flow of the menses but make sexual intercourse and conception impossible, 'are apprehended by the women being spread open so that they are able to be seen by sight and probed by touch'. He recommends surgical intervention as the cure.[37] Again, John's use of the passive voice obscures agency here, but in his chapter on uterine suffocation it becomes clear who is to do this observation and manual manipulation of the female patient. He suggests that one of the signs that venomous fumes from the uterus have reached the vital members (heart, lungs, etc.) and caused the uterus to withdraw is that 'the mouth [of the womb] is found *by the midwives* to be twisted'.[38] Midwives (*obstetrices*) are likewise mentioned as the manual operators in his chapter on childbirth. Although, as I will argue later, it seems unlikely that a professionalized corps of midwives existed in twelfth-century Salerno (I believe John is using the term in a generic way simply to refer to female attendants), John makes it clear that women are, in fact, needed for visual and manual inspection of the female genitalia.

John of Saint Paul's gynaecology is both more substantive and more engaged than that of his predecessors in twelfth-century Salerno. But by that fact it also shows the very real social limits to male gynaecological and obstetrical practice. Interestingly, right in the middle of his chapter on uterine suffocation, John inserts a justification for male medical intervention from the Latin translation of

[36] Johannes de Sancto Paulo, *Breviarium*, MS Additional 16385, f. 55r–v: 'Fluxus nimis menstruorum fit ex habundantia humorum, uel ex subtilitate eorum et acumine uel ex largitate aut scissura uenarum, uel exitus fetus antequam animetur. Scinduntur etiam uene ex nimia compressione in partu. Fiunt etiam ibi emorroides *que uisu et tactu cognoscuntur.* Si aperiatur os uulue cum enargalia in quibus cum dolor augmentatur rubea effluit humiditas. Cum autem quiescit, deffluit humiditas quasi fex uini aliquando alba, aliquando nigra. Cum augmentatur fluxus sanguinis et durat sequitur macies, fastidium, mutatio coloris et tumor pedum ydropisis. Cognoscuntur autem humores habundantes per colorem menstruorum et per colorem panni menstruari desiccari.' My emphasis.

[37] Johannes de Sancto Paulo, *Breviarium*, MS Additional 16385, f. 58r: 'Impeditur quoque conceptio et partus et muliebria ex clausum [*sic*] uulue, et dicuntur clause mulieres. Clauduntur quoque a panniculis uel pinnaculis. i. testiculis a foris ibi coherentibus, aut ipsis patentibus. Pulpa uel membrana innascitur in medio sinu mulieris aut etiam in hoc sinu patente: orificium matricis clauditur. Quando pinnacula aforis sibi coherent, impediuntur menstrua mulieres ad usum ueneriorum et ad purgationem et ad conceptionem. *Apprehenduntur hec omnia patefactis mulieribus ut uisu uideantur et tactu probari possunt.* Curentur autem cirurgia.' My emphasis.

[38] MS Additional 16385, f. 56r: 'Svffocatio matricis est ablatio hanelitus per uuluam. Contingit mulieribus maritatis que a coitu in longum abstinent et uiduis ut breuiter dicam ex diuturna retentione menstruorum et continentia spermatis hec passio accidit. Dum enim per malam et uenenosam qualitatem sperma aut menstrua immutantur: fumus uenonosus ab eis resolutus. nobilia membra percutit cerebrum, scilicet cor, epar, et matrix contrahibut. *et ab obstetricibus os distortum reperitur.*' My emphasis.

the Greek Metrodora text, *Diseases of Women*: 'Women are ashamed to confess [their diseases] out of embarrassment. Therefore, let reason reveal what shame conceals.'[39] This statement seems incongruous here (certainly it would have been more appropriate at the opening of the gynaecological section), yet I think John places it here because, having just listed the symptoms of this severe disease and the difficulty of diagnosis, he is emphasizing the need for frank discussion of the one disease that most intimately links women's sexuality with health.[40] Later, in the chapter on itching of the pudenda, which can lead to a chronic desire for intercourse, John frankly recommends that widows masturbate to relieve themselves and that virgins use what is in essence a medicated dildo.[41] Thus, John seems to see the problem of shame as *women's* problem; it is the male practitioner's reason, his enlightened ability to speak rationally about disease, that will aid women in overcoming their inability to speak about the diseases of the reproductive and sexual organs and thus seek the necessary treatment from learned physicians.

Close examination of Salernitan male writers' works on medical practice thus demonstrates both the extent and the limits of male gynaecological practice in the twelfth century. In addition to his *Practica* and his commentaries on the basic textbooks of medical instruction (the so-called *Articella*), Archimattheus wrote a tract on medical etiquette. He warns the (male) physician 'above all not to gaze upon the wife, daughter or female servant with a lascivious eye; for they obscure the mind of the physician while he is working, and they alter the sense of God cooperating, and they make the physician annoying to the patient and make him less confident in himself'.[42] Archimattheus is drawing, of course, on an ethical tradition that can be traced back to the Hippocratic Oath. But just as in ancient Greece, these precepts against exploiting the privacy of the patient's household did not prohibit consultation on the ills of the female members of the household. It was precisely because Salernitan male practitioners also treated women that they recognized the importance of taking the sex of the patient into account in their diagnoses (Archimattheus himself claims to have written a text on the difference in heat between men and women)[43] and it was

[39] MS Additional 16385, f. 56r: 'Verecundantur femine confiteri propter turpitudinem. Ratio itaque pandat quod uerecundia celat'.

[40] Omitting reference to virgins, John emphasizes that this condition occurs either in married women who have long been deprived of intercourse or in widows. He implies that it is caused by retention of *both* the menses and women's own seed, not either/or as most other writers would stress.

[41] MS Additional 16385, f. 57r: 'Quedam enim mulieres tantum patiuntur in uulua pruritum ut coitum uiri concupiscere uideantur. Tepescat ergo curatione hoc uicium. Vidua: immittat sibi manum et alleuiabitur. Pro uirgine autem fiat aliquod molle simile membro uirili de nitro et cera et nasturtio. Diligentur trita et subiciatur donec pati poterunt.'

[42] Hermann Grensemann, 'Die Schrift *De adventu medici ad aegrotum* nach dem Salernitaner Arzt Archimatheus', *Würzburger medizinhistorische Mitteilungen* 14 (1996) 233–51, at p. 242.

[43] This treatise has not yet been discovered. Archimattheus refers to it in his commentary on Johannitius's *Isagoge*; see Hermann Grensemann, ed., *Archimathei Salernitani, Glossae in Isagogas*

because they were called on to advise on aspects of women's particular diseases that they incorporated gynaecological material into their textbooks of practical medicine.

AUTHORIAL GENDER AND THE GENESIS OF THE *TROTULA*

The most important Salernitan achievement on women's medicine was not, of course, the few brief chapters embedded in these general textbooks, but rather the three specialized texts that would later be combined into a single compendium, the so-called *Trotula* ensemble.[44] Two of the three texts, *On Women's Cosmetics* and *The Book on the Conditions of Women*, originally circulated anonymously. The third text, *On Treatments for Women*, actually has a clear and consistent attribution in the manuscripts, but I wish to treat it as 'anonymous' for the moment in order to demonstrate how close analysis can, in fact, give us independent information on the structuring of gendered knowledge production and practice of women's medicine. Although *Women's Cosmetics* is somewhat removed from my main concern with gynaecology and obstetrics, I include analysis of it here both because 'women's medicine' was defined in Salerno as including cosmetics (see the discussion of *Treatments for Women* below) and because it provides a superb example of how and why male practitioners appropriated the practices of women.

On Women's Cosmetics

Of the three original Salernitan texts on women's medicine, only the original *Women's Cosmetics* gives a clear sense of an authorial personality. The preface is an elegant construct that lays out the author's motives for writing:

As Hippocrates says in the book he composed on the science of prognostication, 'Everyone who through the study of the art of medicine desires to gain either glory or a delightful

---

Johannitii: Ein Kursus in mittelalterlicher Physiologie nach dem Codex Trier Bischöfliches Priesterseminar 76A und dem Codex Toletanus Archivo y Biblioteca Capitulares 97–14 (Hamburg 2004), electronic publication: <http://www.uke.uni-hamburg.de/institute/geschichte-medizin/index_18229.php> accessed 6 June 2005, p. 49.

44 My edition of the *Trotula* ensemble (Green, *Trotula*) presented a much developed, mid 13th century version of the text. Here, I am discussing exclusively the original versions of the three independent texts. Although these remain unedited, I have established through exhaustive philological analysis which manuscripts present the earliest versions of the texts—which, as the philologist's maxim *juniores non semper deteriores* reminds us, is not necessarily the same thing as being the earliest extant copies. All citations that follow, therefore, come from the manuscripts that present the best early versions of the texts. The same system of paragraph numeration is used for the texts cited here as in my published edition of the *Trotula* ensemble. For a full survey of the *Trotula* manuscript and textual tradition, see Green, 'Development'.

multitude of friends, to the same degree let him take pains to furnish his understanding with the precepts of prudent men', lest in [the eyes of] those individuals looking to the art of healing he be found defenseless and unskilled. But if he neglects to do this, instead of glory and fame he will earn shame and infamy, instead of friends he will gain for himself so many enemies. Thus also it will come to pass that, in front of those in the forum by whom he ought to be greeted and called 'physician', he is ridiculed publicly and he is not called 'physician' by them. In consideration of this fact, I fortified my understanding with those precepts of women whom I found to be clever in the art of cosmetics so that I would be found learned [*doctus*] in all things pertaining as much to the adornment of the face as to the other members. Thus, to whatever noble or even common woman who seeks from me something of this artifice I should know how to offer counsel appropriate to her status and means, and she would succeed in obtaining the best result. But because, as Persius says, 'for you to know is nothing, unless another knows what you know', consequently I wish to commend to writing and to render into a succinct treatise some novel things concerning this artifice. And so, let what I have in my mind come to the knowledge of others.[45]

Grammatically, there is only one indicator of gendered authorship in the entire text—the masculine verbal form *doctus* here in the preface. Yet the whole picture of medical practice the anonymous *Women's Cosmetics* author paints suggests a world of men. Learned enough to be able to cite the *Satires* of the ancient Roman Persius as well as the Hippocratic *Prognostics*, the author offers in the preface a high rhetorical justification for his work, arguing that the ideal physician (referred to exclusively by masculine forms) must be as learned as possible in all aspects of medicine if he is to win public acclaim.

The whole preface is, in essence, an argument why a field of knowledge so completely feminine in subject matter should nevertheless be a suitable component of the learned male physician's repertoire. Yet far from reflecting a picture of the accumulated wisdom of male medical practitioners, our author

---

[45] *Women's Cosmetics 1*, Prague, Knihovnà Metropolitní Kapituli, Cod. м–20, s. xiii med. (Italy) f. 49rb: 'Ut ait Ypocras in libro suo quem de prognosticorum scientia composuit, 'Omnis qui medicine artis studio seu gloriam seu delectabilem amicorum copiam consequi desiderat, rationem suam regulis prudencium adeo munire studeat, ne in singulis ad artem medendi spectantibus inermis reperiatur et rudis'. Quod si facere neglexerit loco glorie et fame, dedecus et infamiam, loco amicorum, plures quam sibi inquirat inimicos. Sicque efficietur, ut a quibus in foro salutari deberet et medicus appellari eis rudiculum fiat in publico et [neque] ab eis medicus nuncupatur. Huius in circuitu rationis ego regulis mulierum quas in artificiali decore faciendo facetas inueni meam [ms: m^i eam] rationem muniui [ms: minui], ut in singulis tam ad ornatum faciei quam ceterorum [ms: ceterum] membrorum mulierum doctus reperiar, ita vt cuillibet mulieri nobili seu etiam gratcie de huiusmodi artificio aliquid a me quereti iuxta sui qualitatem et modum conuenientis suum adhibere consilium ut et ego laudem et ipsa exoptatum ualeat consequi effectum. At quoniam ut ait Persius: 'Scire tuum nichil est nisi te scire hoc sciat alter', uolo itaque que de hoc artificio noui literis commendare et in compendiosum scriptum redigere. Quo mediante quod in mente habeo in aliorum ueniat noticiam.' The prologue to the *Women's Cosmetics* as edited in Benton, 'Trotula, Women's Problems', p. 53, conflates versions 1 and 3; in *Women's Cosmetics 3*, a second masculine verbal adjective was added. The references to Hippocrates and Persius are, respectively: *Prognostica*, translation attributed to Constantinus Africanus, preface, printed in *Articella* (Venice, 1492), f. 40r; Persius, *Saturnalia* 1:27: 'scire tuum nihil est nisi te scire hoc sciat alter'.

shows that this picture is really a palimpsest. He admits he has appropriated some of his knowledge of cosmetics from women themselves—some of which he gained from personal observation (including a certain Sicilian woman's cure for mouth odour problems) and some from recording descriptions that he heard (particularly the practices of 'Saracens'). The author, in fact, never claims that a particular therapy is his own (although just after the Sicilian woman's cure for mouth odour he adds another remedy whose use and efficacy he personally endorses).[46] Indeed, the rest of the text, though well-organized and heavily cross-referenced, seems to bear out this impression of feminine—or at least empirical—origin. Reading as if they were first-hand accounts from knowledgeable practitioners, the prescriptions are extremely detailed. Far more than a simple series of 'mix these ingredients and apply', the text often goes into close detail on how ingredients are to be prepared, cooked, rubbed, dried, stored, and used. The author even goes into the bed chamber, explaining how a woman is to anoint her face, hands, breasts, and genitalia (internal and external) with a special scented water and powder prior to intercourse. She is also to use these same preparations to wash the face, armpits, and genitalia of her partner.

True, the text has no doctrinal or, aside from the preface, strong theoretical components, though this is perhaps not surprising since there was no prior tradition of rationalized cosmetics on which he could draw.[47] It is clear, nevertheless, that the author is now laying claim to the empirical knowledge he has collected as proof of his general medical learning. The author maintains a constant presence throughout the text, reminding the reader continually of the order of his argument with frequent cross-references to therapies already described: 'as I have said', 'as I said before', 'the powder which I recommended before', etc.[48]

The *Women's Cosmetics* author appears, then, to be a well-educated male who identifies fully with the ancient ideal of the physician as a public figure who seeks not wealth but glory and 'a great multitude of friends'; his success resides in his reputation for learning and this he can earn only through hard study or, in the present case, close observation of and conversation with skilled female

---

[46] *Women's Cosmetics* 1, Prague, cod. M-20, f. 51r: 'Item si mulier parum de folio lauri et pauxillum de musco sub lingua teneat, licet multum fetoris in se habeat nunquam ab aliquo percipietur eius grauis anelitus. Vnde laudo ut mulier die ac nocte et maxime quando debeat cum aliquo iacere, sub lingua teneat. Siue ipse habeat grauem odorem siue non, ea bonus augmentatur.' The form *laudo* is the only time the first person is used other than in the preface and editorial cross-references.

[47] In this respect, *Women's Cosmetics* differs markedly from the *On Cosmetics* attributed to Richardus Anglicus (late 12th/early 13th century) and that attributed to Arnau of Vilanova (d. 1311), both of which would offer at least some minimal physiological rationalization for the causes of certain skin disorders.

[48] The cross-referential phrases he uses are 'ut predixi', 'ut supradixi', 'ut superius diximus', 'precipimus', 'ut dixi' (five times), 'ut superius dixi', 'ut supradictum est' (the only passive cross-reference), 'quem [sc. pulverem] superius fieri docui', 'aliquod eorum que dixi ad dealbandam faciem', and 'pulverem quem superius dixi'. He also recommends a particular procedure ('laudo', a phrase also used in the preface).

practitioners. Knowledge of cosmetics, this author implies, is simply one more field in which the (male) physician must gain mastery, so that he never be found 'defenseless and unskilled' even in the eyes of women, of whatever social class, who might come to him for cosmetic advice. Far from rejecting women's cosmetics as a private concern of interest only to women themselves, distant from the public concerns of men, the author asserts that the male physician's social stature will be enhanced when he has this field of therapy at his command. The individual woman is still expected to do much of the preparation and all of the application of these therapies: the preparation of mixtures is started by the physician (the reader), yet the woman is to carry out the rest herself. It is the knowledge, the instruction, that comes from the male physician.

Women's Cosmetics thus constructs an image in microcosm of Salernitan medical society. The inscribed (ideal) audience is male physicians not dissimilar from the author himself: they subscribe to the same ideal of the learned physician that he does; they have the same vision of medicine as a learned art, and the same image of themselves as lauded practitioners. The author acknowledges both the existence and the value of 'the precepts of women learned in this art', yet it is he who makes this knowledge useful. The implications of this text for our understanding of the historical situation of twelfth-century Salernitan women are two-fold. First, even though women are learned (i.e. experienced) practitioners of the art of cosmetics, once appropriated by this male author, women's expertise is made irrelevant. Second, as potential patients, women are now dependent on male practitioners as the repositories of the knowledge that they need 'to obtain the best result' in their cosmetic undertakings. The preface implicitly excludes women from the audience, since if women could gain this knowledge for themselves there would be no need to seek the advice of learned (male) physicians. *Women's Cosmetics* is not a text written for women to read for themselves, to fortify *their own* understanding with the precepts of prudent men (or women). It is a text written for men who wish, like this author, to maintain privileged access to specialized medical knowledge that can then be dispensed (at a price) to an illiterate or marginally literate populace.[49] Although much of this cosmetic knowledge seems to have originated with women, it is the author's objective that women should now only be able to obtain such knowledge piecemeal—and only by paying for it.

Book on the Conditions of Women

Conditions of Women provides no internal grammatical evidence of its author's gender as had the *Women's Cosmetics*, nor does the author foreground his persona in the text. Still, I think there are several elements which suggest that that persona was male. This text reflects a very different direction of the flow of medical

---

[49] See Chapter 2 below.

knowledge: the male writer is appropriating, not women's empirical knowledge, but other men's *written* knowledge. The text is fundamentally ambiguous about who the intended audience was to be, an ambiguity that would reverberate throughout the text's long life in the centuries to come.

Conditions of Women was actually composed in two principal stages. The original 'rough draft' of the text bears no preface. Rather, it launches immediately into an explanation of how women's colder bodily temperament in relation to men, as well as the fact that they do not engage in physical labour to the same extent as men, means that their bodies cannot expel all the superfluous humours that accumulate. This is the reason why Nature created for them a special purgation, menstruation. Having provided this general physiological background, the text then moves on to women's menstrual disorders and various other gynaecological and obstetrical conditions. The work is almost entirely composed from material extracted and adapted from other written texts: Constantine the African's translation of Ibn al-Jazzār's *Viaticum* is the main source, although material also comes from one of the early medieval translations of the Hippocratic *Diseases of Women 2*.[50] Although several ancient authorities are named here—Hippocrates, Galen, Dioscorides, Justus, and Paul—these references mostly come from the author's main source, the *Viaticum*, and do not reflect his own independent consultation of other books. There is only one practice here that the author personally affirms ('And this medicine I have proved to be useful for many infirmities of the womb'), and even this remedy for uterine movement can be traced back to the Hippocratic corpus.[51] Aside from this one attestation of efficacy, no authorial presence is discernible. (The note that a certain remedy for menstrual retention was 'made for the queen of the Franks' may be reporting hearsay rather than personal experience.)[52] Clearly knowledgeable enough about medicine to make perceptive adaptations of his source texts, this author is also completely 'bookish', drawing his knowledge from other books rather than from his own empirical practices or from dialogue with or observation of other practitioners. There are no 'hands-on' therapies; when the author discusses treatments for uterine suffocation or prolapse, or obstetrical interventions, he is simply prescribing potions or other 'hands-off' therapies. Given everything I have said above about the limits of male gynaecological and obstetrical practice, therefore, as well as the gendered differentials in engagement with literary culture, there is every reason to believe that the author of this first draft of *Conditions of Women* was male. No explicit claim is made in

[50] For a complete source analysis of the *Treatise on Women's Illnesses* (*Tractatus de egritudinibus mulierum*), see Green, 'Development'.

[51] *Treatise on Women's Illnesses*, BNF, MS lat. 7056, *c.*1240–60 (England or N. France), f. 98vb (= ¶63 of the *Trotula* ensemble): 'Et hoc medicamen pluribus matricis infirmatibus utile esse probauimus'.

[52] The remedy itself comes directly from the *Viaticum* and so is not the original therapy of this author or any other Salernitan. See Green, *Trotula*, p. 232, n. 13.

this version to an intended audience, though it was probably meant for other practitioners since it assumes knowledge of compound medicines and some technical vocabulary.

At some point soon afterwards, the *Treatise on Women's Illnesses* was modified to form the more standard version of the text, *The Book on the Conditions of Women*. The vocabulary was changed, often by reverting to the original terminology of the *Viaticum*, and an overlay of theoretical interpretation was added. For example, *Women's Illnesses* had, in explaining how menstruation was the analogue of male nocturnal emissions, stressed the temporal coincidence of sexual maturity in boys and girls; *Conditions of Women*, in contrast, stressed the qualitative and functional similarity of the two purgations. Moreover, here and elsewhere this author/reviser adds an almost poetic, personified sense of Nature's wisdom: 'For always Nature is burdened by certain humours, either in the man or the female; it strives to take off its yoke and it lays aside its burden.'[53] This version of the text provides no more personal empirical knowledge than its predecessor; indeed, the one claim to have personal knowledge of a remedy's efficacy has been eliminated. Rather, *Conditions of Women* is a textual exercise, a refining of a roughly crafted document that was itself extracted from other written texts. The essential similarities between the two versions must be kept in mind, therefore, when we examine the only major new section added to the revised text, its preface.

This begins with a striking allusion to *Genesis* 1.27: 'male and female He created them'. Sexual difference, our author explains, was instituted by God himself as part of His plan to sustain the world He had created. Male and female were created as complementary opposites, each one designed to temper the elemental excesses of the other. Thus, the male's heat has its opposite in the woman's coldness, his dryness in her wetness. This temperamental and humoural balancing is not equal, of course, since the male qualities are the 'more worthy', the female's less so. Moreover, the female, being weaker, suffers more from the processes of reproduction. Then, in a frustratingly ambiguous passage, the author (who, we should remember, is really only a reviser of the text) states his reasons for writing:

Because, therefore, women are of a weaker nature than men, so more than men they are afflicted in childbirth. It is for this reason also that more frequently diseases abound in them than in men, especially around the organs assigned to the work of nature. And because only with shame and embarrassment do they confess the fragility of the condition of their diseases which occur around their secret parts, they do not dare reveal their distress to (male) physicians. Therefore, [because of] their misfortune, which ought to

---

[53] Green, 'Development' p. 132. On this philosophical novelty of personifying nature in late 11th- and early 12th-century southern Italy, see Charles S. F. Burnett, 'Physics before the *Physics*: Early Translations from Arabic of Texts Concerning Nature in MSS British Library, Additional 22719 and Cotton Galba E IV', *Medioevo: Rivista di Storia della Filosofia Medievale* 27 (2002), pp. 53–109, at p. 62.

be pitied and especially for the sake of a certain woman, my soul was incited to provide some remedy for their above-mentioned diseases. Therefore, for the sake of women I sweated with no small labour to gather the better things from the books of Hippocrates and Galen and Constantine, so that I might explain both the causes and the cures of these diseases.[54]

The reviser who transformed the *Treatise on Women's Illnesses* into *Conditions of Women* was, I believe, participating every bit as much as the original author in a masculine culture of medicine. Like his predecessor, the reviser was clearly literate; indeed, unlike his rather clumsy predecessor, he has some sense of Latin style, less 'classical', perhaps, than that of the author of *Women's Cosmetics*, but certainly striving for some elegance. Like his predecessor, he maintains a hierarchy of authority that privileges, next to Constantine the African, the ancients Galen, Hippocrates, Rufus, Dioscorides, and Justus; no contemporary practitioners, Salernitan or otherwise, are mentioned. Like his predecessor, this author is equally distant from the kind of empirical knowledge that would have been gained from personal practice of women's medicine. While the author will cite Galen's cure of an individual woman, for example, he gives no evidence that he himself actually treated women or had gathered information from other active practitioners. The first person is only used twice in this revised version of the text, once in the prologue where the author declares his reasons for writing, and once later in the text to reinforce an assertion about the cause of menstruation.

The interesting question about *Conditions of Women*, therefore, is not whether or not the author (or rather, reviser) was male, but whether he, like the author of *Women's Cosmetics*, intended to address other male practitioners like himself or if, instead, he mentioned women's shame as a rationale for putting the collected knowledge on women's diseases *into women's own hands*. On the one hand, although I have already indicated that women's literacy in Salerno (and throughout southern Italy) seems to have been minimal, there were *some* literate women and perhaps the 'certain lady' our author refers to may have been not simply the text's inspiration but its original intended recipient. On the other hand, as we have seen, this topos of women's shame has a very long history and was not always used to imply that gynaecological learning needed to be transferred into women's hands. The Latin Metrodora translation, which we know was circulating in southern Italy, offered a rearticulation of the problem of

---

[54] *Conditions of Women 1*, Oxford, Magdalen College, MS 173, s. xiv in. (England?), f. 246v: 'Quia ergo mulieres debilioris sunt nature quam uiri, ideo plus uiris in partu molestantur. Hinc etiam quod in eis frequentius habundant egritudines quam in uiris, et maxime circa membra officio deputata nature. Et quoniam ipse sue condicionis fragilitatem uerecundia et rubore fatentur egritudinum suarum que circa partes secretiores eueniunt, medicis non audent angustias reuelare. Earum ergo miseranda calamitas et maxime cuiusdam mulieris gratia animum meum sollicitat ut contra predictas egritudines earum prouideam sanitati. Vt ergo ex libris Ypocratis, Galieni, Constantini pociora decerperem labore non minimo mulierum gratia desudaui. Vt et causas egritudinum et curas exponerem cum causis.'

women's shame, one that John of Saint Paul would readily grab onto when he was writing his own medical textbook later in the century, yet neither the Latin Metrodora nor John made claims to female audiences.

In fact, the author of *Conditions of Women* implies that it is not only in front of men that women are ashamed. Female birth attendants are instructed not to look the parturient in the face, 'because many women tend to be ashamed of being seen during birth'.[55] If I have understood it correctly, therefore, the gist of the author's assertions about women's shame in the preface is not that he wishes to offer women a manual which they can read privately as an alternative to consulting a male physician, but rather that he wishes to better inform male practitioners about the details of women's diseases so that they might better aid their female patients. To judge from Petrus Musandinus's exploitation of the text for his own masterwork, his *Practica*, the author achieved his goal.

This exclusion of women from the audience of *Conditions of Women* is further reinforced by the grammar of the text. The author does not actually address himself either to this 'certain lady' or to women in general. There are no second-person addresses that create a conversation between an experienced practitioner ('I') and an immediate, specific audience ('you'). Nor, apparently, does the author speak directly to female practitioners: the single reference to midwives (*obstetrices*) refers to them in the third person.[56] There is, in fact, a distinct 'hands-off' character to the text. Therapeutic instructions are almost universally couched in terms of 'let the woman be given' or 'let this unguent be applied'. This may, it is true, reflect the fact that the author is for the most part regurgitating instructions he has found in his source texts. But considering to what lengths the author went to adapt *other* aspects of his sources, it is notable that there has been no perceptible shift in how the author has chosen grammatically to couch the scenario of practice.

---

[55] *Conditions of Women 1*, ¶92, Magdalen MS 173, f. 252v: 'Mulieres que assistunt ei non respiciant eam in uultu, quia multe mulieres solent esse ut uerecunde in ipso partus uisu'. The *Treatise on Women's Illnesses* had explicitly called the attendants midwives (BNF, MS 7056, f. 99vb: 'Ad latus eius sint obstetrices, nec aspiciant uultum eius quia sepe pudor nocet'). This echoes, though perhaps only coincidentally, Muscio's *Gynaecia* ([Muscio], *Sorani Gynaeciorum*, p. 23): 'faciem suam retrorsus [obstetrix] avertat, ne pariens verecundia se concludat'.

[56] *Conditions of Women 1*, ¶93, Magdalen MS 173, f. 252v: 'Si puer egreditur non eo ordine quo deberet, ut si tibia uel brachium prius exeat, assit obstetrix cum parua manu et suaui, et intincta manu cum decoctione fenugreci et seminis lini, reponat puerum et conuertat ad locum suum, ad rectum suum ordinem'. This distancing from midwives is true of *Conditions of Women 2*, too, which adds two further references, ¶116: 'Postea die partus iminente, adaptet se mulier ut moris est, et cum magna cautela obstetricum fiat ei sternutacio constrictis naribus et ore obturato, ut maxima pars uirtutis ad matricem tendat. Deinde detur ei muscillago decoctis, fenugrecum uel lini.' ¶118: 'Item sunt quedam phisica remedia quorum uirtus est occulta, que ab obstetricibus facta sepe contulerunt. Hec sunt: Teneat paciens in dextra magnetem, et confert.' In the proto-ensemble, where the chapters on infant care are added (¶¶124–7), wet-nurses (*nutrices*) are also referred to in the distant third person. This reference is, of course, an exact quotation from Rhazes. On the fifteenth-century Middle English text for women, *Sickness of Women 2*, which similarly fails to address women directly in the body of its text, see Chapter 4 below.

I would like to suggest, therefore, that the author's grammatical situating of himself and his intended audience reflects the fact that both he and they are distanced from the hands-on treatment of women. I suggest, in other words, that despite its preface *Conditions of Women* is really addressed not to the concerned laywoman but to male medical practitioners. It tells the healer not what he should do but rather what he should have done and what the patient should be told to do ('let her do this', 'let her do that'). In fact, there are very few second-person forms and active imperatives directed to the practitioner. Most of the ones that do appear come at the opening of recipes: 'Take . . . Mix . . .'. As soon as the recipes get to the point of actual application, however, the grammar shifts back to passive forms: 'Let this be applied . . . let this be inserted . . . let this be given to drink.' Thus, to the extent that there is a implied 'you', a specific partner in dialogue, this 'you' is never asked to do hands-on treatment. This inscribed reader is expected to already have basic medical knowledge: to know what a 'humour' or a 'faculty' or a 'virtue' is, to know how to prepare such compound medicines as *benedicta* or *oximel* or *diaciminum* or *rosata novella*.[57] *Conditions of Women* is not, therefore, intended for amateurs, for use as a 'self-help' manual by women in their own homes. Neither, however, does it assume that the reader will do all the therapeutic manipulations him/herself. The passive forms all assume an unexpressed agent who will be doing the actual hands-on applications and manipulations.

Conditions of Women thus presents a paradox: it is a text written ostensibly because women do not wish to show their diseases to male physicians, but it is written *as if* it were to be used by men. Whether actually written by a man or not, *Conditions of Women* comes out of male-generated and male-controlled textual traditions. And it reflects a male point of view, literally, in keeping its hands off the female body.[58]

Treatments for Women

The third *Trotula* text, the *Treatments for Women* (*De curis mulierum*), presents none of these even subtle hints of male authorship or a male perspective on the practice of women's medicine. It is neither bookish, on the one hand, nor does it portray a constant physical distancing from the female patient's body. It has no ancient pedigree, bearing no traces of direct influence from ancient Greek or medieval Arabic or Latin texts. The most simplistic of the three *Trotula* texts in terms of its organization and Latin style, the *Treatments for Women* has no learned features whatsoever. On the contrary, it is quite strikingly disorganized,

---

[57] Cf. Green, *Trotula*, pp. 193–204.

[58] As I argue in Chapter 2, the imbedding of the male perspective on the female body in *Conditions of Women* explains why it could be so readily adopted by male readers in later centuries without any significant alteration.

jumping from remedies for sunburn to urinary incontinence, from hair lice to snake bites. As these topics suggest, it defines 'women's medicine' quite broadly: encompassing not only diseases or conditions of the female genitalia, but also social concerns of women including cosmetics, care of children, and even diseases of the male genitalia. The text has no preface explaining its genesis, declaring its purpose, or laying claim to a particular audience. The midwife is never mentioned as a third party to whom instruction must be given nor is she evoked as the 'you' to whom the text is addressed; indeed, the term 'midwife' (*obstetrix*) is never used. Nor is this a handbook of self-treatments for laywomen; the text is clearly meant for medical specialists.

Practices are attributed to others in only a handful of instances. 'Certain unclean and corrupt prostitutes' are credited with (or rather blamed for) a harmful method for faking virginity, which is reported in a disapproving third person. Similarly, 'the ladies' (*domine*) are credited, with more enthusiasm, for a proven remedy for softening and bleaching the hair. There are also third-person references to the Salernitan masters Copho (who is credited with certain anatomical views on the links between the uterus and brain, as well as a special medicinal powder), the Ferrarii, and Trota.[59] All the other remedies—including the obstetrical procedures—are described in the first person ('we use', 'we mix', 'we apply') or in simple imperatives (used most frequently in the cosmetic recipes). These suggest that there is no intermediary between the practitioner who is reading the text (who presumably is meant to identify with the 'we' of the narrational voice) and the female patient, even for the most intimate manual procedures. Even the treatment of certain disorders of men use this same 'we' form, suggesting that these authors have no more difficulty touching the organs of men than of women.[60] In other words, in nearly every case, the medical therapies described in the text are meant to be performed by the reader. Unlike *Conditions of Women* and all the gynaecological chapters in the male Salernitans *practicae*, this is 'hands-on' women's medicine.

For example, in the chapter on perineal tear and uterine prolapse caused by incompetent assistance in childbirth, the author describes how the vagina and the anus become a single canal, through which the womb falls out and hardens. At the beginning of the chapter, the author takes the reader into her confidence:

---

[59] Manuscripts of the *Treatments for Women* 1 and 2 and of the proto-ensemble variously spell her name as Trota, Trotha, Trotta, or Trocta. The latter two spellings would have been normative in Salerno itself, but I have adopted 'Trota' as it is the most common form in the texts. The reference to the 'Ferrarii' *may* reflect a textual corruption; the only known medical practitioners with that name date from several decades after the presumed composition of the text.

[60] *Treatments for Women*, ¶¶144 (on fat men), 152 (on extrusion of the anus), 153 (on anal pain), 154 (on swelling of the penis), and 157 (on bladder stone). Interestingly, the description of Master 'Matheus Ferrarius's' cure of bladder stone in a particular male patient implies that 'Ferrarius' had someone else do the actual manipulation: ¶159, OBL, MS Digby 79, s. xiii in. (England and Italy?), f. 109r: 'lapidem *extrahi fecit suggendo* . . . circa peritoneon *fecit inungere* cum unguento aureo'.

There are some women to whom in giving birth things go wrong, and this happens on account of the inadequacy of those assisting. But let this observation remain our secret among women.[61]

The author then continues with a detailed therapy:

We apply to the womb warm wine in which butter has been boiled, and we diligently foment the womb until it becomes soft, and then gently we replace it. Afterwards, we sew the rupture between the genitals and the vagina in three or four places with a silk thread. Then we apply to the vagina a linen rag the size of the vagina, having first anointed it with pitch. This makes the womb retract on account of its foul smell, for pitch stinks. We cure the rupture with a powder made of comfrey, that is of *consolida maior*, or mouse-ear hawkweed which is the same thing; also, cinnamon should be sprinkled on the powder. Let the woman be placed [*collocetur*] in bed so that her feet are higher than her head, and there let her carry out all her business for eight or nine days or as long as necessary. There let her eat, there let her urinate and defecate and do the other things which we are accustomed do. Also, we make her abstain from all foods that generate indigestion and from all things which bring on coughing. Also, it is necessary to know what ought to be done for them in birth [the next time]. Let a rag be prepared in the shape of an oblong ball and let it be placed in the anus so that in each effort of pushing out the child this is firmly applied to the anus, lest there be [another] dissolution of continuity of this sort.[62]

There are four sites of agency in this passage. The first agent is the author (who may, as we shall see later, be a group rather than an individual): 'we apply', 'we foment', 'we replace', 'we sew'. The second agent is the person (or persons) who put the woman in her bed, i.e. the unexpressed agents behind the passive verb *collocetur*. The third agent is the patient herself: although confined to her bed, she is the 'agent' of the eating, toileting, etc., that she carries on in her bed. Finally, there is the unexpressed agent who attends the next birth, supporting the anus so another fistula or rupture does not occur.

These four loci of agency paint a scenario of practice that speaks volumes about the gendering of medical practice described in this text. At the centre of

---

[61] *Treatments for Women* 1, MS Digby 79, f. 108r: 'Sunt quedam quibus in pariendo male accidit, et hoc propter defectum astancium. Sed istud nostrum cum mulieribus sit secretum'.

[62] *Treatments for Women* 1, ¶149, MS Digby 79, f. 108r: 'Quedam namque sunt quibus uulue et ani fit in unum et idem foramen concursus, et istis exit matrix et indurescit quibus in reponendo subuenimus in hunc modum. Matrici apponimus uinum calidum in quo bullierit butirum, et fomentamus diligenter quousque matrix mollis efficiatur, et tunc suauiter reponimus. Postmodum rupturam que est inter pudenda et uuluam in tribus uel. iiij. locis svimus cum filo serico. Deinde uulue apponimus pannum de lino ad uulue quantitatem, dum modo pice illiniatur. Hoc autem facit matricem retrahi propter sui fetorem, pix namque fetida est. Rupturam sanamus cum puluere facto ex simphito, id est consolida maiori uel anagalli quod idem est, et cinnamomo superspargendo puluerem. Collocetur ista in lecto ita ut pedes superiores capite appareant ibique suas omnes expleat operationes per. viij. uel per. ix. dies uel quantum necesse fuerit. Ibi manducet, ibi egerat et cetera que consueuimus facere. Hanc etiam abstinere facimus ab omnibus indigestionem generantibus et ab omnibus que fuerint quod tussis causa. Hoc etiam sciendum est qualiter eis in partu sit subueniendum. Paretur itaque pannus in modum pile oblonge et ponatur in ano ad hoc ut in quolibet conatu eiciendi puerum firmiter istud ano apponatur, ne fiat huiusmodi continuitatis dissolutio.' The concept of 'dissolution of continuity' refers to any break in the 'fabric' of the body.

the scene, of course, is the female patient. She, after all, is the *raison d'être* for the text and neither her gender nor her sex is in question. The gender of the first agent, the author-practitioner, is equally clear, though it is determined not by her bodily sex but by her social gender. If all that I have thus far suggested about male practitioners *not* having access to the female genitalia is true, then this person touching, rubbing, sewing, *manipulating* the female genitalia must be female. But why, if she is a female who has unmediated access to the female body, does there seem to be a different agent assisting with the subsequent birth? If the authorial voice is a female medical practitioner, is she not then a midwife? It would seem not, since *Treatments for Women* is in no sense a *midwife's* practical manual—at least if we hold to traditional interpretations of midwives as being the normative attendants at childbirth. At the beginning of this chapter, the author has already mentioned that there are other birth attendants out there. Even if some of them are incompetent (as she impolitically implies), she assumes that they will continue to practise. In fact, it is possible that our author does not consider *normal* birth within the province of her medical practice. Aside from very brief instructions on how a woman *having difficulty* giving birth should be bathed, suffumigated and then made to sneeze, normal childbirth is not a topic this author feels a need to discuss. The author sees herself (and her audience) as concerned with women's *diseases*, with pathological conditions, and not necessarily with all manners of attendance on female patients.

Multiple medical agents can be grammatically 'sighted' elsewhere in the text. As with the unspecified person or persons who put the woman with the prolapsed uterus in her bed, the presence of manual assistants can be indirectly discerned. In contrast to *Conditions of Women*, the passive jussive subjunctive ('let this be done') is used very rarely in *Treatments for Women*, in fact only five times beyond the passage I have already discussed: 'Let a perforated chair be prepared' (when a woman suffering from infertility needs to be suffumigated), 'let her be washed with the water of the previous bath' (again, as part of a fertility treatment), 'let a bath be prepared and let [the woman] be put into it' (as an aid in delivery), 'let [the patient] be washed twice daily for three or four days' (after having been treated for haemorrhoids),[63] 'let herbs be cooked and let the pudenda be fomented'. This last is the only instance where manual application to the genitalia is described in terms of 'let this be done' (i.e. let someone else besides the practitioner/reader do it). In this case, that 'someone else' is the patient herself; the recipe in question is a vaginal constrictive, which the woman must herself apply immediately before intercourse. Similar self-treatment also explains the use of the passive in a treatment for sanies mixed with menses: 'Before [this sack filled with medicaments] is tied on [to the genitals], it should be warmed

---

[63] The patient here may be male or female. The chapter begins by saying that both women and men suffer from haemorrhoids and, unlike other conditions like strangury, there is no distinction here between treatments for men and treatments for women.

by the fire between the hands.' The patient performs her own application in two other instances as well (both in active mode): when the woman is to apply to her face an ointment 'we' have prepared, and when a sexually experienced woman is to place leeches into her vagina in order to fake the blood flow of defloration.

Manual assistants make only one explicit appearance in the text. In describing how a woman giving birth to a dead child needs to be bounced about on a sheet, the author specifies that 'we make four young people [*iuuenes*] hold the four corners of the sheet' and 'we make them forcefully pull the opposite corners', the Latin leaving ambiguous whether these 'young people' are female or male.[64] In any case, the references to manual assistants, whether explicitly mentioned or only grammatically inscribed, and to self-treatments by the woman herself at home, make it clear that the author does not see herself as the sole attendant on her patients, waiting to perform every necessary manual labour. She is a healer whose job it is to cure. One of the main objectives of the text is to describe her active, immediate role in the care of patients, a role which is tangibly reflected in this persistent couching of instructions in the active voice.

The other main objective of the text is to draw the reader into alliance with the author, to make her her student and colleague. As I have already mentioned, the author of *Treatments for Women* does not sustain use of the 'we' mode throughout the entire text. In another chapter on uterine prolapse only second-person imperative and active jussive forms are used. Yet here the therapy is equally hands-on, the practitioner being instructed to place a support in the vagina and tie it on with bandages passing over the hips. The juxtaposition of the first-person statements with the second-person imperatives, therefore, sets up a correspondence between author and presumed readers: just as it is the author herself who touches the womb, who foments it and replaces it, who sews the rupture and applies pitch to the vagina, so she assumes her audience will have this same unmediated access to the bodies of their female patients. This is in complete contrast to *Conditions of Women*, which for uterine prolapse only recommended external applications to the abdomen, baths, or orally administered remedies. When that author talked about the womb needing to be replaced, he had it done (in the passive) by a disembodied hand.[65] The use of the first-person plural throughout most of *Treatments for Women* creates a veritable elision of author

---

[64] *Treatments for Women* 1, ¶16, MS Digby 79, f. 107v: 'Eis sic optime subueniemus que in pariendo mortuum laborant. Ponimus parientem super lintheolum et facimus .iiij. iuuenes tenere .iiij. angulos, et parientis capite aliquantulum eleuato, ab oppositis angulis fortiter trahere lintheolum facimus et statim pariet'. Although the physical strength to toss a pregnant woman might make male attendants seem more likely, a 13th-century verse rendition of the *Trotula* interprets these attendants as female: Charles Daremberg (ed.), *Liber de secretis mulierum*, in De Renzi, *Collectio Salernitana*, 4:1–38, p. 17, lines 515–18: 'Aut in linteolo forti ponat parientem, / Quatuor et teneant sua cornua tot mulieres / Fortiter; heque trahant huc illuc concutientes/Erecto capite; pariet sic protinus illa.'

[65] *Conditions of Women 1*, ¶56, MS Magdalen 173, f. 250v: 'Primo autem matrix egressa restituatur manu apposita proprio loco'. Cf. *Treatise on Women's Illnesses*, which simply uses the passive voice: 'Si uero matrix foras eat, intus reponatur.'

and reader, making the author and the reader as one: 'I do this, and of course, you will do this, too.' This is the *societas*—the alliance between master and pupil not immediately in physical proximity to one another—that the written medium could uniquely create.

The implication of all these features of *Treatments for Women* is that, whether or not it was *written down* by a woman, it embodies a female voice—or, more precisely, a female hand and eye—that could view and touch the female body from the intimate perspective that, normatively, only other women could have had. *Treatments for Women* was, moreover, apparently intended for female readers who would have this same kind of unmediated access to the bodies of their female patients. In other words, it appears to have been written down to provide a more permanent and concrete mechanism for the transmission of knowledge from woman to woman than the oral forms that had traditionally served the needs of Salernitan women. This is a rather astounding scenario given what we know—or rather, don't know—about women's literacy at Salerno in this period. What is most surprising about this text, therefore, is that it exists at all. For the text posits a community of female readers who would be able to rely on this text for instruction, a community of women fully engaged with literate medicine.

'AS IF SHE WERE A MASTER': TROTA OF SALERNO

About a third of the way into *Treatments for Women*, the 'voice' of the text shifts briefly from recounting the cures 'we' perform to a specific case history. The topic of the chapter is 'wind in the womb' (*ventositas matricis*), a condition that can occur when 'women receive wind through the vagina which, once it has entered into the right or left side of the womb, generates such windiness that [the women] appear to certain people as if they were suffering from an abdominal or intestinal rupture'.[66] A young woman was about to be cut or operated on (or, more probably, cauterized) for what was thought to be an internal rupture.[67] But then Trota was called in 'as if she were a master' (*quasi magistra*) and she was 'completely astonished', though whether at the severity of the young woman's condition or the incautious diagnosis by her caretakers is unclear. Suspecting that the surgery/cautery was not needed, Trota took the young woman home with her

---

[66] See Monica H. Green, 'Reconstructing the *Oeuvre* of Trota of Salerno', in *La Scuola medica Salernitana: Gli autori e i testi*, ed. Danielle Jacquart and Agostino Paravicini Bagliani, Edizione Nazionale 'La Scuola medica Salernitana', 1 (Florence: SISMEL/Edizioni del Galluzzo, 2007), 183–233, for an edition of this chapter from the original *Treatments for Women*. For a more developed stage of editorial intervention, see Green, *Trotula*, ¶151.

[67] The Latin text is unambiguous—*deberet incidi* (she needed to be cut)—though, if this reading is correct and means something more invasive than simple scarification, it would be most amazing since abdominal surgery was almost unheard of in the Middle Ages. Michael McVaugh has kindly pointed out to me that the verb might originally have been *incendi* (to be burned), which would refer to the more plausible practice of external cautery.

'so that secretly she could determine the cause of her illness'. Trota determined that what had initially been diagnosed as rupture or distension of the intestines was instead 'windiness' of the womb. In other words, it was a uterine, not an intestinal condition.[68] The text then recounts the details of Trota's 'hands-on' therapy—involving repeated baths, plasters on the abdomen, and massaging. Needless to say, Trota cured her perfectly and sent her on her way, unburned, despite the severity of her condition when she found her.

This Trota is the sole named female healer in any of the three *Trotula* texts; the only other women referred to, as we have seen, are the 'Saracen women' mentioned in *Women's Cosmetics* and the 'unclean and corrupt prostitutes' and 'the ladies' whose practices are noted in *Treatments for Women*. In fact, aside from one Berdefolia *medica*, who died in 1155 and who is mentioned in a calendar of the deceased in one of Salerno's parishes,[69] Trota is the sole named female healer we can associate with any phase of Salerno's extraordinary period of medical activity in the twelfth century. The anecdote of Trota's cure of the young woman with *ventositas matricis* confirms what we have already noted as the most distinctive aspect of women's medicine as practised by women: she can touch her female patient's genital area. It was Trota herself, the text makes clear, that not only made the diagnosis, but took the young woman home with her; it was she who put the patient in a bath of mallow and pellitory-of-the-wall, she who 'frequently rubbed her limbs in order to soften them', she who made and applied a plaster for her belly. Trota's success, therefore, is ascribed not simply to her keen diagnostic skills, but to her command of the manual and pharmaceutic knowledge that produced effective medical results. In claiming that she was called in 'as if she were a (female) master', the author of *Treatments for Women* accords Trota the highest prize a physician could win within the Salernitan 'medical marketplace': acknowledgement of expertise by those 'in the forum by whom [s]he ought to be greeted and called "physician"'.

Such a reputation could hardly have been built on a single cure. On the contrary, it is clear that Trota was by no means limited to 'women's medicine' but was rather a healer of considerable range. She was, in fact, a 'master' in the same way many of her male peers were: she, too, wrote a general *Practica* of medicine, a compendium of her many therapies for conditions as diverse as cosmetic problems, hair lice, burns, cancer, frenzy, eye problems, sprained foot, excessive sweat, snakebite, toothache, scrofula, spleen problems, depilatories, and haemorrhoids. She seems in particular to have developed considerable competence in ophthalmology and gastro-intestinal disorders.[70] A

---

[68] This distinction would be lost in later deformations of the text as it evolved in the *Trotula* ensemble; cf. Green, *Trotula*, ¶151 and the notes thereto.

[69] Carlo Alberto Garufi, *Necrologio del Liber confratrum di S. Matteo di Salerno*, Fonti per la Storia d'Italia, 56 (Rome: Tipographico del Senato, 1922), p. 62.

[70] Note that, in the anecdote in *Treatments for Women*, Trota is called in at the point when the young woman was still believed to have a gastro-intestinal affection. There is nothing, therefore, to

further witness to Trota's *oeuvre* is the series of excerpts from her writings that were incorporated into a massive late twelfth-century compendium of the writings of seven major Salernitan physicians called simply *Treatment of Ill-nesses*. At least in the eyes of this compiler, Trota had a stature very nearly equal to that of the masters Johannes Afflacius, Copho, Johannes Platearius, Petrus Musandinus, Bartholomeus, and Ferrarius whose work was set alongside hers. By virtue of being a female practitioner, however, she, like the other Salernitan women, had the opportunity to acquire an expertise in women's diseases and cosmetics that her brother practitioners never did. Her *Practica* (at least in the abbreviated form we still have it) begins with gynaecolog-ical disorders, while beauty treatments constitute a notable portion of the text.[71]

Trota is the consummate empiric. She has recipe after recipe for every ailment: nearly forty remedies for eye diseases, more than fifty for digestive disorders. She lists the ingredients with care (often noting possible substitutes or alternate names) and she is sometimes quite scrupulous in detailing each step of preparation, noting how long a preparation should be left to dry in the sun, what the signs are when a preparation is thoroughly cooked. What she hardly ever does, however, is explore the causes of disease. Of the seven writers used by the compiler of the great Salernitan compendium, *Treatment of Illnesses*, only she never appears in the first section of the text on 'universal' diseases: that is, the topic most demanding of the physician's rational and dialectical skills, the differential diagnosis and treatment of fevers. Her only concession to theory is the occasional incorporation of the humoural concepts of 'hot' and 'cold' causes. The exceptions prove the rule. In addressing a certain eye condition, she notes that sometimes on account of a blockage of one of the nostrils, the humour which ordinarily should exit from the nostril instead goes toward the eyes and causes them to tear or to excrete a putrid substance.[72] This condition is unusual, however, in that it does not have a name, meaning that she cannot refer to it by her usual formula: 'For X [name of disease], take Y.' It is equally rare to find Trota describing the physiological

---

warrant confining Trota within the label 'midwife'. For a summary of the contents of the *Practica*, see Green, 'Trota's *Oeuvre*'.

[71] This foregrounding of women's medical concerns in the extant *Practica* may be the work of a later editor. Indeed, the gynaecological and obstetrical treatments were the only parts of the *Practica* that one late medieval copyist of the text was interested in (OBL, MS Rawlinson C 506, s. xv, England). Already in the early 13th century, Trota's reputation outside of Salerno was primarily associated with cosmetics; see Green, 'Trota's *Oeuvre*'. See also Chapter 5 below on how Trota/'Trotula's' reputation was circumscribed to expertise in 'women's secrets' in the later Middle Ages.

[72] Conrad Hiersemann, *Die Abschnitte aus der Practica des Trottus in der Salernitanischen Sammelschrift 'De Aegritudinum Curatione'. Breslau Codex Salern. 1160–1170*, inaugural dissertation, Leipzig 1921, p. 10, lines 23–5: 'Quibusdam contingit, ut ex op[p]ilatione unius naris ascendat hu[mor], qui solebat decurrere per nares et venit ad o[culos] et inde liquefiunt o[culi], vel putredo decurrit per o[culos]'.

effect of a therapy. In a remedy for tooth pain, she explains the vapour to be applied to the affected tooth works by dissolving and drawing out the rheum which causes the pain.[73] On one occasion, she also addresses prognostic signs: green vomit, she says, unless it is caused by a medicine, is always a sign of death.[74] These three excursions into therapeutic and prognostic rationalizing are notable precisely because they are unique. The three unusually detailed chapters on difficulty of conception, which explain at some length the causes and symptoms of infertility in both men and women, were borrowed from a male writer, Copho, and are thus not representative of Trota's own explanatory system.[75]

The other major work that can be ascribed to Trota provides both parallels and differences, for while it displays many of the characteristic features of the *Practica* and her excerpts in the Salernitan compendium, *Treatment of Illnesses* (for example, a similar pharmacopeia, the general absence of theory, and general topical disorder), it seems also to show her work at a more advanced, one might even say mature level of development.

This additional witness for Trota's work as a medical practitioner is none other than the *Treatments for Women*. Although above I treated it as an anonymous text, it is in fact attributed to Trota already in the earliest manuscripts. (It was, of course, this attribution which led the person who fused the three Salernitan texts on women's medicine together to attribute the whole ensemble to Trota, who then morphed into the eponymous 'Trotula'.)[76] As I have indicated, Trota clearly did not limit her practice to 'women's medicine'; she was a generalist *par excellence*. Yet *Treatments for Women* reflects only a small fraction of her competence, focusing on conditions of the genitalia, cosmetics, and a few sundry other topics. Nevertheless, her practices seem to have evolved: in remedies found in both Trota's *Practica* and *Treatments for Women*, or in the Salernitan compendium *Treatment of Illnesses* and *Treatments for Women*, we find the same basic procedures and an overall correspondence of *materia medica*. But the descriptions of therapeutic manoeuvres seem to be more lengthy and precise in *Treatments for Women*, and there is occasionally the addition of some kind of *rationale* for a procedure. Thus, for example, whereas both the *Treatment of Illnesses* chapter on uterine prolapse and that in *Treatments for Women* prescribe that pitch be rubbed onto the protruded uterus, only in the latter treatise is there the added note that 'This makes the womb retract on account of its foul

---

[73] Hiersemann, *Abschnitte*, p. 14, lines 29–33: 'Item de dolore dentium auferendo et mitigando. Accipe semen cassilaginis et porri equaliter et super carbones ardentes pone embotum et per cannam emboti fumus perinde egrediens super dentem patientem ab infirmo recipiatur. Hic enim fumus reuma, quod dolorem facit, mirabiliter dissolvit et educit et ipsum mitigat'.

[74] Hiersemann, *Abschnitte*, p. 15, line 44–p. 16, line 2: 'Viridis vomitus, nisi fiat ex medicina, semper signum mortis, et in omni etiam purgatione pessimus est viridus color, nisi fiat ex medicina, quia et in fluxu et in urina et in vomitu et in sputo'.

[75] See Green, 'Trota's *Oeuvre*'.   [76] See Green, 'Development'.

smell, for pitch stinks.' In other words, *Treatments for Women* now engages
with the common *theoretical* understanding that the uterus is capable of sensing
odours and being drawn to or fleeing away from good or bad smells.[77] While
obviously Trota herself could have evolved on her own in both her practices and
in her engagement with the theoretical discourses of anatomy and physiology,
as I will explain below, I think *Treatments for Women* offers evidence of her
association with the male Salernitan master, Copho, who is believed to have
been an important innovator in bringing the practices of Arabic medicine to the
Salernitans.

If *Treatments for Women* has so many obvious parallels with Trota's *Practica*
and is actually attributed to her in the manuscripts, why not accept the attribution
as correct? The reason for crediting the text, not to Trota herself, but to some
anonymous third party is twofold. First, as we saw, Trota is cited within the text
in the third person while most of the rest of the text is voiced as a first-person
plural account ('we do'). Second, three times within the earliest form of the text,
we find *English synonyms* being used for the names of diseases or therapeutic
plants.[78] *Treatments for Women* thus probably reflects a text, not as Trota herself
wrote it down, but as it was transcribed from the oral accounts of one or more
of Trota's students who could recount vividly Trota's famous cure of the woman
with *ventositas matricis* but still, later in the text, give another (and different)
treatment for 'wind in the womb'.[79] That Trota was still alive when the text was
written down seems to be indicated by the colophon at the end of the oldest
extant copy: 'All these things here noted have been proved, Trota as witness'
(*Probata hec omnia hic notata, teste Trota*), a claim certainly suggesting that the
text had Trota's personal imprimatur.[80] *Treatments for Women* reflects, then, the
evolution of Trota's cures, the presence of one or more students who carried
on her distinctive traditions in practising women's medicine, and the power
of her reputation to attract attention from far outside the confines of Salerno
itself.

Trota was not alone among Salernitan practitioners in earning this kind
of 'international' attention, of course. Although the 'Northmen' who came to
southern Italy first as mercenaries, then as conquerors, and then as settlers in
the eleventh and twelfth centuries were mostly Normans or Franks, Englishmen
travelling to Salerno and other parts of southern Italy, especially to seek out new
learning, are documented ever since Adelard of Bath came in search of 'studies

---

[77] See Green, *Trotula,* pp. 22–31.

[78] As noted in Green, 'Development', pp. 136–7 and 166, while we cannot be 100% sure that
these were in the *original* draft of the text, the three English words—*or deformations that show their
earlier presence*—do appear in all extant copies. See also Green, *Trotula,* pp. 155 and 227.

[79] See Green, *Trotula,* ¶165.

[80] MS Digby 79, f. 114r. A later copy that shows the text at a slightly later stage of development
ends with the phrase 'Exspliciunt Experimenta Atrote' (Here end the tried-and-true remedies of
Trota); Cambridge, Clare College, MS 12, s. xiii med. (England), f. 227v.

of the Arabs' in the early twelfth century. At least one Englishman, a certain Augerius, settled in Salerno, his sons Robert and William still owning a castle there in 1104.[81] Diplomatic ties between southern Italy and Normandy and England continued right through the end of the twelfth century: both Eleanor of Aquitaine and her son Richard the Lion-hearted are said to have stopped there on their journeys to the Holy Land, and in 1177, after some back-and-forth negotiations, Eleanor's daughter (and Richard's sister) Joanna married William II of Sicily. Thus it is not surprising that, in almost every case, the earliest extant manuscripts we have of Salernitan writings tend to be of English or Norman origin. Perhaps other English or Norman women travelled to Salerno, too, and absorbed the local culture of medicine: in her *Lay of the Two Lovers*, the later twelfth-century Anglo-Norman poet Marie de France has her protagonist refer to a female relative she has in Salerno, 'who has been there for more than thirty years and who has practised the art of physic so much that she is well-versed in medicines'.[82] Although Marie cannot be referring to Trota (who was almost certainly of Lombard origin), Trota had more than enough fame in her own right in England and northern France, being lauded as a cosmetic authority and even viciously parodied by the thirteenth-century French poet Rutebeuf, whose humour would not have worked, of course, had not Trota already been so famous.

Trota was, therefore, as close to being the female equivalent of a *magister* as twelfth-century Salerno probably could have produced. But we should also remember how much she had in common with her fellow Salernitan female practitioners. Her *Practica* is in no sense a learned tract on medicine and it makes no claims to situate itself in a larger tradition of medical writing. Its sheer disorder (and that of *Treatments for Women*, too, which may well be reflective of Trota's manner of oral training), shows Trota to be on the margins of literate medicine. She has learned the standard names of diseases,[83] she understands the etiological concepts of 'hot' and 'cold' and she differentiates her treatment accordingly. Although her writings have no obvious logical structure, she has some sense of the linear nature of her text for she will on occasion refer back to a remedy she has already recounted. She even refers to one of her therapies in the *Practica* as a *doctrina*, a formal teaching.[84] But overall Trota has not seized upon (and perhaps never recognized) the possibilities of the medical book: the possibility

---

[81] Cava de' Tirreni, Badia di Cava, Arca XVII, doc. 114 (an. 1104), in which Robert and William identify themselves as sons 'of the late Augerius who came from the province of Britain' (*quondam augerii qui fuit ortus ex p[ro]uincia brictania*).

[82] *The Lais of Marie de France*, trans. Glyn S. Burgess and Keith Busby (Harmondsworth/New York: Penguin, 1986), p. 83. There is no reason to think that Trota herself was English. The name Tro(c)ta has nowhere been documented in England for this period and it certainly wasn't introduced into England by the Normans; see Green, 'Development', pp. 153–4.

[83] It is notable that Trota does not use the colloquial names for menses, etc., that are documented in the *Treatise on Women's Illnesses*.

[84] Trota, *Practica*, cap. 66: 'et hec est nostra doctrina in tali egritudine' (i.e. anal bleeding).

to impose order on random material, to abstract commonalities and juxtapose them in order to speculate on the causes of disease or the ways in which the healer might best understand them. Perhaps we might imagine that her failure to cite traditional authorities like Hippocrates or Galen or Dioscorides indicates a confident sense that her remedies need no buttressing of 'authority'—they work because she has tested them. But I sense, rather, that Trota was in fact genuinely unconnected to the formal modes of medical discourse developing around her at Salerno.

This is all the more surprising since, as I have hinted at above, she seems to have some particular association with the male practitioner, Copho, from whom she apparently borrowed three chapters on infertility. He, in turn, seems to have borrowed at least once from her, for we find her description of vaginal swelling in his *Practica*. Copho is cited in *Treatments for Women* both as the 'author' of a powder that should be used for the skin condition, impetigo, and as the source of the teaching that sternutatives (substances the provoke sneezing) are good for facilitating labour: 'For as Copho says, the members are shaken to such an extent by the sneezing that the cotyledons are ruptured, that is, the ligaments by which the infant is tied to the womb.'[85] This echoes exactly the way the cotyledons were described in the dissection manual, *Anatomy of the Pig*, which has been attributed to Copho. Copho is also the first Salernitan author to refer to the practices of 'the women of Salerno' (*mulieres Salernitane*). True, he is somewhat stingy with his praise. He rejects the Salernitan women's remedy for worms in the belly in favour of his own: whereas the *mulieres* use a mixture of cumin, pepper, laurel seed, and pomegranate in a base of wine and salt water, 'we, however, give *hieralogodion* [a compound medicine made from colocynth and other imported ingredients] mixed with rain water; nothing is better'.[86] But his disagreements never descend to disdain; he is just as capable of acknowledging that some of these women's cures can free the patient from disease (*liberare*), the same verb he uses for his own successful cures.

Copho never actually refers to Trota by name nor does his gynaecological and obstetrical practice fully accord with hers; as we saw above, he recommends therapies for uterine prolapse quite at odds with elements of Trota's practice.[87] Nevertheless, the associations between these two writers are so close that it is likely that they were contemporaries. Indeed, they may have been even more than that: in 1112 we find a document recording a transference of property in Salerno from 'Zoffus, called "the pagan", son of Count Lando, and his wife Trocta, daughter of the late Peter the cleric' to the Benedictine abbey of the Holy

---

[85] See Green, 'Trota's *Oeuvre*'; cf. Green, *Trotula*, ¶139.

[86] Copho, *Practica*, ed. De Renzi, *Collectio salernitana*, 4:482.

[87] Given Trota's concern to avoid inducing cough in cases of uterine prolapse (a recommendation with which modern biomedical physicians would agree, given the pressure it induces on the pelvic floor), she certainly could not have endorsed Copho's recommendation to provoke sneezing as a therapeutic method!

Trinity in the hills just outside of Salerno.[88] Neither this Zoffus (an early spelling for an unusual name that would later stabilize as 'Cioffus') nor this Trocta are explicitly identified as medical practitioners here, yet both of them seem to be related or have personal ties to physicians. The joint property ownership we find in this document would certainly mirror the kind of intellectual exchange the healers Trota and Copho seem to have established.

This exchange, of course, had its limits as Trota would remain only on the boundary of literate medicine. Indeed, we can well ask what motivated her to write down her cures in the first place. From Copho's *Practica* straight through the end of the century, Salernitan writers claimed to write because they were motivated by didactic intent: either their students have begged them to set down their teachings in writing or, perhaps out of impatience, their students sometimes take up the task and assemble their master's teachings themselves. Copho (or rather the 'editor' who is writing for him) claims that he composed his *Practica* because he believed that 'the learned practitioner of this profession' ought not be ignorant of the natural properties of the body that lead it toward health or disease.[89] A work called *The Method of Healing* claims to be composed 'from the mouth [i.e. the oral teachings] of Chopho and from his own and his students' writings'.[90] Neither extant copy of Trota's *Practica* bears a preface that laid out her reasons for writing, and we can only guess at her motives. I suspect that she dedicated her practices to writing because, as her contemporary Copho was making clear, that was what 'masters' did to establish their authority.

An empirical practitioner of broad experience and deep understanding of medicinal substances and their preparations, for her the medical book never seems to have become more than a repository for individual therapies which could be (and probably were) transmitted just as effectively if less permanently through oral instruction. Clearly, as both the anecdote in *Treatments for Women* and the very genesis of that text by someone who had travelled hundreds of miles to compile her cures show, Trota did succeed in establishing her stature 'in the forum' as an empiricist. But as a theorist who could impart *doctrinae* to students, she had no impact at all. Aside from the compiler of the Salernitan compendium *Treatment of Illnesses*, no Salernitan author would ever again cite her by name. She was, in the end, only 'as if' a master.

[88] Cava de' Tirreni, Badia di Cava, Archivio, arca XIX, doc. 38 (June 1112). For further details on Zoffus/Cioffus, see Green, 'Trota's *Oeuvre*', pp. 204–7.

[89] Copho, *Practica*: 'doctus istius professionis artifex ignorare non debet istis in naturali proprietate existentibus humanum corpus' (ed. De Renzi, *Collectio Salernitana*, 4:439).

[90] Copho, *Methodo medendi*, CTC, MS R.14.31(904), s. xii ex., f. 39r: *a chophonis ore suisque et sociorum suorum scriptis*. The author identifies himself only as 'N', which may be his initial or simply an abbreviation for the generic *nomen*. Constant J. Mews, 'Orality, Literacy, and Authority in the Twelfth Century Schools', *Exemplaria* 2 (1990), 475–500, rightly stresses the genesis of most 12th-century scholastic texts out of oral debate and teaching. The written text is really only the epiphenomenon of all these other face-to-face interactions.

There were no completely separate worlds of 'male medicine' and 'female medicine' in twelfth-century Salerno. Both men and women practised medicine, and both male and female practitioners treated patients of the opposite sex. They shared common assumptions about basic physiology and about the power of herbs and other substances to cure specific afflictions. Men were not completely ignorant of women's medical practices: besides Copho, several male physicians acknowledged the practices of the *mulieres Salernitane* and a few were even familiar with such female practices as the use of vaginal constrictives.[91] Nevertheless, medical practice and medical education were decidedly gendered: while it is clear that male Salernitan practitioners diagnosed and treated female patients for gynaecological conditions, 'female medicine' is distinguished both by its greater hands-on involvement with female patients and, Trota aside, by its complete non-involvement in a larger community of literate medicine, which extended to include medical writers far distant from Salerno both geographically in space and chronologically in time. Indeed, Trota's position as a female boundary-crosser is made all the more unique by the apparent absence of any broader audience of female readers (let alone a cadre of female writers) in twelfth-century Salerno. *Women's Cosmetics*, as we have seen, was not intended for direct use by women, while *Conditions of Women*, although bearing a claim that it was meant for women's benefit, neither addressed them nor even drew on direct empirical experience of treating women. *Treatments for Women*, in turn, although clearly couched as instructions from a group of female practitioners addressing others who will have the same unmediated access to the female body, was generated not by any local Salernitan demand for specialized gynaecological literature for women, but by the interests of a visiting English person eager for a text to take back home. Even with Trota's *Practica* there is no indication that it was addressed to women. It is quite possible that that once sizable tome never had any particular purpose other than to serve as Trota's public assertion of her stature as a *magistra*—an equal of her male peers who likewise asserted their 'mastery' by writing general compendia of their cures.

What is remarkable about women's medicine in twelfth-century Salerno is that at this one moment in time, not simply did women have considerable expertise in the properties of various medicinal substances and medical practices, but it was *acknowledged* that they had such expertise. One of Copho's students, Johannes Platearius, noted in his general *Practica* how the *mulieres Salernitane* treated pustules of the penis with cabbage leaves, just as Trota described in

---

[91] Several of these were described in Trota's *Treatments for Women* (¶¶190–5 and 231), but similar substances are described by Master Salernus and alluded to by John of Saint Paul, who recognizes them as a cause of lesions of the penis (*Breviarium*, Book IV, cap. *De uulnere uirge et tumore testium*, BLL, MS Additional 16385, f. 52: 'Vvlneratur uirga ex acutis humoribus qui cum urina purgantur. autem fit uulneratus ex sanguine. Fit autem aliquibus dum coeunt cum mulieribus que puluerem constrictiuum in uuluam ponunt ut strictiorem uuluam habent').

Treatments for Women.[92] The Salernitan textbook on *materia medica*, the *Circa instans*, recounted no less than twenty different practices of the *mulieres*, such as how they give white poppy, mixed with their 'first milk', to infants in order to induce sleep, or how they make little wafers from pellitory-of-the-wall, water, and flour in order to treat painful urination.[93] Similarly, the compiler of the Salernitan compendium *On the Treatment of Illnesses* recognized the value of Trota's empirical work as a complement to the writings of her more book-learned male peers. This was especially true of her gynaecological and obstetrical knowledge, made more valuable by her access to the female body: the compiler foregrounded her manually interventionist therapies for uterine prolapse and difficult birth, not even bothering to include the minimalist discussions on these topics from his male sources beyond Johannes Afflacius's comments on how to avoid miscarriage.[94] A French visitor to Salerno in the middle or later decades of the century, Bernard of Provence, could readily record the empirical practices of the *mulieres*, citing their practices more often than even Hippocrates or Galen. The stories of Orderic Vitalis and Marie de France claiming that there were accomplished medical women at Salerno were clearly true.

All these texts, moreover, together with the exceptional testimony of the *Treatments for Women*, show a moment when actual *dialogue* between female empirical traditions and male rational traditions occurred: whether the married couple Zoffus and Trocta of 1112 is our pair of medical colleagues Copho and Trota or not, it is clear that at the very moment in the first half of the twelfth century when medicine was discovering the transformative possibilities of the written word, it was still engaged enough with its oral, empirical traditions to allow space for female authority. This moment of *rapprochement* between male and female medical traditions passed, however, leaving no permanent effect. While the male writers of the second half of the century would continue to write general *practicae* and other works on medical therapy, their main intellectual energies shifted not to reconciling the collective empirical knowledge of Salernitan practitioners with the therapeutics they found in their latinized Greek or Arabic authorities, but to searching for more universal rational truths. Women's empirical practices became irrelevant to the enterprise of rational medicine at the end of the twelfth century and it is little wonder that in their many lengthy commentaries on theoretical medicine, male writers such as

[92] Green, *Trotula*, p. 44. Platearius's other reference to the *mulieres* is his description of how they use leek juice to abort the so-called 'brother of the Lombards' (also called *arpa* and perhaps referring to uterine moles).

[93] I am in the process of collecting these and all the other references to the *mulieres Salernitane* in medieval medical literature; currently, the list runs to some five dozen entries.

[94] See Green, 'Trota's *Oeuvre*', where I document that a major portion if not all of the unattributed portions of the gynaecological and obstetrical material in the Salernitan compendium *Treatment of Illnesses* may come from Trota.

Archimattheus, Bartholomeus, and Maurus make no mention of the Salernitan women at all.[95]

We might well wonder what women's medicine would have looked like in later centuries if, instead of appropriating the practices of their female counterparts but then ignoring the women themselves, male Salernitan physicians had instead invited the *mulieres Salernitane* to join them in their enterprise. A late fifteenth-century library catalogue of the charterhouse of Salvatorberg near Erfurt intriguingly lists a medical florilegium entitled 'The medical disputations of Trotula on all the parts of the body made to the envy of the masters.'[96] Perhaps this is a reference to a complete copy of Trota's *Practica*, whose full extent we are now only able to guess at. Equally interesting is this cataloguer's depiction of 'Trotula' as a woman who could hold her own in disputations with male masters. Such an image of 'disputing women' is not rare in the later Middle Ages, at least as a literary conceit,[97] and it echoes intriguingly Orderic Vitalis's account of the *sapiens matrona* whom the Norman monk, Ralph the Ill-Tonsured, encountered in Salerno on his travels.[98] Yet it is one of the ironies of women's history that the same gender system of twelfth-century Salerno that kept men at a distance from the bodies of their female patients was equally powerful in keeping women away from the traditions of education and philosophical discourse that might have generated a women's medicine that was both empirically *and* rationally informed. Trota's contemporary, Hildegard of Bingen (1098–1179), could approach such a combination of empiricism and rationalism in her own medicine both because of her access to the literate traditions of Benedictine monasticism (including the well-stocked libraries of nearby male monasteries) and because of a powerful, independent conception of herself as a vehicle for God's word.[99] Trota, all

---

[95] My thanks to Faith Wallis and Danielle Jacquart, who are working, respectively, on the commentary traditions of Bartholomeus and Maurus, for confirmation of this point. On Archimattheus, see Archimatheus Salernitanus, *Erklärungen zur hippokratischen Schrift Prognostikon. Nach der Handschrift Trier Bischöfliches Priesterseminar 76*, ed. Hermann Grensemann (Hamburg 2002/rev. 2004), at <http://www.uke.uni-hamburg.de/institute/geschichte-medizin/index_18229> accessed 7 October 2006; and *idem, Glossae in Isagogas*.

[96] Bayerische Akademie der Wissenschaften, *Mittelalterliche Bibliothekskataloge Deutschlands und der Schweiz*, 2. Band: Bistum, Mainz, Erfurt (Munich: C.H. Beck'sche, 1928), p. 439: *Excepciones trocule artis phisice facte ad invidiam magistrorum de omnibus partibus corporis.*

[97] Helen Solterer, *The Master and Minerva: Disputing Women in French Medieval Culture* (Berkeley: University of California Press, 1995).

[98] See n. 23 above.

[99] See Florence Eliza Glaze, 'Medical Writer: "Behold the Human Creature"', in Barbara Newman, ed., *Voice of the Living Light: Hildegard of Bingen and her World* (Berkeley: University of California Press, 1998), pp. 125–48; and Laurence Moulinier, ed., *Beate Hildegardis Cause et cure*, Rarissima mediaevalia, 1 (Berlin: Akademie Verlag, 2003). Rather than being compared with her extraordinarily learned contemporaries Hildegard and Heloise of the Paraclete (d. 1164), Trota would perhaps better be likened to the holy women of the 13th century and later, those who had far less command of Latin and relied heavily, or entirely, on their Latinate scribe/confessors to render their thoughts into writing. Close structural and linguistic analysis of such texts often shows how heavy-handed such scribal/editorial impositions could be. See, for example, Catherine M. Mooney, 'The Authorial Role of Brother A. in the Composition of Angela of Foligno's Revelations', in E. Ann

the evidence suggests, briefly enjoyed similar status as an authority within the community of Salerno and, more enduringly, within the larger community of Norman France and England. Yet neither Hildegard's nor Trota's engagement with medicine was sufficiently strong to generate any female successors. Their respective intellectual patrimonies may have lived on among women in local oral traditions, but if either woman spawned a tradition of female writing on medicine, they did so without leaving a trace.

Matter and John Coakely, eds., *Creative Women in Medieval and Early Modern Italy: A Religious and Artistic Renaissance* (Philadephia: University of Pennsylvania Press, 1994), pp. 34–63; and Else Marie Wiberg Pedersen, 'The In-carnation of Beatrice of Nazareth's Theology', in *New Trends in Feminine Spirituality: The Holy Women of Liège and their Impact*, ed. Juliette Dor, Lesley Johnson, and Jocelyn Wogan-Browne, Medieval Women: Texts and Contexts, 2 (Turnhout: Brepols, 1999), pp. 61–79. In Trota's case, her extant works (for better or worse) show little editorial imposition of order or style, though *Treatments for Women* does, from time to time, achieve a certain simple elegance.

2

Men's Practice of Women's Medicine in the Thirteenth and Fourteenth Centuries

Nor did she have any scruples about showing him every part of her body as freely as she would have displayed it to a woman, provided that the nature of her infirmity required her to do so.[1]

Boccaccio, *The Decameron* (1349–51)

Boccaccio's description of the ravages of the Black Death in Florence in 1348 is one of the most memorable we have, precisely because of his acuity in depicting the collapse of social order. One casualty of the chaos of this first great wave of the plague was sexual propriety: a patrician woman would now deign to show her body to a male servant, 'provided that the nature of her infirmity required her to do so'. Given Boccaccio's succinct (and I believe accurate) insight into the problem of sexual shame in medical practice, we may find it surprising that well before the onslaught of the Black Death in the mid fourteenth century, men had successfully expanded their gynaecological care of women beyond the levels we witnessed in twelfth-century Salerno. The Salernitan texts on women's medicine—now combined into a single ensemble called the *Trotula* and owned (as we shall see) by the same elite Latinate physicians, surgeons, clerics, and other litterati who read and used Latin medical texts in general—played a key role in establishing this competence.[2] Granted, thirteenth- and fourteenth-century physicians' and surgeons' interests in women's health could be described as timid, with little innovation 'outside of the box' of the nosological categories or therapeutic traditions they had inherited from their Arabic sources. The fact that

---

[1] Giovanni Boccaccio, *The Decameron*, trans. G. H. McWilliam, 2nd edn (New York: Penguin, 1995), p. 55.

[2] In this chapter, I begin to refer to the three specialized Salernitan texts on women's medicine as the *Trotula* treatises, using that term both to refer to the treatises generically and to their combined form, the *Trotula* ensemble. Briefly, the so-called *Trotula* ensemble was created (probably near the end of the 12th century) by fusing the *Conditions of Women*, the *Treatments for Women*, and *Women's Cosmetics* (in that order) together into a single compendium. Over the next century, several different editors (probably working independently) modified this new compendium, adding recipes, shifting the order of others slightly, subtly emending the language. In all, there are fifteen different versions of the texts. For full details, see Green, 'Development'.

no new specialized gynaecological texts were composed for over one hundred years after the *Trotula* is itself testimony to the lack of intellectual energy invested in this field. Nevertheless, we find tentative signs of a growing confidence.

Looking for 'innovation' in medieval medicine may seem a modernist and anachronous endeavour when dealing with an intellectual system that valued authority and considered successful synthesis and emulation of one's predecessors to be a laudable goal. Yet, as I will argue, there are two areas of engagement with women's health where we can see the growing expertise of male practitioners. Here, the distinction between internal medicine (the province of the physician) and surgery (which took as its task care of the surface of the body and the rectification of lesions, growths, and fractures) becomes important. Control of diet and prescription of drugs, on the one hand, involved a very different kind of interaction with the patient than the hands-on work of surgery, on the other. Among physicians, male involvement with women's health rarely moved much beyond intervening in cases of menstrual difficulties, certain uterine conditions, and fertility problems and, to a far lesser extent, offering recommendations for difficult birth. This was all a 'hands off' kind of gynaecology similar to the Salernitans. Yet suddenly, in the early fourteenth century, physicians connected to the medical school of Montpellier (which, along with Bologna and Paris, had long since superseded Salerno as the chief centre of medical teaching in Europe) began to make expanded claims to be able to diagnose and treat infertility. This would in fact be the major focus of male physicians' gynaecological concerns right into the fifteenth century and would serve as the opening wedge for their expanded competence in women's healthcare. For surgeons, we find a slow progression rather than a sudden leap, a gradual adding on by a series of writers who (with one exception) do not seem to have systematically problematized women's medicine *per se*. In the twelfth century, surgical involvement with women's particular conditions was limited to the breasts; late in the following century, surgeons' attention turned to the female genitalia, and then only as a delayed reaction to the influence of their Arabic authorities. Obstetrical intervention developed somewhat differently: although not explicitly incorporated into surgical writing until after the mid fourteenth century, already *c.* 1300 there are signs that males were turned to for aid in obstetrical emergencies. Despite these different trajectories of physicians' and surgeons' involvement with women's health, both areas show an increased confidence among male medical practitioners in claiming expertise in women's health.

That said, Boccaccio's passing remark is revealing because it captures the key, though usually unarticulated, *barrier* to the expansion of male practice of women's medicine: the problem of sexual shame. As at Salerno, so throughout the rest of Europe social conventions about female honour and male–female relations, while never excluding men from either speculating about or actually practising medicine on female patients, did significantly complicate the practice of women's medicine by men. We have no lack of evidence that men were involved in women's healthcare on a general level throughout the high and late

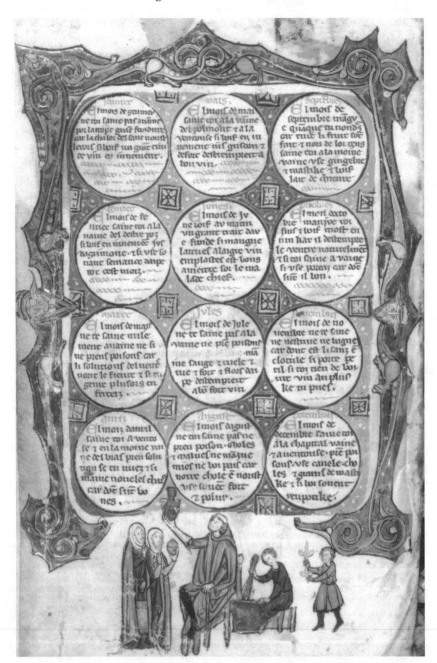

FIG. 2.1 Set of month-by-month health rules in a beguine's psalter; in the lower margin, two women take their urine to a male physician for examination.

medieval periods. From the Salernitan Peter Borda who was identified in 1086
as the personal physician of Sichelgaita, widow of the Norman lord Robert
Guiscard, all the way up to the end of the medieval period, male practitioners
can be readily identified who treated and served as personal physicians to queens,
duchesses, and other noblewomen. Indeed, from the fourteenth century on, it
would probably be difficult to find a high-ranking woman who was *not* attended
by a male practitioner at some point in her life. Nor was it just aristocratic women
who employed men. Throughout southern Europe, we find heads of households
as well as religious institutions entering into contracts with physicians or surgeons
to provide them with regular medical care. These would often specify that care
was to be provided for the women and children of the family, and we have
numerous documentary cases where female patients, both adults and children,
were indeed cared for by male practitioners. Iconographically, this normativeness
of male medical practice is seen in such unexpected contexts as a beguine's psalter
from Belgium *c.*1300, which has a set of month-by-month health rules, and,
in the lower margin of the same page, two women shown taking their urine

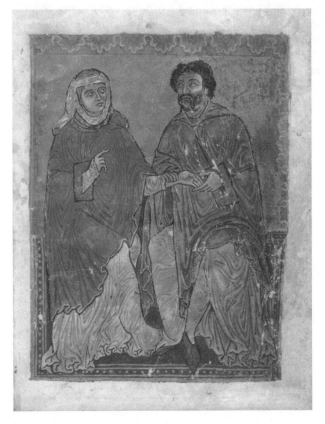

FIG. 2.2 Male physi-
cian taking female
patient's pulse.

to a male physician for examination (Fig. 2.1).[3] An early fourteenth-century Viennese beguine, Agnes Blannbekin, describes as quite normative how one might go to the marketplace to seek out an apothecary for medicaments, just as one would go to a victualler for food or a merchant's shop for various goods. She also describes as quite routine her experience of being phlebotomized by a male bloodletter.[4] A collection of medical texts from early fourteenth-century Germany made, apparently, as a personal manual of practice for one Gotefridus, includes a handsome depiction of a male physician taking a female patient's pulse (Fig. 2.2).[5] This richly clothed, obviously well-off woman shows how male medical ministrations could be delivered without any compromising unveiling or undressing.

Even this image, however, with patient and practitioner locked in direct eye contact, is suggestive of the dangers. If taking a woman's pulse was problematic, how much the more complicated must any kind of gynaecological examination have been? The seeming irreconcilability of the problem of shame and any cross-sex practice of gynaecology has sustained the modern myth that medieval gynaecology was an exclusively female preserve. Yet the problem of shame in the practice of gynaecology was an issue not only for women but for men as well. Male practitioners both clerical and lay were cautioned about the dangers of involvement with women and, on occasion, men might express more discomfort about cross-sex practice than women. For the sake of both men and women, therefore, the problem of sexual shame in cross-sex medical practice was solved by employing female intermediaries to perform the visual and manual tasks that the male physician or surgeon could not or would not do.

'AND THESE THINGS SUFFICE CONCERNING THE CONDITIONS OF WOMEN': THE *TROTULA* AND ITS EUROPEAN AUDIENCES

It is a reflection of the Salernitan achievement that the gendering of twelfth-century literate medicine was to persist, for it was out of Salerno that a scholastic,

---

[3] Cambridge, Fitzwilliam Museum, MS 288, *c.*1300, f. 6v. On this manuscript, see Judith Oliver, *Gothic Manuscript Illumination in the Diocese of Liège (c.1250–1330)*, 2 vols., Corpus of Illuminated Manuscripts from the Low Countries, 3 (Leuven: Uitgeverij Peeters, 1988), vol. 1, p. 100; vol. 2, pp. 246, 250–1, 285; and pl. 15. Beguines were women who usually lived apart from their families and did not marry, devoting themselves to a pious life of devotion and work without the limitations of formal religious vows.

[4] Ulrike Wiethaus, 'Street Mysticism: An Introduction to *The Life and Revelations* of Agnes Blannbekin', in *Women Writing Latin from Roman Antiquity to Early Modern Europe*, vol. 2: *Medieval Women Writing Latin*, ed. Laurie J. Churchill, Phyllis R. Brown, and Jane E. Jeffrey (New York: Routledge, 2002), pp. 281–307, at 297 and 301.

[5] BLL, MS Arundel 295, s. xiv in. (Germany), f. 256r. Like many other male physicians of the period, Gotefridus also took responsibility for diagnosing pregnancy; he includes a treatise *De signis conceptus* in the manuscript.

text-based, *learned* medical tradition was born, a tradition that from its very inception was gendered masculine. It was at Salerno that the commentary traditions began on, first, a mid eleventh-century medical compendium, Gario-pontus's *Passionarius*, and soon after on the *Articella*, a collection of introductory texts that served as the foundation for medical curricula in universities all over Europe. It was also at Salerno that basic texts on *materia medica*, diagnosis, and even medical ethics were composed, many of which (such as the pharmaceutical treatises *Circa instans* and the *Antidotary of Nicholus*, or the text on urines by the Salerno-trained Giles of Corbeil) would prove the standard manuals in their fields for over two centuries. It was also in the southern Italian Kingdom of Sicily that the formal learning that the Salernitans had honed would first be made the standard by which medical licensing was judged.[6] In other words, all the features that had most characterized the work of male medical practitioners in Salerno—their literacy, their grounding in grammar, rhetoric and logic, their engagement with philosophical principles, and the social confirmation of their stature by licensing procedures—would define the learned medicine of the later medieval universities. And these, of course, were the exclusive preserve of males.[7]

The *Trotula* never became 'school' texts: while we can associate them with various university masters and college libraries, it cannot be claimed that women's medicine ever became a formal element of learned medical instruction. But then neither did many other elements of practical medicine. Rather, it was on the day-to-day level of medical practice, the actual encounters with real patients, that the practising physician or surgeon needed some guidance about how to diagnose, prognose, and then treat women's diseases. While medical writers continued the Salernitans' practice of incorporating gynaecological and some obstetrical chapters into their general medical textbooks, the *Trotula* functioned for many practitioners as their chief guide to a more detailed understanding of the conditions that particularly afflicted women.

We can never know, of course, the full number of copies that once existed. But whatever their representativeness, the seventy-six extant Latin manuscripts of the gynaecological *Trotula* texts that date from before 1400 (including a unique Latin verse adaptation) together with sixteen witnesses of manuscripts that are no longer extant, present an imposing body of evidence.[8] Of this total, about one-fifth bear witness to at least one individual or institution that owned them up through the fourteenth century (see Appendix 1). In so far as we can name the owners,

---

[6] See Chapter 1 above.

[7] Although not addressing medical culture, Ruth Mazo Karras, *From Boys to Men: Formations of Masculinity in Late Medieval Europe* (Philadelphia: University of Pennsylvania Press, 2003), provides a detailed account of how masculinity was forged among students in medieval universities.

[8] In all, I have now identified 131 extant Latin copies of the *Trotula*, 133 if we include a 13th-century Latin verse adaptation and a 15th-century Latin and English prose adaptation. For the purposes of my discussion in this chapter, I only count manuscripts written or documented before 1400 and only those containing one or both of the two gynaecological treatises or the full *Trotula* ensemble.

the Latin *Trotula* were owned exclusively by men. The monk Walter of Saint George (fl. *c.*1286) donated two copies of the *Trotula* to the Benedictine Abbey of St Augustine's at Canterbury, and at least four of his brethren followed suit in the next century. University men similarly favoured institutions with which they were associated. William Rede (*c.*1315–85), Bishop of Chichester and a noted astronomer, distributed some 250 books among six different Oxford colleges, giving a collection of mostly Salernitan texts including the *Trotula* to New College where we know medicine was actively being studied at least from the fifteenth century and possibly before.⁹ Simon Bredon (d. 1372), also an astronomer and sometime physician to Elizabeth de Burgh, Lady of Clare, donated his copy to Merton College.¹⁰ Henry Whitfield, who held degrees in arts, medicine, and theology, and was an ordained priest and fellow of Queen's College, gave his copy to Stapledon Hall (later Exeter College) in 1383 or 1387. In Paris, both Gerard of Utrecht (d. betw. 1326 and 1338), a theologian, and Jacques de Padua, master of arts, medicine, and doctor of theology (fl. 1342–53), bequeathed their copies of the *Trotula* to the Sorbonne. Although from the fourteenth century on surgeons were more likely to use the texts in vernacular translation,¹¹ we can find copies of the Latin *Trotula* in the hands of such men as a late thirteenth-century Florentine surgeon named Sinibaldus and Bernat Serra (d. 1338), surgeon to Kings Jaume II and Alfons III of the Crown of Aragon. Ecclesiastical institutions and university and college libraries also owned copies, many of them acquired as testamentary bequests. We find a copy at the hospital of Rothenburg ob der Tauber in Bavaria and one in the hands of the canons of the cathedral of Laon in Picardy, who had a long tradition of medical practice at the local hospital of Notre-Dame. And as we have already seen, even a medical layman like Charles V of France had a copy of the Latin *Trotula* on his library's shelves. In fact, the only notable group who show no interest in the *Trotula* are those northern Italian physicians most thoroughly wedded to the Arabic authorities that began to infiltrate the university curricula in the latter half of the thirteenth century; their non-interest in the *Trotula* was due not to their dismissal of female physiology and pathology as an important area of knowledge, but rather to their sense that the work of Salerno had been superseded by the richer theoretical and empirical works of Rhazes, Avicenna, and others. In their own writings, they show just as much interest in offering care to their female clientele as physicians elsewhere.¹² The *Trotula* texts, therefore, or other works

⁹ See R. W. Hunt, 'The Medieval Library', in *New College Oxford, 1379–1979*, ed. John Buxton and Penry Williams (Oxford: Wardens and Fellows of New College, 1979), pp. 317–45, esp. pp. 332–4.

¹⁰ On Bredon's connection to Elizabeth de Burgh (herself an owner of medical books though not, apparently, of the *Trotula*), see Green, 'Possibilities', pp. 23, 50, and 57–8.

¹¹ See Chapter 4.

¹² Save for two 15th-century collections of excerpts (see Chapter 6 below), I have found no evidence for the circulation of the Latin *Trotula* in Italy after the beginning of the 14th century, though the texts take on new life (and a new audience) in the form of two Italian translations. On Bolognese physicians' involvement in gynaecological care and speculative research on women,

that covered comparable subject matter, were owned by every sector of literate society that we usually associate with Latinate medicine in the Middle Ages.

For manuscripts of the *Trotula* having no ownership information, we can reasonably speculate about owners' identities and the intent with which they would have used a treatise on women's medicine by examining the patterns of content and form of the codices as a whole. Although in two, possibly three cases such codicological analysis raises the possibility of female use (see Chapter 3 below), the majority of Latin codices look very similar to the volumes of known male ownership—not, of course, because the same litany of texts was being copied over and over again (in only two cases can it be shown that one manuscript is a direct, text-for-text copy of another),[13] but because similarly motivated readers throughout western Europe wanted to incorporate these unique texts on women's medicine into their own handbooks.[14]

Most frequently, the *Trotula* texts are placed squarely within the mundane, pedestrian world of daily medical practice: they are surrounded by texts on urines, pulses, *materia medica,* medical ethics, pharmaceutical weights and measures, prognostics, some medical astrology, and, overwhelmingly, simple general therapeutics. Oxford, Pembroke College, MS 21 can be taken as an example. Written in England towards the end of the thirteenth century, it begins with Constantine the African's treatise on stomach ailments, and then moves on to John of Saint Paul's work on uncompounded medicines ('simples') and Richard the Englishman's *Anatomy.* A brief excerpt from the medical poem *Schola Salernitana* follows, then Richard's rules for interpreting urines (especially those of women), a regimen for maintaining health, then a tract on the nature of the semen (male as well as female). Next come works on preparation of medicinal foods and drinks, the preparation of plasters, prognostic signs, the Salernitan *Conditions of Women,* and then the short tract attributed to the Salernitan Archimattheus that instructed the physician how he should behave when entering the patient's household. The volume concludes with works on urines and the proper doses of medicines, another regimen, a study of laxative medicines, and a tract on diet. Pembroke 21 is clearly a practising physician's handbook, comprising all the principal features of medieval medical practice: diagnosis (particularly by urines), prognosis, and therapy (particularly by controlled diet and medicines). The addition of more short texts and recipes in the fourteenth and fifteenth centuries shows that the book continued to serve its role as a much-used

see Nancy G. Siraisi, *Taddeo Alderotti and His Pupils: Two Generations of Italian Medical Learning* (Princeton: Princeton University Press, 1981), pp. 278–9 and 282–3.

[13] The two 'couples' are OBL, MS e Musaeo 219, s. xiv in. (England) and its apograph Oxford, Merton College, MS 324, s. xv[1] (England); and Oxford, Pembroke College, MS 21, s. xiii ex. (England) and its apograph OBL, MS Ashmole 399, c.1298 (England).

[14] The *Trotula* were largely effective in rendering obsolete the bulk of the early medieval gynaecological corpus; see Green, *The 'Trotula'.* Hence, when a 13th- or 14th-century reader wanted a work on women's medicine, it was to the *Trotula* that he most frequently turned.

reference. The impression codices such as this give, therefore, is that the *Trotula* was used predominantly by professional medical practitioners in the course of their day-to-day practice of diagnosing, prognosing, and prescribing therapies.

A second category of reader was surgeons or individuals with a particular interest in surgical learning. Twelve of the seventy-six extant codices from the late twelfth through the fourteenth century, plus one lost manuscript that was held at Titchfield Abbey by around 1400, have a distinctly surgical character or are known to have been owned by surgeons. The earliest extant copy of any of the *Trotula* texts, a late twelfth-century manuscript made in southern France contains, in addition to the proto-ensemble of the *Trotula*, a text on phlebotomy and cupping, one on cautery, and Copho's anatomy of the pig.[15] In the mid thirteenth century, a Latin versifier in England rendered the whole *Trotula* ensemble, together with the surgical works of Roger Frugardi (*c*.1170) and Roland of Parma (*c*.1230), and a general text on methods of healing into a long poem on medical practice.[16] The *Trotula* is also paired with the surgical works of Roger, Roland, and Bruno of Longobucco (writing in 1253) in a late thirteenth- or early fourteenth-century pamphlet from northern Europe.[17] An Italian manuscript from the latter part of the thirteenth century includes, after the intermediate version of the *Trotula* ensemble (the most expansive form of the compendium), an anonymous compilation drawn from Galen and Avicenna of remedies of particular utility in surgical practice; this is then followed by further medicines and unguents excerpted from various authors including the probable scribe and owner of the manuscript, a Florentine surgeon named Sinibaldus.[18] A manuscript from the first half of the fourteenth century now in Basel has as its three main texts a tract on eye diseases by the Arabic authority 'Alī ibn 'Isa, the standardized *Trotula* ensemble, and Lanfranc's *Larger Surgery*, rounded out by smaller texts on medicines, weights and measures, and various recipes and disease regimens. That the compiler (or commissioner) of this manuscript may have been a cleric is suggested by the presence of Secundus's apophthegms and by the Franciscan Herman the Friar's historical chronicle.[19] One fourteenth-century German manuscript shows the compiler's particular interest in urogenital disorders, with its several tracts on kidney and bladder

[15] BLL, MS Royal 12.E.XV, s. xii ex. (France?). This manuscript would later be owned by the English king Edward IV (r. 1461–83), though whether his particular interest was in the *Trotula* as opposed to some other contents cannot be determined.

[16] BNF, MS lat. 8161A, s. xiii med. (England); ed. Charles Daremberg, in *Collectio Salernitana ossia documenti inediti, e trattati di medicina appartenenti alla scuola medica salernitana*, ed. Salvatore De Renzi, 5 vols. (Naples: Filiatre-Sebezio, 1852–9; repr. Bologna: Forni, 1967), 4: 1–176.

[17] BLL, MS Additional 18210, s. xiii ex./xiv in. (N. Europe).

[18] Florence, Biblioteca Laurenziana-Medicea, Plut. 73, cod. 37, s. xiii² (Italy).

[19] Basel, Öffentliche Universitätsbibliothek, MS D II 9, s. xiv (Italy?). The presence in this manuscript of the *Tabula antidotarii* of Armengaud Blaise (Arnau of Vilanova's nephew), written *c*.1305 in Montpellier, may suggest some associations with that medical school. On the significance of Secundus's work, see Chapter 5 below.

stones.[20] A fourteenth-century English manuscript demonstrates equal interest in human surgery and the care of dogs and horses.[21] A late thirteenth-century male surgeon (*cyrurgicus*) owned a copy of the standardized ensemble alongside Isaac Israeli's work on diets and Richardus Anglicus's anatomy; the manuscript then passed to the cathedral of Laon in the early fourteenth century where it continued to be annotated for several decades.[22] Perhaps the largest surgical and gynaecological compendium produced in the Middle Ages was a volume commissioned by a cleric, Richard de Fournival (d. before 1260), a poet, physician, and high church official of Amiens.[23]

A third, very different codicological context can be found in a manuscript of early fourteenth-century composition, a collection of preacher's texts and minor medical works. It situates the first two-thirds of the *Trotula* ensemble amid excerpts from Thomas of Cantimpré's mid thirteenth-century encyclopedia of learning for preachers, *On the Nature of Things*, some texts on poetic metrics, several short treatises on urines and prognostics, Petrus Alfonsi's *Clerical Discipline* (an early twelfth-century text that was often culled for anecdotes and folk tales that could be incorporated into sermons), and finally, added gradually over time, a series of short sermons. The original owners are unknown, but two monks, Heinrich and Friedrich, both of them rectors, jointly owned the manuscript in the later fourteenth century and, around 1400, they donated it to the Premonstratensian monastery of Mildenfurth in Thuringia.[24]

Finally, there are what could be called 'scientific' codices, which place the *Trotula* next to texts of natural philosophy: works on the elements, the heavens, astronomy, mathematics, and other aspects of science. Most of these volumes combine natural philosophical and medical texts in a way which suggests that, in addition to their need for astrological materials to aid in regular medical prognostications, owners of the *Trotula* texts occasionally considered themselves adept in the ways of science in general, not simply medicine. Some of the natural-philosophical associations of the gynaecological treatises came out of rather different concerns than a strict interest in women's health; I will have more to say about these in Chapter 5.

Just as the codicological context of the *Trotula* was always changing, so too did the substance of the texts themselves. The *Trotula* were subject to a whole

---

[20] Munich, Bayerische Staatsbibliothek, Clm 570, s. xiv[1] (Germany).

[21] OBL, MS Ashmole 1427, s. xiv[1] (England).

[22] Laon, Bibliothèque Municipale, MS 417, s. xiv in. (Italy). Incorporated into the manuscript later was a list of prebends in Laon, held predominately by Italian canons, between 1284 and 1314.

[23] On Fournival and his book, see Appendix 1 below, item 35; Green, 'Handlist I', pp. 157–8; and Monica H. Green, 'From "Diseases of Women" to "Secrets of Women": The Transformation of Gynecological Literature in the Later Middle Ages', *Journal of Medieval and Early Modern Studies* 30 (2000), 5–39, p. 20.

[24] Jena, Thüringer Universitäts- und Landesbibliothek, MS El. q. 17, s. xiv[1] (Germany). The *Trotula* appears on ff. 52vb–59va. My thanks to Dr. Bernhard Tönnies for sharing with me a draft description of this manuscript from his forthcoming catalogue of the Jena manuscripts.

variety of editorial interventions that produced a total of fifteen distinct versions between the twelfth and late thirteenth centuries. The manipulations, in form and in content, that the *Trotula* texts underwent are too numerous to survey here, but examination of a few subtle changes can help us better understand how male practitioners addressed (or studiously avoided) the challenge of cross-sex practice of women's medicine.[25]

Two aspects of the Salernitan gynaecological treatises would, one would think, have been problematic for the dozens (perhaps hundreds) of male readers of these texts: first, Trota's *Treatments for Women*, written as if by a female teacher speaking to a female audience of practitioners, had assumed that its audience could engage in the same 'hands-on' medical practice that its author(s) freely engaged in. How did male readers 'read themselves' into the 'we' that touched, massaged, sewed and in other ways manipulated the female body? Second, vague though it was, the *Conditions of Women* preface raised the troubling prospect that because women's shame prevented them from speaking freely to male physicians, the latter might be poorly qualified to serve women's health needs. As we shall see, neither issue was openly addressed.

The problems raised by Trota's *Treatments for Women* were ignored in two ways: either by reading the text and ignoring the problematic scenarios of 'hands-on' practice, or by ignoring the text altogether. As noted in the previous chapter, male writers normally employed passive forms or jussive subjunctives ('let this be done') when referring to 'hands-on' aspects of gynaecological diagnosis or treatment. Although one would think that the text of *Treatments for Women* would need to be modified to shift all the active verbs ('we do', 'we mix', 'we apply') into passive forms, no such systematic editing ever took place, either when the text circulated independently or when it was combined into the larger ensemble. Apparently, male readers (assuming they read these passages closely) were able to do 'simultaneous translation', taking themselves out of the communal 'we's' of the text and instead reading these instructions as if they were posed as injunctions for an attendant—'let this be done'. In a few cases, the 'we' did in fact disappear: for example, in ¶149 on ano-vaginal fistula and prolapse, where the author had originally referred to 'the other things which we are accustomed to do' as part of the general toileting the patient should perform in bed, by the time we reach later versions of the ensemble the 'we' has disappeared, having undergone significant deformation as the text matured.[26] Perhaps more revealingly, in that same chapter the original author had admitted that the condition was caused by the inadequacies of the women assisting. But

[25] On the major transformations of the *Trotula*, see Green, 'Documenting'. We cannot yet say whether the kinds of editorial interventions or careless errors we find in many copies of the *Trotula* (cf. Green, *Trotula*, pp. 52–8) are more frequent than in other kinds of medical texts, since so few have yet been critically edited.

[26] In the standardized ensemble, the most developed form of the text, the passage reads 'there [in bed] let her defecate and let her do all the customary things' (*ibi egerat et omnia assueta faciat*).

she asks that this should not be mentioned publicly, presumably so as not to air this dirty laundry outside the community of women. Already by the time we get to the second version of the text, however, the sentence reads: 'But this thing, you know, is kept secret among women [*Sed istud nosti quod cum mulieribus sit secretum*]'. As revised, the statement seems to be spoken from outside the community of women, in effect exposing women's secret to men.

For the most part, I suspect that the *Treatment for Women*'s 'we's' were never systematically revised because there was never any systematic rethinking of how this 'women's medicine' might be employed by men. Indeed, I suspect that more often readers ignored the whole text. Take, for example, a large volume, British Library, MS Sloane 1610, the bulk of which was written early in the fourteenth century. It contains the group of introductory theoretical tracts known as the *Articella*, plus Giles of Corbeil's poems on pulses and urines, an anatomical work attributed to Galen, Isaac Israeli's works on diets, fevers, and urines, and Ibn al-Jazzār's medical encyclopedia, the *Viaticum*. In other words, this has the full curriculum for the study of medicine as it was structured at Paris.[27] Later in the century, another hand added, into a blank space left by the original scribe, the full text of *Conditions of Women* followed by the chapter on impediments to conception from Archimattheus's *Practica*, both of which he seems to have copied out of an early thirteenth-century copy from England that also had a complete copy of the second version of *Treatments for Women*.[28] Yet the scribe of these addenda in Sloane 1610 (who was probably also the owner of the manuscript) copied only a single chapter from Trota's work: the one describing how widows, nuns and vowesses suffered from their sexual continence and how they should be treated (¶141). Why copy just this one chapter and omit such sections of *Treatments for Women* (which likewise had no parallel in *Conditions of Women*) as treatments for perineal tear or uterine prolapse? It seems likely that for this scribe/owner, who added copious notes elsewhere in the manuscript on urines and fevers, the hands-on aspects of women's medicine were simply irrelevant. As a physician, he was primarily interested in material that would aid him in his tasks of diagnosis and prescription of regimen or drugs to control health. Actually touching the female body was not part of his job. When push came to shove, it was the 'hands-on' material of *Treatments for Women* that most often was left on the wayside of transmission.

In fact, only one medical compiler in this period, the thirteenth-century author Gilbertus Anglicus (Gilbert the Englishman, fl. 1230–40), systematically incorporated any of *Treatments for Women*'s unique obstetrical or 'hands-on'

---

[27] BLL, MS Sloane 1610, s. xiv (northern Europe). On the Paris curriculum, see Danielle Jacquart and Françoise Micheau, *La médecine arabe et l'occident médiéval* (Paris: Maisonneuve et Larose, 1990), ch. 5.

[28] BLL, MS Sloane 1615, c.1220–40 (S. France). For *Conditions of Women*, the scribe seems to have collated the Sloane 1615 copy with a copy of the standardized ensemble.

gynaecological material into his own work.[29] Gilbert's large *Compendium of Medicine* culled material from several twelfth and early thirteenth century writers.[30] He drew heavily on Trota's *Treatments for Women* for his chapters on vaginal constrictives, uterine prolapse, various obstetrical conditions, and cosmetics. His failure to credit these borrowings to Trota conforms to his omission of the names of his other sources (most importantly, the Montpellierain writer Roger de Barone and the Italian surgeon, Roger Frugardi). Gilbert's appropriation of Trota's *Treatments for Women* nevertheless shows a keen eye for the originality of her therapies.

As was his wont throughout the *Compendium*, Gilbert used the relevant chapters of Roger de Barone's *Practical Medicine* for the basic structure of his gynaecological chapters. He begins to deploy Trota's material when he comes to the topic of 'wind in the womb' (*ventositas matricis*). He opens with the material from Roger de Barone, but then incorporates ¶151 from Trota's *Treatments for Women*. Gilbert suppresses Trota's name from the anecdote of her cure and recasts the account as a straightforward prescription of what any (male) practitioner should do. Intriguingly, Gilbert readily appropriates Trota's hands-on bathing and massaging of the female patient as part of her cure by recasting them into passive forms: 'Let a bath be made from a decoction of mallow . . .', 'Let the limbs and soles of the feet be frequently rubbed.' And he says nothing about the practice of taking the patient into his own home to perform this cure.[31] Gilbert appropriates other elements of the 'hands-on' therapies from *Treatments for Women*, though rather amazingly, he becomes quite cavalier (or perhaps simply inattentive) about *not* recasting some instructions into more cautious passive forms. Thus, in the chapter on ano-vaginal fistula (¶149), he tells his reader that *you* should sew the rupture with red thread and that *you* should then apply a fine linen cloth, smeared with pitch, onto the reconstructed perineum.[32] He expands upon the several

---

[29] It may be no coincidence that the one writer who continued to disseminate Trota's work should have been English given the clear patterns of circulation of Salernitan texts in England; see Chapter 1 above. One other exceptional use of Trota is Francesco da Piedemonte (d. 1320), who incorporated her instructions for ano-vaginal fistula (¶149) into his *Supplementum*; here, he claims he has learned the procedure *ab experto*. Franciscus de Pedemontium, *Supplementum in secundum librum secretorum remediorum Ioannis Mesuae, quae vocant De appropriatis*, in *Supplementum in secundum librum Compendii secretorum medicinae Ioannis Mesues medici celeberrimi tum Petria Apponi Patavini, tum Francisci de Pedemontium medicorum illustrium* (Venice: Iunta, 1589), Summa IIII. Quartae particulae sectionis primae, cap. 17: De cura accidentium, quae sequuntur partum (f. 101ra–b).

[30] Gilbert's *Compendium* has not been edited since it was first printed in 1510 in Lyons. I therefore cite from the earliest extant manuscript, Brugge, Openbare Bibliotheek, MS 469, an. 1271, ff. 1r–244v, which I have collated against three other early manuscripts.

[31] Gilbert's cautious appropriation of this cure contrasts strikingly with that of a 15th-century French translator of the *Trotula*, who sees no problem in a male physician taking a female patient into his home. See Chapter 4 below on this *Regimen for Ladies*.

[32] Brugge, MS 469, f. 205vb: 'Post modum rupturam que est inter pudicum circulum et naturam femineam in. iii. uel iiii. locis sues cum filo serico. Deinde nature appones pannum delicatum, pice linitum, hoc facit matricem retrahi propter fetorem. Pix enim fetida est'.

remedies in *Treatments* for pain after birth, inserting a long digression on how the uterus delights in holding and retaining the foetus, mourning when it looses it, and also why, based on its anatomy, the uterus is so desirous of intercourse.

There is much in *Treatments for Women* that Gilbert does not exploit: he skips over the chapter on treating nuns, widows, and vowesses for the consequences of their celibacy (a topic which, as we have seen, interested other users of the text); he omits the instructions for slimming down fat women or plumping up thin ones to aid conception; and he makes no use of Trota's material on diseased fluxes from the womb. Yet given how little attention the hands-on treatments of Trota's text would receive from other medical compilers and copyists, it is striking how thoroughly Gilbert exploits the unique cures to be found in *Treatments for Women*. In fact, Gilbert seems to have readily colluded with the more subversive aspects of *Treatments for Women*. He not simply adopts but expounds upon the patriarchally questionable instructions for 'restoring' virginity, adding an unapologetic justification for their presence: 'Sometimes virgins are corrupted, whence their 'door' is widened as plainly happens in sexually experienced women, and they suffer repudiation and perpetual disgrace, or they are fated for divorce, in which there is danger both to men and to women'.[33] He incorporates the instructions for shrinking and deodorizing an overstretched, foul-smelling vagina from *Women's Cosmetics* and then incorporates all the vaginal 'restoratives' from *Treatments for Women*, even the one that Trota had rejected as an inefficient practice of 'unclean' prostitutes. Finally, apparently drawing on the Salernitan writer John of Saint Paul, he recommends surgical intervention if the vagina is *too* tight (though like John he does not clarify who is to do this surgery).[34]

Gilbert's retention of so much that was unique about Trota's interpretation of women's medicine is thus itself unique. Given how widely disseminated the *Trotula* ensemble as a whole would be, it is striking how poorly the independent *Treatments for Women* circulated. There is only one complete extant copy of what seems to have been the original version of the text (not surprisingly, it is an English manuscript that may have partly been written in Italy), and Gilbert's *Compendium* itself constitutes one of the two other fragmentary witnesses. Gilbert's English origins may well account for his familiarity with the independent *Treatments for Women* and, ironically, his text did more to disseminate Trota's teachings than her original work itself.[35] But the poor circulation of *Treatments for Women*

[33] Brugge, MS 469, f. 199vb: 'Corrumpuntur quandoque uirgines, vnde et ianua ampliatur ut corruptela pateat contingenti et merito repudium patiuntur et in sempiternum dedecus uel diuorcium in utrisque periculum tam uiri quam mulieres sortiuntur'.

[34] Brugge, MS 469, f. 200rb: 'Et si nimis stricta est cum humidis emplasmetur et unguentis ampliabitur, aut si necesse est beneficio cyrurgie ei opitulabitur'. On John of Saint Paul, see Chapter 1 above. On gynaecological surgical procedures, see below.

[35] Gilbertus's *Compendium* was apparently used in university circles in late 13th and early 14th century Paris (there exist at least two *pecia* exemplars among the twenty-seven extant copies of the text), and many other copies (for example, several at Oxford colleges) are quite standardized in format, suggesting mass production.

cannot account for the failure of other thirteenth- or fourteenth-century writers to recognize the originality of Trota's text since, as we have seen, the *Trotula* ensemble—which had incorporated *Treatments for Women* at its core—was fully formed by 1200 and was circulating widely. Even when they had the full (if somewhat modified) text of *Treatments for Women* right in front of them, most male practitioners seem to have ignored its original features.

It is perhaps not surprising, therefore, that no editorial adjustment or elaboration was made to the preface of *Conditions of Women*—the opening text of the *Trotula* ensemble—where, as we have seen, the author used women's shame as a central element of his justification for writing the text: women are ashamed to bare their ills to a physician, *therefore* there was need for him to compile a handbook describing women's diseases and their cures. This statement could have readily backfired to serve as an argument for women's shunning male physicians altogether and taking control of the text. Indeed, a French translator would make precisely that argument sometime in the early or mid thirteenth century.[36] Yet remarkably, male readers seem to have been oblivious to the suggestion, however oblique, that their gender ill-suited them for gynaecological practice: the passage was never rewritten by a single scribe, it was never deleted, and it was never commented upon by a single annotator of the Latin texts. Indeed, when vernacularizing the text for male audiences, most translators just as unproblematically rendered the passage about women's shame and the problem with physicians with no alteration. Only a sole Italian translator omitted the reference to male physicians, thereby implying that 'the problem' was women's only, and even this may be due to unclear phrasing in his Latin original.[37]

Thus, neither editors, scribes, nor readers ever disqualify themselves from the practice of women's gynaecological care yet neither do they elaborate on what the physician's or surgeon's role should be *vis-à-vis* the midwife or other female attendant in the actual treatment of female patients. Indeed, despite the *Trotula*'s wide circulation, very few medical writers in their own work acknowledge the texts' existence or turn to them for learned opinion.[38] Gerard de Berry, an early author of a formal commentary on Ibn al-Jazzār's *Viaticum*, referred to 'Trotula' as an authority on cosmetics, not gynaecology, as did Abbé Poutrel, the alleged author of a French surgical text from *c.*1300.[39] The other thirteenth-century user of 'Trotula' was Petrus Hispanus, who made use of *Conditions of Women*

[36] See discussion of the French *Quant Dex nostre Seignor* in Chapter 4 below.

[37] On this Italian translation of the *Trotula*, called *Book on the Secret Conditions of Women*, see Monica H. Green, 'Gender and the Vernacularization of Women's Medicine in Late Medieval and Early Modern Europe' (forthcoming).

[38] 'Trotula's' authority was, however, used in other ways during this period; see Chapter 5 below.

[39] Both may well have been referring to a text of Trota's now no longer extant, for both quote a cosmetic recipe that has thus far never been found as part of either Trota's *oeuvre* or the *Trotula* texts. See Monica H. Green, 'Reconstructing the *Oeuvre* of Trota of Salerno', in *La Scuola medica Salernitana: Gli autori e i testi*, ed. Danielle Jacquart and Agostino Paravicini Bagliani, Edizione Nazionale 'La Scuola medica Salernitana', 1 (Florence: SISMEL / Edizioni del Galluzzo, 2007), 183–233.

and clearly credited 'Trotula' with its views. Yet 'she' is only one among a dozen different authorities he employs for his gynaecological section. The authentic work of Trota makes no appearance at all.

In short, then, although thirteenth- and fourteenth-century physicians readily incorporated the *Trotula* into their medical handbooks, most of them apparently being quite comfortable accepting a female as its author (there are, at any rate, no contestations of her authorship in this period), almost no acknowledgement was made that the embedded author Trota brought *something different* to women's medicine than the dialectical reasonings and 'hands-off' therapeutics normally found in male-authored medical compendia (and, of course, in the male-authored *Conditions of Women*). The *Trotula* could be absorbed into the regular medical practice of learned men so easily because those elements of the texts that raised complicated questions about how gynaecological care was actually to be delivered to female patients were simply ignored.

'AND INNUMERABLE WOMEN CAME TO HIM': PHYSICIANS' EXPERTISE IN FERTILITY

In the margin of a large fifteenth-century French compendium of fertility texts there is a note describing what may have been a not unusual situation:

Master Odo told me that there was once a priest in Montpellier who made marvelous things for conception from the following two substances [a compound medicine called *trifera magna* and the juice of *santio*], and he had a great reputation and even greater fame than the physicians of Montpellier. And innumerable women came to him and they became pregnant by using these two remedies.[40]

Just who this priest (or even 'Master Odo') was is not clear, but it hardly matters.[41] The priest's success in alleviating the fertility problems of 'innumerable women' is simply one among many instances of a striking upsurge in the high and later medieval period of medical concern to enhance fertility. Richard the Englishman, writing in the late twelfth or early thirteenth century, describes in

---

[40] BNF, MS lat. 7066, f. 12v: 'Magister Odo dixit mihi quod erat unus presbyter in Montepessulano qui ex istis duabus receptis sequentibus [*sc.* triffere magne et succi santionis] faciebat ad impregnacionem mirabilia, et habebat maximum nomen et maiorem famam quam medici de Montepessulano, et ipsum ibant quamplurime mulieres et impregnabantur cum remediis istis duobus'. *Trifera magna* was a compound medicine that employed opium and various herbs, gums, and spices; one of its chief uses was to help women conceive by purging the menses. I have not yet been able to identify *santio*.

[41] This Master Odo is identified earlier in the manuscript as Odo de Credulis. Ernest Wickersheimer, *Dictionnaire biographique des médecins en France au Moyen Age*, 2 vols. (1936; repr. Geneva: Librairie Droz, 1979), 2: 584, identifies an Odon de Credolio as a clerk and physician who witnessed an act for Philip I *c.*1086–90. The coincidence of names is striking, but the university of Montpellier was not founded until a century later so one must wonder where Odo came by his title 'master'.

his *Practica* how all the medical powers of the Salernitan physicians were called on to treat the sterility of the Queen of Sicily. He was no doubt referring to King William II's English bride Joanna (1165–99), who had married at age eleven or twelve and then had to suffer the ignominy of twelve years of sterility until her husband's death in 1189.[42] Richard considered medical treatment of infertility futile, but his pessimism was apparently not shared. From the humble women who sought out the advice of the priest in Montpellier all the way up to queens, noblewomen and urban elites of Europe, both women and their male kin often aggressively sought assistance in reproduction from a variety of sources. A fourteenth-century practitioner in the southern French town of Manosque, a certain Antoni Imbert, was convicted of having promised (but failed) to cure women's infertility by magical means.[43] His crime, of course, was not in being a man treating women, but in being a fraud and a dabbler in magic. It is a measure of the success of more learned male practitioners that a man like Antoni did not cause more scandal than he did. When called upon to bring their skills to bear on fertility problems, the physicians of Salerno and Montpellier, and elsewhere in Europe, readily complied and, when they were successful, were dearly prized.

Late antique and early medieval gynaecological texts had always had one or more brief chapters on aids to conception, but aside from Muscio's rather general statements that infertility could be caused by either structural defects of the genitals or general disease conditions, these consisted only of a few remedies, with no theorizing of causation. It is to the Salernitans that credit goes for giving infertility a permanent place in the nosological canon of western medicine. Separate chapters on infertility can be found in the writings of all the Salernitan masters—from Trota to Copho, Bartholomeus, Salernus, and Petrus Musandinus—while one anonymous writer late in the twelfth century wrote a short tract specifically devoted to the topic.[44] Several Montpellier masters of the fourteenth century would then pick up the topic, elaborating on it considerably.

A wonderful story involves the most famous of Montpellier's medical masters, the great Catalan physician Arnau of Vilanova (d. 1311). Around 1304 or 1307,

---

[42] Richardus Anglicus, *Practica*, in BAV, MS Pal. lat. 1253, s. xiii[2], f. 85v. On Joanna (who would bear a living heir in her second marriage but then go on to die in a later childbirth), see D. S. H. Abulafia, 'Joanna, Countess of Toulouse (1165–99)', *Oxford Dictionary of National Biography* (Oxford: Oxford University Press, 2004), online edition: <http://www.oxforddnb.com.library.lib.asu.edu:80/view/article/14 818> accessed 15 May 2005.

[43] Joseph Shatzmiller and Rodrigue Lavoie, 'Médecine et gynécologie au moyen-âge: un exemple provençal', *Razo: Cahiers du Centre d'études Médiévales de Nice*, no. 4 (Nice: Faculté des Lettres et Sciences Humaines, Université de Nice, 1984), 133–43; see also Joseph Shatzmiller, *Médecine et justice en Provence médiévale: Documents de Manosque, 1262–1348* (Aix-en-Provence: Publications de l'Université de Provence, 1989), pp. 176–83.

[44] On infertility in general Salernitan compendia, see Table 1.1 above. The anonymous text *Inprimis considerandum* has clear similarities with other Salernitan writings on infertility, esp. in its stress on the four elemental imbalances that can cause it. There is much more here about the *signs* of each type of infertility in women, including the nature of their sexual response. Whether it was written in response to Joanna's infertility is unclear as it makes no allusions to specific cases.

while visiting Marseille (apparently to denounce some heretics before a papal commission), he was asked by the families of Elzéar of Sabran (1285–1323) and Delphine de Puimichel (1282–1360) to diagnose the fertility problems of this noble couple who lived in the nearby town of Apt. They had been married since 1300 but, having secretly taken a joint vow of chastity, they were not, unsurprisingly, producing heirs. They let Arnau in on their secret and he complied by pretending to treat them for two weeks, when in fact he used the time to discuss spiritual matters with them. There was a great assembly of physicians in Marseille at this time, and Arnau presented the couple's case before them, claiming that Elzéar had three different impediments to conception while Delphine was afflicted with four. By cleverly diagnosing both of them, he ensured that their marriage could not be annulled and they could continue in their chaste ways.[45] This tale (which in the form we have it was probably not written down until the mid 1390s) might be dismissed as typical hagiographic exaggeration were it not for the fact that there are no fewer than seven fertility texts that begin to circulate from Montpellier in the fourteenth century, five of which would come to bear Arnau's name. Most of the attributions are clearly spurious, but as the story of Delphine and Elzéar shows, they are not entirely fantastic in depicting Montpellier as the most important centre for the diagnosis of infertility.

The work most likely to be an authentic composition of Arnau is little more than a table laying out, in a dialectical form, a whole host of impediments to conception. Despite its brevity, it makes clear why sterility should be a proper object of diagnosis by a learned physician. It opens with a statement very characteristic of Arnau's epistemological view that the actual composition of any given individual's humoural temperament could only be known by experience, not by reason. In this case, Arnau offers nothing by way of therapy, but his successors would soon fill that gap.[46]

The relative chronology of the other Montpellierain fertility texts is not entirely clear, but comparison of four of them can give some sense of the development of the field over the course of the fourteenth century as well as the increasing sense that the conditions of the female body were indeed amenable

---

[45] Jacques Cambell, *Vies occitanes de Saint Auzias et de Sainte Dauphine, avec traduction française, introduction et notes* (Rome: [Pontificium Athenaeum antonianum], 1963), pp. 160–3; my thanks to Rosalynn Voaden for alerting me to this fascinating story and allowing me to consult her copies of the *Vitae*. The Occitan lives were translated from earlier Latin versions, but the story of Arnau appears in Delphine's life, for which, unfortunately, the Latin original has been lost. Neither Arnau nor this episode of the medical diagnosis appears in the canonization proceedings of the two saints. Interestingly, Delphine's confessor at the end of her life, Durand André (fl. 1360–75), was a physician as well as a priest; whether he had anything to do with the elaboration of the story of Arnau is unknown.

[46] See the reproduction of part of the *Compilatio de conceptione* from BNF, MS lat. 6971, s. xv, f. 70r-v in Peter Biller, *The Measure of Multitude: Population in Medieval Thought* (Oxford: Oxford University Press, 2000), plate 5. On the authenticity of the work, see Michael R. McVaugh, *Medicine Before the Plague: Practitioners and Their Patients in the Crown of Aragon, 1285–1345* (Cambridge: Cambridge University Press, 1993), pp. 203–4.

to rational examination.[47] Perhaps the earliest was the *Treatise on the Sterility of Women* which, although attributed to Bernard of Gordon (d. 1308), is probably the work of one of his students. Offering no theory of the causes of sterility nor citing any authorities, the *Treatise* follows closely the schemes employed by the Salernitans; it categorizes female sterility according to the predominant complexional characteristics: too much heat, cold, humidity, or dryness. The most extended regimen found here is said to have been prepared specifically for the countess of nearby Rodez, 'who was as if numbed and sterile due to [both] frigidity and humidity'.[48] For the countess's condition as well as all the others, this author enumerates in close detail various therapies involving baths, unguents, fumigations, controlled diet, etc.

A second treatise, also simply called a *Treatise on Sterility* and variously attributed to Arnau and other Montpellierain physicians, was certainly in circulation by the middle of the century.[49] Adopting an Aristotelian perspective, this author attempts to reframe the problem of infertility as more than a simple disease category; instead, it is a failure of the very function for which the reproductive organs were created: generation. Thus, *all* diseases of the genitalia become the concern of the expert on infertility and, in fact, we find here most of the standard gynaecological and andrological topics that were addressed in the Arabic encyclopedias and their Latin descendants. This approach makes for rather bizarre results as, for example, when uterine suffocation is seen as a cause of sterility, even though the author explicitly acknowledges that what often causes the suffocation is the fact that the woman is a virgin or widow—*and therefore is not having sexual relations at all!* The poorly developed logic of the text seems to have been unapparent to the author, for he closes the text with proud assertions of the efficacy of his remedies: for the past six or seven years, he says, he has proved the value of his treatments, among others on a noble woman in Lomagne who, though she had been sterile for thirteen years, was able to conceive within two months with the aid of his regimen.

---

[47] Besides the texts discussed here, there are two other texts attributed to Arnau—one with the incipit *Complementum coitus est sanitas trium membrorum principalium*, the other called a *Consilium contra sterilitatem*—plus a work attributed to Johannes Pataranus (Jean Pataran, fl. 1375–82), *Regimen de conceptione in complexione flegmatica*, an elaborate regimen of sixteen different elements (diet, drinks, baths, etc.) laid out in detail under separate headings which is extant in two 15th-century copies. All remain unedited.

[48] Pseudo-Bernard, *Tractatus de sterilitate mulierum*, edited by Montero Cartelle in Pedro Conde Parrado, Enrique Montero Cartelle, M.ª Cruz Herrero Ingelmo, eds., *Tractatus de conceptu; Tractatus de sterilitate mulierum*, Lingüística y filología, 37 (Valladolid: Universidad de Valladolid, 1999), p. 150: *Ordinacio facta pro comitissa rut(h)enensi que era[t] quasi stupida et sterilis de causa frig[iditatis] et hum[iditatis]*. As I have argued elsewhere, this passage identifying the Countess of Rodez as the recipient of the regimen may reflect the original form of the text, not a later variant as Montero suggests; see my review of Conde Parrado *et al.* in *Speculum* 77, no. 2 (April 2002), 496–98.

[49] Enrique Montero Cartelle (ed.), *Tractatus de sterilitate: Anónimo de Montpellier (s. XIV). Attribuido a A. de Vilanova, R. de Moleris y J. de Turre*, Lingüística y Filología, no. 16 (Valladolid: Universidad de Valladolid and Caja Salamanca y Soria, 1993).

The third text, the *Treatise on Conception*, has no personal anecdotes or attestations of efficacy, though the author does open his text with the assertion that the remedies here 'were experienced [that is, observed to be efficacious] by me many times'. The text also shows, in its intensely formalized rationalism, how the topic of infertility has now become a suitable area for the dialectical inquiry of scholasticism; the attributions to, once again, Arnau and also to Jean Jacme (d. 1384), a chancellor of the medical school of Montpellier, and (most plausibly) Pierre Nadilz (fl. 1369–74), personal physician to Charles II, king of Navarre, are certainly appropriate.[50] Despite an egalitarian admission that either the male and the female can be the cause of infertility, the author immediately claims that most of the impediments come from the woman and it is only these that he will address. He moves beyond the anonymous author of the *Treatise on Sterility*, however, in looking more closely at anatomical or physiological defects of the uterus and its adnexa. He also goes much further into the bedroom, prescribing not simply a precoital laxative, but also the employment of specific sexual techniques to be used by the male to promote simultaneous climax and hence conception.

All these three texts, together with Arnau's *Compilation on Conception*, readily show how a kind of gynaecology could be developed without any direct examination of the female genitalia, either in the living patient or in postmortem autopsy.[51] The author of the pseudo-Bernard *Treatise on the Sterility of Women* mentions diagnosis by, among other signs, the pulse, urine, the colour of the menses, and 'a notable colour around the genitalia, both in front and behind'. His listing of the latter two factors in the same breadth as the pulse and urine—which were archetypically the diagnostic preserve of the physician—might imply an expectation of direct observation, yet he also includes level of sexual desire and 'quick emission of seed', information which could only have come from the patient's report.[52] Aside from this, none of the authors mentions examination of the genitalia, either internal or external.[53] The author of the *Treatise on*

---

[50] Edited under the title *Tractatus de conceptu* by Conde Parrado, in Conde Parrado, *Tractatus de conceptu*, pp. 47–89. My own opinion is that perhaps the editor has been too hasty in dismissing the authorship of Pierre de Nadilz. His name is found in four of the seven extant manuscripts (including the earliest) in contrast to Arnau and Jean, whose names are attached to the text twice and once, respectively.

[51] All three anonymous authors assume the existence of a female seed, but none of them mentions the female testicles, let alone makes any claims about their shape, size, or function. A description of the female testicles had been available in Latin since the late 11th century, when Constantine the African translated the *Theorica* of 'Alī ibn al-'Abbās's encyclopedic text (see Monica H. Green, 'The *De genecia* Attributed to Constantine the African', *Speculum* 62 (1987), 299–323; repr. in Green, *Women's Healthcare*, Essay III), and all Salernitan anatomical writers mentioned them.

[52] Pseudo-Bernard, *Tractatus de sterilitate mulierum*, p. 130. In his *Lilium medicine*, Bernard of Gordon explains how the physician should ask the woman to bring him her menstrual rag so that he can assess its colour; *Lilium medicine* (Naples: Franciscus de Tuppo, 1480), f. 185ra.

[53] I have found no clear evidence of the use of the vaginal speculum in medieval Europe prior to the 15th century. See Chapter 6 below.

Conception attributed to Pierre de Nadilz can readily recommend recourse to a surgeon if a wound or aposteme or other lesion is impeding conception, but he feels no need to explain in detail what such lesions might be or how they occur. When direct applications on the female genitalia are required, 'the midwife' (*obstetrix*) suddenly appears to serve as the necessary eyes and hands.[54] Yet all three authors are equally confident that they have developed a real science of infertility, and that the proof of their correct understanding lies in their effective treatments.

Where did they get such confidence? It was not, I believe, simply from musing on the opinions of their written authorities, nor from speculative abstraction of the 'principles of science' that characterized their medical learning. A treatise called *Interrogations on the Treatment of Sterility*, apparently of later fourteenth-century origin, itemizes forty-one points on which the physician needs to acquire information in order to determine the cause of sterility and pinpoint some method of intervention.[55] It is clear from the phrasing of the forty-one points that this is *an interrogation of the woman*: is she too fat? is she old or young? has she been for a long time with her husband? has she ever been pregnant before? has she ever miscarried? Importantly, the physician asks for the woman's own perceptions of her body: does she feel herself to be hot or cold? does she menstruate at the proper time? does she feel that her uterus has descended below its neck? does she feel in intercourse that the male's semen is hot or cold? Only a few of the questions solicit information about the male partner, and all of these (e.g. 'Is his penis too long or too short?') could be answered by the woman herself. This text, therefore, is neither a theoretical disquisition about what *might* be the cause of infertility nor a series of abstract therapies. It is literally a guide for conducting a patient interview.

It would be interesting to think that the case of Delphine and Elzéar really was the principal stimulus for the development of Montpellierain speculations on infertility, making it all the more unfortunate that we do not have a better chronology for the composition of these texts. But whether there was some particular provoking historical event or not, the Montpellier masters chose an unwittingly fortuitous moment to develop this expertise. European population levels had been growing at unprecedented rates in the previous three centuries, a demographic phenomenon that has been attributed to multiple factors. While academic interest in population was spurred by the adoption of Aristotelian

---

[54] On the surgeon, see *Treatise on Conception*, p. 84. There are two references to the midwife in the *Treatise on Sterility* attributed to Raymund, and six in the *Treatise on Conception* attributed to Pierre de Nadilz.

[55] The text is edited in Enrique Montero Cartelle and María Cruz Herrero Ingelmo, 'Las *Interrogaciones in cura sterilitatis* en el marco de la literatura médica medieval', *Faventia* 25, no. 2 (2003), 85–97. This same text also appears as part of one of William of Brescia's *consilia* in a 15th-century Munich manuscript; see Erich W. G. Schmidt, *Die Bedeutung Wilhems von Brescia als Verfasser von Konsilien. Untersuchung über einen medizinischen Schriftsteller des XIII.–XIV. Jarhhunderts*, inaugural-dissertation (Leipzig: Emil Lehmann, 1922), pp. 22–5.

science in the mid thirteenth century (and so was primarily a strictly intellectual debate),[56] fertility became a major social concern after the depopulation caused by the famines of the second decade of the fourteenth century and, all the more so, after the continuing devastations of the Black Death from the middle of the century on.[57] Increased attention to infertility—one might even say disproportionate attention to it—would characterize gynaecological writings through the end of the Middle Ages. The Englishman John of Gaddesden's medical *summa*, the *English Rose* (*Rosa anglica*), for example, which may have been written right around the time of the great famines of 1315–17, treated infertility as the chief disease of women, under which all others were subsumed.[58] By the fifteenth century, whole codices were being filled with texts on fertility, while newly composed works, usually addressed to powerful patrons, portrayed knowledge of fertility as one of the highest achievements of medical science.[59] Master Odo's claim that an anonymous priest, with his simple fertility remedy, could outperform even the physicians of Montpellier was thus no small boast.

'DISEASES. . .WHICH PROPERLY PERTAIN TO SURGEONS': SURGERY OF THE GENITALIA

While male physicians looked after women's menstrual regularity, examined their urine, assessed their pulse, and intervened medicinally in their fertility problems, surgeons were primarily concerned to treat conditions of the surface of the body and the repair of wounds, dislocations, fractures, and fistulae. They did not engage in 'exploratory' procedures of the thoracic or abdominal cavities, and most of what we now think of as the mainstay of gynaecological or obstetrical surgery (ovariectomies, myomectomies, and abdominal hysterectomies) would have been impossible, indeed inconceivable, for them. That said, there was still considerable *potential* room for the development of gynaecological and obstetrical surgical interventions. That these did not develop, or did so only slowly, confirms what we have already suspected from the Salernitan evidence: while the male medical gaze or even the male medical touch was not universally forbidden, neither was it completely free.

The female breast was, surprisingly given its later history as a focus of erotic concern, unproblematically included in the definition of what constituted the male surgeon's territory. This is apparent already in the earliest Latin surgical writings of the twelfth century when, after nearly a thousand-year hiatus, surgical

---

[56] Biller, *Measure of Multitude*. See also Chapter 5 below for this larger interest in generation.

[57] William Chester Jordan, *The Great Famine: Northern Europe in the Early Fourteenth Century* (Princeton, NJ: Princeton University Press, 1996).

[58] John of Gaddesden, *Rosa anglica practica medicine a capite ad pedes noviter impressa et perquam diligentissime emendata* (Venice: Bonetus Locatellus for Octavianus Scotus, 1502).

[59] See Chapter 6 below.

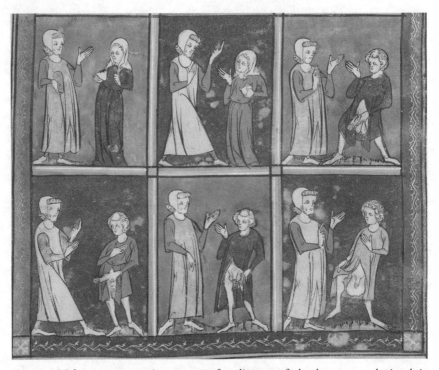

FIG. 2.3 Male surgeon treating women for diseases of the breasts, as depicted in a thirteenth-century French translation of Roger Frugardi's *Surgery*; note also the unproblematic representation of the male genitalia in the other four scenes.

writing was revived in western Europe. Although we find no discussion of breast diseases in the writings of male Salernitan masters until we reach John of Saint Paul near the end of the century, a surgeon perhaps of Salernitan origin, Roger Frugardi, composed a comprehensive Latin surgery around the year 1170 that included three chapters on diseases of the breasts. These addressed abscesses, cancer, and inverted nipples (which particularly afflicted primaparae, preventing them from nursing). Roger's work is important because it seems to come out of his own surgical practice, owing almost nothing to any text that had gone before it. An illustrated French translation from the middle of the thirteenth century demonstrates clearly how Roger's precepts were to be put into practice: amid ninety-six quite lavish illustrations of various therapies described in the *Surgery*, two women show lesions of their breasts to a male surgeon (Fig. 2.3).[60]

---

[60] The best study of the illustrations in BLL, MS Sloane 1977 is Helen Valls, 'Studies on Roger Frugardi's *Chirurgia*', PhD dissertation, University of Toronto, 1995.

Conditions of the female breast would remain a standard feature of surgical writing for the rest of the Middle Ages (see Table 2.1). The exception is Bruno of Longobucco (d. 1286), who came from Calabria in southern Italy but emigrated to Bologna where he apprenticed under the famed practitioner and teacher, Ugo Borgognoni of Lucca (fl. 1205–40). In 1253, Bruno wrote his *Surgery*, in which he included nothing at all on women's breasts; on the contrary, all he had was an updating of Albucasis's chapter (similar to Constantine's) on fatty male breasts, when they grew large 'like women's . . . which nature abhors'.[61] Bruno's peculiarity in omitting the female breasts can be seen by contrasting him with Theodoric of Lucca (*c.*1210–98), who was Ugo Borgognoni's own son. Theodoric drafted his *Surgery* in several stages between 1243 and 1266, initially adhering closely to the teachings of his father, but gradually adding other material including much of Bruno's text. Theodoric added some discussion of cancer of the female breast in his general chapter on cancer, plus a brief note about apostemes in the female breast which were caused by, among other things, coagulation of the milk. William of Saliceto (1210–76/80), who also studied with Ugo in Bologna, went into even further therapeutic detail, for example by specifying the exact size and firmness of certain tumours and the specific veins to be incised in treatment.[62]

By the time we reach Lanfranc of Milan (d. before 1306)—who, as a student of William, completed the Bolognese dynasty of surgical writers—knowledge of the character and proper treatment of the various diseases of the breast could be something about which a practitioner boasted in order to differentiate himself from the ignorant rabble. Lanfranc, in discussing the special treatment needed for bloody apostemes of the breasts (caused when the menstrual blood that should be converted into milk fails to do so), describes a remedy with which he himself has cured such apostemes in a single day. But then he warns against the dangers of a different kind of medicine:

I saw a noble woman who had an aposteme of blood and I instructed her to apply the remedy described above. A certain lay [unlettered] surgeon rejected this and he applied upon [the aposteme] a maturative which, however much he applied, so much the more did the [bloody] matter multiply. Nor did this surgeon wish to listen to my counsel. And the friends of the sick woman preferred to listen to the counsel of that lay surgeon than to mine. Seeing this, I withdrew, and I predicted that the woman would become manic.

61 Susan P. Hall, *The 'Cyrurgia magna' of Brunus Longoburgensis: A Critical Edition*, DPhil thesis (Oxford University, 1957), p. 280; the identification of Albucasis as Bruno's source here is hers. My thanks to Michael McVaugh for checking his notes on Hall's dissertation. For biographical information and other details on the surgeons discussed in the following pages, see Michael R. McVaugh, 'Surgical Education in the Middle Ages', *Dynamis: Acta Hispanica ad Medicinae Scientiarumque Historiam Illustrandam* 20 (2000), 283–304.

62 William of Saliceto, *Chirurgia* (Piacenza: Joannes Petrus de Ferriatis, 1476).

Table 2.1. Gynaecological and Obstetrical Contents of Medieval Surgical Texts[a]

Condition	Con[b]	Alb	Rog	Rol	Bru	The	Sal[c]	Lan	Mon[d]	Cha
Breasts										
[fatty breasts in men]	X	X	—	—	X	X	—	X	X	X
cancer of the breast	—	—	X	X	—	—[e]	X	—	X	—[f]
breast abscesses	—	—	X	—	—	—	—	—	—	—
apostemes of breasts	—	—	—	—	—	X[g]	X	X	X	X
induration of the breasts	—	—	—	—	—	—	—	—	X	—
ulcers of the breasts	—	—	—	—	—	—	—	—	X	—
fistula of the breasts	—	—	—	—	—	—	—	—	X	—
hardness due to retained milk/coagulation of the milk	—	—	—	—	—	X	X	X	X[h]	X[i]
insufficiency of milk[j]	—	—	—	—	—	—	—	—	X	—
inverted nipples	—	—	X	X	—	—	—	X	X	—
hairy growths from the nipples	—	—	—	—	—	—	—	—	X	—
excessive growth of breasts in young women	—	—	—	—	—	—	—	X	X	X
Genitalia[k]										
cold and humidity of the womb	—	X[l]	—	—	—	—	—	—	—	—
hermaphrodites	X	X	—	—	X	—	—	X	—	X
polyps and warts	X	—	—	—	—	—	[X]	—	—	—
fleshy growths[m]	—	X	—	—	—	—	[X]	X	X[n]	X
closed 'mouth' of the uterus/vagina[o]	X	X	—	—	—	—	—	X	X	X
aposteme of the vagina	X	X	—	—	—	—	—	—	X[p]	—[q]
excessive openness of the vagina	—	—	—	—	—	—	—	—	X	X[r]
titillation of the vagina	—	—	—	—	—	—	—	—	X	—
priapism	—	—	—	—	—	—	—	—	X	—
prolapse and extrusion of the uterus through the vagina	—	—	—	—	—	—	—	—	X	X
elevation of the uterus until it compresses the organs of respiration	—	—	—	—	—	—	—	—	X	—

Table 2.1. Continued

Obstetrics										
extraction of the foetus and afterbirth[s]	X	X	—	—	—	—	—	—	—	X
complete rupture of the perineum in women	—	—	—	—	—	—	—	—	X	—
partial rupture of the perineum	—	—	—	—	—	—	—	—	X	—

[a] Con = Constantinus Africanus (d. before 1098/99); Alb = Albucasis (10th century, translated into Latin before 1187); Rog = Roger Frugardi (*c*.1170); Rol = Roland of Parma (*c*.1230); Bru = Bruno da Longobucco (writing in 1253); The = Theodoric of Lucca (writing between 1243 and 1266); Sal = William of Saliceto (writing between 1268 and 1275); Lan = Lanfranc of Milan (writing in 1296); Mon = Henri de Mondeville (writing *c*.1310); Cha = Guy de Chauliac (writing in 1363).

[b] Constantine completed only capp. 1–43 of his translation of the surgical book of al-Majūsī's *Kāmil as-Sīnā'a*; this included the chapter on male breasts but not those on the genitalia. The rest of the translation was completed in 1113–14 by John the Saracen and Rusticus of Pisa, but this fuller version had a very limited circulation.

[c] William puts most of his material on the female genitalia in his general *practica*, the *Summa conservationis*; wherever the latter material involves surgical treatments, I have included it below in brackets.

[d] For all of Mondeville's chapters except that on apostemes of the breasts, we have nothing but the chapter headings of a part of his *Surgery* that he planned to write but never completed (Tract. III, doctr. iii, which would have treated conditions in a head-to-toe order). I include him in this table, however, precisely because his outline shows that he *envisaged* the diseases of women in a far more comprehensive and detailed way than any of his predecessors.

[e] Theodoric has no separate chapter on cancer of the breast, but embeds his discussion of it in his general chapter on cancers.

[f] Chauliac does not devote a separate chapter to breast cancer, though he mentions it as one of the more common forms of the disease in his chapter on cancrous apostemes; Guy de Chauliac, *Inventarium sive Chirurgia magna*, ed. Michael R. McVaugh, with Margaret S. Ogden, 2 vols. (Leiden: Brill, 1997), vol. 1, pp. 97–8; cf. p. 122.

[g] Theodoric treats apostemes of the breasts and the penis in the same chapter without, however, explaining why they should be related.

[h] In his table of contents to Tract. III, doctr. iii, Mondeville lists three separate chapters on *coagulatio, caseatio*, and *congelatio* of the milk in the breasts, yet in his discussion of apostemes in Tract. III, doctr. ii, cap. xviii, he had said that they were all the same thing (p. 498: *Notandum, quod caseatio, congestio, coagulatio, conglobatio lactis sunt idem*). In his list of chapter headings to the unfinished Tract III, doctr. iii, he also listed a chapter on pain due to abundance of milk.

[i] Chauliac discusses *coagulacio* of the milk in his section on apostemes (*Inventarium*, 122.16–22). Later (366.33–40), he mentions that, normally, excess or paucity of milk is treated by physicians, but 'for the sake of instruction' he adds a recipe to draw out and dry up the milk.

[j] Insufficient milk was normally seen as a medical problem, i.e., one to be addressed by the physician rather than the surgeon.

[k] I list only those conditions that are specifically said to occur in the female genitalia.

[l] This chapter is included in Albucasis's general section on cauterization, where he recommends cauterization of the abdomen for uterine cold or humidity when its disrupting fertility or normal flow of the menses.

[m] In the case of Albucasis, and following him, Mondeville and Chauliac, they seem to be talking specifically of an enlarged clitoris; the Latin term used is *tentigo*, and in the anatomical sections of both Mondeville and Chauliac it is clearly understood as a normal part of the female anatomy (Chauliac explicitly likens it to the male prepuce). In other cases, the piece of flesh is said to hang from the uterus or the vagina, and there is very little evidence that, aside from texts derived from Albucasis, the clitoris was normally recognized in medieval anatomy. It is mentioned neither in the Latin *Trotula* nor any of its vernacular translations with the possible exception of one French version; see Chapter 4 below.

Table 2.1. Continued

  ⁿ Mondeville speaks of *caro quae videtur virga juxta vulvam* ('flesh which looks like a penis close to the vagina').

  ᵒ The term 'hymen' is never used by any of these authors nor is it clear that all of them were referring to the vaginal tissue that is often found in women. I am therefore reluctant to reduce all these conditions to the modern category of 'imperforate hymen'. These medieval authors speak of *clausum os* (Constantine), *caro superaddita in orificio* (Mondeville), *clausio* which can appear as either *caro addita* or a *pellis* (Chauliac). Lanfranc speaks of *both* orifices potentially being closed: both that at the entrance to the vagina and that at the mouth of the uterus. Both conditions require surgical intervention, though the latter can sometimes prove incurable.

  ᵖ Mondeville identifies not simply *apostema vel exitura* as a kind of vaginal lesion, but also *pustulae, nodus,* and *haemorrhois.* I have included them all under the heading 'apostemes' since, lacking Mondeville's own descriptions and any other corroborating testimony, we cannot know how Mondeville differentiated them. What is important to stress, rather, is that he recognized a variety of conditions of the female genitalia that required surgical intervention.

  ᑫ Chauliac includes *et vulve* in his chapter heading to apostemes of the penis (*Inventarium*, p. 130), but while he says the cure of both these conditions is similar to that for apostemes of the testicles, he in fact says nothing specific about how the female genitalia are to be treated.

  ʳ Chauliac identifies his single recipe as one to constrict the *uterus* (*Constringitur matrix*, in *Inventarium*, p. 388) though his source, Avicenna, had identified it as a vaginal constrictive.

  ˢ In Albucasis and Chauliac, these two topics are treated in separate chapters.

And on the third day after my withdrawal she did become manic and, with the frenzy firmly established, she died.[63]

  The normativeness of such practice can also be seen in William of Brescia's (fl. 1274–1326) two separate *consilia* (personalized diagnoses and prescriptions, often conducted via correspondence) on the treatment of breast diseases in the female relatives of his elite male clients. In one case, he diagnosed (apparently for a fellow physician) a case of breast cancer, characterized by the heat, pain, throbbing pulse of the veins, and blackened or yellowish colour of the breast. In another, both the sister and the niece of one correspondent were suffering from hardness that remained in their breasts after treatment for an aposteme.[64] William went on to serve as personal physician to a series of four different popes in the late thirteenth and early fourteenth century, which shows that expertise in breast diseases, if hardly the centre of one's practice, in no way impeded a male physician's successful career. The only negative sentiment connected to treatment

  [63] Lanfranc of Milan, *Cyrurgia*, in *Cyrurgia Guidonis de Cauliaco. et Cyrurgia Bruni, Teodorici, Rolandi, Lanfranci, Rogerii, Bertapalie* (Venice, 1519), f. 294va. A maturative is a kind of medicine that causes a lesion to 'mature' and erupt through the skin. Lanfranc includes many anecdotes like this in his text.

  [64] Schmidt, *Bedeutung Wilhems von Brescia*, at pp. 12–13. Originating in the later 13th century in Italy, *consilia* summarized the symptoms, prognosis and a prescribed therapy for individual patients, thus providing us with the closest medieval approximation of the modern medical case history. Many of these were written for or about women of the middle and upper classes that formed the bulk of these physicians' clientele. The genre of the *consilia* cannot be considered straightforward 'case histories' in the modern sense, however, since these were often written for patients the physician had never seen. See Jole Agrimi and Chiara Crisciani, *Les 'consilia' medicaux*, translated by Caroline Viola, *Typologie des sources du moyen âge occidental*, fasc. 69 (Brepols: Turnhout, 1994); and Siraisi, *Taddeo Alderotti*, pp. 273 ff.

of breast conditions that I have found is the worry that the surgeon might incur infamy from *too interventionist* a therapy: cancer in particular was thought to yield rarely to the needed treatment (complete excision) and Guy de Chauliac, writing in 1363, explicitly recommended that the surgeon avoid the threat to his reputation that involvement with such hopeless cases would bring.[65] Although the breasts rarely became the subject of specialized examination by medical writers (the only specialized treatise is a fifteenth-century Italian text, which is probably largely derived from a Latin source),[66] the later thirteenth- and early fourteenth-century northern Italian surgeons seem not to have followed in the textual footsteps of their Arabic sources but charted new territory—a development that would have been impossible had they not actually been regularly treating breast conditions (and so female patients) in their clinical practices.

The genitalia, on the other hand, the conditions of the labia, clitoris, vagina, and uterus, were more problematic for the surgeon's inspection and touch. Although, as we have seen, the Salernitan physician John of Saint Paul had alluded to surgical incisions to open up an obstructed vagina,[67] his contemporary Roger Frugardi never mentioned the female genitalia at all, and neither of Roger's commentators—Roland of Parma (writing *c.*1230), or the so-called 'Four Masters Gloss' (written soon after Roland)—expanded into this area. Although Bruno of Longobucco and Theodoric began to exploit some elements of Abulcasis's surgery in the mid thirteenth century, neither paid any attention whatsoever to his chapters on an enlarged clitoris or vaginal obstruction and apostemes.[68] Bruno did, it is true, include 'Alī ibn al-'Abbās's discussion of hermaphroditism, noting that both the male hermaphrodite and the female one (their 'primary sex' being determined by where they urinated) needed to be treated by cutting off whatever parts were 'in excess'. The fact that such individuals were already of ambiguous sex apparently made surgical intervention on a 'female' acceptable.[69] Elsewhere, however, Bruno signalled the problematic

[65] Guy de Chauliac, *Inventarium sive Chirurgia magna*, ed. Michael R. McVaugh, with Margaret S. Ogden, Studies in Ancient Medicine, vol. 14, I and II (Leiden: New York, 1997), vol. I, p. 122, lines 12–15. Neither Roger Frugardi, Theodoric, or Lanfranc had been optimistic that any cure was possible, especially if the cancer had advanced beyond the early stage.

[66] Aside from independently circulated excerpts from such writers as Avicenna, the only known treatise on the breasts was composed in Italian in the 15th century and entitled *The Very Beautiful Treatise on Diseases of the Breasts* (*Tractatus pulcherrimus de passionibus mamillarum*). Although probably drawn from the work of a physician (it describes no surgical interventions), it is found in both of its two extant copies amid surgical treatises. See Monica H. Green, 'Medieval Gynecological Texts: A Handlist', in Green, *Women's Healthcare*, Appendix, pp. 1–36, at p. 34.

[67] See Chapter 1 above.

[68] Even more detailed summaries of gynaecological surgery could be found in the third book of Avicenna's great encyclopedia of medicine, the *Canon*. Again, both Bruno and Theodoric made use of Avicenna, yet both ignored his gynaecological material.

[69] Cf. a case from Perelada, in north-eastern Catalonia, from 1331 where a woman who 'could not fulfil her conjugal debt nor conceive nor bear a child' was examined, in the presence of a lady of the town, by a male surgeon. She was found to have a male penis and testicles. McVaugh, *Before the Plague*, p. 206.

nature of dealing with the normal female genitalia: when he came to discuss the problem of bladder stones in the female patient, he retained Albucasis's instructions that one should employ a female assistant to perform the necessary examination and incision if treatment involved touching the vagina.[70]

By the time we come to William of Saliceto and his student Lanfranc of Milan (writing in 1268–75 and 1296, respectively), the Arabic authorities began to have a more pronounced effect. What distinguishes William and Lanfranc (who later practised in Paris) was that they both attempted to bring surgery more tightly into conformity with the precepts of internal medicine. William did so by authoring complementary texts on both internal medicine (a general *practica*) and surgery, making it all the more intriguing why he put some material into one text rather than the other. In the *Surgery*, which he wrote first, besides the material on the breasts mentioned above, he presents nothing specific to the female genitalia: a chapter headed 'On [anal] polyps, condylomas, and haemorrhoids in the anus and vagina' in fact says nothing whatsoever about the latter organ.[71] William seems to have no more experience with surgical treatment of the female genitalia than his predecessors. Yet in his general *practica*, we find the now normal array of gynaecological headings (including a chapter on infertility almost four times longer than any other section) as well as a category hitherto unseen in Latin surgeries: 'On sores [*ragadie*] in the uterus and the opening of the penis and the thing which is called *furfur*, that is, excess flesh growing in the mouth of the uterus which sometimes is prolonged and sometimes shortened, and it is not prolonged except in the summer and it shortens in the winter.'[72] William

---

[70] Bruno's adaptation of Albucasis's text is in fact very interesting, since Albucasis had stipulated that a eunuch or female practitioner should perform the procedure whether or not the woman was a virgin or married. Bruno, in contrast, permits the *medicus* or a *medica* (the eunuch having disappeared) to perform the incision if the woman is still a virgin, since in this case the procedure involves inserting a finger only into the anus. For sexually experienced women, a female practitioner (*medica*) 'or, if you cannot find any woman sufficiently learned in the affairs of women, any midwife (in her place)' should palpate the stone by inserting a finger into the vagina. For Bruno, see Bruno, *Cyrurgia*, ed. Hall, p. 309; for Albucasis, see *Albucasis on Surgery and Instruments. A Definitive Edition of the Arabic Text with English Translation and Commentary*, ed. and trans. M. S. Spink and G. L. Lewis (London: The Wellcome Institute of the History of Medicine, 1973), pp. 420–2.

[71] William of Saliceto, *Chirurgia*, cap. xlv, *de ficis condilomatibus et emoroydis in ano et uulua* (leaves are unnumbered). No critical edition of William's *Surgery* has been made, so I cannot say whether the words '*et uulua*' are original or not, nor how the first version written in Bologna in 1268 differs from the second written in Verona in 1275. For the latest information on the circulation of Saliceto's work, see Jole Agrimi and Chiara Crisciani, 'The Science and Practice of Medicine in the Thirteenth Century According to Guglielmo da Saliceto, Italian Surgeon', in *Practical Medicine from Salerno to the Black Death*, ed. Luis García-Ballester, Roger French, Jon Arrizabalaga, and Andrew Cunningham (Cambridge: Cambridge University Press, 1994), pp. 60–87.

[72] William of Saliceto, *Summa conseruationis* (Piacenza: Johannes Petrus de Ferriatis, 1476), Bk I, cap. clxviii. *De ragadiis in matrice et apperitione uirge et rei que nominatur furfur. i. caro addita orta in ore matricis que quandoque prolongatur quandoque abreuiatur. et non prolongatur nisi in estate et abbreuiatur in hyeme* (leaves are unnumbered). Also unusual is William's inclusion of chapters on vaginal constrictives and abortifacients. William displays an uncommon (and uncommonly

was clearly using Avicenna as a source here, yet in several respects William has moved far beyond his Arabic authority. Not simply has he combined what had been three separate topics in Avicenna (*ragadie* or vaginal tears, *furfus* or a penis-like growth of excess flesh, and *bothor* or genital warts or pustules), but whereas Avicenna had simply said that a mirror, placed against the outside of the vagina, could be used to check for internal tears, William adds that a *cuffa* (a type of cupping glass) can be used to better view into the vagina.[73] Likewise, when he comes to treating these vaginal sores, he says explicitly that 'the vagina should often be inverted with a large *cuffa* so that it is made manifest to the physician [*medico*] by sight how much and in what way he needs to operate on the afflicted place'.[74] Treatment involves, among other things, use of a heated iron to cauterize the lesions.

Now, it has been recognized by several scholars how unusual William is in his emphasis on testing 'the ancients' against his own experience.[75] He is in no way challenging Avicenna's observations here, but his very specific instructions about using a *cuffa* do indeed suggest that he has gone well beyond a mere re-mouthing of his authoritative text to a clinical practice directly on the genitalia of female patients. Clearly, William has not single-handedly overturned traditional views on the impropriety of male touch of the genitalia. In his chapters on uterine suffocation (where he mentions masturbation of the afflicted woman), on testing for virginity, and on several aspects of childbirth, the midwife is still the necessary intermediary who touches the female patient's body. But William now suggests that an important boundary has been crossed: it is acceptable for the male practitioner—even one as well situated as William was in northern Italian society—to inspect and treat the female genitalia as long as he touches her not with his own hands but with instruments.

In Lanfranc's case, his medical training induced him to think more speculatively than anyone before him about female physiology as it related to surgical conditions. Thus, for example, after going into a surprising amount of detail near the beginning of his *Surgery* on the generation of the embryo, taking pains to differentiate (following Aristotle) between male semen and the female

---

pragmatic) interest in sexuality throughout the text; see Helen Lemay, 'William of Saliceto on Human Sexuality', *Viator* 12 (1981), 167–81.

[73] William of Saliceto, *Summa conseruationis*, Bk I, cap. clxviii, *De ragadiis in matrice*: 'et si ponatur sub mulierem speculum coram uulua eius et aperiatur uulua eius uel inuersetur cum cuffa absque scarificatione confetur super illud quod in speculo representabitur et apparebit in eo, significabit super ragadiae formam et figuram et earum malitiam'.

[74] *Ibid.*: 'sepe inuersetur uulua cum cuffa magna ut manifestetur medico per uisum quantum contra infirmititatem operatur et qualiter'.

[75] Agrimi and Crisciani, 'Science and Practice'; Nancy G. Siraisi, 'How to Write a Latin Book on Surgery: Organizing Principles and Authorial Devices in Guglielmo da Saliceto and Dino del Garbo', in *Practical Medicine from Salerno to the Black Death*, ed. Luis García-Ballester, Roger French, Jon Arrizabalaga, and Andrew Cunningham (Cambridge: Cambridge University Press, 1994), pp. 88–109.

contribution of menstrual blood, he then clarifies why this is relevant to surgery: if a limb is amputated, bone (which comes from male seed) never grows back, but flesh (which comes from blood and regenerates daily) does. Similarly, he explains in more detail than any prior surgeon how there are certain arteries and veins that carry the menstrual blood up to the breasts, where it is converted into milk.[76] When this process fails, either because of the excessive quantity or the poor quality of the blood, breast abscesses are generated.

Even more strikingly, Lanfranc's thorough reading of his Arabic authorities (and, no doubt, the example of his teacher, William of Saliceto) emboldened him to reincorporate aspects of Albucasis's and Avicenna's gynaecological surgery. Although he doesn't provide separate headings, he does include the anatomy of the uterus (it is like a penis inverted) and he addresses wounds of the uterus (those caused by a spear or sword are always fatal, while those caused by 'something hard' entering the vagina are usually amenable to cure if they are still recent). In his therapeutic section, Lanfranc includes a chapter on removing any skin-like growths that obstruct the vagina or cervix; 'correcting' the superfluous growths of hermaphrodites; and excising excessive growths 'that hang from the vagina' with which some women are accustomed to play the part of men with other women. Surprisingly, virtually none of this new material is coming verbatim from Albucasis or Avicenna; even though they had both addressed these topics, Lanfranc seems to be describing procedures and tools that he has employed himself. In other words, although neither William nor Lanfranc has uttered a word about how their surgical practices seem to have taken a radical new step beyond the territory carved out by their predecessors Roger, Roland, Bruno and Theodoric, they have in fact added certain aspects of gynaecological surgery permanently to the learned male surgeon's repertoire.

Henri de Mondeville, who placed great emphasis on the surgeon's need to know anatomy, included a detailed description of the uterus and adnexa in his *Surgery*, on which he was working in Paris *c*.1310 but left incomplete. In the planned Third Doctrine of his Third Treatise, Mondeville had dedicated chapter 21 to the diseases of the uterus and the adnexa. His list of diseases of the female genitalia is truly breathtaking, for far beyond his Latin predecessors—beyond even his Arabic authorities Albucasis and Avicenna—Mondeville itemized twenty-three different diseases of the female genitalia that were within the surgeon's purview.[77] None

---

[76] The existence of these veins had already been postulated by Galen, and had been described by one of the 12th-century Salernitan anatomical authors; see Rebecca Flemming, *Medicine and the Making of Roman Women: Gender, Nature, and Authority from Celsus to Galen* (Oxford: Oxford University Press, 2001); and George Washington Corner, *Anatomical Texts of the Earlier Middle Ages* (Washington, DC: Carnegie Institution of Washington, 1927), p. 84.

[77] Henri de Mondeville, *Chirurgia*, in *Die Chirurgie des Heinrich von Mondeville (Hermondaville): nach Berliner, Erfurter und Pariser codices*, ed. Julius Leopold Pagel (Berlin: August Hirschwald, 1892), p. 340.

of these, to be sure, are obstetrical conditions: Mondeville continues to see the surgeon's work as lying in the excision or repair of excessively growing or damaged flesh, though he also envisions surgical intervention in such gynaecological conditions as 'wind' in the uterus, prolapse,[78] and uterine suffocation. Mondeville may perhaps have imagined that the surgeon would be involved in birth after the fact: in his chapter 29 on the perineum, Mondeville included, as two of five conditions afflicting that anatomical structure, both complete and partial rupture in women. Rupture of the perineum could conceivably be due to rape or sexual violence (a story in the thirteenth-century Spanish *Cantigas de Santa Maria*, for example, tells a horrific tale of a man who cut open his wife when she took a vow of virginity and refused to have sex with him). Its most common cause, however, is childbirth and it thus seems likely that Mondeville is the first surgical writer to identify this quite common obstetrical affliction since Trota had described it in the twelfth century.[79]

Unfortunately, we don't know how Mondeville proposed to *treat* any of these conditions, nor how he suggested male surgeons should negotiate with midwives or other female assistants in examining or manipulating the female patient's genitalia. Mondeville never completed this part of his *Surgery* and we have no other evidence to reconstruct his clinical practices. It would seem, however, that he was not alone in seeing the surgeon's province expanding. Writing in 1363, the other great French surgical synthesizer Guy de Chauliac claimed that 'the diseases of the parts of the pelvic region which properly pertain to surgeons' include 'diseases of the uterus, such as obstruction of the vagina [*clausio*] and its enlargement, enlarged clitoris [*tentigo*], extraction of the foetus and the afterbirth and the [uterine] mole; . . . and prolapse of the uterus'.[80] Obstruction of the vagina and an enlarged clitoris (or some kind of fleshy growth) had, of course, been made standard items in the surgeon's repertoire more than half a century earlier. And Mondeville had at least planned to include uterine prolapse, a topic that had been addressed by physicians ever since Salerno. Yet Guy is the

---

[78] It is actually surprising that uterine prolapse remained a 'medical' condition, to be treated primarily by potions, plasters, etc., instead of a surgical condition. The use of trusses and other mechanical supports as described by Trota are most akin to the remedies that surgeons used for hernia and anal prolapse. For more on the differences in treatment of hernia and uterine prolapse, see the Conclusion below.

[79] Although modern incidence rates from the West are misleading given the frequency now of Caesarean births and pre-emptive episiotomies, in countries where hospital births and surgical interventions are less readily available, obstructed labour, the principal cause of perineal tears (up to and including full vesico-vaginal or ano-vaginal fistulae), occurs at rates ranging from 0.96 to 18.3% per 100 live births; see the World Health Organization report by Carmen Dolea and Carla AbouZahr, 'Global Burden of Obstructed Labour in the Year 2000', <http://www.who.int/healthinfo/statistics/bod_obstructedlabour.pdf>, accessed 4 October 2006. Since these conditions are more common among women bearing their first child in the teenage years (a trait shared with many medieval European women, particularly in southern Europe), the latter statistics might well be comparable to incidences in medieval Europe.

[80] Guy de Chauliac, *Inventarium*, p. 368.

first surgical author to include any element of obstetrics, despite the powerful influence for over one hundred years of the *Surgery* of Albucasis, who had dedicated his longest sections on women to precisely that topic.

'HOW THE MIDWIFE OUGHT TO BE INSTRUCTED': THE BEGINNINGS OF OBSTETRICAL SURGERY

In all, Albucasis had devoted a total of ten chapters of his *Surgery* to women's conditions, three of which addressed obstetrical procedures. Avicenna, too, had included three detailed chapters on obstetrical interventions that employed surgical techniques. The long time lag between the availability of these two works in Latin translation (both had been translated by Gerard of Cremona before 1187) and the first mention of obstetrics by a surgical writer in 1363 shows how powerful the sexual division of labour was in regard to hands-on treatment of the female genitalia. Yet both these great Arabic authorities had in fact laid out a model for how the male surgeon could play a role in childbirth. For Albucasis, the midwife (*obstetrix*) was unquestionably subordinate to the surgeon: 'How the midwife ought to be instructed' is the rubric he uses to introduce the first of his obstetrical chapters and Guy himself seems to have taken to heart this presumption that the male surgeon should rightly serve in a supervisory capacity. Interestingly, although Guy (like Albucasis) makes clear that it is the midwife who is administering fomentations and unctions and other aids to ease the birth, when he comes to the use of instruments to extract the dead foetus, his verbal forms shift to the passive. He also uses a passive form in describing the excision of the living foetus from its dead mother. Guy cites no personal experiences of attendance at birth so we cannot be entirely sure how extensive his own involvement with childbirth or midwives may have been. But there is other evidence that the taboo that had kept male surgeons marginal to the birthing process was slowly breaking down.

Right around the same time that Lanfranc, prior to his exile to France, would have been formulating his new vision of surgical science writing in northern Italy, we find several copies of Albucasis's *Surgery* that incorporate the series of sixteen foetus-in-utero figures that had originally accompanied Muscio's late antique *Gynaecology*.[81] Muscio's work had fallen into desuetude by the early thirteenth century and may have been considered no more than a curiosity even by those few, like Richard de Fournival, who continued to have the whole text

---

[81] Abulcasis's text in its Latin form enjoyed a healthy circulation particularly in southern Europe (it is currently known to exist in thirty-three copies) and was translated into Old French, Hebrew, and Occitan; it was also translated directly from Arabic into Catalan in 1313. Five Latin manuscripts incorporate the Muscio figures, the four earliest all coming from Italy in the 13th or early 14th century. See Chapter 3 below for further discussion of the use of the Muscio figures as instructional aids.

copied. The star of Albucasis's surgery, in contrast, was rising. The latter text had, ever since its original composition in Arabic, been accompanied by illustrations of surgical instruments, an illustrative tradition that carried through into most of the thirty-three surviving copies of the Latin text. Yet aside from a couple of early manuscripts that add scenes of cautery or a procedure to reduce spinal dislocation, there was no anatomical or clinical iconographic tradition such as the one found in the French translation of Roger Frugardi cited above. It must have seemed very fortuitous indeed, therefore, when manuscript illuminators in Italy in the late 1200s realized that the Muscian figures conformed quite well to the instructions in Albucasis's text for addressing the different kinds of foetal malpresentation. With their often vibrant colours, the foetal images would have signalled to the owners of these manuscripts that knowledge of obstetrical interventions was as much a part of the learned surgeon's repertoire as reducing dislocations or treating head wounds. One manuscript, now in Budapest, not only incorporates the Muscian figures, but also, on the page presenting Albucasis's description of extraction of the dead foetus, depicts a heart-rending scene of (to judge from her attire) a queen lying near death and a male physician giving instructions from his book.[82]

Interests in obstetrical surgery were also rising in another respect, one in which Christian Europe went beyond even what the Arabs had described. This had its origin, not among surgeons (or any other kind of medical practitioner), but among theologians and priests. Beginning apparently in the early eleventh century, clerics began to discuss the merits of excising the living foetus out of its mother's womb when she had died before or in childbirth. By the twelfth century, injunctions were being pronounced that the foetus must be removed in such cases, in order that it might be baptized and its eternal life saved. Since there was no expectation that the foetus would survive much beyond baptism, these 'Caesarean births' could hardly be deemed 'medical' procedures.[83] Nothing in

[82] Budapest, Eötvös Loránd Tudomány Egyetem Könyvtára (University Library), MS lat. 15, *c.*1300 (Italy), f. 26r (*olim* 24r); other figures in the image include a female attendant standing near the woman's head and, at her feet, a male figure (surgeon?) who seems to be seeking advice from the seated physician. The foetus-in-utero figures appear at the end of the text on f. 46v. For reproductions, see Eva Irblich (ed.), *Abū'l Qāsim Halaf Ibn 'Abbas al-Zahrāuī, Chirurgia. Faksimile und Kommentar* (Graz: Akademische Druck- und Verlagsanstalt, 1979), plates 9 and 11. My deepest thanks go to Jocelyn Wogan-Browne who examined the manuscript itself for me when I was unable to obtain suitable reproductions from the library.

[83] What we now call Caesarean section should really, for the medieval period, be referred to by the more technically accurate legal term, *sectio in mortua*, 'cutting open of the dead woman'. Beside the concern with baptism that I discuss here, there was also debate about whether a dead woman could be interred in consecrated ground if she had an unbaptized foetus within her. Again, however, this was a theological, not a medical question. A thorough assessment of these varying motives has yet to be done; see the literature reviewed in Monica H. Green, 'Bodies, Gender, Health, Disease: Recent Work on Medieval Women's Medicine', *Studies in Medieval and Renaissance History* 3rd ser., 2 (2005), 1–49. On the 13th-century development of the idea of limbo, which gave some sort of 'salvation' even to unbaptized infants, see Donald Mowbray, 'A Community of Sufferers and the Authority of Masters: The Development of the Idea of Limbo by Masters of Theology at the University of Paris (*c.*1230–1300)', in *Authority and Community in the Middle Ages*, ed.

the early ecclesiastical records suggests that surgeons (or even midwives, for that matter) were specifically charged with performing the procedure. Nevertheless, the procedure began to attract the attention of physicians and surgeons by the late thirteenth century. A manuscript of Avicenna's *Canon* made in Paris in the last quarter of the century includes, at the head of the chapter on the anatomy of the uterus, an image of a male physician directing two midwives in the performance of a Caesarean section (Fig. 2.4).[84] The illuminator has gone beyond the obstetrical practices of Avicenna's text which, although greatly detailed, had only described means to remove the dead child from its still living mother; the life of the child was, by itself, of no concern to Avicenna and hence we find, in terms of surgical recommendations, only vaginal procedures of extraction being offered.[85] The illuminator of this Latin manuscript, in contrast, depicts a scenario that reflected the new Christian concerns with extraction of the living foetus

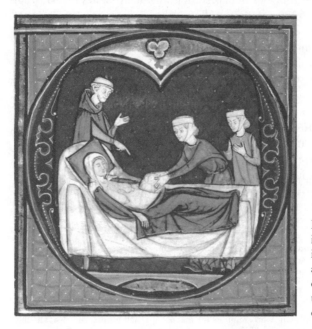

Fig. 2.4 Male physician instructing two midwives in the performance of a Caesarean section on a dead mother, from a later thirteenth-century copy of Avicenna's *Canon*.

Ian P. Wei, Donald Mowbray, and Rhiannon Purdie (Stroud: Sutton, 1999), pp. 43–68. On the role of midwives in Caesarean births, see Chapter 3 below. On the complicated genesis of the name 'Caesarean birth', see Renate Blumenfeld-Kosinski, *Not of Woman Born: Representations of Caesarean Birth in Medieval and Renaissance Culture* (Ithaca, NY: Cornell University Press, 1990), pp. 143–53.

    [84] Besançon, Bibliothèque Municipale, MS 457, s. xiii[3/4] (Paris), f. 260v.

    [85] Avicenna, *Liber canonis* (Venice, 1507; repr. Hildesheim: Georg Olms, 1964), f. 367rb: 'occupatus sis in vita matris et non occuparis in vita fetus'. In addition to various potions, pessaries, and uterine injections, Avicenna also recommends use of a special instrument to open the cervix; he then details procedures for embryotomy.

through incision of the dead mother's abdomen. The image in this quite deluxe manuscript of Avicenna's masterpiece, moreover, depicts the social scenario we would expect its literate male readers to have considered normative: the male physician is not himself touching the dead mother but rather is instructing the two midwives. The point is clear: it is *his* responsibility to supervise, theirs to do the manual labour.[86] Bernard de Gordon, writing in 1305, referred in passing to a procedure (*artificium*) of opening the mouth of the dead mother (so that the foetus could continue to breathe) and having her belly opened to extract the foetus. He gives no details on where the incision was to be made or any other specific surgical information. Yet other sources confirm that male practitioners were increasingly involved in such procedures. A preacher in Florence, also in 1305, notes with pride how he called in four doctors and midwives to extract a foetus when its mother died.[87] A legal case from Marseille in 1331 describes how, when a woman named Boneta died in childbirth, the attending midwives sent for a male barber 'who was experienced in this [procedure]' so that he might extract the living child from its mother's womb. The earliest known image of a male surgeon performing a Caesarean section with his own hand appears in a mid fourteenth-century Venetian copy of a French life of Caesar.[88]

When in 1296 Lanfranc laid out his detailed description of the field of surgery and the duties of the surgeon, he identified, after invasive procedures like phlebotomy and cutting for bladder stones, and reconstructive procedures like repairing wounds or broken bones, a third task of removing superfluous growths: polyps from the nose, for example, or warts or a sixth finger. Included in his list was the removal of any flesh that closed off the vagina.[89] The frequency with which a surgeon in the late thirteenth or fourteenth century might have actually been called upon to open a closed vagina may have been not much greater than

---

[86] In her study of images of Caesarean birth found in manuscripts of the lives of the Caesars (i.e. a non-medical context), Blumenfeld-Kosinski, *Not of Woman Born*, argued that in 13th- and 14th-century copies only female attendants are present, while in 15th-century manuscripts male practitioners are not only present but are now wielding the knife. Midwives disappear or are relegated to the background. The data I present here pushes that transition back by at least a century.

[87] Bernard de Gordon, *Lilium medicine* (Naples: Franciscus de Tuppo, 1480), f. 192 va. On the testimony of Giordano of Rivalto, a Dominican friar of Santa Maria Novella in Florence, see Katharine Park, *Secrets of Women: Gender, Generation, and the Origins of Human Dissection* (New York: Zone Books, 2006), pp. 64–5.

[88] The Marseille case can be found in Archives Départmentales des Bouches-du-Rhône, 3B 27, case no. 6; my thanks to Dan Smail for bringing this important case to my attention. The image of the male surgeon performing a Caesarean section, unfortunately rather damaged (Venice, Biblioteca Nazionale Marciana, MS Fr. Z. 3 (224), s. xiv med) is reproduced in Blumenfeld-Kosinski, *Not of Woman Born*, p. 75.

[89] Lanfranc, *Cyrurgia*, f. 168va: 'Per tertiam intentionem superfluum remouendo scrophulas capitis et colli: et aliarum partium extirpando catharactas: vngulas: pannum: sebel: carnem superfluam: polipum ex naso: porros et verrucas: ficus atrices: et condilomata superfluitatem hermafroditis: folliculum clause vulue: sextum digitum et multas alias superfluitates remouendo humano corpori non decentes'.

the number of times he was asked to cut off a sixth finger. But when a situation arose needing the intervention of a surgeon, they seem to have risen to the task. An account from the early fourteenth century tells the following story:

In a town near Bern . . . a woman lived for ten years with a man. Since she could not have sex with a man, she was separated [from her partner] by the spiritual court. In Bologna (on her way to Rome), her vagina was cut open by a surgeon, and a penis and testicles came out. She returned home, married a wife, did hard [physical labour], and had proper and adequate sexual congress with her wife.[90]

Perhaps it is too convenient for the narration that the surgery happens to be performed in Bologna, the veritable capital of surgery at the time. But we know of a similar case from Catalonia from just about the same period; in that case, no 'cure' was effected but it is notable that is was a *surgeon* who was called in to examine this woman who 'has a male penis and testicles like a man' and various other abnormalities of her genitalia.[91] The statistical probability that surgeons may have been presented with cases of hermaphroditism was probably just as high then as it is now: an estimated 1.728 cases for every 100 live births.[92] The teachings of Lanfranc and others on repairs of genital lesions or growths may thus have been as relevant as most other rare but potentially debilitating conditions.

But such gynaecological and obstetrical conditions as vaginal lacerations (whether from birth or forced intercourse), fistulae, and prolapsed uteruses were probably not rare at all. A story from fourteenth-century northern Italy reminds us how severe women's suffering must have been. Among the miracle stories collected during the canonization proceedings of the Tuscan saint, Chiara of Montefalco, in 1318–19 is the story of Flore Nicole. She suffered from 'a horrible infirmity in her womb, namely, that her womb had exited outside her body'. In her testimony, she recounted how 'because of the extreme pain, she wished to have her womb cut [out] with a knife'. She suffered thus for three years. Her mother, seeing how severely she was afflicted, suggested that Flore pray to Saint Chiara 'that she liberate you from this infirmity or kill you'. Saint Chiara did of course (as is the nature of miracle stories) cure her, but Flore's testimony provides us with one other crucial detail: asked if she had 'made medicines' for her condition, she responded 'many, and they seemed to harm her and do no good. And beyond that she consulted many physicians'.[93] It is notable,

---

[90] *Annals of the Friars Minor of Colmar* (1308–14), as cited in Miri Rubin, 'The Person in the Form: Medieval Challenges to Bodily "Order"', in *Framing Medieval Bodies*, ed. Sarah Kay and Miri Rubin (Manchester: Manchester University Press, 1994), pp. 100–22.

[91] McVaugh, *Before the Plague*, p. 206.

[92] For modern biomedical understandings of hermaphroditism, see Anne Fausto-Sterling, *Sexing the Body: Gender Politics and the Construction of Sexuality* (New York: Basic Books, 2000); she notes that her estimates (p. 53) will vary depending on the local gene pool.

[93] Ernesto Menestò (ed.), *Il Processo di canonizzazione di Chiara da Montefalco* (Regione dell 'Umbria: La Nuova Italia, 1984), pp. 395–6. Flore's mother's corroborating testimony appears on pp. 431–2.

therefore, that even though Flore herself envisaged her real need to have surgical intervention—cutting with a knife—she only consulted physicians (*medicos*) who, as we have seen, had long since been willing to offer various non-surgical treatments for her kind of condition. In fact, it may be that gynaecological surgery developed because patients or their kin insisted that surgeons bring the same skills to women's afflictions that they brought to men's.[94]

Surgeons' hesitating entry into gynaecological and obstetrical conditions can be contrasted with the extraordinary developments they made in male urological surgery in this same period. The illustrator of the thirteenth-century French translation of Roger Frugardi's *Surgery*, discussed above in relation to its depictions of the female breast, had no compunctions about graphically depicting the male genitalia when the text moved to detailed examination of wounds, cancers, and swellings of the penis and testicles (Fig. 2.3 above). Operations for inguinal hernia in particular (a condition nearly unique to men because of the anatomical structure of the male genitalia in relation to the abdominal wall) were discussed in excruciating detail, becoming a point of controversy between practitioners who offered different methods. Surgical techniques varied from simple trussing to cauterization to excision of one of the testicles.[95] In other words, there was no reticence about dealing with the sexual organs as such. It was only the female sexual organs that proved an inhibiting factor and, as we have seen, even here male surgeons seem to have only gradually become emboldened by the confident pronouncements of their Arabic authorities.

When the plague struck in the first great pandemic of 1347–9, learned medicine had established itself as a major intellectual and social presence throughout much of western Europe. Whereas intellectuals as late as the eleventh century were still debating whether medicine was anything more than a mechanical art, by the mid fourteenth century it was taught formally at at least one-third of Europe's universities, often as one of the higher faculties alongside theology and law. This prestige extended to practitioners even on the margins of university culture. Surgical writers, only some of whom had university affiliations, attempted to claim that they, too, had authoritative textual traditions; they had produced works of considerable sophistication that circulated widely both in their Latin originals and in numerous vernacular translations. In Spain, France, Italy, Germany, and England, to varying degrees learned practitioners were licensed, granted municipal appointments, and served as expert witnesses in court. This enormous prestige survived the crisis of the Black Death more or less unscathed, largely because the expectations made of such practitioners were not that they could *cure* every condition

[94] See the story of Dulceta of Marseille below.

[95] Michael R. McVaugh, 'Treatment of Hernia in the Later Middle Ages: Surgical Correction and Social Construction', in Roger French, *et al.*, *Medicine from the Black Death to the French Disease* (Aldershot: Ashgate, 1998), pp. 131–55.

presented to them, but rather that they could explain the condition and make acceptable predictions about the possibility of cure. There is no reason to believe that these expectations were any different in the area of women's medicine.[96]

How, then, might we imagine scenarios of such cross-sex practice of gynae-cology? One of the manuscripts mentioned before as an example of the new later thirteenth-century focus on generation merits discussion again. This codex, Ashmole 399, includes an inserted bifolium of images that predates the rest of the manuscript by about a quarter of a century.[97] Whether it was originally part of another codex or circulated alone is unclear. What is clear is that it presents, in a striking series of images, a learned perspective on women's health and women's relations to their male healers. The first four images (on the recto and verso sides of folio 33) depict the disease of uterine suffocation: its major symptom (a falling as in epilepsy, but without that disease's characteristic foaming at the mouth), its likely victims (widows and virgins), its seemingly lethal effects (an afflicted woman, thought to be dead, is laid out on her bier ready for burial, with her servants wailing around her), and its therapy (fumi-gations to the genitalia and foul odours to the nose).[98] The next two images (on the recto of folio 34; fig. 2.5) show a different practitioner, or at least the same one coming on a different day: his clothing is of a different colour than that of the male physician in the first sequence. Here, no scrolls are added that might have incorporated some explanatory text. The upper image shows a woman in her sick bed, with three distressed attendants by her side. The physician, who has just examined her urine, drops the urine glass, apparently a gesture foreboding her imminent death. The lower image on that page depicts, it has been suggested, either an anatomy scene of the deceased woman or an embalming.

The final two images (on the verso of folio 34; Figs 2.5 and 2.6) shift subject matter again: I believe they are meant to depict the scenario of practice that the author of the Salernitan *Women's Cosmetics* envisioned. In the upper image, five women stand in line waiting their turn to be seen by the physician seated in front of them. The first woman gestures toward her hair; the second toward her face; the third, holding a vial, gestures back toward the fourth who seems to be troubled by bad breath, a wisp of foul vapours coming out of her mouth. The fifth, with money bag in hand, suffers from blackened teeth. Every

---

[96] On the question of medical efficacy, see the Conclusion below.

[97] On the dating of the inserted bifolium (s. xiii³/⁴), see O. Pächt and J. J. G. Alexander, *Illuminated Manuscripts in the Bodleian Library*, Oxford, vol. III British School (Oxford: Clarendon, 1973), p. 41. Pächt and Alexander date the rest of the manuscript as *c*.1292, but Malcolm Parkes points out that there is a mark following the date 1299 in the calendar, which was a way for scribes to indicate the Easter following. This would give a date of 1298 for these portions of the manuscript. (My thanks to Dr Parkes for sharing with me a draft of his paper, 'The Mappa Mundi at Hereford: Report on the Handwriting and Copying of the Text', and for generously taking the time to examine the manuscript with me in 2003.)

[98] These four images of the uterine suffocation case are reproduced in Green, *Trotula*, pp. 28–29.

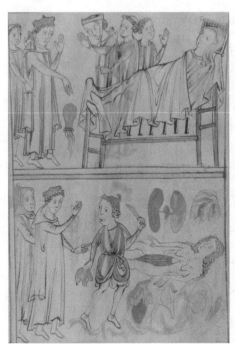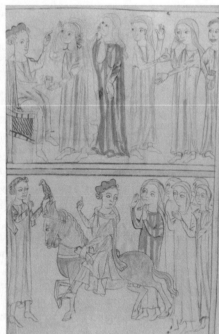

FIGS. 2.5 AND 2.6 Illustrations of women's medical encounters, from England, third quarter of the thirteenth century.

single one of these conditions had been addressed in the Salernitan *Women's Cosmetics*. In the lower image, the physician is taking his leave (apparently to go hawking), with the women mourning his departure. As the author of *Women's Cosmetics* had promised, he has earned 'glory [and] a delightful multitude of friends'. This single bifolium comes closer than anything else known in medieval Europe to a narrative of women's encounters with the medical profession. It may, indeed, have been created precisely as a kind of advertisement for the services that a physician trained in the Salernitan tradition had on offer. The male physicians never touch the woman; even in death, it is only a surgeon or barber (depicted as a buffoonish rustic) who touches the body. Rather, with his finger lifted in the classic gesture of instruction, the male physician doles out his learning, expecting that either some female attendant or the woman herself will carry out the necessary applications or procedures.

The ubiquity of male practice of gynaecology can be gauged by the surprisingly rare instances where female patients or gynaecological conditions are deliberately excluded from discussion. After the composition of Gariopontus's *Passionarius* in the eleventh century, hardly a single general medical encyclopedia did not address conditions of the female reproductive organs in at least perfunctory fashion. Those that did not can often be traced to religious communities that housed no women.[99] These cases stand out precisely because they are so rare. John de Greenborough (or Grandborough, d. after 1383), for example, spent, according to his own testimony, more than thirty years attending to the sick at the male Benedictine house of St Mary's in Coventry. In and around a copy of Gilbert the Englishman's *Compendium of Medicine*, he made copious notes of his own cures and those he had read in the books of 'English, Irish, Jewish, Saracen, Lombard, and Salernitan physicians'.[100] One of the few areas where he omitted commentary was the gynaecological section where, unsurprisingly given his exclusive clientele, he has nothing whatsoever to say. In contrast, another English cleric, John Mirfield (d. 1407), was preparing an even more sizable compendium of medical knowledge for the hospital of Saint Bartholomew in London. Mirfield, never pretending to any originality as a medical writer, drew upon the readily available works of Gilbert and such surgical authorities as Roger Frugardi and Lanfranc. There was no skimping whatsoever on the gynaecological material: all of Roger Frugardi's and Lanfranc's material on conditions of the breasts was synthesized here; all of Gilbert's and Lanfranc's chapters on gynaecological conditions were incorporated. Mirfield even included topics like procedures to 'restore' virginity and contraceptives which, one would think, would be quite problematic for a cleric to approve—as in fact they were, for the latter topic appears in cipher in at least one of the extant manuscripts.[101] Obstetrical chapters included aid in difficult birth and means to expel the dead foetus, both of which may have been important at Saint Bartholomew's since, included among the poor and sick whom it took into its walls, there were pregnant singlewomen who had 'done amiss' (and who may have been particularly desirous to 'restore' their virginity).[102]

---

[99] In addition to the case of John de Greenborough, noted below, a monastic context similarly seems to explain why one copy of the Middle English translation of Gilbert made in the latter half of the 15th century was systematically purged of all references to women and children; see Faye Marie Getz, *Healing and Society in Medieval England: A Middle English Translation of the Pharmaceutical Writings of Gilbertus Anglicus* (Madison, Wisconsin: University of Wisconsin Press, 1991), pp. li–lii. None of the other dozen copies of this same translation are similarly expurgated; on the contrary, the gynaecological section went on to have a significant independent career (see Chapter 4 below). A French translation of Roger Frugardi's *Surgery* made in the 15th century seems likewise to have deliberately omitted the three chapters on diseases of women's breasts; cf. Valls, 'Studies on Roger', p. 207.

[100] BLL, MS Royal 12.G.IV, s. xiii ex. (England), with later notes by Greenborough, f. 187v: 'a practicis phisicorum Anglie Hibernie Iudeorum Saracenorum Lumbardorum et expendebat multa in medicos circa compilationem illarum medicinarum'.

[101] I have consulted the copy of Mirfield's *Breviarium Bartholomei* in BLL, MS Harley 3, s. xiv ex. (England). Interestingly, Mirfield is deriving his constrictive remedies from an undetermined source; only two of them derive from the Salernitan *Treatments for Women* and even then not directly.

[102] J. Gairdner (ed.), *The Historical Collections of a Citizen of London in the Fifteenth Century*, Camden Society, n.s. 17 (London, 1876; repr. New York: Johnson Reprint Corp., 1965), pp. viii–ix.

Most of these transformations in male gynaecological practice had begun well before the major demographic catastrophes of the fourteenth century: the famines that devastated northern Europe between 1314 and 1317, and the Black Death itself. But the latter catastrophe in particular may have been doubly influential in solidifying the changes and (as we will see in Chapter 6) perhaps even hastening the rate of change. Boccaccio clearly saw the plague as altering how physical exposure of the female body to male gaze was to be negotiated, and it may not be irrelevant that the bubonic plague (which Guy de Chauliac had himself survived) often manifests itself by large necrotic swellings of the lymph nodes, including those in the groin.[103] Secondly, because of the hitherto unthinkable mortality of the pandemic, the 'science of generation' took on an urgent social import far beyond the intellectual curiosity it had previously elicited.[104] The formulation of new logical understandings of infertility by the Montpellierain physicians and the growing confidence of Bolognese surgeons and their heirs in their skill in treating structural defects of the female genitalia that impeded conception—as well as what seems to be surgeons' increasing concern to become knowledgeable about emergency obstetrical interventions—all prepared them, long before the awful onslaught of the plague, to claim competence in certain areas of women's medicine.

'AN UNSPOKEN RULE OF LAW': MALE PRACTITIONERS AND FEMALE PATIENTS

According to a collection of miracle stories gathered for the canonization of Saint Louis of Toulouse, around the year 1297 a poor young woman in Marseille named Dulceta suffered from a prolonged labour with a foetus dead *in utero*. A midwife extracted what she could, but some material remained lodged in Dulceta's vagina and she remained an invalid for two years thereafter, having to pull her bedclothes over her with her teeth because she had no use of either

Importantly, the descriptions of both St Bartholomew's and Thomas Spital, which performed the same function, stress the importance of protecting these women's privacy and reputations.

[103] Guy's account of his own experience (*Inventarium*, 117.35–119.35) is one of our most important medical descriptions of the pandemic from the period. He differentiated between the disease that swept Europe in 1348 (of which he had already distinguished a rapid, pulmonary form from a slightly slower one that produced swellings in the armpits and groin) and a slightly differently manifesting condition in 1360. In case of the latter, he noted that instead of afflicting the populace in general, it targeted 'many rich and noble people and innumerable children, and few women'. Had there been any obvious difference in the manifestation of the earlier pandemic by sex, we can assume that he or some other commentator would have mentioned it. Modern controversy over how the great pandemic of the Black Death should be classified in biomedical terms continues. I find persuasive the evidence of modern DNA techniques to confirm the presence of the plague bacillus, *Yersinia pestis*, in 14th-century remains. See most recently Michel Drancourt, *et al.*, 'Yersinia pestis Orientalis in Remains of Ancient Plague Patients', *Emerging Infectious Diseases*, Feb. 2007, <http://www.cdc.gov/EID/content/13/12/332.htm> accessed 10 February 2007.

[104] I discuss concerns with generation more fully in Chapter 5 below.

her hands or her feet, suffering from worms growing in sores on her thighs and buttocks, and 'stinking so badly that scarcely anyone could stand to be near her'.[105] Although Dulceta would eventually be cured (of course) by the sainted Louis, prior to the saint's intervention her husband sought out a male surgeon to extract the retained material. The surgeon agreed to do it, but only on condition that the husband or others of his kinsfolk be present. The account does not suggest that Dulceta herself feared compromising her virtue by having a male surgeon see and touch her genitalia; rather, she feared the inevitable pain of the surgical intervention. It was then, after more than two years of suffering, that she prayed to Saint Louis for aid.

As we saw in Chapter 1, ever since the Hippocratics it had been suggested that *women's* shame in baring their ills had been the biggest impediment to their receiving proper medical care. Yet as Dulceta's story reminds us, it is not sufficient only to ask if women were willing to accept the ministrations of male practitioners. Clearly, women's acquiescence, even if given with some reluctance, was necessary for there to be any male practice of gynaecology. But something else was necessary, too: the acquiescence of men. Dulceta's story shows that decisions of medical care may have been made by male kin as much as by women themselves; in this case in particular, not simply was Dulceta herself bedridden, but her husband was a full twenty-five years older than her and may have been accustomed to making all the major decisions in the family. Moreover, in depicting the male surgeon's reluctance to operate without a chaperone, Dulceta's story shows that notions of shame or compromised honour in cross-sex medical practice may have been generated as much by men as by women themselves.

Neither the developments in medicine nor those in surgery we surveyed above had by themselves eliminated the social problems surrounding the male-practitioner/female-patient encounter. The rhetoric of women's shame continues, as does a sexual division of medical labour. The segregation seems to have been strongest in the Kingdom of Naples. Southern Italy had a tradition of medical licensing going back to 1140, when King Roger of Sicily first decreed that those wishing to practise in his kingdom must present themselves to 'our officials and judges' for examination.[106] During the reigns of the Angevin monarchs Charles II (r. 1285–1309), Robert I (1309–43, including the regency of his son Charles of Calabria, 1318–24), and Joanna I (1343–81), 3670 licences to practise medicine or surgery were copied into notarial registers of the Kingdom

---

[105] *Processus Canonizationis et legendae variae Sancti Ludovici O.F.M., Episcopi Tolosani, Analecta Franciscana*, vol. 7 (Quaracchi/Florence: Fratri Collegii S. Bonaventurae, 1951). The canonization proceedings consist of testimony from Dulceta herself (who speaks of the paralysis and the worms), her husband, the midwife who attended the birth, and perhaps a friend or neighbour who attests to the stench of her lesions (pp. 165–9). None of these personal testimonies tells of the surgeon, who is instead described in a book of St Louis's miracle stories (p. 301).

[106] See Chapter 1, n. 24 above.

of Naples.[107] Licences to practise surgery were given to twenty-three women, a tiny proportion of the total, yet these few documents offer powerful evidence of the social forces that kept women in medical practice. At least thirteen of the women are licensed specifically to treat female patients, usually for conditions of the genitalia. (The breasts, which as we have already seen, were regularly treated by male surgeons, are mentioned only once.)[108] Beginning in 1321, we see the first explicit rhetorical justification for specialized female practice of women's medicine. Francisca, wife of Matteo de Romano of Salerno and an acknowledged illiterate, was given a licence at Naples on the grounds that 'although it should be alien to female propriety to be interested in the affairs of men lest they rush into things abusive of matronly shame and incur the first sin of forbidden transgression, nevertheless . . . the office of medicine is expediently conceded to women by an unspoken rule of law, mindful that by honesty of morals women are more suited to treat sick women than men'.[109] The licence of Maria Incarnata, who was approved for practice by Queen Joanna in 1343, similarly states that 'females, by their honesty of character, are more suitable than men to treat sick women, especially in their own diseases'.[110] As late as 1404, women in southern Italy are still being licensed 'because females are more suitable to treat women than men'.[111]

As powerful as this logic of women's modesty is in leading to the conclusion that *of course* women should take care of other women's conditions—hearkening back to the story of Agnodice—in fact female modesty was not the overwhelming motive force behind the social structuring of women's medical care throughout the rest of Europe. No strict sexual segregation on the southern Italian model, with its separate (and apparently tiny) cadre of female practitioners, was observed anywhere else in Europe. Even Jacoba Felicie in Paris may have argued for the need for female practitioners because she came from a small town in Provence which, at the time, was under the same rulership as the Kingdom of Naples. In any case, it is clear from the testimony given

[107] Raffaele Calvanico, *Fonti per la storia della medicina e della chirurgia per il regno di Napoli nel periodo angioino (a. 1273–1410)* (Naples: L'Arte Tipografica, 1962). Although not published until after the War, Calvanico made his transcriptions prior to 1943 when the bulk of the Neapolitan archives were destroyed. The total of 3670 licenses includes some duplicates. Women's licenses account for thirty-four of this total, i.e. less than 1.0%; eliminating duplicates we have evidence for twenty-three female practitioners. Calvanico in some cases only reproduces a summary of the license, so it is not always clear what the precise terms of the women's mandates were.

[108] The one case where treatments of women's breasts are specifically mentioned is the licence of Margherita of Naples, from 1313–14; Calvanico, *Fonti*, item 3534, p. 256.

[109] Calvanico, *Fonti*, item 1451 (with duplicate licenses in items 1872 and 1874).

[110] Calvanico, *Fonti*, item 3571.

[111] Francesco Pierro, 'Nuovi contributi alla conoscenza delle medichesse nel regno di Napoli negli ultimi tre secoli del medioevo', *Archivio Storico Pugliese* 17, fasc. 1–4 (1964), 231–41, citing the license of Donna Cusina di Filippo de Pastino, who was granted permission to treat 'wounds, ulcers, apostemes, pains, fatigues, diseases and illnesses and other diverse sicknesses and sufferings' of women.

at her trial in 1322 that she was treating both women and men, and as was noted in the Introduction above, the university masters who were accusing her of illicit practice gave no credence whatsoever to her argument for same-sex practice.

Nevertheless, it may well be that the university masters of Paris preferred to avoid the discussion altogether, not because they thought Jacoba's argument 'frivolous' and 'worthless' (which is what they claimed), but precisely because they knew that the encounter between male practitioner and female patient *was* problematic. Not simply could a private encounter impugn the woman's honour, it could also threaten the reputation of the male practitioner himself. One continuing strand of polemic against cross-sex medical practice was directed against male clergy. In 1114, King Henry I of England wished to appoint Faritius, the abbot of Abingdon, as archbishop of Canterbury. The bishops of Salisbury and Lincoln thereupon objected that it was unseemly to have as archbishop anyone who inspected women's urine (*non debere archepiscopum urinas mulierum inspicere*). Faritius is, in fact, known to have attended upon Henry's queen, Matilda, when she gave birth in 1101, and his fellow bishops apparently felt that this pollution alone was sufficient to disqualify him from the archbishopric.[112] Hildebert of Lavardin (d. 1133/4), bishop of Le Mans, suggested that physicians were regularly exposed to three great temptations: women, ambition, and greed.[113] Similarly, a twelfth- or thirteenth-century condemnation of the hypocrisy of monks lays out the particular dangers of monks practising medicine:

Moreover, not only do they routinely inspect the urine of men but also—for shame!—the urine of women, too; and making up a story from the pulse of the vein whether death will come soon or health, they deceive the sick person. What, I ask you, is this religion, or rather insane obstinacy, that causes a young woman to consult a young monk, her alone with him, about the secret diseases of her genitals . . . ?[114]

To be sure, there is obviously an element of this diatribe that touches on concerns about the pastoral care of women. The intimacy necessary to provide spiritual guidance to a woman was also recognized as fraught with dangers of temptation or, at the very least, as giving rise to unseemly gossip.[115] Indeed,

---

[112] Edward J. Kealey, *Medieval Medicus: A Social History of Anglo-Norman Medicine* (Baltimore and London: Johns Hopkins University Press, 1981), pp. 18–19 and 69.

[113] Louis Dubreuil-Chambardel, *Les médecins dans l'ouest de la France aux XIe et XIIe siécles* (Paris: Secrétaire général de la Société française d'histoire de la médecine, 1914), pp. 184–5.

[114] *Tractatus Beati Gregorii Pape contra religionis simulatores*, in Marvin L. Colker (ed.), *Analecta Dublinensia: Three Medieval Latin Texts in the Library of Trinity College Dublin* (Cambridge, MA: Medieval Academy of America, 1975), p. 38.

[115] Constant J. Mews, 'Introduction', in *Listen, Daughter: The 'Speculum virginum' and the Formation of Religious Women in the Middle Ages*, ed. Constant J. Mews (New York: Palgrave, 2001), pp. 1–14, alludes to recognition of this problem of 'excessive familiarity between the sexes'

it was in large part concern about the potentially compromising treatment of female patients that motivated various injunctions by Dominican authorities to control the medical practices of the preaching friars.[116] The starkest evidence that contact with female patients was thought to be actively corrupting is from male Cathar medical practitioners in southern France; they may, indeed, in some cases have turned female patients away for precisely the reason that they feared women's corrupting influence.[117]

For most male practitioners, however, the threat of involvement with women was to their professional reputation rather than their souls. Various medical writers followed the lead of the Hippocratics and the Salernitan Archimattheus in warning male physicians, cleric or lay, to shun any sexual involvement with females in the patient's household lest they compromise their professional judgement. The Italian surgeon Lanfranc asserts that the good practitioner 'should not presume to regard the woman of the house of the sick man with an impertinent look, nor should he talk with her in counsel unless it is necessary for treatment'.[118] The mid fourteenth-century English surgeon John Arderne more conservatively advises the surgeon not to 'look too openly on the lady or the daughters or other fair women in great men's houses, or kiss them, or touch their breasts, or their hands, or their private parts, lest he anger the lord of the house'.[119] As with statements about women's shame, of course, there was clearly a certain amount of rhetorical formulicity here. Yet the social context of medical practice was, to some extent, largely unchanged since Hippocratic times: the medical practitioner (particularly the physician) had no office or clinic but rather came into the patient's household when his services were needed. Arderne's advice to surgeons identifies the potentially injured party not as the women whose sexual propriety might be compromised, but as the male head of the household whose honour was at stake. The dynamics, therefore, are as much between men (the physician and his real client, the male head of house) as between male practitioners and female patients. Which brings us back to the real import of Dulceta's case: the husband needed to be willing to allow

---

in the context of 12th-century pedagogical manuals for women (p. 6), though to my knowledge the issue of the parallels between the roles of priests and physicians has never been explored. The 'closet' confessional now so archetypical of Catholic churches did not come into regular use until the Council of Trent (1545–63).

[116] Angela Montford, 'Dangers and Disorders: The Decline of the Dominican *Frater Medicus*', *Social History of Medicine* 16, no. 2 (2003), 169–91.

[117] Peter Biller, 'Medicine and Heresy', in *Religion and Medicine in the Middle Ages*, ed. Peter Biller and Joseph Ziegler, York Studies in Medieval Theology, 3 (York: York Medieval Press, 2001), pp. 155–74, at pp 171–2.

[118] Lanfranc, *Cyrurgia*, Tract. I, doctr. 1, cap. ii, f. 167va: 'Mulierem de domo egri visu temerario respicere non presumat: nec cum ea loquatur ad consilium nisi pro vtilitate cure'.

[119] John Arderne, *Treatises of Fistula in ano*, in *Treatises of Fistula in Ano, Haemorrhoids and Clysters by John Arderne*, ed. D'Arcy Power, Early English Text Society o.s. 139 (London: Oxford University Press, 1910; rpt. 1968), p. 5. To my knowledge, Arderne is the only surgical writer to specify avoidance of the female breast.

a male surgeon to operate on his wife and the surgeon needed to set the conditions under which he would do so without being accused of impropriety. Dulceta, at least as the story is recounted to us, feared additional pain, not shame—something she had already suffered dreadfully for years in her invalid condition.

Despite the Salernitan *Conditions of Women*'s expression of concern that women did not wish to show the diseases 'of their more secret place' to male physicians, and despite a variety of other evidence, ranging from oblique remarks to full out polemics, that similarly reflected the general sense that male inspection of the female genitalia—or even discussion of them—breached the norms of propriety and threatened both men and women with ignominy, women's medicine did, in fact, become a regular part of the average male practitioner's practice well before the collapse of the social moral order noted by Boccaccio. Only in southern Italy do we find evidence that concerns for women's modesty trumped the claims of men's learning: it is only there that we find women, despite their illiteracy, being licensed to practise surgery with the explicit argument that they are more suitable to treat women than are men.[120] Elsewhere, women did practice medicine (as we will see in more detail in the following chapter), but not with the same mandate to care for female patients exclusively. With rare exceptions, male practitioners never, not even in southern Italy, disqualified themselves as caretakers of female patients, since they could always use females as *assistants* when ocular inspection or manual intervention was needed. Rather than taking the assertion of women's shame in the *Conditions of Women* preface as an injunction against their practice, male healers seem to have taken it as an argument for their need to come to the patient interview armed with a text that already explained women's diseases for them, saving them and their patients an embarrassing interrogation. The treatment of women's unique disorders had become more a matter of delicate negotiation than complete taboo. The Latin *Trotula*, as well as the gynaecological and obstetrical material to be found in other texts, thus served as a validation for men's claims to expertise in women's medicine.

Part of that delicate negotiation of male gynaecological and obstetrical practice, ironically, necessitated leaving open a space for women's continued involvement as caretakers of other women. With no successful resolution of the problem of sexual shame or the social impropriety of male contact with women's bodies, visual or tactile, the world of medical guilds, licensing, and university training constructed by men still required women's participation if male

---

[120] Even this social validation of women's suitability to care for other women did not preclude a male practitioner like Francesco da Piedemonte (d. 1320), court physician to Robert the Wise of the Kingdom of Naples, from composing highly detailed work on women's diseases and obstetrics in the context of his general *practica*. Francesco had served in 1308–9 as an examiner of the Neapolitan female surgeon Lauretta, whom he deemed to be suited for practice even though she was *ydiota*, 'illiterate'.

practitioners were to treat the wives and daughters of their male clientele. Male practitioners needed female assistants who would implement the therapeutic procedures they prescribed and, obviously, they needed acquiescence from female patients themselves. Women had a real, and not always passive, place in the masculinized world of literate medicine. But it was not an equal one.

3

Bruno's Paradox: Women and Literate Medicine

At the present time, what ought to be judged even more indecent and horrible [than medical practice by illiterate men] is that vile and presumptuous women usurp and abuse this art, women who, although they have faith [in what they are doing], have neither art nor understanding. [The *Book for*] *Almansor* tells us that those who exercise this art [of surgery] for the most part are illiterates, rustics, and fools, and because of their stupidity diseases of the worst kind are generated in people which may even kill the patients. For they do not practice wisely or from a sure foundation [of knowledge] but they do so casually, not knowing at all the causes or the names of the infirmities they claim to be able to cure.

Bruno of Longobucco, *Surgery* (1253)[1]

When the Italian surgeon Bruno of Longobucco used female practitioners as the ultimate example of the dangers of illiterate medical practice, he was setting a rhetorical precedent that would be followed for centuries. Here, Bruno elaborates on a general condemnation of illiterate practice he found in one of his Arabic authorities, Rhazes, by adding the specific comment about female practitioners, whom Rhazes had not mentioned at all. Yet later, when Bruno had to describe how to treat bladder stones in a sexually experienced female patient, he followed one of his other Arabic authorities, the Spaniard Albucasis, in acknowledging that it was necessary to employ a female healer (*medica*) or, 'if you cannot find any woman sufficiently learned in the affairs of women', a midwife (*obstetrix*) to carry out the procedure.[2]

Bruno's paradox—his desire to dismiss all female practitioners as ignorant and his simultaneous recognition that his own capabilities as a medical practitioner

---

[1] Susan P. Hall, 'The *Cyrurgia Magna* of Brunus Longoburgensis: A Critical Edition', DPhil thesis, Oxford University, 1957, p. 4; my thanks to Michael McVaugh for sharing with me portions of his transcription of Hall's dissertation before I was finally able to consult it myself. This quote is the full context of the passage I cited in the Introduction. The name 'Almansor' refers to Rhazes's treatise known in Latin as the *Liber ad Almansorem*, Book VII (on surgery), cap. 1.

[2] Hall, *Cyrurgia magna*, p. 309. See Chapter 2 above.

were compromised without them—brings us again to the fundamental question that medical knowledge on the female body makes pressing: if women are involved at any level in the medical care of other women, or even just of themselves, then the gynaecological and obstetrical lore embodied in medical books can only be made effective if it is somehow passed back to them. As we saw in Chapter 2, Bruno was alone among all major Latin surgical writers in omitting not only the female genitalia but also women's breasts from the scope of the male surgeon's art. Yet ignoring women as patients was not a viable option for a practitioner wishing to earn the 'glory and fame' promised to successful learned healers by the Salernitans. Even Bruno recognized that at times he had to deal with women and thus defer to social norms that prevented him from touching their genitalia.[3] Whether Bruno liked it or not, a woman's hands and eyes were necessary. The question not only for Bruno but for all literate males was how much knowledge had to be ceded to women along with the responsibility for touching and viewing the female patient. The question for us is whether that knowledge was expected to come from books.

From women's perspective, of course, there may have been no automatic privileging of knowledge that came from books over that of experience or oral tradition. It is quite clear that much medical practice, among both men and women, was even at the end of the Middle Ages still based on oral instruction, apprenticeship, or individual empiricism; to the degree this was true, differentials in literacy would have had little effect in limiting women's medical practices. Yet it would be going too far to imagine women functioning, as practitioners and as patients, in a world in which men's knowledge, opinions, and practices—and their books—were completely irrelevant. The evidence of the previous chapter shows that male practitioners, however limited their clinical experience, were indeed claiming for themselves authoritative knowledge over certain aspects of women's medicine: they were being consulted for menstrual disorders, for uterine pain, for infertility, even at times for difficult birth. Male practice of women's medicine was therefore never irrelevant and it constituted at least part of the world in which women, both as patients and as practitioners, had to function. The possibility that women might share in the literate culture of men, or create a separate one of their own, is thus key to determining how far literate medical knowledge was gendered.

Female practitioners could be found throughout the 'medical marketplace' of western Europe from the thirteenth to fifteenth centuries. Their full and equal participation in the world of medical books, however, would have required full and equal participation in the world of literate education, something that never

---

[3] Indeed, Bruno also acknowledges some *mulieres sagaces* who treat inguinal hernia in their children with a truss; Hall, *Cyrurgia magna*, pp. 278–79. He says this in the context of criticism of other types of hernia treatments, thus acknowledging (implicitly) the efficacy of the women's treatment.

happened given women's exclusion from the universities and other venues of secondary education. As we have already seen, no female medical authors are known from the Middle Ages beyond Trota of Salerno and Hildegard of Bingen in the twelfth century, and a handful of writers of medical recipes at the end of the medieval period. Yet women were not universally illiterate and may have been active medical *readers*. Women's ranges of literate skill must therefore be plumbed to assess the possibility that female practitioners might have participated in literate medical culture as direct readers of medical texts. Moreover, if we can see women as in any way 'quasi-literates'—individuals without full literacy who nevertheless needed the learning in books to exercise their social functions (whether as medical practitioners or as mothers or household and estate administrators)—we need to assess possible aural and visual reception of the learning embodied in books. As we shall see, despite the rising levels of literacy among certain classes of women from the thirteenth century on, patterns of women's literacy did not map onto their patterns of medical practice.

WOMEN AS HEALERS: THE RANGE OF MEDICAL PRACTICES

In testimony at her trial in 1410, the surgeon Perretta Petone claimed that 'many women' like her were practising all over Paris.[4] While she may have been exaggerating for rhetorical effect, Perretta was certainly right that she was not alone as a female in medical practice. From the famous surgeon Hersende, who accompanied St Louis on Crusade in 1250 and who would later marry a Parisian apothecary, to various Jewish eye doctors in fifteenth-century Frankfurt, to phlebotomists at the French Dominican nunnery of Longchamp, to Muslim midwives at the royal court of Navarre—whether they were surgeons or oculists, barbers or herbalists or simply 'healers' (*metgessa, medica, miresse,* or *arztzatin*), women were almost always among the range of practitioners that offered their services in the western European medical marketplace from the twelfth through fifteenth centuries.[5] Although the number of women who take on the epithet

---

[4] Geneviève Dumas, 'Les femmes et les pratiques de la santé dans le "Registre des plaidoiries du Parlement de Paris, 1364–1427"', *Canadian Bulletin of Medical History/Bulletin canadien d'histoire de la médecine* 13 (1996), 3–27, at p. 22. In her study of working women in late 13th- and early 14th-century Paris (i.e., a century before Perretta was practising), Janice Archer estimates that on average about 10 female barbers were practising in Paris any given year between 1297 and 1300 (9% of all *barbier(e)s*), 8 *mirgesses* (21% of *mire(sse)s*), and 3 *ventrieres*. See Janice Marie Archer, 'Working Women in Thirteenth-Century Paris', PhD dissertation, University of Arizona, 1995, pp. 123 and 259–60. No comparable documentary data exist from the early 15th century to enable a comparison.

[5] Bibliography on female practitioners published up through 2003 can be found in Monica H. Green, 'Bodies, Gender, Health, Disease: Recent Work on Medieval Women's Medicine', *Studies in Medieval and Renaissance History*, 3rd ser. vol. 2 (2005), 1–46, and the works cited therein.

'healer' and even surgeon was in decline by the beginning of the fifteenth century, apparently because of the increasing effectiveness of licensing enforcement and the growing power of male-controlled guilds to limit practice by members' wives and daughters, in other fields women can still be found practising at the end of the medieval period in ancillary capacities to their practitioner husbands, taking over their workshops and apprentices when widowed.

The fact that we can identify and name a few hundred women who practised medicine in high medieval Europe should not, however, lead us to believe that women practised universally nor that they practised at comparable levels with men. In collective studies on medical practitioners generally, women never make up more than 1.5 per cent of the total.[6] Such numbers are suspect for several reasons, but the fact remains that we may never be able to assess the full extent of medieval women's medical practice since, all too often, women fall through the evidentiary cracks of the documentation that survives. The few women whom we can identify often show up because they are widowed (and therefore emerge from the legal shadow of their husbands), because they chose to step into the male world and request a licence to practise, or because, not having been licensed, they were caught and brought up on charges. Nevertheless, the existence of additional women can be inferred by considering that at least five institutional or social spaces were left for their existence in the structures of medieval medical practice and gender segregation: (1) as caretakers of each other in the context of all-female religious institutions; (2) as healers brought into such institutions because they would not threaten cloistered women's chastity; (3) as medical attendants both in hospitals and private households, where the 'caring' tasks of domestic service often extended into 'curing' ones; (4) as wives and daughters of male practitioners who engaged in the 'family business'; and finally, (5) as midwives. As with Bruno, even polemical condemnations of female practitioners and begrudging acknowledgements of their necessity in day-to-day care help point us to spaces that our evidence cannot yet fill in.

The context of the cloister would presumably have created the need for two kinds of medical attendance: care of the sick in general and care of the 'voluntarily unwell', the inmates who were regularly let blood as part of a ritualized procedure established for monastics in the early Middle Ages to avoid lethargy and inhibit lust. The office of the infirmarian/infirmaress had been established by the Benedictine *Rule* in the sixth century and seems to have been included in most monastic structures throughout the Middle Ages. The fifteenth-century rule

---

On Hersende and the barber-surgeons at Longchamp, Jeanne de Crespi (d. 1349) and Macée de Chaulmont (d. 1489), see Ernest Wickersheimer, *Dictionnaire biographique des médecins en France au Moyen Age*, 2 vols. (1936; repr. Geneva, Librairie Droz, 1979), respectively, vol. 1, pp. 294–95, and vol. 2, pp. 505 and 532. On the Muslim midwives in Navarre, see Maria Narbona-Cárceles, 'Woman at Court: A Prosopographic Study of the Court of Carlos III of Navarre (1387–1425)', *Medieval Prosopography* 22 (2001), 31–64.

6 Green, 'Documenting'.

book of the Dominican house of St Katharina's in Nuremberg, for example, devotes a whole chapter to the duties of the infirmaress, who is depicted at the bedside of one of her patients (Fig. 3.1).[7] Monastic communities were peculiar, however, in regularly *creating* a group who demanded medical attention through the periodic practice of phlebotomy.[8] Writing to Heloise in the twelfth century, Peter Abelard advised not only that the convent should have an infirmarian and an infirmary stocked with all necessary medicaments for treating the sick, but also that 'there should be some woman [in the nunnery] experienced in blood-letting, in order that it not be necessary for a man to come among the women for this purpose'.[9] The strictly enclosed English anchoresses addressed by the author of the *Ancrene Wisse* were told that they needed to be bled four times a year or more often if needed; the twelfth-century nun, Hildegard of Bingen, laid out a detailed regimen for bloodletting, scarification and cautery in her own medical writing.[10] Neither male nor female communities necessarily relied on one of their own to perform these functions and evidence for specialized phlebotomists within female institutions remains rare: the two Dominican phlebotomists from the French house of Longchamp, for example, are known to us only because they happen to be identified as such in the obituaries of the house. Nevertheless, it seems likely that more evidence for this kind of medical practice within nunneries will surface.

The possibility that some of the practitioners coming into the cloister may have been women constitutes the second 'space' for female medical practitioners. St Augustine, writing to a group of nuns in Hippo (in modern-day Tunisia) in the late fourth or early fifth century, had urged them to consult male physicians when necessary and it is clear that this option was still employed in the High Middle Ages.[11] Yet since contact with males was seen as inherently threatening to female chastity (both of body and reputation), which was paramount to nuns' identity, some level of female medical care was needed. Consider the case of the order of the Poor Clares. Clare had originally, in the early part of the thirteenth century, wanted to establish her female foundation on the same model of poverty

[7] Johannes Meyer, *Buch der Ämter*, Bloomington, University of Indiana, Lilly Library, MS Ricketts 198, s. xv, f. 50r. Reproduced by courtesy of the Lilly Library, Indiana University, Bloomington, Indiana.

[8] Mary K. K. H. Yearl, 'The Time of Bloodletting', PhD dissertation, Yale University, 2005. Yearl argues (pp. 93–103) that there was no difference in the rationale or procedures for letting blood in female vs. male monastics. She does not explore the question of the personnel needed to perform this habitual procedure.

[9] Peter Abelard, Letter VII, as cited in Monica H. Green, 'Books as a Source of Medical Education for Women in the Middle Ages', *Dynamis: Acta Hispanica ad Medicinae Scientiarumque Historiam Illustrandam* 20 (2000), 331–69, at p. 342.

[10] Bella Millett and Jocelyn Wogan-Browne (eds. and trans.), *Medieval English Prose for Women: From the Katherine Group and 'Ancrene Wisse'*, rev. ed. (Oxford, Clarendon, 1992), pp. 140–141; Laurence Moulinier (ed.), *Beate Hildegardis Cause et cure*, Rarissima mediaevalia, 1 (Berlin: Akademie Verlag, 2003), pp. 159–70.

[11] St Augustine, *Rule for Nuns*, as cited in Green, 'Books as a Source', p. 341.

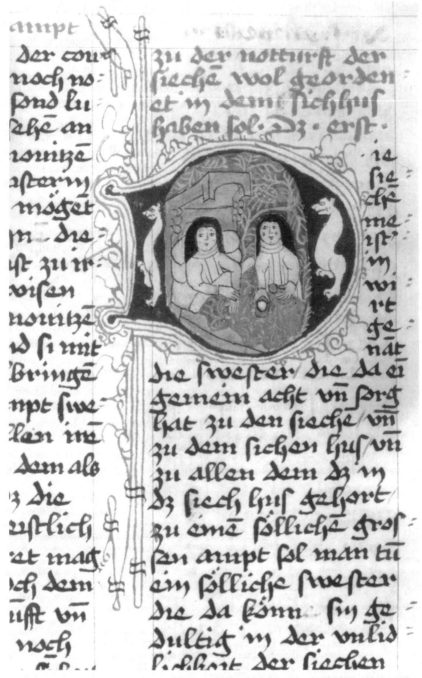

FIG. 3.1 Depiction of a monastic infirmaress in a manuscript owned by the Dominican convent of St Katharina's in Nuremberg. Johannes Meyer, *Buch der Ämter*.

and public begging that St Francis had for his friars, yet very quickly the Poor Clares became the most strictly enclosed female order in Europe, with elaborate architectural structures to ensure that the nuns neither saw nor were seen by the parishioners with whom they shared their church or by others.[12] When Pope Innocent IV wrote a new rule for the Poor Clares in 1247, he stipulated that no abbess ought to permit bloodletting more than four times a year, 'unless manifest necessity requires that it be more. Nor may [the nuns] receive bloodletting from an outsider, especially a man, when it can be conveniently avoided'. For serious illnesses, however, Innocent readily allowed both male physicians and phlebotomists to enter the house, provided they were at all times accompanied by 'two appropriate companions'.[13] Thus, while there was some expectation that routine phlebotomy was to be done in-house for the same reasons that Abelard had identified, there was also reliance on the skills of male healers for grave conditions.[14]

Nevertheless, the employment of male practitioners continued to prove problematic. In a ruling pronounced by the Order's Cardinal Protector in 1297, where the assumption of male medical practice was also made, there was the added stipulation that 'when the Sisters need to be let blood or be treated medically in their secret places [*in locis secretis*]', *female* phlebotomists and healers (*minutrices et medice*) should be allowed to enter the convent. Two or three mature nuns were to supervise them, in order to ensure that there were no private discussions on the sly, a provision no more onerous than others meant to avert private conversation.[15] A similar assumption of both male and female medical practice was made in an 'admonition' to some Dominican nuns in Germany in 1259, who were told that 'Secular physicians shall in no manner be admitted into the cloister nor shall they sit with the sisters in the doorways or on the stoops.... [I]f it is necessary that secular physicians be consulted, let this be done by messengers and let the person who is sick be described according to her age and the type and duration of her illness or, if it is possible, let go-betweens handle this in the window but, as was said, let them not

---

[12] Caroline A. Bruzelius, 'Hearing is Believing: Clarissan Architecture, *c.*1213–1340', *Gesta* 31, no. 2 (1992), 83–91.

[13] 'The Form of Life of Pope Innocent IV (1247)', in *Clare of Assisi: Early Documents*, ed. and trans. Regis J. Armstrong, rev. ed. (Saint Bonaventure, NY: Franciscan Institute Publications, Saint Bonaventure University, 1993), pp. 118–19. The injunction to avoid male phlebotomists was repeated by, for example, a house of Poor Clares in Barcelona; see Green, 'Books as a Source', at p. 342.

[14] For evidence on nuns' employment of male practitioners in general, see Green, 'Books as a Source'; and Katrinette Bodarwé, 'Pflege und Medizin in mittelalterlichen Frauenkonventen', *Medizinhistorisches Journal* 37 (2002), 231–63.

[15] P. Benv[enuto] Burghetti, 'De regimine Clarissarum durante saec. XIV', *Archivum Francis-canum Historicum* 13 (1920), 89–135, at pp. 113–14. The 1307 version reads nearly identically, adding only the stipulation that these female practitioners be of good reputation and upright behaviour (*si clare fame fuerint et honeste conversationis et vite*, p. 126). My deepest thanks to Angela Montford for alerting me to this and the following source.

enter. And let this likewise be observed concerning women who profess the art of surgery or medicine'.[16] Whether these rules were as much concern to the religious women themselves is unclear; when Clare wrote her own rule in 1253 in response to Innocent's, she made no mention whatsoever about the provision of medical care. Nevertheless, such rules show quite clearly the belief that female practitioners were in regular enough supply that nuns could be expected to rely on their ministrations. The institution of female monasticism thus created two 'spaces' for female practitioners, one inside monastery walls and another just outside them.

A third 'space' for women in medical practice has as its closest modern analogue the nurse, though we should not imagine any specific or uniform training in medicine that such women received. The beguines of the Low Countries, for example, loose coalitions of women living together but taking no formal religious vows, took their origin from women who tended to lepers in the late twelfth and early thirteenth centuries; as the movement grew and expanded through the Low Countries and beyond, tending to the sick became one of the distinguishing occupations of these women who relied primarily on their own labour, rather than charitable endowments, for their upkeep. Similarly, many hospitals (which were more 'hostels' or poor houses, really, than the centres of advanced medical care that we now associate with the word) were being founded throughout Europe from the late twelfth century on; serving them were religious orders of Hospitallers, who often included nursing sisters.[17] In the secular realm, large households may have had individuals with special responsibilities for caring for the sick. The French dowager queen, Blanche of Navarre (d. 1398), for example, had in her household two women who looked after the sick: Symmonete, 'who attends to the sick' (*qui sert les malades*) and who was also Blanche's personal chambermaid, and the wife of Morelet, Blanche's litter-bearer (her own name is never given), 'who looks after the sick' (*qui garde les malades*). The late fourteenth- and early fifteenth-century French writer, Christine de Pizan, recommends to

---

[16] E. Ritzinger and H. C. Scheeben, 'Beitrage zur Geschichte der Teutonia in der zweit-en Hälfte des 13. Jahrhunderts', *Archiv der deutschen Dominikaner* 3 (1941), 11–95, at pp. 29–30.

[17] On the beguines' medical works, see Walter Simons, *Cities of Ladies: Beguine Communities in the Medieval Low Countries, 1200–1565* (Philadelphia: University of Pennsylvania Press, 2001), pp. 39–40 and 76–78; on the Hospitallers, see Jessalynn Bird, 'Medicine for Body and Soul: Jacques de Vitry's Sermons to Hospitallers and their Charges', in Peter Biller and Joseph Ziegler, eds., *Religion and Medicine in the Middle Ages*, York Studies in Medieval Theology, 3 (York: York Medieval Press, 2001), pp. 91–108; and *eadem*, 'Texts on Hospitals: Translation of Jacques de Vitry, *Historia Occidentalis* 29, and Edition of Jacques de Vitry's Sermons on Hospitallers', in Peter Biller and Joseph Ziegler, eds., *Religion and Medicine in the Middle Ages*, York Studies in Medieval Theology, 3 (York: York Medieval Press, 2001), pp. 109–34. On married women who tended the ill, see Sharon Farmer, 'The Leper in the Master Bedroom: Thinking Through a Thirteenth-Century Exemplum', in *Framing the Family: Narrative and Representation in the Medieval and Early Modern Periods*, ed. Rosalynn Voaden and Diane Wolfthal (Tempe, AZ: Arizona Center for Medieval and Renaissance Studies, 2005), 79–100.

prostitutes that they might give up their dissolute ways and turn to care of the sick as a way to earn a living.[18]

Whereas these 'nurses' were usually unmarried, the fourth space for female medical practice was open to married women. Women of artisanal classes sometimes participated in 'the family business', working alongside their husbands, fathers, and sons, and carrying on their practice as widows after their husbands' deaths. This same pattern seems to have been true of the 'craft' subfields within medicine, that is, surgery, barbery, and pharmacy, and even at times general medicine. Stephanie, daughter of a thirteenth-century physician in Lyons named Etienne de Montaneis, is herself called a *medica*.[19] Katherine *la surgiene* of London was identified in 1286 as the daughter of Thomas the surgeon and sister of William the surgeon.[20] In the southern French town of Manosque in the early fourteenth century, the surgeon Fava is married to the patriarch of a Jewish medical family, Astrugus, and has a son and two grandsons who also practice the family trade.[21] Around the turn of the fifteenth century Marie de Gy practised as a healer in Dijon both before and after the death of her husband, a barber.[22] Viewing medical work as a 'family business' explains the cases when women 'suddenly' enter into medical practice after their husband dies.[23]

Medicine may have been so much of a 'family business', in fact, that it led surgeons and barbers to engage in 'occupational endogamy', that is, the marrying off of their daughters to men in the same trade. Take, for example, the late fourteenth- and early fifteenth-century English family of the Bradmores. John and Nicholas Bradmore were brothers, both practising surgery in London—John apparently with somewhat more success as he served as royal surgeon throughout the reign of King Henry IV (1399–1413) and acquired considerable amounts of property. A third male surgeon in the Bradmore dynasty is John's son-in-law, John Longe, the son of a butcher, to whom John Bradmore would leave a massive Latin surgical compendium that he had composed.[24] The women who

---

[18]   Green, 'Possibilities'.

[19]   Wickersheimer, *Dictionnaire*, 2:747; cf. 1:142. Interestingly, in one of the glosses on Justinian's *Digest*, there is a reference to the daughter of a physician in Lyons who was 'renowned for her knowledge of various kinds of doctrine' (*hodie apud nonnullos observatur, ut ipse filiam quandam medici Lugdunensis vario doctrinae genere praeditam noui*); v. *instituerit*. (I owe this reference to Timothy Sistrunk.) Whether Stephanie is the same as the woman the glossators refer to cannot yet be determined. Still, it forms an intriguing parallel with Boccaccio's story of Gillette of Narbonne (for which, see below).

[20]   Carole Rawcliffe, *Medicine and Society in Later Medieval England* (Phoenix Mill: Alan Sutton, 1995), p. 188.

[21]   Joseph Shatzmiller, *Médecine et justice en Provence médiévale: Documents de Manosque, 1262–1348* (Aix-en-Provence: Publications de l'Université de Provence, 1989), pp. 150–51.

[22]   Wickersheimer, *Dictionnaire*, 2:538.

[23]   On the general problem of identifying female practitioners only when they are widowed, see Green, 'Documenting'. See also the case of Jeanne la Poqueline discussed in the Conclusion below, who encountered difficulties setting up a practice when her husband abandoned her instead of dying.

[24]   For more on Bradmore's book, see Chapter 6 below.

connected this family together included John Bradmore's daughter, Agnes, who married John Longe, and Agnes Woodcock, Nicholas Bradmore's apprentice, whom he held in sufficient regard to bequeathe a red belt with a silver buckle and 6s. 8d. in his will of 1417.[25] Although Agnes Bradmore/Longe would take a stonemason as her second husband (probably in the early 1430s, by which point she was a well-propertied middle-aged woman), it is not far-fetched to imagine that earlier in her life she had practised as a surgeon alongside her father, her uncle, or her first husband. The images of the male and female surgeons working in tandem, which may have been produced in London right when the Bradmores and Longes were active (Figs. 3.2 and 3.3), help us imagine how the two Agneses in these households might have served in similar capacities, cupping and lancing both male and female patients. To be sure, there may have been some sexual division of labour within these household units.[26] Medieval women's work has often been found to be intermittent, characterized by low skill levels (*vis-à-vis* those of men) and often low status, tied very much to their other domestic duties, and very often combined with a variety of other types of work.[27] The female surgeon or barber depicted in Figures 3.2 and 3.3 is doing the cupping and lancing, while male figures earlier in the same sequence perform more invasive surgical procedures.[28]

The final 'space' left open for female medical practice is the one we would assume was most heavily populated: midwifery. Yet it is surprisingly difficult to identify professional midwives between the late antique period, when Caelius Aurelianus, Theodorus Priscianus, and Muscio were writing their gynaecological texts for *obstetrices* and *medicae*, and the thirteenth century, when the word again began to have professional connotations. Indeed, in many areas no women can be identified taking on 'midwife' as a professional title until well into the fifteenth century. The reasons for the thin documentation for midwives are several and

[25] S. J. Lang, 'John Bradmore and His Book *Philomena*', *Social History of Medicine* 5 (1992), 121–30; and 'The *Philomena* of John Bradmore and its Middle English Derivative: A perspective on Surgery in Late Medieval England', PhD dissertation, University of St Andrews, 1998. On Agnes Woodcock, see Rawcliffe, *Medicine and Society*, p. 188.

[26] Writing in 1296, the surgeon Lanfranc had taken his fellow male surgeons to task for leaving phlebotomy, scarifying, cauterizing, and the use of leeches to barbers and women out of their own disdain for manual labour; Lanfranc of Milan, *Cyrurgia magna*, in *Cyrurgia Guidonis de Cauliaco. et Cyrurgia Bruni, Teodorici, Rolandi, Lanfranci, Rogerii, Bertapalie* (Venice, 1519), ff. 166va–210vb, at f. 168va.

[27] Green, 'Documenting', which draws on the formulations of Maryanne Kowaleski, 'Women's Work in a Market Town: Exeter in the Late Fourteenth Century', in *Women and Work in Preindustrial Europe*, ed. Barbara A. Hanawalt (Bloomington: University of Indiana Press, 1986), pp. 145–64.

[28] OBL, MS Laud misc. 724, *c*.1400. The date applies only to the sequence of illustrations on ff. 94r to 97v; the Latin texts in the manuscript were written later. See Kathleen L. Scott, *Later Gothic Manuscripts 1390–1490*, 2 vols., *A Survey of Manuscripts Illuminated in the British Isles*, general ed., J. J. G. Alexander, VI (London: Harvey Miller, 1998), vol. 1, plates 106–7; vol. 2, cat. no. 15, pp. 75–77. A collection of Middle English texts, BLL, MS Sloane 6, s. xv$^{2/4}$, presents similar images of male and female practitioners, with the female similarly doing only cupping and lancing.

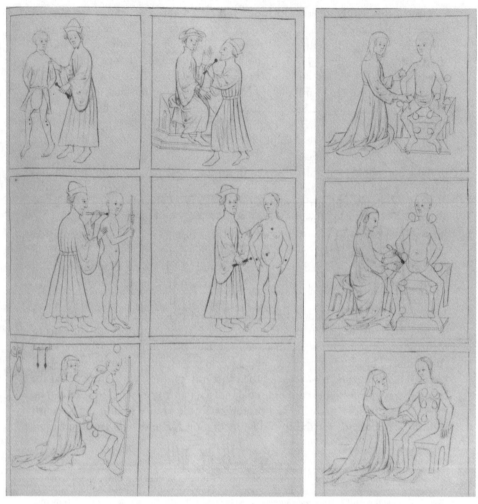

FIGS. 3.2 AND 3.3 A female barber or surgeon cupping and lancing male and female patients. In the remaining series of images (which number 32 in all) a male practitioner performs more invasive procedures.

are in part due to difficulties in identifying occupations for medieval women in *any* field of work. However, I have come to believe that the silence of the evidence—a silence that is found across western Europe throughout all different kinds of documentary materials—is itself testimony that midwifery emerged (or rather, re-emerged) as a profession only slowly between the thirteenth and fifteenth centuries. I will return to the genesis of midwifery as a profession later since, as the field most likely to have led to a *feminine* birth of gynaecology, it merits closer analysis. For now, the possibility that women might have been widely engaged with medical practice has been established. The question that remains is, if literacy proved key to the developing professional identities of male physicians, surgeons, barbers, and apothecaries (as we saw in the Introduction and Chapter 2), did it function the same way for women?

WOMEN AS READERS: THE LIMITS OF LITERACY

The literacy of practitioners

On the third day of the *Decameron*, as his elite band of travellers flee the plague in Florence, Giovanni Boccaccio has the lady Neifile tell the story of Gillette of Narbonne, the daughter of a *famoso medico* named Gerard of Narbonne. When the king of France falls ill, Gillette goes (admittedly with ulterior motives) to cure him. When he hesitates to believe she is capable of such a cure, she responds: 'Sire, you disdain my art because I am young and a woman; but let me remind you that I am not healing you with my own knowledge, but with the aid of God and with the knowledge of Master Gerard of Narbonne, who was my father and a famous physician while he lived'.[29] Boccaccio, at least, was able to envision a learned physician's daughter absorbing her father's knowledge, but even in this story Gillette neither makes a living off her knowledge nor is there any clear indication that she has studied her father's books. For women who had no personal ties to university-trained masters, the learning of the universities was impossibly out of reach. But women, as we have seen, were not the only practitioners who moved on the peripheries of university culture. Jewish and Muslim males, as well as most Christian surgeons, barbers, and apothecaries were likewise excluded and, as I have argued in the Introduction, literacy and book-use was the closest thing to an equalizing factor these other male groups had *vis-à-vis* their more formally educated brethren. The surgical writers of the twelfth through fourteenth centuries recognized the potential of the written word not simply to grant to surgery the stature of a *scientia*, but also to grant to surgeons the benefit of a *societas* larger than the personal bonds created between a single master and his students. And they were not disappointed in this hope, for the wide circulation of their works in Latin and the vernaculars proves that

---

[29] Giovanni Boccaccio, *The Decameron*, terza giornata, novella nona, ed. V. Branca (1992), available online at <http://www.brown.edu/Departments/Italian_Studies/dweb/> accessed 9 October /2004. No Gerard of Narbonne is mentioned in the standard reference work on medieval French medical practitioners (Wickersheimer, *Dictionnaire*), though see n. 19 above. There is also documentary evidence that a 15th-century Neapolitan woman, Costanza Calenda, the daughter of the subprior of the University of Naples, studied at the university there; see Paul Oskar Kristeller, 'Learned Women of Early Modern Italy: Humanists and University Scholars', in *Beyond Their Sex: Learned Women of the European Past*, ed. Patricia H. Labalme (New York: New York University Press, 1984), pp. 91–116, at pp. 102–3.

textual communities did indeed form around their highly crafted assertions of authoritative knowledge.

One example of such a textual community of surgeons can be found in the London family of the Bradmores, whom we have already met. The more successful of the two surgeon brothers, John Bradmore, is not known to have had any university education yet he was fully Latin-literate, having composed his own surgical textbook in Latin. When he prepared his will in 1412, he listed three books: a 'black paper book' of unspecified contents that he left to his brother Nicholas, his 'black book of surgery' that he left to a fellow surgeon, Philip Brychford, and his magnum opus, his massive surgical compilation, which he left to his son-in-law, John Longe. These four male surgeons made up their own small 'textual community', with Bradmore's gifts in death probably merely cementing book-sharing habits they had engaged in during his life. Did the women of the household belong, too? Could Agnes Bradmore/Longe read her own father's Latin composition?

It seems unlikely. Looking over all five 'spaces' left open for female medical practice—medical practice by cloistered women themselves, by women brought into the cloister to preserve nuns's chastity, by beguines and nursing sisters working in hospitals, by married women working alongside male kin, and, finally, by midwives—we find both differences and commonalities. Some women would have practised largely independently of men, others either side-by-side or under the supervision of them. Some worked for money, others for spiritual reward. But while some (like the nuns) would have had clear advantages in terms of their potential to relate to literate medicine, all, I will argue, failed to see that potential materialize. What differentiated women from male practitioners was that whereas many men may have been able to draw on their clerical, notarial, or mercantile backgrounds for training that helped them engage with the increasingly literate culture of medicine, female practitioners would rarely have had such advantages. It is not surprising, therefore, that there is very little positive evidence for female practitioners' engagement with literate medicine in Latin or any other language.

The in-house phlebotomists in nunneries, for example, even if they regularly deferred to male practitioners for more serious conditions, might be seen as a potential audience for basic works on phlebotomy, Egyptian days (a list of days when bloodletting should be avoided), or anatomy. Yet to date, hardly any medical texts have been found in female monastic libraries and few of these rise above the level of recipe collections.[30] Similarly, beguinages and hospitals are notably impoverished in terms of medical literature; often, the only books we

---

[30] Green, 'Books as a Source'; Bodarwé, 'Pflege'. Exceptions are the Dominican convent of St Marien in Lemgo, which owned a collection of texts in Latin and Low German on plague, phlebotomy, charms, herbs, and care for the dead; and OBL, MS Bodley 9 (SC 1851), s. xv$^{2/4}$, which contains brief texts on the four humours, perilous days, and phlebotomy alongside prayers written for nuns. It may have been owned by the nuns of Canonsleigh, Devon. (My thanks to Stephanie Volf for this latter reference.)

can find are devotional works, especially texts on the art of dying well. As we saw in the last chapter, the beguine's psalter incorporating a basic regimen for monthly living (Fig. 2.1 above) showed her deferring to a male physician for analysis of her urine and, apparently, preparation of medicines in his shop. Of the phlebotomists and *medice* imagined by the Cardinal Protector in his 1297 rule for the Poor Clares we as yet know nothing, though we can probably assume they were no more literate than the nuns they ministered to (and probably much less so). Of the other women in professional medical practice, the evidence is mixed.

One of Perretta Petone's contemporaries in early fifteenth-century Paris was Phelipe La Chomete who, early in life, had been deemed to be 'ingenious and inclined to do medicine' and so she was 'put in a place to learn it and there she became very experienced'.[31] Whether Phelipe's training involved book learning is not explicitly stated, though the fact that she came to serve in the household of the Duchess of Burgundy may suggest that she did in fact have some of the literate skills that aristocratic women would have expected in their attendants. Social class may also be predictive of some level of literacy in the famous case of Jacoba Felicie in Paris in 1322, who described herself as *nobilis* and was consistently referred to even by the hostile medical faculty as *domina Jacoba* ('Lady Jacoba'). To be sure, there is nothing in Jacoba's trial records to confirm that she was literate or owned books (her accusers declare her *illiterata*), but the detailed descriptions of how she took pulses and examined urines certainly indicates her close familiarity with the practices of book-learned physicians.[32] Similarly, women like the *phisica* Mayrona, a Jewish practitioner in the southern French town of Manosque in the late fourteenth century, may have been literate since she also practised as a moneylender which would require a certain level of numeracy if not also some literacy. The literacy of women in Jewish communities (where medical practice was one of the few acceptable trades) seems to have been somewhat higher, on average, than that of Christian women, so it is no surprise to find a Jewish woman, Alegra, wife of a Jewish tailor in Majorca, in possession of a medical book.[33]

More often, however, we have no evidence to confirm women practitioners' literacy one way or the other. Indeed, some female practitioners, such as several surgeons licensed to practise in the southern Italian Kingdom of Naples between 1309 and 1345, are explicitly identified as *ydiota*, 'illiterate'. This includes the surgeon Raymunda de Taberna, who was licensed in 1345 by Queen Joanna of Naples 'lest [women] incur any shameful compromising of their matronly modesty' by being treated by men. Raymunda is examined by Joanna's surgeons

---

[31] Guy Llewelyn Thompson, *Paris and its People Under English Rule: The Anglo-Burgundian Regime 1420–1436*, Oxford Historical Monographs (Oxford: Clarendon, 1991), p. 153, n. 19.

[32] See the Introduction, above.

[33] On Jewish women's literacy, see Green, 'Possibilities', pp. 12–13.

and is found to be qualified to treat cancers, simple wounds, and fistulae. While Raymunda's illiteracy is unremarkable in comparison to other female practitioners, what *is* remarkable is that she is just as illiterate as they despite the fact that her brother (the only male relative with whom she is identified) is a notary![34] As with Jacoba, the term *ydiota* may have been used in the narrow sense of 'not literate in Latin',[35] but we have no evidence to assume even Raymunda's vernacular literacy.[36] In fact, besides Perretta Petone in Paris, the only clear cases of ownership of a medical book by a woman who made some kind of specialty out of medical practice is a *livre de sirurgie* (a book of surgery, or possibly medicine in general) that was willed to Symmonete, one of the medical attendants in the entourage of the widowed queen of France, Blanche of Navarre, and a French herbal that was owned by Isabelle of Portugal, the queen of France (d. 1471), who earned a reputation for her medical ministrations to the poor.[37] It is likely, of course, that other female practitioners might be added to this list if we had fuller documentation on them. Perhaps Isabelle le Mairesse of Tournai, who had borrowed a medical book (*un livre de médechine*) from one master Jehan de Maulcachiet in 1389, worked as a practitioner who, like Perretta, recognized the importance of the knowledge contained in medical books even if she could not own one herself.[38]

A further indication that female practitioners' literacy might be under-represented is the fact that, as we have seen, many women practising medicine are known to have been related, by birth or marriage, to male practitioners. As such, they may have shared in whatever literate culture their fathers or husbands had access to. However, as the profession of medicine became more and more masculinized, fewer women may have been able to lay claim to even these rights of inheritance. This exclusion had perhaps always been true of the wives and daughters of physicians (Gillette's story notwithstanding), who never

[34] The documents are collected in Raffaele Calvanico, *Fonti per la storia della medicina e della chirurgia per il regno di Napoli nel periodo angioino (a. 1273–1410)* (Naples: L'Arte Tipografica, 1962), items 1413, 1451 and 1872, 3071 (cf. 3195), 3226, 3598, and 3643.

[35] Herbert Grundmann, 'Litteratus-illiteratus: Der Wandel einer Bildungnorm vom Altertum zum Mittelalter', in Grundmann, *Ausgewählte Aufsätze, 3: Bildung und Sprache*, Monumenta Germaniae Historica Schriften 25:3 (Stuttgart: Hiersemann, 1978), pp. 1–66; Brian Stock, *The Implications of Literacy: Written Language and Models of Interpretation in the Eleventh and Twelfth Centuries* (Princeton: Princeton University Press, 1983), pp. 28–30.

[36] To my knowledge, no studies have yet been done of the circulation of vernacular medical texts in 14th-century southern Italy. It is thus not clear whether any material was available that Raymunda or her fellow *ydiota* practitioners *might* have read in the vernacular. The first woman to be identified as *ydiota* is Lauretta, wife of Giovanni di Ponte da Saracena Calabra, who in 1308–9 was residing in Santa Maria. She was examined by the learned Neapolitan physician, Francesco da Piedimonte, who found her to be 'in the cure of the diseases of stones, apostemes and external wounds [. . .] learned in curing the said diseases, even though she is unlettered [*ydiota*]' (Calvanico, *Fonti*, item 1413, p. 156).

[37] On Symmonete, see Green, 'Possibilities', pp. 51–2. Blanche had given her other medical book to her lady-in-waiting, Jehanne de Rouieres, in 1396.

[38] Green, 'Possibilities', pp. 10 and 55.

would have been able to approximate their male relative's university learning. Constantia, daughter and universal heir of Master Petrus Fica, doctor of arts and medicine in the Sicilian town of Trapani, was bequeathed all his books at his death in 1433, yet of the twenty-three or more that were medical, all were in Latin. Could she read them and make use of them? Or was she simply bequeathed them on the understanding that these valuable books would later be sold off to generate income or even serve as a dowry for her marriage to another male physician?[39] The same questions could be asked of a woman in Avignon, Leonarde Pauchade, the widow of a barber, who in 1452 willed her deceased husband's entire workshop—from the shaving basins and whetting stones to his books of surgery—to another male barber, Pierre Theurot, as thanks for his cure of her when she was ill.[40] Moreover, it is clear in certain cases that wives were deliberately excluded from inheriting their practitioner husband's or father's medical tools and books. As we have seen, in 1412 John Bradmore willed his massive Latin surgical compendium not to his daughter, but to his son-in-law who, having been the son of a butcher, probably only learned Latin in the context of his surgical apprenticeship. Several decades later in Valencia, an apothecary willed all his movable goods to his wife *except* 'the things and tools that I have of my apothecary's art, and the books that I have of this art'.[41]

This deliberate exclusion of the apothecary's wife from her husband's profession shows that the growing legal and social impediments to women's medical practice were having an effect. Valencia, we will recall, was the city that had passed an ordinance in 1329 forbidding women to engage in any medical practice other than treating women and children and, even then, prohibiting them from administering potions.[42] While neither this ordinance nor similar ones elsewhere proved effective in driving women completely out of medical practice, the fourteenth-century developments eradicated the (at least nominally) egalitarian legal status of female practitioners that had been established in the thirteenth century. These new legal impediments coincided with older discursive practices (like Bruno's) that branded women as categorically unfit to practise medicine. Thus, aside from midwives, there was no *positive* category of 'female medical practitioner' that was ever created separate from the feminine form of physician, surgeon, barber, or apothecary. Even Pierre Dubois's famous call in 1309 to create a corps of female physicians and surgeons to take the message of Christianity into 'heathen' lands saw such women as the companions of their physician and

---

[39] Henri Bresc, *Livre et société en Sicile (1299–1499)* (Palermo: Centro di Studi Filologici e Linguisitici Siciliani, 1971), document 67. Petrus stipulates that if Constantia does not abide by the terms of his will, all his goods are to go to the pious society of San Domenico.

[40] Wickersheimer, *Dictionnaire*, 2:535 and 663; and Broomhall, *Women's Medical Work in Early Modern France* (Manchester: University of Manchester Press, 2004) p. 25.

[41] Will of Pere Torres, 7 July 1458; see Green, 'Books as Sources', p. 356, n. 74.

[42] See the Introduction above.

surgeon husbands, not as a separate female profession.[43] There is, in short, no evidence that female practitioners *identified with each other* or in any way banded together to secure their literate training.[44] To the extent that female practitioners may have engaged with the world of literate medicine, therefore, it was probably because they absorbed the new professional standards of literacy from the male practitioners to whom they were related. How often those personal ties to literate medicine trumped women's gendered exclusion from basic literate education is unclear. In Perretta's case, although she stresses that she learned medicine from several different relatives (her phrasing leaves it unclear whether they were male or female), her actual ability to engage with the culture of literate medicine remained minimal.

The literacy of midwives

I have deferred analysis of midwives and their literacy precisely because theirs was the field of medicine over which women had the closest thing to a monopoly. If there was any ideal match between a group of female practitioners and a particular kind of medical literature, one would think it would be midwives and works on women's medicine. Yet as we have seen, other kinds of female medical practitioners seem to have had only tenuous and irregular connections to literate medicine. Why should we expect midwives to be different? In fact we should not expect them to be different, for two reasons that show how differently women were affected by the literate revolution in medicine.

Although we generally think of midwifery as a timeless profession, the evidence (or rather, non-evidence) suggests that there were few specialist midwives in medieval Europe prior to the thirteenth century. Midwives in Antiquity and Late Antiquity—the professionalized ones referred to in Roman law, admonished in Christian edicts, and memorialized in statues and inscriptions—had been sustained by the concentrations of population in Mediterranean urban centres and by a medical system that not only granted them a broad mandate over both obstetrics and gynaecology but also valued their literacy. This professionalized corps of midwives was the intended audience of the late antique North African writers Theodorus Priscianus, Caelius Aurelianus, and Muscio. Like so many aspects of specialized urban life, including other medical specializations, these professional, literate midwives seem to have largely disappeared with the contraction of urban life in the western Mediterranean.

[43] Pierre Dubois, *De recuperatione Terre Sante. Traité de politique générale*, ed. Ch.-V. Langlois (Paris: Alphonse Picard, 1891), p. 62: 'Isti medici et cerurgi uxores habeant similiter intructas, cum quarum auxiliis egrotantibus plenius subveniant'.

[44] As both Green, 'Books as a Source', and Bodarwé, 'Pflege', have shown, this is true even of monastic contexts where the concentration of female literates would have been highest. Whatever Hildegard of Bingen's intentions were in compiling her great *Physica* in the 12th century, it had no apparent effect in generating a continuing medical textual community of nuns.

What never disappeared was female attendance at birth. Rather, the responsibility for attendance at birth (and for maintenance of the medical lore that needed to go with it) seems to have been dispersed across a generalized mass of neighbours and kinswomen, none of whom would necessarily have more skill, knowledge, or authority than others aside from the stature that advanced age conferred.[45] The Latin word *obstetrix* ('she who stands by') was of good classical lineage and remained available for use throughout the Middle Ages in both theological and legal contexts. However, aside from the German *Hebamme* (literally, 'nurse who lifts' [the baby]) which is documented already from the eighth century,[46] the vernacular forms of the word—*ventrière, bajula, matrone, midwif, vroedvrauw, levatrice, partera, madrina, commare* or *comadre*—and, more importantly, the use of the epithet as an occupational title for individual women, are not documented before the latter half of the thirteenth century and even then quite rarely.[47] For example, in the thirteenth-century French romance *Silence*, where the birth of the cross-dressing heroine is a major part of the plot, nowhere is a specific term for 'midwife' used to refer to the kinswoman who assists the birth by herself or any others who might normally have been called in.[48] Similarly, many of the new hospitals being founded from the late twelfth century on stipulated in their rules that, in addition to pilgrims, the poor, and the infirm, they were to take in poor pregnant women and allow them to give birth there. Yet it is not until 1378 that we find our first evidence for the employment of a midwife to care for any of these hospital births.[49] Moreover, even when vernacular words for 'midwife' begin to come into use, many are notoriously imprecise since they are frequently interchangeable with the words for 'wet-nurse', 'godmother', and even just 'woman'. This fluidity of terms is exasperating for the historian—is this *commare* a midwife or a godmother? Is that *bajula* a wet-nurse or a birth attendant? The Catalan scholar Montserrat Cabré i Pairet has seized on this terminological fluidity and argued that it reflects the fact that most of women's

[45] Obviously, this is a very simplified narrative, since I am glossing over the fact that early medieval Europe was a conglomeration of different ethnic groups, all of which no doubt had their own traditional birth practices.

[46] On uses of *Hebamme*, see *Deutsches Wörterbuch von Jacob und Wilhelm Grimm* <http://www.dwb.uni-trier.de/index.html> accessed 9 October 2004.

[47] See Green, 'Bodies', pp. 14–17. My survey of the standard historical dictionaries finds that the French *meraleresse* is first documented in 1267, and *ventrière* c.1300; the Castilian and Catalan *ama, comare, matrona, madrina,* and *partera* in the 15th century; the Dutch *hevemoeder* and *vroedemoeder* (or *vroedvrauw*) in the 14th century; and the Danish *jordemoder* in 1510. My thanks to, respectively, Montserrat Cabré, Orlanda Lie, and Ann Marie Rasmussen for the Spanish, Dutch, and Danish citations. Obviously, written witnesses to these terms will appear well after they came into oral usage.

[48] Heldris of Cornwall, *Silence: A Thirteenth-Century French Romance*, trans. Sarah Roche-Mahdi (East Lansing: Michigan State University Press, 1992).

[49] On Julienne, the first attested midwife employed by the Hôtel-Dieu in Paris, see Danielle Jacquart, ed. *Supplément* to Ernest Wickersheimer, *Dictionnaire biographique des médecins en France au Moyen Age* (Geneva: Librairie Droz, 1979), p. 195. For more examples of the 'non-appearance' of midwives, see Green, 'Bodies'.

medical practices came out of their daily activities *as women*.[50] 'Midwife' is not simply a medical function but a social role. The *commare* may be present not simply at the birth, but also serve the social and religious role of godmother at the baptism (which the mother herself would not attend since she was still lying-in after the birth). When a midwife becomes a 'professional', she potentially puts herself outside these communal ties by engaging in a mercenary relationship.

This general dispersal of midwifery skills throughout the community of women would explain why we find so few women claiming the occupational title 'midwife' for themselves. 'Spontaneous' creations of midwives may have been brought about by new concentrations of population that could sustain full-time birth attendants. Thus, it is probably not just an accident of documentary survival that the earliest women we can identify in France to take on *ventrière* as an occupational label were in Paris, the city that by the end of the thirteenth century had the largest population in Europe. Even in circumstances of population density, however, there was no automatic pressure for midwives to emerge *as a profession*. In thirteenth-century Douai, for example, a town perhaps a tenth of the size of Paris but still with a dense enough population base to support a couple of professional midwives, we find no indication that 'midwife' was recognized alongside other female occupations like baker, butcher, or spinner.[51] Similar results are found in a variety of other cities where women's occupations have been surveyed. In later fourteenth-century Avignon, a city then with a post-plague population of *c.*30,000, we likewise find no women taking on the professional title of midwife although they readily identified themselves as fruitsellers, candle-makers, and carpenters.[52] In fact, in no instance prior to the fifteenth century have midwives been documented in the proportions we would expect in relation to their demographic demand. As late as the mid fifteenth century, a French archdeacon inspecting various parishes outside of Paris, Jean Mouchard, was still finding parishes that had no midwife.[53]

---

[50] Montserrat Cabré i Pairet, 'Nacer en relación', in *De dos en dos: Las practicas de creación y recreación de la vida y de la convivencia*, ed. Marta Beltran i Tarres (Madrid: Hora y Hora, 2000), pp. 15–32. Even in Germany, the simple term *Amme* (nurse) continued to be used to refer to birth attendants through the end of the Middle Ages. See, for example, the German translation of some Muscian obstetrical excerpts in Leipzig, Universitätsbibliothek, MS 1192, an. 1434–40 (eastern Germany), ff. 263v–264v.

[51] On Douai, see Ellen E. Kittell and Kurt Gueller, ''Whether Man or Woman': Gender Inclusivity in the Town Ordinances of Medieval Douai', *Journal of Medieval and Early Modern Studies* 30 (2000), 63–100.

[52] Joëlle Rollo-Koster, 'The Women of Papal Avignon. A New Source: The *Liber divisionis* of 1371', *Journal of Women's History* 8 (1996), 36–59, who documents 113 women using at least thirty-five different occupational titles. A comprehensive survey of notarial and legal records in late medieval Marseille has similarly found a range of professional titles taken on by women, but few nameable midwives prior to an unusual court case in 1403. See Monica H. Green and Daniel Lord Smail, 'The Trial of Floreta d'Ays (1403): Jews, Christians, and Obstetrics in Later Medieval Marseille,' *Journal of Medieval History* (forthcoming).

[53] Annie Saunier, 'Le visiteur, les femmes et les ''obstetrices'' des paroisses de l'archidiaconé de Josas de 1458 à 1470', in *Santé, médecine et assistance au moyen âge, Actes du 110ᵉ Congrès National*

Mouchard's register of inspections of these parishes is remarkable for another reason. When he found that a parish had no midwife, he often ordered that the women of the parish should *elect* one.[54] This is a remarkable injunction, for it implies not only that a midwife can be 'made' by election (as opposed to years of apprenticeship) but that, like churchwardens or town officials, everyone in the predetermined group of 'citizens' (in this case, all women of the parish) are not simply empowered to chose, but also to be chosen. The issue of 'election' aside, Mouchard's search for midwives reflects the culmination of a 200 year process in France, where there was probably some combination of professionalization from within the community of women and pressure from external forces that demanded that someone serve the *function* of the midwife in the community.[55] In 1215, the Fourth Lateran Council had dictated that laypeople should be better instructed in the basic elements of the faith; one concern was that they be instructed how to perform emergency baptisms lest a newborn who died soon after birth lose its chance at eternal life. Initially, these instructions were only for laypeople (i.e., the parents), which in itself confirms that professional midwives were not normatively thought to be present at all births. Beginning in the early fourteenth century, however, midwives were singled out for special instruction and came under the scrutiny of ecclesiastical synods, bishops, and local parish priests. Perhaps the earliest legislation is a statute from the archdiocese of Paris in 1311 stipulating that every village should have a sworn midwife; not surprisingly, our earliest references to specific *matrones jurées* come from Paris about two decades later.[56] By 1365, we find instructions for

---

des Sociétés Savantes, Montpellier, 1985, Section d'histoire médiévale et de philologie, 2 vols. (Paris: Editions du C.T.H.S., 1987), 1:43–62, which identifies 116 midwives in the parishes to the south of Paris. Regarding fecundity levels, Christiane Klapisch-Zuber finds upper-class women in Florence who survived their child-bearing years carrying on average eleven pregnancies to term; see 'Le dernier enfant: fécondité et vieillissement chez les Florentines XIVe–XVe siècles', in *Mesurer et comprendre: Mélanges offerts à Jacques Dupaquier,* ed. Jean-Pierre Barder, François Lebrun, and René Le Mée (Paris: Pressed Universitaires de France, 1993), pp. 277–90. Thus, the *potential* need for midwives' services must have been great.

[54] In some cases, apparently because the parish was so small, he noted that there was no midwife but then left it at that.

[55] How much the ecclesiastically supervised appointment of midwives was replicated outside of France is not yet clear. In England, no records of ecclesiastical appointments have been found from before the 16th century. In Germanic-speaking territories, a separate process of professionalization began in the early 14th century, when municipalities began to appoint midwives to attend to the needs of poor women in their communities. This process did not, however, initially entail formal licensing of midwives generally, which did not begin until the 15th century, the first references to midwives' oaths occurring in 1417. The earliest known instance in the Low Countries is a midwives' ordinance from Brussels in 1424. In southern Europe, where no regulation has been attested prior to the 16th century, midwives remain difficult to identify well through the 15th century. See the literature cited in Green, 'Bodies'.

[56] Kathryn Taglia, 'Delivering a Christian Identity: Midwives in Northern French Synodal Legislation, *c.*1200–1500', in Peter Biller and Joseph Ziegler, eds., *Religion and Medicine in the Middle Ages*, York Studies in Medieval Theology, 3 (York: York Medieval Press, 2001), pp. 77–90; Jacquart, *Supplément*, pp. 65 and 202. Unfortunately, we do not know exactly what the midwives

diaconal visitations of parishes (such as Jean Mouchard would perform a century later) which included the task of selecting midwives and having them sent to the bishop's court where they were to take an examination (of what kind is not clear) and swear an oath; they would then obtain a certificate confirming their formal approval.[57]

The effect of the disappearance and then slow re-emergence of midwives in their relation to literate medicine is that midwives, as a profession, were cut off not only from knowledge of their predecessors but from their predecessors' texts. There is no evidence that the late antique works of Theodorus Priscianus, Caelius Aurelianus, or Muscio continued to circulate in women's hands in the early Middle Ages, nor can female ownership be documented when these works briefly took on new life from the eleventh through early thirteenth centuries. This early medieval disruption of literary tradition as it supported professional identities was, of course, true of all medical fields. But whereas the physicians in twelfth-century Salerno could take up the Hippocratic *Prognostics* and find an image of the learned physician on which they could model themselves while surgeons from Roger Frugardi on could pick up Constantine the African's and later Albucasis's surgical writings and find works that defined the scope of their field and methods of practice, there were no midwives reading ancient texts on gynaecology or obstetrics to re-create a vision of their profession.[58] Rather, the purview of the midwife's profession was defined *for* them by male literates. Lost in the process was any sense that midwifery was a literate profession or that its scope had once extended well beyond attendance at childbirth alone to encompass all of women's medicine as it related to the reproductive organs.

Writing in the 1230s in Magdeburg, the Franciscan friar and encyclopedist Bartholomew the Englishman defined a midwife as 'a woman who possesses the art of aiding a woman in birth so that [the mother] might give birth more easily and the infant might not incur any danger . . . She also receives the child as it emerges from the womb'.[59] Bartholomew's description of midwifery as an 'art' suggests that midwifery was already seen in his day as a specialized occupation, not just a relatively undifferentiated body of knowledge shared generically among women. Bartholomew did, of course, like any other well-trained cleric, have a rich tradition of biblical and canon law references to midwives to draw on, so there remains the suspicion that his is just a 'dictionary definition' rather than

were to 'swear' to; midwives' oaths from the 15th and 16th centuries have them swear to uphold good Christian morals and to provide care to poor women as well as the rich.

[57] Saunier, 'Le visiteur'.

[58] As I note in the Conclusion, female midwife writers of the early modern period would look back to classical figures or biblical midwives for precedents. Although much more professionalized in their own day, they had no knowledge of their predecessors in the late antique or medieval period.

[59] As quoted in Michel Salvat, 'L'Accouchement dans la littérature scientifique médiévale', *Senefiance* 9 (1980), 87–106, at pp. 90–1, 101.

an observation made from contemporary practices. A decade later, however, the Dominican friar Thomas of Cantimpré envisaged *obstetrices* as a category of practitioners who could actually be rounded up and given instruction from priests. I will return later to Thomas's little catechism for midwives (which he largely cribbed from Muscio), but here it is important to note that Thomas included this material precisely because he worried that competent midwives were so hard to find. In his own autograph copy of his text, he included several recipes for assisting birth that the priest could use himself when 'a midwife knowledgeable in the science of obstetrics cannot be found'.[60] Indeed, the fact that Thomas thought his spare obstetrical gleanings from Muscio's late antique text to be superior to any knowledge midwives would have gained through their own experiences says a great deal about the *perception* of midwives' knowledge in the thirteenth century. By the time midwives were re-emerging as specialist birth attendants, most aspects of *gynaecology*—theory, diagnosis, prescription of treatment for uterine conditions, menstrual dysfunctions, infertility—had already passed over into the province of male physicians. It would not be until the middle of the fifteenth century that anyone would rediscover the full text of Muscio's *Gynaecology* with its preface explaining the need for a text midwives could read and understand, and its unambiguous validating of literacy as the chief qualification of the expert midwife. The German physician who for a moment considered translating the work mused that if rendered into the vernacular, it surely would be a 'treasure to midwives'.[61]

In sum, then, there were no more social pressures pushing midwives toward literacy than there were for their sister practitioners in other fields. To the extent that we can identify individual midwives prior to the fifteenth century, they do not seem to be regularly married to men in the medical trades; in this respect, they differed from female surgeons and barbers.[62] There would be little occasion, therefore, for the increasing emphasis on literacy among general medical practitioners to 'rub off' onto midwives's own sense of professional identity. Rather, if midwives were literate, it seems to have been coincidental rather than a prerequisite of their work. Of the known husbands of French midwives, several were of a social class or engaged in professions that would have necessitated literacy. Asseline Alexandre, who attended the births of the Duchess of Burgundy in the 1370s, was married to a bourgeois of Paris.[63] Pierrette de Bouvile, who was the sworn midwife in the 1460s in the village of Arpajon (south of Paris), was married to a man who served as a churchwarden and assisted

---

[60] Thomas of Cantimpré, *Liber de natura rerum*, Bk I (Berlin: W. de Gruyter, 1973), p. 76.

[61] See Chapter 6 below on Johannes Hartlieb.

[62] Of the thirty-six French midwives identified by Jacquart, a husband's profession is known in four cases; none was a medical practitioner. In contrast, of the four female barbers whose husbands' occupations are known, all are barbers. Of the 116 midwives identified by Saunier in Jean Mouchard's registers, none was related to a medical practitioner.

[63] Jacquart, *Milieu*, p. 50.

with ecclesiastical justice and the rendering of accounts in the parish.[64] And there were no doubt some exceptional individual practitioners, such as Bourgot L'Oubliere, who served as both midwife and gardener to the French queen in the early fifteenth century, whose social situation may have made their literacy more likely.[65] Most French midwives, however, when we know anything about their background, come from artisanal families whose literacy levels were probably low, women like Catherine Lemesre in Lille, who was married to a baker, or Chandellier in Dijon who was married to a painter.

Thus, even though childbirth was a universal event throughout Europe, and even though it was clearly considered normative for a woman to have assistance from other women at birth, we cannot assume that midwives necessarily always existed as a medical *profession* that would be the obvious and automatic 'target audience' for works dealing with women's health. Aside from Trota's *Treatments for Women* (which was a training manual for women's medicine generally, not just obstetrics), midwives did not write handbooks for the instruction of other midwives as male surgeons did for other surgeons. In fact, as we will see in Chapters 4 and 6, until the composition of a mid fifteenth-century Italian text by the physician Michele Savonarola, midwives *per se* were never identified as the direct readers of any of the vernacular texts on women's medicine addressed to female audiences. It is not surprising, therefore, that no known licensing requirements demanded midwives' literacy prior to the sixteenth century.[66] The process of 'professionalizing' midwives—lifting them above the realm of common women by virtue of their specialized knowledge and skills—was slow and erratic. With no professional handbooks of their own, with no trace of guilds or formal apprenticeships, and with nobody prior to mid fifteenth century even raising the idea that midwives with books in their hands would be a good thing, it is not surprising that, in contrast to the increasing frequency of depictions of both saintly and secular women holding or reading books, there are no literary or visual depictions of midwives that allude to their literacy.[67]

The literacy of lay women

If, as I have suggested, no group of female medical practitioners, not even midwives, seems to have developed as a *specialized* audience for literate medicine, then if we are to find any women reading medical literature at all it will have to be among the general laity. Recent studies on Christian women's literacy have not only demonstrated that it was growing at a rapid pace in the high and later medieval periods, but that it was developing in particularly distinct ways. What we find is a 'typically feminine' pattern of book ownership, a pattern that shows works of individual religious instruction (Books of Hours, psalters,

---

[64] Saunier, 'Le visiteur', at p. 52.   [65] Thompson, *Paris and Its People*, p. 159.
[66] See the Conclusion below.   [67] Green, 'Books as a Source'.

breviaries, saints' lives, guides for moral living, etc.) constituting the majority of books owned by women, while romances and other bellettristic literature come in at a distant second, sometimes surpassed by historical chronicles or general encyclopedias. Ownership of medical books by women can be documented only intermittently: a mere forty-four women from the twelfth century through the beginning of the sixteenth.[68] Between Trota and Hildegard in the twelfth century, and a collection of remedies that Anne de Croy, Princess of Chimay, had compiled in 1533, only two women can be identified as medical authors: Regina Hurleweg and Anna Gremsin, both of whom seem to have compiled sizable collections of remedies in fifteenth-century Germany.[69] Other women can be identified as 'authoresses' of individual remedies, but whether they were themselves responsible for setting them into writing is unclear.[70]

The types of medical texts women owned (when, that is, their contents are not obscured behind such vague rubrics as 'livre de médecine') tend to be regimens, herbals and simple recipe collections. There seems to have been no cultivation of an ethos of women's duties that required possession of medical texts. Women who owned medical books rarely gave them as gifts or willed them to other women. Indeed, only four examples of such exchanges among women are known.[71] There is no evidence, in other words, that medical books played the same social function in constructing 'proper' feminine roles as did Books of Hours and psalters, which were frequently exchanged among women and which would be used in elementary tutoring to inculcate proper gender roles in female and male children, as well as for their more obvious function as handbooks for daily prayer.[72]

[68] These data, as well as a survey of scholarship on women's literacy up through 1999, can be found in Green, 'Possibilities'. The list published there is here modified as follows: I omit the ninth-century Theutberga (item 16) from the present count as she predates the period under discussion. The second Jeanne de Chalon (item 24) needs to be removed: Jacques Paviot, 'Les livres de Jeanne de Chalon, comtesse de Tonnerre (v. 1388–v. 1450)', in *Au cloître et dans le monde: Femmes, hommes et sociétiés (IXe–XVe siècle)*, ed. Patrick Henriet and Anne-Marie Legras (Paris: Presses de l'Université de Paris-Sorbonne, 2000), pp. 247–56, has demonstrated that the three medical books thought to have been owned by Jeanne were in fact acquired by her nephew some years after her death. Three other women should be added: Isabelle of Portugal, Duchess of Burgundy (1397–1471); Louise of Savoy (1476–1531), Duchess of Angoulême; and Anne de Beaujeu (1461–1522), Duchess of Bourbon and, for a time, regent of France.

[69] Green, 'Possibilities'.

[70] As I point out in 'Possibilities' and 'Books as a Source', the humble medical recipe might yet prove an important genre of women's composition. See also the Conclusion below.

[71] Green, 'Possibilities', Table 1, items 7–8, 19–21, and 41–42. The fourth case is Charlotte of Savoy (d. 1483) who passed on at least two of her medical books to her daughter Anne de Beaujeu. We also have a case of a medical text apparently commissioned by a woman for her daughter: a treatise on the virtues of rosemary said to have been prepared in 1338 at the behest of Jeanne of Valois for Philippa of Hainault; see Green, 'Possibilities', p. 65. As I will suggest below, moreover, I suspect that there was a small 'exchange market' of texts on women's medicine that is not attested in the present data on ownership.

[72] Sandra Penketh, 'Women and Books of Hours', in Jane H. M. Taylor and Lesley Smith, eds., *Women and the Book: Assessing the Visual Evidence* (London: British Library, 1997), pp. 266–80. For

Wealth and social status were the great dividers among female literates, but their common gender increasingly united them in terms of the languages they commanded. None of the causes of increased female literacy in the High Middle Ages altered the inaccessibility of Latin, which since at least the eighth century had been a learned tongue that required years of formal training. Whereas literacy in Latin had been more or less equitable between men and women up through the twelfth century (for the simple fact that, aside from Old English, it was functionally the only written language with its own corpus of texts), after the twelfth century the gender differential became more pronounced.[73] Training in Latin has been called a male puberty rite, a term which aptly captures the ways in which grammar school training (and, for adolescent males after the twelfth century, university education or professional training in notarial schools and royal chanceries) socialized boys *as boys*.[74] Women's near universal exclusion from grammar schools, and their total exclusion from the universities meant that they had no *formal* route to obtain an identical Latinate education as boys.

When the *Trotula* texts were composed in twelfth-century southern Italy, Latin was still the only language that most people, if literate, would be 'literate' in. The vernacular languages, both Romance and Germanic, were just beginning to develop a corpus of literary texts and there was very little in any vernacular tradition, aside from Anglo-Saxon, on medical topics. We have already seen, of course, that *Treatments for Women* and perhaps *Conditions of Women* assumed female audiences in their earliest Latin versions. Unfortunately, whatever copies there were in the twelfth century have been lost.[75] Of the thirteenth-century Latin manuscripts, the majority (as we saw in Chapter 2) were owned by men or suggest use by readers associated with the universities, religious institutions, or professionalized medical practice. There are three manuscripts, however, that do not fit the patterns of masculine use. Two of them are copies of the standardized ensemble, the most well-developed and 'polished' version of the *Trotula* ensemble. Although this version of the text is the one most closely

a parallel study from southern Europe, see Judith Bryce, 'Les Livres des Florentines: Reconsidering Women's Literacy in Quattrocento Florence', in *At the Margins: Minority Groups in Premodern Italy*, ed. Stephen J. Milner (Minneapolis: University of Minnesota Press, 2005), pp. 133–61.

[73] Although some evidence exists of nuns using Anglo-Saxon for medical recipes (Green, 'Books as a Source'), women were not the normative audience for Anglo-Saxon medical texts. R. A. Buck, 'Women and Language in the Anglo-Saxon Leechbooks', *Women and Language* 23, 2 (Fall 2000), 41–50, argues that the female patient is mostly spoken about rather than spoken to.

[74] Walter Ong, 'Latin Language Study as a Renaissance Puberty Rite', *Studies in Philology* 56 (1959), 103–24; Marjorie Curry Woods, 'Rape and the Pedagogical Rhetoric of Sexual Violence', in Rita Copeland (ed.), *Criticism and Dissent in the Middle Ages* (Cambridge: Cambridge University Press, 1996), pp. 56–86.

[75] The earliest extant copy of *Conditions of Women 1* dates from the 14th century; the earliest of *Treatments for Women 1* and *2* date from the 13th century. As is often the case in manuscript transmission, 'later' versions of the texts (in this case, the proto-ensemble, whose earliest copy dates from the end of the 12th century) are found in the earliest extant manuscripts.

associated with university circles, these two copies resist such categorization. One, now in Glasgow, is physically the smallest of all the extant manuscripts of the text, measuring less than six by four inches. If anything, it more resembles the Books of Hours that women were associated with than the larger compendia of practical or theoretical texts in which we usually find the *Trotula* embedded. Moreover, it is found here with only one other text: a brief work on helpful or harmful foods, a work that could be used quite easily by a layperson to regulate their diet. The one other copy of the *Trotula* that shares the Glasgow manuscript's distinctive readings is now in Poland; here, the *Trotula* appears as the only text in a small pamphlet, a presentation as unusual in its isolation as the Glasgow copy is in its size.[76] Were women the original owners of these two copies of the text? There is nothing to prove it, but the possibility is intriguing.

The third anomalous Latin manuscript, likewise in an unusually small pamphlet, is a late thirteenth-century copy of *Women's Cosmetics 3*, a version that altered the text so that it could speak directly to a female reader/user.[77] The text is presented here with a copy of Pietro d'Abano's 1295 treatise on physiognomy, which is itself highly unusual in being the first physiognomic text to elaborate systematically on female as well as male characteristics (previous writers having focused primarily on men). In fact, any sort of pairing of cosmetics and physiognomy is unusual, which suggests that the combination of these two texts may have had some appeal to a female reader interested not only in understanding the artifice of beauty but also in interpreting the signs of character that external bodily features betray.[78] While hardly offering conclusive proof, the codicological character of these three manuscripts falls far enough outside the normative patterns of masculine reading to raise the possibility that a few women may, on occasion, have been among the direct readers of the Latin *Trotula*.[79]

[76] Two copies of the standardized ensemble—Glasgow, Glasgow University Library, MS Hunter 341 (U.8.9.), *c.*1270–1320 (N. France), pp. 1–70, and Wrocław (Breslau), Biblioteka Uniwersytecka, MS 2022 (*olim* R 291; I F 184), s. xiii², (Germany), ff. 153ra–164ra have approximately 150 readings that they share with none of the seven other contemporary copies of the text. See the apparatus to Green, *Trotula*, passim.

[77] BNF, MS lat. 16089, s. xiii ex. This is in fact the only copy of *Women's Cosmetics 3* that maintains the *tu* references consistently. The others tend to revert back to an assumption that a practitioner who is not the direct user of the cosmetics is the reader. On this version of the text, see Green, 'Development', pp. 142–3.

[78] The same pairing of Pietro's physiognomic text with a cosmetic text (perhaps this same version of the Salernitan *Women's Cosmetics*) seems also to be found in a now lost manuscript that had been owned by Amplonius Ratinck in Erfurt in the 14th century (see Appendix 1, item 56). On Pietro's text, see Walton O. Schalick, 'The Face Behind the Mask: 13th- and 14th-Century European Medical Cosmetology and Physiognomy', in *Medicine and the History of the Body: Proceedings of the 20th, 21st and 22nd International Symposium on the Comparative History of Medicine, East and West*, ed. Yasuo Otsuka, Shizu Sakai, and Shigehisa Kuriyama (Tokyo: Ishiyaku EuroAmerica, 1999), pp. 295–312. Schalick finds that there is little interplay between cosmetic and physiognomic literatures, making the pairing of these two texts all the more significant.

[79] Aside from the three manuscripts being discussed here, the Latin *Trotula* appears as the sole text in only one other copy: Hamburg, Staats- und Universitätsbibliothek, Cod. med. 798,

The end of the thirteenth century represents the approximate point at which Latin ceased to be a language in which most literate women felt comfortable. The only female authors in Latin after 1300 are such religious figures as Angela of Foligno, Catherine of Siena, and Birgitta of Sweden, whose revelations or letters were *dictated in the vernacular* and then rendered into Latin by their scribe/confessors.[80] We may assume that the female booksellers who supplied books to students and faculty of the University of Paris in the thirteenth and fourteenth centuries were more than minimally literate in Latin, and women throughout Europe continued to read some Latin in their prayerbooks.[81] But for both the bourgeoisie and more privileged lay and religious women, the late medieval period saw more and more movement away from Latin toward the vernacular, to the point that by the fifteenth century even nuns who were expected to know the liturgy could often not properly recite it in Latin.[82] Indeed, the general assumption that women could not read Latin (or could not understand it even if they could read it) becomes a common rhetorical justification for translating.[83] For most

s. xv¹ (Germany), pp. 23–79, where it would soon be bound together with a copy of the Latin pseudo-Albertus Magnus, *Secreta mulierum*, and a Dutch translation of the *Trotula*.

[80] Ulrike Wiethaus, 'Street Mysticism: An Introduction to *The Life and Revelations* of Agnes Blannbekin', in *Women Writing Latin from Roman Antiquity to Early Modern Europe*, vol. 2: *Medieval Women Writing Latin*, ed. Laurie J. Churchill, Phyllis R. Brown, and Jane E. Jeffrey (New York: Routledge, 2002), pp. 281–307.

[81] Mary A. Rouse and Richard H. Rouse, 'The Book Trade at the University of Paris, *c.*1250-*c.* 1350', in Rouse and Rouse, *Authentic Witnesses: Approaches to Medieval Texts and Manuscripts* (Notre Dame, Indiana: University of Notre Dame Press, 1991), pp. 259–338; Marjorie Curry Woods, 'Shared Books, Primers, Psalters, and the Adult Acquisition of Literacy among Devout Laywomen and Women in Orders in Late Medieval England', in *New Trends in Feminine Spirituality: The Holy Women of Liège and Their Impact*, ed. Juliette Dor, Lesley Johnson, and Jocelyn Wogan-Browne, Medieval Women: Texts and Contexts, 2 (Turnhout: Brepols, 1999), pp. 177–93.

[82] See Penelope D. Johnson, *Equal in Monastic Profession: Religious Women in Medieval France* (Chicago: University of Chicago Press, 1991), pp. 146–7. See also Jeanne Krochalis, 'The Benedictine Rule for Nuns: Library of Congress, MS 4', *Manuscripta* 30 (1986), 21–34, regarding an English translation of the *Rule* made, perhaps, by a nun, but from a French rather than a Latin original. The late 15th-century rule for the nuns of St Agnes in Freiburg mentions the presence of Latin books, but these seem to be for the use of the priest who ministers to the nuns. See Karl Christ, 'Mittelalterliche Bibliotheksordnungen für Frauenklöster', *Zentralblatt für Bibliothekswesen* 59, nos. 1/2 (Jan./Feb. 1942), 1–29, esp. p. 25. For the use of German instead of Latin in nuns' correspondence, see Debra L. Stoudt, 'The Production and Preservation of Letters by Fourteenth-Century Dominican Nuns', *Mediaeval Studies* 53 (1991), 309–26. For the use of Italian, see Katherine Gill, 'Women and the Production of Religious Literature in the Vernacular, 1300–1500', in *Creative Women in Medieval and Early Modern Italy*, ed. E. Ann Matter and John Coakley (Philadelphia: University of Pennsylvania Press, 1994), 64–104.

[83] Jocelyn Wogan-Browne, Nicholas Watson, Andrew Taylor, and Ruth Evans, eds., *The Idea of the Vernacular: An Anthology of Middle English Literary Theory, 1280–1520* (University Park, PA: Pennsylvania State University Press, 1999), pp. 120–22; Katherine Zieman, 'Reading, Singing and Understanding: Constructions of the Literacy of Women Religious in Late Medieval England', in *Learning and Literacy in Medieval England and Abroad*, ed. Sarah Rees Jones (Turnhout: Brepols, 2003), 97–120.

women, therefore, the Latin–vernacular gulf was very real, with the result that works written in the vernacular were more likely to meet the needs of a female audience.

Finally, we should remember that even when rendered into the vernacular, medical texts did not automatically become accessible to readers. Often emulating the learning of the universities, their use may have required induction into the logical systems that underpinned their modes of explanation. Thus, for example, when the physicians and surgeons of Paris were examining Perretta Petone in 1410, they asked her whether celery and hyssop were hot or cold.[84] Perretta's French book, 'full of many good remedies' (*bon contenues plusieurs beaux remedes*) though it was, was probably nothing more than a simple collection of recipes that never explained *why* celery or hyssop or any other substances worked the way they did. Whether for reasons of cost, social access, or intelligibility, the sizable corpus of French medical literature that existed in early fifteenth-century Paris was inaccessible to her. I will return to the topic of vernacularization and its effects on the gendering of women's medicine in the next chapter. Before moving away from Latin, however, we need also to explore ways women might get access to Latin learning other than by reading it.

WOMEN AS HEARERS: PASTORAL CONCERNS AND THE ATTENTIVE MIDWIFE

In Heinrich von dem Türlin's early thirteenth-century tale *The Crown*, the fictitious Queen Ginover asserted her disbelief of 'that which I have often heard read' from a book of medical theory.[85] The particular theory that concerned her had been the allegedly colder nature of women vs. men, a central element of medieval theories of sexual difference that had opened *Conditions of Women*. As we will see later, evidence for women's reactions to the content of medical and scientific lore on the female body is extraordinarily rare. But what concerns us here is not the content of these views but the manner in which Ginover is said to have encountered them: she *heard* them being read.

As with Queen Ginover, a possible scenario for the transmission of the lore embodied in the Latin *Trotula* and other gynaecological texts was not

---

[84] Laurent Garrigues, 'Les Professions médicales à Paris au début du XVe siècle: Praticiens en procès au parlement', *Bibliothèque de l'École des Chartes* 156 (1998), 317–67, at p. 342. Perretta said incorrectly that celery was cold, and that hyssop was sometimes hot, sometimes cold. The *Circa instans*, the leading herbal authority, identified both as hot and dry in the third degree; see Hans Wölfel, *Das Arzneidrogenbuch 'Circa instans' in einer Fassung des XIII. Jahrhunderts aus der Universitätsbibliothek Erlangen. Text und Kommentar als Beitrag zur Pflanzen- und Drogenkunde des Mittelalters* (Berlin: A. Preilipper, 1939), pp. 8–9 (*apium*) and 62 (*ysopus*).

[85] Heinrich von dem Türlin, *The Crown: A Tale of Sir Gawein and King Arthur's Court*, trans. J. W. Thomas (Lincoln, Neb. and London: University of Nebraska Press, 1989), p. 40.

women's direct reading of the texts but oral transmission by men who could more readily deal with the Latin and who would, presumably, have offered this knowledge to women via extemporaneous translation into the vernacular. Unlike the present-day West, where most reading is done individually and silently, well into the later Middle Ages reading was often an aural, communal activity.[86] Reading aloud to groups of women (or mixed groups of men and women) is well documented from literary sources.[87] Moreover, although we think of the twelfth century as a great age of women's Latin literacy—from religious women like Heloise, Hildegard, and Herrad of Landsberg to secular women like Adela of Blois and Ermengard of Narbonne—recent researches suggest that even at this point women's relationship to Latin learning was often not direct but relied on instruction by a Latinate male.[88] Two texts from the mid thirteenth century suggest how this scenario might have been played out for medicine.

First is a Latin verse rendition of the *Trotula* texts made, perhaps, in England or France. Part of a series of versified texts which, taken together, form a general surgical compendium, the two tracts on, respectively, women's diseases and cosmetics are followed by a four-book tract on surgery and a final section on medical etiquette and theory.[89] The *Trotula* texts, like the four surgical sections, were written with second-person references addressed to the *lector*, the reader, and were undoubtedly intended primarily for male surgeons or physicians literate enough to appreciate the cadences of the Latin verse. Women are involved only as a secondary, aural audience. Echoing the preface to *Conditions of Women* but turning its traditional topos of women's shame in a new direction, the first poem declared its purpose:

And because a great multitude of diseases very often afflict the womb, hence it is opportune (since there is very often necessity) and decent (since women are ashamed to speak openly to a male physician [*medico*]) that there be a treatise to show to matrons, from which,

---

[86] Paul Saenger, *Space between Words: The Origins of Silent Reading* (Stanford: Stanford University Press, 1997); Joyce Coleman, *Public Reading and the Reading Public in Late Medieval England and France* (Cambridge: Cambridge University Press, 1996).

[87] Coleman, *Public Reading*.

[88] See, for example, Morgan Powell, 'The *Speculum virginum* and the Audio-Visual Poetics of Women's Religious Instruction', in *Listen Daughter: The 'Speculum virginum' and the Formation of Religious Women in the Middle Ages*, ed. Constant J. Mews (New York: Palgrave, 2001), pp. 111–36, esp. pp. 131–2, who documents how the widely circulating Latin *Mirror of Virgins*, a guide to monastic life for women, was owned primarily by male clerics in order to guide women in their profession. He plausibly speculates that instruction would be given by extemporaneous translation into the vernacular.

[89] *Liber de secretis mulierum*, in BNF, MS lat. 8161A, s. xiii med. (England), ed. Charles Daremberg in *Collectio Salernitana ossia documenti inediti, e trattati di medicina appartenenti alla scuola medica salernitana*, ed. Salvatore De Renzi, 5 vols. (Naples: Filiatre-Sebezio, 1852–59; repr. Bologna: Forni, 1967), 4:1–38. Although the editor identifies the separate sections as seven 'books' of a single treatise, in the manuscript itself only the four sections on surgery are grouped as a coherent, numbered unit.

these matters having been heard (*talibus auditis*), they would be able to determine what the remedy for their health is.[90]

Women, then, are expected not to be the readers of this text but its auditors. The author of this Latin verse *Trotula* surely had in mind lay women in general when s/he spoke of 'matrons' and imagined that they would be treating their own gynaecological disorders. Even so, one has to wonder how effectively the contents of this text could be conveyed to women. The fact that only one copy survives is not much evidence of its success.

A second text composed around the same time shows that it was not only physicians or surgeons who took it upon themselves to instruct women. Sometime before 1244, the Dominican friar Thomas of Cantimpré, by then the subprior of the Dominican house in Leuven, completed his massive encyclopedia of Christian knowledge, *On the Nature of Things*. The first book covered human anatomy and, after examining the process of conception and the development of the embryo, Thomas included a summary of obstetrical procedures derived ultimately from Muscio's *Gynaecology*. There are two significant elements in Thomas's choices in presenting this material, both of which show his sense that if textual communities among midwives did not yet exist, they should. First, he presented these instructions as being the teachings of Cleopatra, a 'physician of queens' (*medica reginarum*), to her daughter. This was not sheer invention. Thomas was not using Muscio's original *Gynaecology* but rather an abbreviated version, the *Non omnes quidem*, that had circulated since the eleventh century as the third in a sequence of three texts whose opening section was the *Gynaecology of Cleopatra*. By deliberately linking the introductory prologue about this *medica reginarum* and her daughter with the obstetrical sections from Muscio, Thomas showed how important it was for him to lay claim to a feminine source.[91]

Having situated two female characters with a suitable mistress–apprentice relationship into his 'frame' of the text, however, Thomas then somewhat surprisingly initiated a rhetoric of female practitioners' ignorance that, like Bruno's, was to have echoes for centuries to come. Twice, both in introducing the excerpt and concluding it, Thomas explained why he had included it:

Also in birth it ought to be noted that if the child comes to the gate [i.e., the birth canal] before birth so disposed that it lies on its side or its back, or it puts forth its feet below and its head above, then it is born with difficulty and with effort and danger to both its mother and itself. Midwives are able to deal with this danger, at least those who are experienced. But alas! Few are to be found, and hence many children are miscarried and are unable to be born alive, and consequently are not reborn to [eternal] glory.

---

[90] *Liber de secretis mulierum*, ed. Daremberg, vol. 4, p. 1 (my emphasis). Similarly, the second section claimed to teach the art of cosmetics to whomever was dissatisfied with their appearance, 'especially women' (*ibid.*, p. 25).

[91] On the use of female authorship for strategic purposes, see also Chapter 5 below.

And again:

These things we have diligently added to our book because of the danger of miscarriages and the ignorance of midwives. And we hope, as do all those who ought
to counsel souls subject to free will, that by this art [of obstetrics] they might also
counsel as much as they can those who in regard to their own judgement and power
of will are least able to help themselves, that they might be able to avoid eternal
darkness. We urge, therefore, and we wish that they call together some more discreet
midwives and instruct them privately, and through them others might more easily be
instructed.[92]

Thomas's concern for the 'care of souls' and the need to educate midwives
was no idiosyncratic idea. As we have seen, by the thirteenth century, secular
clergy had increasing obligations to instruct those who might need to perform
an emergency baptism on a newborn baby. Concern with the infant's soul went
so far as to demand that if the pregnant woman died in labour or through some
other cause, the foetus was to be removed by surgical excision.[93] Moreover,
although clearly concerned with baptism, Thomas's focus on midwives may also
have come from his unusual involvement in the pastoral care of women and his
awareness of the plight of poor birthing women.[94] In his early years, prior to his
conversion to the Dominican order, Thomas had been a student and colleague
of Jacques de Vitry, an ardent advocate of both the beguines and the hospital
movement. Jacques himself did not discuss this, but one feature common to
many hospitals was the allowance that they could take in poor, pregnant women
and accommodate them not only for the birth itself but also for the subsequent
lying-in period.[95] As noted above, we have no indication that any of these
institutions employed women formally designated as 'midwives', but it may well
be that Thomas recognized that preachers had the opportunity to select out of
the undifferentiated women who assisted at births those 'most discerning' and
capable of being educated.[96]

[92] Thomas de Cantimpré, *Liber de natura rerum*, ed. H. Boese, vol. 1 (Berlin/New York: Walter
de Gruyter, 1973), Book I, cap. 76, pp. 75–6.

[93] Although recommendations for surgical extraction of the foetus can be traced back at least to
the early 11th century, the level of pastoral concern seems to have risen markedly after Lateran IV
in 1215. On Caesarean section, see Chapter 2 above.

[94] Thomas wrote or co-wrote four lives of holy women, more than any other medieval writer.
Intriguingly, he seems to been particularly perceptive to the pain and dangers of childbirth: his most
common metaphor to describe someone in intense pain is to liken their cries to a woman labouring
in birth.

[95] For example, one of the hospitals that Jacques singled out for praise was Sancto Spirito of
Sassia, just outside Rome. Its *Rule* stipulated that care be extended to poor pregnant women;
Patrologia latina 217, 1129–58, at col. 1146A. Simons, *City of Ladies*, p. 78, notes that beguines
were specifically prohibited from assisting at births, legislation which itself suggests that they were
doing precisely that.

[96] In contrast to later French instructions that parish midwives are to be elected by the women
of the parish, Thomas grants the priest that power of selection.

Thomas's *Nature of Things* became an extraordinarily popular work: there are dozens of Latin manuscripts, plus translations into Dutch and German.[97] The obstetrical instructions were excerpted from his encyclopedia and circulated both independently in Dutch and as an embedded addition to a Dutch translation of the pseudo-Albertus, *Secrets of Women*, a peculiar natural-philosophical compendium on generation composed in Latin toward the end of the thirteenth century. The Dutch *Secrets*, made in the first half of the fourteenth century, was in turn translated into French, and from French into Italian.[98] In the *Secrets* text, Thomas's loose catechistic 'frame' of a mother's instructions to her daughter midwife was transposed into a direct second-person speech that the mother gave to her daughter; the male reader could in turn simply recite this off the page to any listening midwife.[99] In the French and Italian translations, the *Secrets* text tended to be owned by surgeons and physicians, and even in the Low Countries it is evident that surgeons were particularly interested in the obstetrical lore: a Dutch translator of Lanfranc's Latin *Surgery*, which (as we saw in Chapter 2) had radically expanded the conceptualization of female physiology and disease as it related to surgery, turned to the Dutch *Secrets of Women* precisely for the additional information it provided on obstetrics.[100]

Thomas's precepts clearly served, then, to inform not only priests and confessors but also surgeons about matters they, at some level, were responsible for supervising. Yet we should not fail to note the profound irony in the popularity of these translations of an abbreviation (of an abbreviation) of

[97] There was also a translation into French, but not of the book which included this obstetrical section.

[98] On the circulation of the *Liber de natura rerum*, see Thomas Kaeppeli and E. Panella, *Scriptores Ordinis Praedicatoris Medii Aevi*, Bd. 4 (Rome: S. Sabina, 1993), pp. 344–55; and Christian Hünemörder and Kurt Ruh, 'Thomas von Cantimpré OP', in *Die deutsche Literatur des Mittelalters: Verfasserlexikon*, rev. ed., ed. Kurt Ruh *et al.*, 10 vols. (Berlin: De Gruyter, 1978–1999), vol. 9 (1995), coll. 838–51. For the independent transmission of Thomas's obstetrical instructions in Dutch, see Monica H. Green, 'Medieval Gynecological Texts: A Handlist', in Green, *Women's Healthcare*, Appendix, pp. 1–36, at p. 33; for the Dutch, French, and Italian translations of the *Secrets of Women* where Thomas's text is embedded, see Green, 'Traittié', p. 151 and *passim*.

[99] In Glasgow, University Library, MS Ferguson 241, s. xv in. (France), f. 69v, the passage begins: 'On puet aidier a vne femme a l'enfanter pour les merres et enfans garantir. Et adce pueent a sagir et a prendre les sages dames sy comme Allex Patrix [a corruption of 'Cleopatra'] qui fut la plus sage dame du monde de medechine. Et aussy a prist de che mestier a sa fille en disant ainsy: "Entre vous femmes quant l'enfantement appert ne soies mie honteuse. Car il touche a vous vies. Quant vne femme est trop grosse et trop chargie de char et de craisse ou que sa porte est trop estroitte ou entortillie dedens, c'est grant peril a l'enfanter. Aussy quant la teste est trop grosse ou que l'enfant vient deuant la porte tout mort crosu et contrefait. Ch'est grant peril entre vous sages dames. Escoutes et aprenes vne doctrine profitable quant l'enfant appert a la porte par la teste."'

[100] Joris Reynaert, '*Der vrouwen heimelijcheit* als secundaire bron in de Zuid-Nederlandse bewerking van de *Chirurgia Magna* van Lanfranc van Milaan', in *Verslagen en Mededelingen van de Koninklijke academie voor Nederlandse Taal- en Letterkunde* 111, no. 1 (2001), 165–188.

Muscio's obstetrics.[101] Now completely divorced from the original context where these spare instructions for correcting foetal malpresentations had been eludicated by a rich explanatory framework of general anatomy, physiology, and pathological theory, neither priests nor surgeons could have been aware that they were passing back to midwives teachings that had been meant originally for midwives to read for themselves.

WOMEN AS VIEWERS: TEACHING BY SHOWING?

We know that many of the most luxuriously illustrated psalters, Books of Hours, and even volumes of romance from later medieval Europe were produced for women, and we have a much better understanding now of how text and image could work together dynamically to allow 'double readings'—textual and visual—both subtle and literal.[102] Images clearly often served as pedagogic supplements to texts that were actually read *to* women by men. Already in the twelfth century, for example, the first medieval treatise devoted to the female monastic life, the *Mirror of Virgins*, was composed—and clearly came to function—with precisely this gendered scenario of use in mind. All but one of the Latin manuscripts have (or were intended to have) the cycle of illustrations meant to show how contemplation of vice and virtue could lead to spiritual purity; these Latin manuscripts were owned primarily by men or male religious houses and were apparently meant to be *read by men* who would then use the accompanying images to instruct women. Only when the text was translated into the vernacular and came to be used for *private* reading by women did the illustration cycles drop out of the manuscripts.[103]

That images could also be used to educate women about medicine seems possible, but such does not seem to have been the case. Childbirth, for example, was a commonly illustrated theme in medieval manuscript books: works such as illustrated Bibles in various languages show highly detailed scenes depicting the births of, say, John the Baptist or the Virgin Mary; French histories depict the birth of Julius Gaius Caesar by Caesarean section; household objects in northern Italy offer a variety of scenes of childbirth in order to enhance the reproductive

---

[101] The Latin obstetrical instructions from the Muscian *Non omnes quidem* also circulated in England under the English title 'A proscesse for women that ben in trauel of childryn and how the mydwyffe shal do helpe'; OBL, MS Bodley 591 (SC 2363), ff. 107v–109r. This is followed by obstetrical excerpts from Petrus Hispanus's Latin *Thesaurus pauperum*, then more charms and recipes in English for the same.

[102] Michael Camille, 'Seeing and Reading: Some Visual Implications of Medieval Literacy and Illiteracy', *Art History* 8 (1985), 26–49.

[103] Morgan Powell, 'The Mirror and the Woman: Instruction for Religious Women and the Emergence of Vernacular Poetics, 1120–1250', PhD dissertation, Princeton University, 1997, esp. chapter 2.

success of patrician women.[104] But these scenes, aside from the 'Caesarean' images, almost never depict the height of labour or any medically specific information. To the extent that such images were 'educational', it was primarily to instruct women in the virtues of fertility and the importance of lineage.[105] Gynaecological literature, for its part, whether in Latin or the vernacular, was decidedly impoverished in visual imagery.

That had not always been the case. The late antique author Muscio had conceived of his *Gynaecology* as an illustrated text: it was to have an image of the uterus, identifying all its major parts, and a sequence of foetus-in-utero figures, originally fifteen in number, to show both the normal presentation of the foetus (head-first) and the several abnormal presentations that automatically demanded the intervention of the midwife. Although Muscio had said that the uterine image was included 'so that each part might be known and its furthest limits can be easily understood',[106] he did not explicitly say why the foetal images were important other than to speak about 'positions' (*schemata*) in which the foetus might be found. He certainly never implies that they were included to make up for any literacy deficiencies in his audience (he had, after all, listed literacy as the first and most important requirement of the midwife), and there is no indication that other parts of the text that might have benefited from illustrations (such as the detailed description on embryotomy) had ever been illustrated. Nevertheless, the foetal images proved their own attraction and began to circulate independently of the full *Gynaecology* in the thirteenth century.[107]

Their re-uses give a sense of the changing audiences for obstetrical information, for like the rest of the late-antique inheritance of gynaecological literature the foetal images survived because they passed through male hands. One case is an unusual manuscript produced in France in the middle decades of the thirteenth century. This situates a compendium of five gynaecological texts (including two different versions of the *Trotula*) amid various twelfth- and

---

[104] See, for example, the exquisite birth scenes reproduced from a 15th-century German Bible in Britta-Juliane Kruse, *Verborgene Heilkünste: Geschichte der Frauenmedizin im Spätmittelalter*, Quellen und Forschungen zur Literatur- und Kulturgeschichte, 5 (Berlin: Walter de Gruyter, 1996). For depictions of Caesar's birth, see Renate Blumenfeld-Kosinski, *Not of Woman Born: Representations of Caesarean Birth in Medieval and Renaissance Culture* (Ithaca, NY: Cornell University Press, 1990). For Italian household objects, see Jacqueline Marie Musacchio, *The Art and Ritual of Childbirth in Renaissance Italy* (New Haven and London: Yale University Press, 1999).

[105] Elizabeth L'Estrange, *Holy Motherhood: Gender, Dynasty, and Visual Culture in the Later Middle Ages* (Manchester: Manchester University Press, 2008).

[106] [Muscio], *Sorani Gynaeciorum vetus translatio latina*, ed. Valentin Rose (Leipzig: Teubner, 1882), p. 8.

[107] For a general overview of the circulation of Muscio, see Ann Ellis Hanson and Monica H. Green, 'Soranus of Ephesus: *Methodicorum princeps*', in Wolfgang Haase and Hildegard Temporini, general editors, *Aufstieg und Niedergang der römischen Welt*, Teilband II, Band 37.2 (Berlin and New York: Walter de Gruyter, 1994), pp. 968–1075. The depiction of the uterus is known in only two manuscripts, one from the 9th century, the other from the early 13th.

early thirteenth-century texts on surgery and general medicine.[108] Clearly, this compiler's interests in women's medical conditions were intense: there are more marginal addenda alongside the gynaecological chapters of Richard the Englishman's *Practica*, for example, than any other part of that text. Included in the lower margins of several pages of the pseudo-Cleopatra text are the Muscian foetal illustrations. Another instance of the recycling of the images is a Hebrew manuscript from the late fourteenth or early fifteenth century that situates the images next to a chapter on difficult birth apparently extracted from a larger Hebrew medical compendium.[109]

Could such illustrations, embedded within these thick volumes of Latin or Hebrew texts, really have found their way into the hands of midwives? It seems unlikely. Rather, these manuscripts, and most of the other re-uses of the Muscian images from the thirteenth through fifteenth centuries, suggest the co-optation of the Muscian material for professional male practitioners. This is how the illustrations were being used in late thirteenth century northern Italy when they were incorporated into copies of Albucasis's Latin *Surgery*, and this is how the illustrations were still being used in fifteenth-century England when they were copied into an extraordinary scroll containing the Latin surgical writings of John Arderne.[110] We also find them incorporated into the handbooks of physicians, from an early fifteenth-century Venetian physician of rather modest importance to the personal physician to the Holy Roman Empress, Eleanor of Portugal, who made his own copy of the *Gynaecology of Cleopatra* together with the foetal images in 1457–8.[111] Perhaps we can imagine that the surgeons or physicians who owned these manuscripts showed the birth images to midwives with whom they worked. The same English manuscript with various scenes of male and female surgeons, for example, includes a depiction of two female birth attendants assisting a woman in the throes of labour, followed by the Muscian foetus-in-utero sequence (Fig. 3.4).[112] The only clear case of the images moving directly into women's hands comes a few decades later when an English compiler incorporated the illustrations, together with the description of foetal malpresentations from the *Non omnes quidem*, into his reworking of an already-Englished gynaecological

---

[108] BNF, MS lat. 7056, s. xiii med. (England or N. France); see Green, 'Handlist I', p. 165.

[109] Ron Barkaï, 'A Medieval Hebrew Treatise on Obstetrics', *Medical History* 33 (1989), 96–119.

[110] On the recycling of the images in manuscripts of Albucasis's *Surgery*, see Chapter 2 above. The scroll is Stockholm, Kungliga Biblioteket, MS X.118, *c.*1425–35. This manuscript, whose text is entirely in Latin, has been tentatively, though to my mind unpersuasively, connected with Philippa de Bohun (d. 1430), who married the king of Denmark, Sweden and Norway in 1406; her date of death alone would make impossible any connection to this manuscript if its composition can be placed, according to Kathleen Scott, as late as 1435. See Scott, *Later Gothic Manuscripts*, vol. 1, plates 261–2; vol. 2, cat. no. 66, pp. 197–9.

[111] Respectively, Montpellier, Bibliothèque de la Faculté de médecine, MS H 277, s. xv in. (Italy, perhaps Venice), owned by an as yet unidentified Venetian physician who was active at least through 1431; and Dresden, Sächsische Landesbibliothek, cod. lat. P.34 (N. 78), an. 1457–58 (copied by physician Hermann Heyms, fl. 1427–72).

[112] OBL, MS Laud misc. 724, s. xv (England), f. 97r.

text, the *Sickness of Women*. This new text, ostensibly addressed to a female audience, would soon be co-opted by surgeons for their own purposes but it did, at least momentarily, put the Muscian foetal images back into the hands of women.[113]

Besides the Muscian images, there were two other illustrative traditions depicting the anatomy and diseases of the female body, neither of which necessarily functioned to teach gynaecology to the marginally literate. One, an abstract diagram of the female genitalia (Fig. 3.5, lower right side), had circulated since at least the twelfth century in the company of several other anatomical diagrams yet is found with gynaecological and obstetrical material only in two manuscripts.[114] The other image is the 'disease woman', a full-length female figure created originally out of a modified 'muscle man' anatomical figure with her belly opened to show the internal genitalia (Fig. 3.6). Although found initially in a thirteenth-century anatomical manuscript from southern France, the figure only became popular in the fifteenth century when labels for various diseases were added. The labels were further expanded with brief bits of text explaining such gynaecological conditions as disorders of the breasts, the causes of infertility, and menstrual irregularity. In essence, the image generated its own text. Of the dozen extant witnesses of the 'disease woman', most situate it in medical or surgical codices (often along with a 'wound man' depicting the various kinds of injuries the human body is subject to, and a 'venesection man' depicting the sites of veins for bloodletting).[115] The 'disease woman' might also be appropriated by clerics. Martin von Geismar (d. 1450), for example, a canon who received his master of arts degree from Erfurt and a licentiate in canon law from Heidelberg, owned a manuscript with the *Trotula*, among other things. On the inside front cover, a fully labelled 'disease woman' is sketched in.[116] Another appearance of the 'disease woman' in a clerical context is in a copy made *c.*1500 of Thomas of Cantimpré's Latin *On the Nature of Things*.[117] For clerics like von Geismar,'

---

[113] I discuss the Middle English *Sickness of Women 2* at greater length in Chapter 4 below. See also Chapter 6 for the re-use of the Muscian images in Eucharius Rösslin's *Rosegarden for Pregnant Women and Midwives*.

[114] Only three extant mss present the female genitalia, the latter two incorporating it with other gynaecological texts: (1) Cambridge, Gonville and Caius College, MS 190/233, s. xii/xiii (England?); (2) OBL, MS Ashmole 399, an. 1298 (England); and (3) LWL, MS 49, *c.*1420 (Germany). The image from the Ashmole ms is reproduced as the frontispiece in Green, *Women's Healthcare*. A fourth manuscript, Pisa, Biblioteca Universitaria, MS Roncioni 99, s. xiv[1] (Italy), presents the male genitalia but not the female.

[115] No thorough study of the 'disease woman' tradition has yet been done. My analyses have located twelve extant copies, of which the earliest is Basel, Öffentliche Universitätsbibliothek, MS D.II.11, s. xiii (S. France), f. 170v.

[116] Kassel, Stadt- und Landesbibliothek, 2° Ms. med. 7, *c.*1435 (Germany). The 'disease woman' figure is reproduced in Monica H. Green, 'Gynäkologische und geburtshilfliche Illustrationen in mittelalterlichen Manuskripten: Sprechende Bilder halfen den Frauen', *Die Waage* 30, no. 4 (1991), 161–7. For more on Geismar, see Chapter 5 below.

[117] Bruges, Bibliothèque de la Ville [= Brugge, Openbare Bibliotheek], MS 411, *c.*1500, f. 259r. This very roughly drawn image is reproduced in Ginger Lee Guardiola, 'Within and Without: The

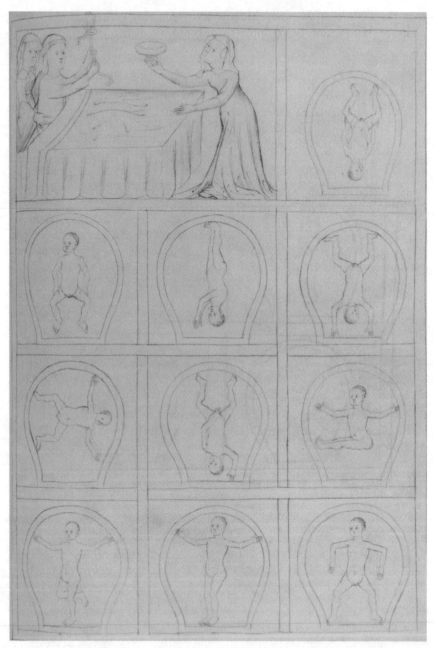

FIG. 3.4 Muscio foetus-in-utero figures with birth scene and two female attendants; these images were incorporated into a large collection of Latin surgical texts, suggesting the interests of an English surgeon in overseeing birth and supervising midwives.

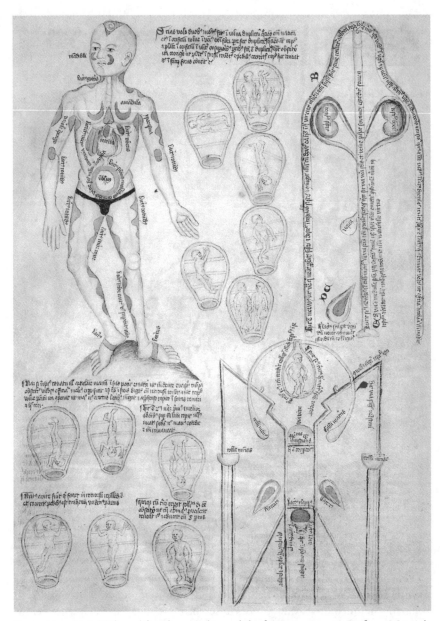

FIGS. 3.5 AND 3.6 Male and female genitalia, and the foetus-in-utero series from Muscio's *Gynaecia*, which spill over onto the following page where they conclude next to a 'disease woman'.

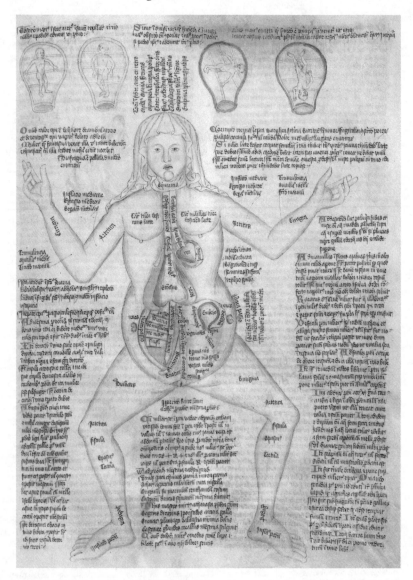

as with Thomas of Cantimpré before him, education of midwives may well have been an ulterior motive, but as we will see in more detail in Chapter 5 below, they had plenty of reasons of their own for wishing to have both texts and images that told of the 'secrets' of women's bodies.

Social and Medical Worlds of the Medieval Midwife, 1000–1500', PhD dissertation, University of Colorado at Boulder, 2002, p. 62.

Figures 3.5 and 3.6 come from a stunningly illustrated manuscript produced in Germany around 1420, the most striking example known of how a cleric might gather together gynaecological and obstetrical material—textual as well as visual—to educate both himself and midwives. Known now as the Wellcome Apocalypse, this large 'picture book' presents the text of the Apocalypse of St John followed by his *vita* and then by a treatise on the art of dying. Then comes a medical section (prepared by a different artist, apparently, but clearly an integral part of the original codex). Here we find images similar to those in the late thirteenth-century Ashmole manuscript discussed in the previous chapter: a 'wound man' depicting the different kinds of injuries that might be inflicted on the human body; the so-called 'Five-Figure Series' (a vein man, artery man, bone man, nerve man, and muscle man); schematic diagrams of the male and female genitalia as well as the sensory organs and the viscera; and the foetus-in-utero series from Muscio's *Gynaecology*, which spill over onto the following page where they conclude next to a 'disease woman'. Images of medical encounters then follow: a caesarean section being performed by a male practitioner; a naked woman with extended belly talking to a woman beside her; a woman consulting with a male practitioner; and male and female attendants inverting a pregnant patient in order to induce vomiting. Scattered over these leaves are several dozen remedies for obstetrical and gynaecological conditions, including instructions for proper lactation.[118] The presence of so much material on women's medicine in what was clearly a *cleric's* manual may seem surprising, but when we recall not only clerical concerns about baptism and the fate of the newborn's soul, but also the fact that priests would often have been summoned to administer last rights to women on the brink of death in difficult labours,[119] the idea that clerics might feel obligated to have some knowledge of childbirth becomes obvious. Add to this the fact that clerics would often have been the more literate members of their communities (especially in more rural settings) and we can well understand why celibate priests, who ostensibly should be most distanced from matters of female anatomy and birth, might in fact have deemed obstetrical knowledge vitally important.

The wealth of illustration that went into the Wellcome Apocalypse only reinforces, however, the visual impoverishment of the rest of the gynaecological manuscript tradition. Aside from three copies of a fifteenth-century Dutch translation that include depictions of pessaries, fumigation stools, and baths, none of the nearly 200 extant copies of the *Trotula*, Latin or vernacular, have any

---

[118] LWL, MS 49, *c.*1420 (Germany). All these images can be found in the Wellcome Library's image databank, available at <http://library.wellcome.ac.uk/>. For analysis, see Almuth Seebohm, *Apokalypse, Ars moriendi, Medizinische Traktate, Tugend- und Lasterlehren: Die erbaulich-didaktische Sammelhandschrift, London, Wellcome Institute for the History of Medicine, Ms. 49* (München: H. Lengenfelder, 1995). Seebohm stresses the didactic purpose and clerical audience of the manuscript.

[119] The manuscript also includes the 'Hippocratic signs' of impending death, again a subject of urgent concern for the cleric who would have to decide when to administer last rites.

kind of illustration meant to elucidate arguments or instructions in the texts.[120] The few elements of illumination the *Trotula* did garner were for decorative rather than pedagogical purposes. A thirteenth-century manuscript copied in Florence has a historiated initial with a women's head, apparently meant to depict the authoress 'Trotula', who is here lauded as a *magistra* who has skillfully chosen the best excerpts from 'the experts of old' on the topic of women's medicine and decoration.[121] Then in the lower margin of this same opening page, a naked woman holds a penis and scrotum meant, no doubt, to suggest 'Trotula's' special expertise in matters of generation.[122] Generation would also be the main theme of the illustration that opened one rather luxurious fourteenth-century manuscript of a French translation of the *Trotula* (now unfortunately destroyed) where, at the beginning of *Conditions of Women*, the illustrator chose to depict the creation of Adam, not Eve, in the historiated letter 'O' that began the text.[123]

Throughout Europe, therefore, gynaecological texts only rarely were presented in such a way that would invite simultaneous visual and textual interpretation, and only in the case of the Dutch *Trotula* and the English *Sickness of Women 2* were these illustrated texts directed specifically at female audiences. The principal manuscript traditions make no concession to the marginally literate. This poverty of illustrative material is in fact true of most medical texts, but that is exactly the point: gynaecological texts assume the same kinds of fully literate audiences that other medical texts do.[124] In surgery, the field most likely to employ images to depict complicated procedures or specialized instruments, there was no reluctance to depict the male genitalia in order to describe detailed treatments

---

[120] See Chapter 4 below for more on this Dutch translation for women. Representative pages from one of the manuscripts are reproduced in Green, *Trotula*.

[121] Florence, Biblioteca Laurenziana, Plut. 73, cod. 37, s. xiii² (Florence), ff. 2r–41r: *Incipit liber magistre Trotu[le] cuius florem legit ex dictis prouidorum Galieni, Auicenn[e], et aliorum peritorum ueterum, in utilit[atem] mulier[um] et pro deco[ra]tione ea[rum], scilicet de fa[cie] et de uu[l]ua ear[um]* ('Here begins the book of Mistress Trotula, whose flower she chose from the sayings of the provident Galen, Avicenna, and other experts of old, on the utility of women and for their decoration, that is, of their face and their vagina'). The scribe and probable owner of this manuscript was one Sinibaldus of Florence. The image is reproduced in Maria Pasca (ed.), *La Scuola medica salernitana: storia, immagini, manoscritti dall'XI al XIII secolo* (Naples: Electa Napoli, 1988), p. 46.

[122] There may have been a tradition of illustrating this particular version of the *Trotula* (the intermediate ensemble), since the one other depiction of the authoress 'Trotula' presents this same version of the text. See Fig. 5.11 below. Use of the detached male genitalia as a symbol of fecundity had a long history in Tuscan regions; see George Ferzoco, 'The Massa Marittima Mural', *Toscana Studies* 1 (2004), 71–105. On 'Trotula' as an authority on generation, see Chapter 5 below.

[123] Turin, Biblioteca Nazionale Universitaria, MS L.IV.25, s. xiv (Italy); this copy of the *Quant Dex nostre Seignor* was destroyed in the library fire of 1904.

[124] Studies such as Peter Murray Jones, *Medieval Medicine in Illuminated Manuscripts*, rev. ed. (London: British Library [by] arrangement with Centro Tibaldi, 1998) would seem to contradict my statement about the poverty of medical illustration, but the often gorgeously illustrated manuscripts (usually anatomical texts, surgical texts, and herbals) that art historians have studied are the exception rather than the norm. They represent only a fraction of the thousands of medical manuscripts still extant from the Middle Ages.

of the male pelvic region. (See Fig. 2.3 above.) Yet even after conditions of the female genitalia were added to surgical texts in the late thirteenth century, no iconographic tradition developed for these new chapters. In fact, the only depictions of the external female genitalia in a medical context are the birth images in a unique copy of Albucasis's Latin *Surgery*, which show semi-nude Muslim women giving birth, and a fifteenth-century copy of a French translation of the same text.[125] Even if this reluctance to depict the female genitalia was due to a particular representational taboo (as it probably was), the fact remains that there were no visual aids available to teach the marginally literate.

We are brought back, then, to the central problem of communicating gynaeco-logical knowledge across gender boundaries. Engagement with lore on women's anatomy and diseases via the medium of the written word or even the paint-ed picture demanded that the knowledge pass, at least momentarily, through men's hands. Such a scenario could only have been at best awkward, at worst self-defeating since it perpetuated the situation that the author of *Conditions of Women* claimed he wished to avoid: women refusing to seek help from males out of shame over the diseases of their 'secret parts'. It was one thing to depend on a male raconteur to orally deliver a poem of romance or epic battles to a mixed audience of ladies and knights in a courtly setting, quite another to expect the same practices of oral delivery to function unproblematically for the trans-mission of information about women's 'private' diseases. Thomas of Cantimpré had recognized this problem in the thirteenth century when he instructed that the priest should gather together a single-sex group of midwives and instruct them *secretly*.[126] While it seems quite likely that literate males, both medical practitioners and clerics, were occasionally the conduit for the transmission of obstetrical teachings to illiterate women, such oral or visual transmission would have still left women dependent upon men and the learning that men could gather (or that they chose to transmit).

[125] Vienna, Österreichische Nationalbibliothek, MS n.s. 2641, s. xiv ex., ff. 12v, 40v–41v, and 43r; this is available in facsimile in Eva Irblich (ed.), *Abū'l Qāsim Halaf Ibn 'Abbas al-Zahrāuī, Chirurgia. Faksimile und Kommentar* (Graz: Akademische Druck- und Verlagsanstalt, 1979); and Metz, Bibliothèque Municipale, MS 1228, s. xv, which was lost in the second World War.

[126] Thomas's discussion of generation and birth is repeated almost verbatim by the English friar John de Foxton in 1408 in his own encyclopedia of human knowledge. However, de Foxton does not repeat Thomas's injunction to round up 'some more discerning midwives' and instruct them, nor does he mention the *Trotula* despite the fact that a copy was available at the library of the York Austin friars where he possibly worked (see Appendix 1, items 12 and 13); see John Block Freidman (ed.), *John de Foxton's 'Liber cosmographiae' (1408)* (Leiden: E. J. Brill, 1988), pp. xxxv–xl, 64. Indeed, de Foxton did not even wish the casual Latinate (presumably male) reader to have easy access to this information on birth: more words from these brief chapters are written in de Foxton's unique cipher than almost anywhere else in the text. For other examples of cipher being used for gynecological and obstetrical information, see John Block Friedman, 'The Cipher Alphabet of John de Foxton's *Liber Cosmographiae*', *Scriptorium* 36 (1982), 219–35.

Moreover, it must be stressed that while the widely circulating encyclopedia of Thomas of Cantimpré as well as the unique Wellcome Apocalypse show a willingness among clerics to share basic obstetrical information, no such generosity seems to have led to the sharing of gynaecological knowledge. Gynaecological texts did not feature as regular items in the libraries of the mendicant orders, which tended to be poorly supplied with medical books in general.[127] While this in itself is not surprising—in the later medieval centuries, mendicants, especially the Dominicans, were increasingly proscribed from providing medical care to the general populace[128]—it does confirm that there were limits to how far clerics would go to transmit gynaecological information to women. In England, only three copies of the *Trotula* are found with religious texts in such a way that would remotely suggest pastoral usage of the text.[129] While it is quite common to find prayers and charms to aid birth in priests' manuals, and also to find birth girdles and other relics to aid birth in the hands of both priests and monks,[130] even in England clerics seem to have ceded strictly physical mechanisms to aid birth to secular medical practitioners.[131]

There were thus two major barriers to women's full engagement with literate medicine. First was their general lack of Latin and their exclusion from the whole system of educational structures, from secondary education on, that promoted acquisition of Latin and the basics of a liberal arts training. Up through the thirteenth century, the Latin-vernacular divide in literacy was more easily bridged and we find a few intriguing examples of manuscripts of the Latin *Trotula* that women might have owned and used for their own private edification. But such women were probably of a very different social

[127] K. W. Humphreys, 'The Medical Books of the Medieval Friars', *Libri: International Library Review* 3 (1954), 95–103. The only copies of the *Trotula* I have documented in a mendicant library are the one John Erghome gave to the Augustinian Priory of York, and Munich, Bayerische Staatsbibliothek, Clm 8742, s. xiii ex./xiv in. (Germany), which was owned by the Franciscan brothers of St Jacob in Munich. Circulation of gynecological texts among monks was, of course, quite different; see Appendix 1. On clerics' very different relationship to the *Secreta mulierum*, see Chapter 5 below.

[128] Angela Montford, 'Dangers and Disorders: The Decline of the Dominican *Frater Medicus*', *Social History of Medicine* 16, no. 2 (2003), 169–91.

[129] These are CTC, MS R.14.30 (903), which was owned by a monk of St Augustine's, Canterbury, the astronomer John of London; OBL, MS Digby 29, a manuscript owned by Richard Stapleton; and MS Digby 75. This last, which dates from 1458, was originally two separate mss: the first is a collection of medical and astrological texts in Latin (including the *Trotula*) to which have been added many medical recipes in Middle English. The second part has priests' manuals, astrological and mathematical texts; it, too, has medical recipes in English. Both parts mix Latin and English, both are written at approximately the same time. The two sections may, therefore, have been brought together by a priest with medical interests.

[130] My thanks to Stephanie Volf and Marilyn Oliva for this information.

[131] Germany is a rather different story in terms of clerical involvement in matters of women's medicine and generation; I will return to this in Chapters 5 and 6 below.

class than the women who actually relied on their medical skills to make a living. Among the latter, limited literacy skills would have been compounded by their lack of professional or functional identities that might have encouraged the development of 'textual communities' around written works on medicine; in this respect, female practitioners differed fundamentally from surgeons and apothecaries, who had begun to form such textual communities in the twelfth and thirteenth centuries, and (as we will see in the next chapter) from male householders and other laymen, who would form their own textual communities in the later Middle Ages. If these obstructing factors shifted, however—if, say, women acquired some level of literacy in their mother tongue and then had the texts in translation, *and* if women somehow found some common ground around which to form textual communities—would that not radically alter the accessibility of gynaecological knowledge and, equally important, the dynamics of the practice of women's medicine?

In fact, some textual communities were already forming among women, not among medical practitioners (who, as I have argued, probably did not form any *collective* identities aside from those imposed on them by ecclesiastical or municipal authorities), but rather among lay women. These included religious and devotional communities—nuns, beguines, anchorites, and so forth—but also, and more importantly for a field of medicine devoted to the generative organs, their lay female relatives who stayed in secular life. Such communities have been repeatedly documented in both northern and southern Europe with increasing frequency toward the end of the Middle Ages.[132] There also existed other female communities (such as women's parish guilds) that may, potentially, have served as arenas for exchange of knowledge and ideas that derived from books.[133] These communities included those that actually read together and those that 'virtually' existed through the exchange of texts and their ideas. These networks of women (who need not all have been literate) gathered primarily around religious texts. But once assembled in a common bond of reading, it was possible that such gatherings could have contributed to the dissemination of medical lore. I think it likely, for example, that the creation of such a female textual community—with a shared sense of what was appropriate and edifying to read—accounts for the surprising (and as yet unduplicated) concentration of medical readers among aristocratic French women in the fourteenth and fifteenth centuries, for whom medical reading had been authorized since Aldobrandino of Siena's mid thirteenth-century composition of

---

[132] This literature has now grown quite huge. Jocelyn Wogan-Browne, "'Reading is Good Prayer': Recent Research on Female Reading Communities', *New Medieval Literatures* 5 (2002), 229–97, offers an excellent summary of the field, especially as it relates to England. For Italy, see Gill, 'Women and the Production of Religious Literature'.

[133] Katherine French, '"To Free Them from Binding": Women in the Late Medieval English Parish', *Journal of Interdisciplinary History* 27, no. 3 (1997), 387–412.

a regimen of health for Queen Beatrix of Savoy.[134] While to date no *documentable* female community has been found around texts specifically devoted to women's medicine, at least some of the vernacularizers of gynaecological literature believed they existed or, like Thomas of Cantimpré, that they could be brought into existence.

---

[134] As noted in Green, 'Possibilities' (pp. 26–32), female owners of Aldobrandino's work cannot be *documented* until the 15th century and it is clear that women never made up the majority of owners. (The dedication to Beatrix is in fact found in only a small percentage of extant copies.) Nevertheless, the French tradition of women's medical reading is decidedly more pronounced than elsewhere. See also the Conclusion below.

4

In a Language Women Understand:
the Gender of the Vernacular

And because women are more ashamed to speak about their diseases to men
than to women, I am composing for them this book in a language they
understand, so that some women will know how to aid others.

Quant Dex nostre Seignor, a French translation of *Conditions of Women*
(thirteenth century)

Women's shame about their diseases, women's reluctance to speak to men,
women's greater comfort with the vernacular. All these would lead us to
believe that the *Trotula*, once rendered into the vernacular, would now pass
directly into the hands of women who could, thereby, take control of their
own health matters and entirely avoid men whether as practitioners or inter-
preters of written Latin texts. The opening claim in this thirteenth-century
French translation of the *Trotula* certainly reinforces our expectations. But
we would be wrong to assume that feminization was the *only* function of
the vernacular. Yes, as we will see, several vernacular translations of the *Trotula*—like the French version above—were indeed meant specifically for women
and were probably used by certain women within their own female textual
communities. But as with the Latin *Trotula*, all *known* thirteenth- through
fifteenth-century owners of manuscripts of the vernacular translations of the
Trotula (and all other vernacular gynaecological texts for that matter) were
male and, as I will argue below, codicological evidence often suggests audiences not far different from those the texts received in Latin. What is novel
about the various vernacular traditions is that because men's and women's
ability to read the vernacular was more equitable, there was more direct contest between them for the use and control of these texts. Indeed, we find for
the first time some evidence that women might object not simply to men
observing their bodies, but to men observing *texts* about their bodies. These
sentiments did not come directly from women—in no case do we have evidence
that women themselves made the translations or even directly commissioned
them—but certain male advocates of women seem to have been attentive to
their concerns.

While vernacularization functioned to challenge or reinforce gender categories, it also had other effects. For men, the process of vernacularization functioned in two ways: it helped broaden who could define themselves as 'professional' while at the same time (and for the same reasons) it lessened the gap between 'professional' and 'lay'. The audiences for Latin gynaecological writings did not, of course, disappear after the fourteenth century. On the contrary, Latin retained its function as the *lingua franca* of the western European university-educated elite right through the end of the medieval period and Latin gynaecological texts continued to circulate among learned physicians and within the Latinate milieux of universities and religious institutions.[1] The vernacular versions of the *Trotula*, rather than appealing to these older audiences, opened up the texts to new, additional male audiences: surgeons, barbers, and apothecaries, but also landed gentlemen, merchants, and noblemen concerned to have self-help knowledge as well as a command of the science of generation. For men aspiring to some sort of professional medical identity, the vernacularized *Trotula* functioned in essentially the same way the Latin texts had: they offered a compendium of information that would aid them when called upon to diagnose and prescribe therapy for their female clients. In fact, the transition to the vernacular for these readers seems to have been less a radical transition than a slow expansion of medical learning into languages beyond Latin. Many of these readers were not completely ignorant of Latin, and we find abundant code-switching between Latin and the vernacular throughout their medical books. The same is true of the lay male readers of the texts, who did not wish to challenge the learning of educated physicians so much as emulate it.

For women, in contrast, vernacularization did not have this same double effect of expanding both professional and lay audiences. I find no evidence for the creation of a textual community of women who identified themselves *as specialists* on women's medicine. Unlike obstetrical texts of the sixteenth century (when the profession of midwifery was more formally organized and when the city councillors of Nuremberg, for example, could assume that all licensed midwives would be able to read), none of the medieval translations of the *Trotula* claim midwives or other female practitioners as their principal intended audience.[2] Nor is there evidence that midwives, for their part, laid claim to the *Trotula* as a defining text of their professional identity in the way surgeons laid claim to the works of Lanfranc or Guy de Chauliac, or apothecaries to the Salernitan

---

[1] See Chapter 6 below on uses of the *Trotula* and other Latin gynaecological literature in the 15th and 16th centuries.

[2] Anna Delva, *Vrouwengeneeskunde in Vlaanderen tijdens de late middeleeuwen*, Vlaamse His-torische Studies 2 (Brugge: Genootschap voor Geschiedenis, 1983), claims, without evidence, that the Dutch *Trotula* she edited (Brugge, Openbare Bibliotheek, MS 593) was made by a midwife for the use of other midwives, a claim vitiated by the fact that the text contains no obstetrical material whatsoever nor are midwives anywhere mentioned. For more on midwives as audiences, see the Conclusion below.

Circa instans or *Antidotary of Nicholus*. Aside from the obstetrical instructions in Thomas of Cantimpré's encyclopedia of learning for secular priests (which were later co-opted into texts that circulated among surgeons), there is no evidence even of question-and-answer texts being written to inform midwives in the basic theoretical precepts of their craft such as have been documented for semi-literate surgeons and barbers.[3] This finding is hardly surprising. As we have seen, prior to the thirteenth century there was no identifiable 'profession' of midwifery, while later, even after attempts at regulation began, such regulations had no widespread effect on standardizing the knowledge expected of midwives. What such regulations did do, apparently, was reinforce the notion that midwives were birth attendants and not specialists in women's health generally, as had been true when Muscio was writing in late Antiquity. Nor does anyone seem to have assumed, as Muscio did, that midwives (or at least some midwives who could train others) were literate and needed written texts to educate themselves. In fact, aside from excerpts of Muscio's *Gynaecology* that circulated in priests' or surgeons' compendia—and so in neither case in a form *directly* accessible to midwives—no medieval text focuses exclusively on obstetrics. Michele Savonarola's mid fifteenth-century *Regimen for the Women of Ferrara*, of which we will learn more in Chapter 6, in covering fertility, childbirth, *and* childcare, addressed the interests of both midwives and their clients—upper-class birthing mothers—a conflation of practitioner and patient interests that would characterize many other early modern 'midwifery' texts. Moreover, in presenting midwives *only* with material on fertility, childbirth, and childcare, Savonarola was also at the forefront of defining *gynaecology* (all of women's other conditions) as something outside women's competence. The vernacular traditions of the *Trotula* and other medieval gynaecological texts stand out, therefore, because if they were addressed to women, they addressed them generically, which in practice meant women in the upper ranks of society.

The twenty-one known translations of the *Trotula* come from most of the areas where the Latin texts circulated. (See Table 4.1.) They date from the late twelfth century through the end of the fifteenth and demonstrate a wide variety of approaches to the texts: from literal translations of the entire ensemble that take a broad view of 'women's medicine', to highly selective and novel recastings of the text(s) to suit very particular purposes. With only two exceptions (a French verse rendition and an English prose translation that both derive from the *Quant Dex nostre Seignor* quoted above), the translations are all independent of one another. We can no more claim a single motivational force, whether personal,

---

[3] Sylvie Bazin-Tacchella, 'Adaptations françaises de la *Chirurgia Magna* de Guy de Chauliac et codification du savoir chirurgical au XVᵉ siècle', in *Bien dire et bien aprandre: Actes du colloque du Centre d'Études Médiévales et Dialectales de Lille III. 'Traduction, transposition, adaptation au Moyen Age', Lille, 22–24 septembre 1994*, t. 14 (1996), pp. 169–88, documents at least ten different catechetical texts in French for surgeons and barbers, all of which convey not simply basic technical information but also certain theoretical information, such as the role of the liver in blood production.

Table 4.1. Medieval Translations of the *Trotula* and their Audiences[a]

Language	Date[b]	Title	Audience[c]
Hebrew	1197–9	*Book on the Hidden Place* (*Sefer ha-seter*)	PM
French	early 13th	*Secrets of Women* (*Secrés de femmes*)	LM + W
French	early 13th	*Quant Dex nostre Seignor*	W
French	mid 13th	*Bien sachiés femmes* (verse)	PM + W?
French	early 14th?	*Si com Aristocele nous dit* (verse)	W
French	mid 14th?	*Li livre de Trocule*	PM
French	15th	*Regimen of Ladies to Aid Them in Their Maladies and Adversities* (*Regime des dames pour leurs aydier en leurs maladies et aduersitez*)	PM
French	15th	*A Treatise on the Many Maladies Which Can Happen to Women, and on Their Secrets Maladies* (*Un traictié de plusieurs maladies qui peuent avenir aux femmes, et de leur maladies secretes*)	PM
Irish	14th	*Cum autur uniuercitatis*	PM
Italian	14th	*The Book on the Secret Conditions of Women* and *Book on the Adornment of Women by Which They May Make Their Bodies Beautiful* (*Libro delle segrete cose delle donne* and *Libro dello adornamento delle donne per che modo debbono fare belli i loro membri*)	PM + LM?
Italian	15th	*A Work of Small Size and Great Utility, Especially for Women* (*Vna opera de picol volume e bona utilitade e maximamente per le done*)	PM
German	15th	*The Flower of Women* (*Flos mulierum/Blume der Frawen*)	PM
German	c.1460–5	Johannes Hartlieb, *The Book Trotula* (*Das Buch Trotula*)	LM
Dutch	14th	*On the Secret Medicine of Women* (*Van heymeliken medicinen in vrouwen/Secreta mulierum*)	PM
Dutch	early 14th	*The Secrets of Men and Women* (*Der Mannen ende Vrouwen Heimelijcheit/Mulierum secreta*) (verse)	PM + LM?
Dutch	15th	*Liber Trotula* (in three redactions)	W, W, PM
English	late 14th/early 15th	*Knowing of Woman's Kind in Childing*	W
English	15th	*The Book of Trotulus* (*Liber Trotuli*)	PM
English	15th	*Secrets of Women* (*Secreta mulierum*)	PM + LM
English	15th	*The Book called Trotela* (ascribed in one copy to the authorship of John of Burgundy)	LM + W?
English	15th	*Book Made by a Woman Named Rota* (in two redactions)	W, PM

[a] For further information on all these translations, see Green, 'Handlist II'; and *eadem*, 'Medieval Gynecological Texts: A Handlist', in *Women's Healthcare*, Appendix, pp. 1–36.

[b] Except in those cases where an exact year is known, all dates refer to centuries.

[c] PM = professional male; LM = lay male; W = women.

institutional, or discursive, for this manifold phenomenon than we can for the Latin tradition. And as with the Latin tradition, moreover, the original versions that left the hand of their vernacular creators could vary greatly from the versions actually used by various audiences.

Despite this diversity, all the medieval translations of the *Trotula* can, I argue, be grouped under three different headings: those meant for professional male readers, those meant for lay male readers, and those meant for female lay readers. A survey of all twenty-one translations is obviously not possible here, so I will do three samplings: first, the French tradition, the longest and fullest series, shows how unstable the gendering of the vernacular could be, professional males winning out over lay women almost immediately after vernacularization began in the thirteenth century; second, a fifteenth-century German translation exhibits the motives for addressing a lay male patron; and third, the English tradition, which begins towards the end of the fourteenth century, provides examples of texts (including but not limited to the *Trotula*) directed to all three types of audiences—in fact, two texts are found in both men's and women's versions. The other vernacular traditions follow these patterns: the sole Irish translation seems to have been meant for professional males with surgical interests, much like the later French tradition. The Italian translations seem to have been meant for and used by both male practitioners and lay males. The Dutch translations most closely parallel the English tradition, some intended for men and others meant for women, with evidence that the latter were also soon co-opted by men.[4] No southern European translations of the *Trotula* are addressed to women, nor, aside from a fourteenth-century Catalan text which is primarily cosmetic, is any other vernacular gynaecological material directed to women in the south prior to Savonarola's text in the mid fifteenth century. In those northern areas where at least some texts are addressed to women, however, we find a veritable gendered tug-of-war, with disputes arising over who should be authorized to read these texts on women's medicine.

'FOR AIDING THEM IN THEIR MALADIES AND ADVERSITIES': GYNAECOLOGY IN FRENCH

The Latin *Conditions of Women*, as we have seen, had already opened the door to the problematics of male practice of women's medicine. Central to this problem was women's reluctance, out of shame, to expose the diseases of their 'private parts' to male physicians. The author of *Conditions of Women* had, however, raised the problem of shame in a quite ambiguous and unresolved way. Was his

---

[4] More details on the Italian and Dutch translations, which are largely passed over here, can be found in Monica H. Green, 'Gender and the Vernacularization of Women's Medicine in Late Medieval and Early Modern Europe' (forthcoming).

text meant for women's direct use so that they did not have to turn to a male physician? Or was it meant to inform the male physician of women's diseases in advance of the clinical encounter, so that he would not have to embarrass the woman with excessive questioning? Editors, copyists, and readers of the Latin *Trotula* seem to have adopted the latter interpretation for, as we have seen, the statement about women's shame is retained, with no alteration, throughout the four centuries of circulation of the Latin texts.[5] This rather unthinking approach to the issue of women's shame and the implied questions it raises for the practice of gynaecology is replicated in several vernacular traditions of the *Trotula* texts. Some translators, however, recognizing the uncomfortable dynamics between men and women at this delicate intersection of conflicting gender boundaries, take the rhetorical possibilities of the *Conditions of Women* preface in a different direction: they add explicit claims that their translations are intended for female audiences. The vernacularization of the gynaecological and obstetrical portions of the *Trotula* thus, unwittingly or not, raised questions that struck at the heart of how gynaecology (and to a lesser extent, obstetrics) was to be practised and who was to claim authority over this body of knowledge.

The earliest translation of the *Trotula* in the area we now call France was not, in fact, into French. In the twelfth century, as we have seen, Latin was still the principal language of most literates and it is rare to find medical texts of any kind in the vernacular.[6] Hebrew, on the other hand, was already gaining status among Jewish men as a language not limited to religious purposes. Between the years 1197 and 1199, an anonymous translator in southern France rendered over two dozen different Latin texts into Hebrew. Besides *Conditions of Women* and *Women's Cosmetics*, he was also responsible for translations of Muscio's *Gynaecology* as well as the Muscian adaptation, *Diseases of Women B*.[7] No direct addresses to female readers or auditors are found in the sections *Conditions of Women* or *Women's Cosmetics* that remain. And while he did couch his translation of Muscio's *Gynaecology* in the form of a dialogue between the biblical heroine Dinah and her father (perhaps to suggest that fathers should be responsible for teaching their daughters about gynaecology?), given Jewish women's low levels of literacy in Hebrew it seems unlikely that these texts would have regularly found a female reading audience.[8] Hebrew was not, of course, a real 'vernacular'

[5] See Chapter 2 above.

[6] Aside from scattered 12th-century recipes in Anglo-Norman, the earliest documented translations of medical texts into a Romance language are several works rendered into Occitan in the early 13th century.

[7] Ron Barkaï, *A History of Jewish Gynaecological Texts in the Middle Ages* (Leiden: Brill, 1998); and Carmen Caballero Navas, 'Algunos "secretos de mujeres" revelados: El *Še'ar yašub* y la recepción y transmisión del *Trotula* en hebreo [Some "secrets of women" revealed: The *She'ar yašub* and the reception and transmission of the *Trotula* in Hebrew]', *Miscelánea de Estudios Árabes y Hebraicos, sección Hebreo* 55 (2006), 381–425.

[8] Ron Barkaï, *Les Infortunes de Dinah: le livre de la génération. La gynécologie juive au Moyen-Age*, trans. Jacqueline Barnavi and Michel Garel (Paris: Cerf, 1991).

but rather a learned, written language in much the same way Latin was. Rather than being concerned to make the *Trotula* (or his other gynaecological texts) directly accessible to women, this translator was concerned to render 'all the erudites' books on theoretical and practical medicine into the Holy Tongue' so that Jews would not have to compromise their religious traditions by consulting Gentile physicians.[9] For him, therefore, *translatio* was an act of religious and cultural appropriation. The needs of a female reading audience had nothing to do with it.

Soon after this Hebrew translator finished his enormous undertaking, spoken Romance vernaculars began to generate large bodies of written literature among Christians, among which medicine figured early and commonly. The second earliest translation of the *Trotula* perhaps originated in France, though the sole known copy comes from French-speaking England. Called *Secrés de femmes* ('Secrets of Women'), this is a rendering of only a few chapters on fertility from the *Conditions of Women*'s urtext, the *Treatise on Women's Illnesses*. The author of this short verse text probably had a mixed audience in mind, for it reads as if it were a sermon addressing married couples, instructing them on how to avoid infertility. The author opens with a harsh condemnation of male homosexuality (whose effects on fertility no other medical writer felt the need to state), and then chides both men and women for arguing with their spouses. Women are clearly in this audience, for not simply does the author tell them that they must obey their husbands, he later switches to a direct address to women in three recipes for aiding conception.[10]

The next two French translations of the *Trotula* would, at least in their explicit audience claims, be addressed directly to women rather than a mixed audience, though when read in their entirety these two texts differ quite considerably in their clues about intended use. A French prose translation of *Conditions of Women*, probably composed in the early thirteenth century, has no documented title in the manuscripts, though we can refer to it by its incipit, *Quant Dex nostre Seignor* ('When God our Lord'). It is the first to seize directly upon the shame topos of the *Conditions of Women* prologue and exploit it to claim a female audience, tying that claim to the choice of the vernacular:

And because women are more ashamed to speak about their diseases to men than to women, I am composing for them this book in a language they understand, so that some women will know how to aid others. They should know well that I have put here the best things which they need for their infirmities that I have found in the sayings

[9] Barkaï, *History*, p. 21.

[10] CTC, MS O.1.20 (1044), ff. 21rb–23rb, for example, f. 22va: 'En lait de anesse laine o tot les somellons / Sor uostre nomblil estreit tres bien le liez / Apres a uostre baron en. i. lit coucherez / Vous et il ensemble uos uolentes facez'. For a fuller description of the text, see Green, 'Handlist II', pp. 89–90.

of Hippocrates and Galen and Constantine and Cleopatra, and here they will discover whence their maladies come and how they will be able to cure them.[11]

The translator clearly imagines a *community* of women who will share knowledge among themselves. True, he does not employ a direct female address: there are no 'you women' references. Nevertheless, in the fullest copy that we have (the others are either fragmentary or deliberately abbreviated),[12] the text is couched in such a way that it could be understood to 'speak' directly to an audience of women charged with taking care of others. Simple second-person-singular imperatives or third-person generics are most commonly used in the instructions throughout the text: *Face se seignier* (have her bled), *prenge l'on* (one takes), *face l'on* (one makes), *mesle l'on* (one mixes), *l'on la puisse metre en la naisance* (one pushes it into the vagina). Another formula is simply to say 'X is good to take for . . .' (e.g., *maoult ualt la mere erbol* [mugwort] *a prendre*). There is nothing to contradict this image of care being provided among a group of women: no physicians are mentioned save a few citations of authorities such as Galen or Hippocrates (all of which derive directly from the Latin text), no intermediaries stand between the reader and the female patient. Admittedly, if the text was ever used directly by women, we have no evidence of it: aside from a single-leaf fragment (whose original format we cannot know), in every copy of the text it is embedded within collections of learned medical treatises, often in Latin. Named owners are known from the fifteenth or sixteenth centuries, and in every case they are male. (See Appendix 1, items 80 and 85–7.) Perhaps *Quant Dex nostre Seignor* circulated originally in the small pamphlets that typify later texts for women; as such, they may have been particularly subject to disintegration and loss. Or perhaps the text had always been intended to be read aloud by male practitioners or other literates to an audience of women. Either way, although the *Trotula* had now been rendered 'into a language women understand', it did not remain in women's hands.

An Anglo-Norman verse adaptation of *Quant Dex nostre Seignor* made around the middle of the thirteenth century (which I will refer to by its incipit, *Bien*

---

[11] BLL, MS Sloane 3525, s. xiv in. (region of Paris), ff. 246vb–247ra: 'Et pour ce ke femes sunt plus huntoses de dire lor enfermetez as homes ke as femes, si lor faz icest livre en language ke eles l'entendent, que les unes sachent les autres aidier. Bien sachent que ie i met del mielz ke lor besoigne a lor enfermetez, que ie ai troué des diz Ypocras et Galien et Costentin et Cleopatras, et ici troueront dont li mal uiennent et comant porront guarir.' 'Cleopatra' had entered this litany of authors in *Conditions of Women 3*, where her name was substituted for Constantine's. This Old French translation is unique in situating all four authorities together.

[12] Only one of the six known copies of this original redaction of *Quant Dex nostre Seignor* (there are also two later redactions that I will discuss below) dates from earlier than the turn of the 14th century. To the four copies listed in Green, 'Handlist II', at pp. 90–1, add now (formerly) Thomas Phillipps collection, MS 1109, s. xiv ex. (England), f. 8r–11v, which was sold by Sotheby's of London in 1965 and whose current whereabouts are unknown; and a 13th-century fragmentary copy in London, Public Record Office, MS E 163/22/2/1, s. xiii (England?), f. 1r–v, which was discovered by Agnes Davis and examined for her master's thesis at Lincoln College, Oxford (2002).

sachiés femmes) reorients the text toward a masculine audience. Like its Old French prose source, this poem starts out with a clear address to women in general:

Know well, women, have no doubt of it, / That here is indeed written [women's] knowledge / Of having children and giving birth, / Of their secrets everything is here divulged . . . Here they [*eles*] will certainly find out / Whence these diseases come and how they are healed.[13]

Already in these opening lines we find the dissonance that will characterize the rest of the text: after the direct address of the first line ('Bien sachiés, femmes') which sets up the impression that women are the intended audience, the author from then on always refers to women as 'they', not 'you'. The second-person addresses (of which there are many) are instead reserved for the reader/practitioner. The several references to what the male healer (*li mire*) should do, all of which are new additions to this verse version of the text, suggest that professional male practitioners, not laywomen, are the real addressees.[14] To be sure, it is possible that *li mire* was meant to include female practitioners as well. Yet the feminine form *miresse* is well attested in medieval French and (rhyming and metrical schemes notwithstanding) it could certainly have been incorporated had this author wished to acknowledge the work of female practitioners.[15] It is clear, however, that the redactor saw medicine as a masculine endeavour. Among his other additions are subtle flourishes that depict both Galen and Hippocrates

---

[13] *Bien sachiés femmes*, edited from CTC, MS O.1.20 (1044), s. xiii[2] (England), ff. 216r–235v in Tony Hunt, *Anglo-Norman Medicine*, 2 vols. (Cambridge: D. S. Brewer, 1994–97), 2:76–107. The quotation here comes from p. 76, lines 1–4 and 11–12.

[14] Besides an added description of Hippocrates as a great *mire* (see n. 16 below), there are six new references to *li mires* in *Bien sachiés femmes*. The first comes in lines 115–16 of Hunt's edition (¶8 of the Latin) which counsels that *li mires* ought to guard against excessively bleeding the patient (*As febletez [li] mires bien se gart, / Kar a tous febles doit bien ovrer par art*). In line 155 (= ¶11 of the Latin), *li bons mires* ('the good physician') is told that he should give a potion of the compound medicine *hierapigra*. In line 545 (¶63 of the Latin), it is said that 'this [remedy] very much profits the physician to do' (*Ice profite mult, se fait le mire fis*), whereas the Old French prose had simply said 'It is good' (*kar ce ualt*). In line 564, another warning is given to the physician (*Parces covient li mires garder les maneres*). In lines 713–14 (Latin, ¶73), the redactor specifies (where neither the Latin nor the French prose had) that Dioscorides is specifically instructing the *physician* (*Dïacorides dit, li mires qui ne faut, / Poudre de finigrec . . .*). In lines 739–40 (Latin ¶75), it is made explicit that it is *the physician* who aids the couple in their infertility (*Si l'un d'els n'i a coupe, donc lor est bien aidans / Li mires par mecines si qu'il avront enfans*). The three other uses of *mire* correspond with the original prose version and refer not to the reader or the ideal practitioner but to specific individuals (a physician who cured a queen of France [line 263, Latin ¶25], the physicians who mistook a suffocated woman for dead [line 383, Latin ¶46], and the physician Justin, one of whose remedies is cited [line 437, Latin ¶49]). (The use of *mire* in line 322 is the modern editor's own emendation and I omit it from discussion here since it has no medieval authority.)

[15] Ellen E. Kittell and Kurt Gueller, ' "Whether Man or Woman': Gender Inclusivity in the Town Ordinances of Medieval Douai', *Journal of Medieval and Early Modern Studies* 30 (2000), 63–100, offer a wonderful analysis of the use of dyadic gendered phrases (e.g., *borgois u borgoise*, *taneres u taneresse*) to include both men and women in occupational and other descriptions. This same usage is found in both Latin and French ordinances about medical practice.

(whose authority was already established in the text) as great teachers of male *scholars*: Galen wrote a book 'which formerly was of great utility to scholars', while 'Hippocrates was the physician who never made a mistake, and who above all faithfully taught his students.'[16] Indeed, if we take away the single word 'femmes' in the opening line and 'eles' in line 11, there is no indication whatsoever that women were meant to read or even hear this text. The shame topos has completely disappeared and there is no suggestion that male practice was in anyway problematic. Moreover, in the one extant manuscript, which in this case dates closely to what was probably the moment of composition, the text is situated amid highly technical French and Latin medical and surgical texts, among which are also several dozen detailed images of the male healer at work.[17] The manuscript concludes with a French tract on confession, which may suggest a clerical owner. This is in fact the same manuscript that included not only some Anglo-Norman verses on cosmetics (which were explicitly addressed to female readers), but also the 'sermon' version of the *Trotula* addressed to a mixed male and female audience. Given their corruptions, it is clear that neither of the two Anglo-Norman renditions of the *Trotula* here is the original copy; we can thus imagine that they circulated in other contexts prior to the creation of this present manuscript.[18] Nevertheless, the internal evidence within the texts—both of which depict women as (at best) the passive listening audience of medical knowledge conveyed by men—together with the professional character of the manuscript, gives us an image of how learning on women's medicine, though rendered 'into a language women understand', may have continued to circulate through male hands.

Male control would, in fact, characterize the circulation of most French gynaecological literature for the rest of the medieval period. The thirteenth-century Old French prose translation, *Quant Dex nostre Seignor*, continued to be used into the fourteenth and fifteenth centuries, yet it was not preserved in its entirety but rather abbreviated in certain characteristic ways.[19] In a fourteenth-century copy now in Paris, the text retains the clear statement in the prologue that it is meant for women, yet it presents only the chapters on menstruation and fertility (a habit of omission whose significance we shall see in the next

---

[16] Hunt, *Anglo-Norman Medicine*, p. 80, lines 117–18; and p. 106, lines 843–4. Hippocrates also appears as a teacher of clerks on p. 106, lines 835–6.

[17] The better part of the manuscript's contents have been published in the two volumes of Tony Hunt's *Anglo-Norman Medicine*. For reproductions of the illustrations, see Tony Hunt, *The Medieval Surgery* (Woodbridge, Suffolk: Boydell Press, 1992).

[18] Hunt, *Anglo-Norman Medicine*, finds it likely, on linguistic grounds, that both texts were composed on the Continent, a further indication that the Anglo-Norman form in which we find them here was not original. The manuscript does, in fact, give the sense that it was made as a 'repository' for valuable texts and not directly as a working manual; it has, besides two different versions of the *Trotula*, two different translations of Roger Frugardi's *Chirurgia* plus the Latin text of the same work.

[19] I discuss this pattern of abbreviation at greater length in Chapter 5 below.

chapter) and it is found among astrological, astronomical, and medical texts in Latin and French, i.e., precisely the kind of context where we have as yet so little evidence of female reading.[20] Later versions of this same translation, which situate the text in similar codicological contexts, would suppress the passage on women's shame entirely. The sole known owner is an otherwise unidentified man from Lille, Baudoin Cauwet, who promised some wine to anyone who returned the book to him should it be lost.[21] It is therefore ironic that what seems to be the final reincarnation of *Quant Dex nostre Seignor* should render it available once again to women. Paragraphs 1–4 of the text (on menstruation) were excerpted, apparently at the end of the fifteenth or at the beginning of the sixteenth century, and worked into a little tract on generation and infertility.[22] Female ownership of the single known manuscript of this version seems plausible, since the codex as a whole is made up of moral and devotional texts of the kind we often find in women's hands. Yet the text has been so whittled away that it can no longer claim to be offering its female owner anything but the most limited knowledge of female physiology or therapy for women's diseases.[23]

Four more French translations would follow the thirteenth-century versions, only one of which seems to have been directed to a female audience. The preface of an incomplete Anglo-Norman verse rendition (which I refer to by its incipit, *Si com Aristocele nous dit*), now extant in a unique early fourteenth-century copy, echoes the shame topos of the Latin *Conditions of Women* in an interesting way. It both seems to claim a female audience and, simultaneously, tries to warn away a male one.[24] This is perhaps already an admission that no such exclusion of male readers was in fact possible, a theme we will see repeated

---

[20] BNF, MS nouv. acq. lat. 693, s. xiii/xiv (France), ff. 181v–183r.

[21] Lille, Bibliothèque Municipale, MS 863, s. xv med. (probably Tournai), f. 2r, 'Ce livre appartient à Bauduin Cauwet, demorant à Lille. Se aucun le treuve ou luy reporte et il luy donra le vin. Cauwet'.

[22] BLL, MS Lansdowne 380, s. xvi in., ff. 269r–271v. The introductory section derives from Redaction II (= ¶¶1–4), but thereafter the text diverges completely from *Conditions of Women* to go into a novel discourse on the causes of infertility. Several remedies (none of which derives from the *Trotula*) follow. The novelty of this redaction of *Quant Dex nostre Seignor* is paralleled and complemented by the redaction of Aldobrandino of Siena's *Régime du corps* which immediately precedes it in the manuscript. Here, the redactor has reworked and drastically expanded Part I, cap. 7 of the *Régime* to create an 'enseignement de medecine' dedicated to sexual relations and addressed to both men and women. See Green, 'Handlist II', p. 92.

[23] For more on the 16th-century trend to address works on fertility to female audiences, see the Conclusion below.

[24] *Si com Aristocele nous dit*, CTC, MS O.2.5 (1109), s. xiv[1] (England), ff. 123rb–124va. The text, which is rather corrupted, opens as follows (lines 1–14): 'As Aristotle tell us in what he writes in his letter to Alexander, it is not right or fitting that [women's] maladies, which hold the body in weakness, are known to everyone. This would not be disclosed to a man: what a woman conceals is so covered up that she scarcely ever wishes to display its extent to any man. For this reason, I am teaching medicine both to the lady and to the maid through which one can privately help oneself without a confidant' (*Si com Aristocele nous dit / En Alisaundre en son ecrit / N'est par reison ne afaitement / Que sues seunt a tote gent / Le[s] maladies que aueniunt / En langor le cors teinunt / A homme icel n'eut ouere / Ke femme cele tant est couere / Ke en vis unkes a nul home / Ke voil mustrer coe*

again. Like the Anglo-Norman versions we have already seen, the codicological context of the single extant copy belies any connection of this text with 'typically feminine' patterns of reading: the manuscript contains not only French tracts on medicine as well as geomancy and other kinds of prognostication, but Latin tracts on astronomy, chiromancy, and natural philosophy, a book of penances, the quite misogynous sayings of the philosopher Secundus, and two texts on human generation as well as a brief tract comparing male and female nature. It may have been owned initially by Robert de Barry, rector of Begelly, Pembrokeshire.[25]

Translations made on the Continent situate the *Trotula* more squarely in medical contexts. One of them, *Le Livre de Trocule*, although extant now only in a single fragmentary fifteenth-century copy, may have been the version owned in the 1370s by the French king, Charles V. Both Charles's copy and the still extant manuscript situate the *Trotula* amid translations of major surgical and medical texts: Lanfranc's *Surgery*, collections of compound medicines, and surgical receipts. Charles's copy was borrowed by a surgeon, one Master Pierre of Montpellier, who seems never to have returned it.[26] Not enough of this version is extant to assess how it handled the passage about women's shame or how it envisaged the gender dynamics of gynaecological practice. Another French translation of the standardized ensemble, however, which may date from the fifteenth century, shows clearly how the claim to be caring for women does not imply that a gynaecological author is actually addressing them.

This translation is called *The Regimen of Ladies for Aiding Them in Their Maladies and Adversities of Conception, Birth, and Otherwise*, and in its preface it dutifully repeats the sympathetic observation that women do not wish to show their diseases to male physicians, closing with the assertion that this collection of remedies is intended 'to console and comfort ladies in their private diseases'.[27] The translation is generally very literal, though the translator has recast many of the instructions into direct second-person addresses (*tu* or *vous*). This 'you' (with whom the reader is expected to identify) is not the woman herself, however, but

---

la sume / Pur ceo aprenne [MS: *aprendre*] *medecine / E a dame et a meschine / Par quei puse priuement / Sei eider sanz afient*). My thanks to Jocelyn Wogan-Browne for her help with this difficult text.

[25] See Appendix 1, item 78.

[26] For a description of the text, see Green, 'Handlist II', p. 93. On ownership, see Appendix 1, items 83–84.

[27] BNF, MS fr. 1327, s. xv med., f. 61r: 'le voulum du Regime des dames pour leurs aydier en leurs maladies et aduersitez tant de la concepcion comme de l'anfentement et aultrement'; f. 61v: 'Et parquoy aussi elles sont appareillées de receuoir plusiers grandes et diuerses maladies et mesmement enuiron le membre secret ou se fait la generacion, car a l'occasion de sa condicion de la frigidite qui est en elles pour la vergoigne que elles ont la face leur en rougist, et pour raison de la maladie que elles ont qui est en lieu secret elles en seuffrent plusgrant angoisse, pource quelles ne losent pas bien dire et reueler aux medecins'; f. 62r: 'pour consoler et esiouyr les dames de leurs priuees maladies'.

the practitioner who treats her, the male physician (*le medecin*).[28] The translator even went so far as to deny that the male physician faced any competition from female practitioners. He suppresses the three references to midwives in *Conditions of Women*, thereby implying that the birth practices described are simply those that women (who are here granted no *professional* identity) use among themselves.[29] Furthermore, and most remarkably, in the anecdote of Trota/'Trotula's' famous cure, 'Trotula' is no longer the name of a famous practitioner but the *name of a disease*, the case history having been turned into a straightforward prescription for therapy: 'It happens that this malady [wind in the womb] is commonly called 'Trotula' as [it is] the chief malady [*maistresse maladie*] and suffering of women'.[30] It is now the male physician who is to take the woman into his home so that secretly he can discern the cause of the disease. In fact, it is quite remarkable how comfortable this translator seems to be with the idea that male practitioners face no problem of access to the female body at all: he does no subtle grammatical dance around the statements about touching or inserting medicines into the female genitalia. All are couched in the same casual 'nous' or 'tu/vous' that characterize the rest of the text. In describing the efficacy of a remedy to get rid of pieces of flesh that hang from the womb because women do not clean themselves sufficiently after intercourse, he confidently claims 'we have indeed witnessed the fact that this gets rid [of the growth]'.[31] Certain subtle elaborations on the Latin text likewise suggest personal experience (or at least an attempt to pretend to have personal experience) of women in childbirth: for example, whereas the Latin *Treatments for Women* had simply said 'There are other women who after birth have an immoderate flow of blood', the French elaborates 'And there are some women who, due to the great pain and labour that they have in giving birth, after the baby is born there issues and gushes forth from the body such a great copiosity of immoderately flowing blood that they think they will die of it'.[32]

[28] Interestingly, in ¶92, where the Latin had gradually become deformed from saying that the women who assist a woman in childbirth should not look the parturient in the face to saying that the *men* who assist should not, the French changes it from 'those [men] assisting' to 'those [men] who are in the house' (BNF fr. 1327, f. 77r: 'Et ceulx qui seront alostel ne la regardent point au visaige car pluseurs femmes sont grandement vergoigneuses en leurs enfentement et apres lenfentement'). The rephrasing seems deliberately to exclude male *medical* attendants.

[29] In ¶116, for example, while the original Latin had read 'Tempore partus imminente, paret se mulier ut mos est, et obstetrix similiter cum magna cautela', the translation simply refers to women taking care of themselves: 'elles doiuent elles gouuerner en grant cautelle' (BNF, MS fr. 1327, f. 79r).

[30] BNF, MS fr. 1327, f. 89v: 'il conuient que telle maladie vulgalement soit appelee Trocula comme la maistresse maladie et douleur des dames'.

[31] *Ibid.*, f. 94r: 'Et telle generacion se depart en faisant fomentacion de la decoccion de aucunes herbes chaudes et la suffumiger souuent car de ce nous auons bien veu le experience car de ce elle sen alloit'; cf. ¶170 in the Latin text. Obviously, the translator is taking on the authorial identity of the 'we' here, but the claim to personal experience is entirely his own.

[32] Compare Green, *Trotula*, ¶147, and BNF, fr. 1327, f. 88r: 'ET AUSSI aucunes dames y a que aloccasion de la grande peine et traueil quelles ont aleur enfentement que depuis que lenfant est nez

The suggestions of male use internal to the text are supported by its codicological context: in the single known manuscript of the *Regimen of Ladies*, it appears with French translations of two of Bernard of Gordon's medical writings (his encyclopedia, the *The Lily of Medicine*, and a treatise on prognostication), both here presented with an emphasis on their utility for surgeons; a highly specialized tract on eye diseases; two brief alchemical tracts; and a plague regimen. Again, no owner is known by name, but this translation of the *Trotula*, as well as the character of the codex as a whole, conforms more to 'male' patterns of medical reading than anything we have yet documented for women. Indeed, it could have just as well been in Latin as in French in terms of its professional character.[33]

Finally, the seventh known French translation of the *Trotula*—not extant in full but bearing the title *A Treatise on the Many Maladies Which Can Happen to Women and on Their Secrets Maladies*—was made in the fourteenth or fifteenth century and likewise seems to address a male audience.[34] I will discuss this translation in more detail below; here it merely needs to be stressed that, like the *Regimen of Ladies*, it appears within a 'professional' context of surgical texts and other technical therapeutic texts, paralleling the circulation of the other later medieval French translations.

Overall, the French tradition of vernacularization of the *Trotula* presents a see-sawing pattern: some translations lay claim to a female audience, while others, although articulating no explicitly gendered audience claims in their prefaces, seem in fact to be putting the texts into the hands of professional male practitioners. The twelfth-century Hebrew translation was made as part of a much broader translation effort to render the latest, most authoritative works of Christian medicine available to Jewish practitioners. There is nothing to suggest any intention to make the texts available specifically to women. In Christian communities, the *Trotula* was initially seen as a source of information that could be exploited both by preachers and by at least one translator who envisaged a female audience (undoubtedly upper-class) that would share the gynaecological and obstetrical information of *Conditions of Women* among themselves. Already by the middle of the thirteenth century, however, this same 'women's text' could be appropriated by a versificator who reconceived the text as a model of *male* medical practice: it has now become a handbook not simply for physicians (*mires*) but also a model for scholars and clerks (*escolers* and *clers*). In the early fourteenth

---

il leur sault et gectent du corps si grant coppiosite de sang inmoderement fluant que elles en cuydent morir'. Similar elaborations of the pain women suffer in birth or other conditions can be found in ¶¶149, 160, 162, 169, 184, 200, 213, 225, and 232. Indeed, there is a certain general tendency to dramatize: the translator interprets ¶217, which in the Latin had simply given instructions on how to cut the umbilical cord of the newborn, into a 'grant deouleur au nombril' that certain children suffer. Nevertheless, many of these elaborations, despite the rhetorical flourishes, suggest personal clinical knowledge.

[33] Latin is, in fact, retained in many of the recipes in the Bernard of Gordon translation.
[34] Green, 'Handlist II', pp. 94–5.

century, the Anglo-Norman *Si Aristotele nous dit* could still appropriate the shame claim to argue for a self-treating female audience, yet all subsequent translations (both the texts themselves and the uses that were made of them in actual codices) claim gynaecology as the province of the male practitioner, particularly the surgeon. The only French version addressed to women after the fourteenth century is the brief late fifteenth- or early sixteenth-century adaptation of the Old French translation, *Quant Dex nostre Seignor*, which is surprisingly similar in intent to the first French text, *Secrés de femmes*: the only material being presented to women is information on how infertility can be managed. The idea that women should be responsible for their gynaecological care beyond fertility interventions seems to have vanished.

Equally important is to stress what these translations, 'male' or 'female', do not do: not one addresses midwives *per se* and not one makes the broadly conceived field of 'women's medicine' of Trota's independent *Treatments for Women* available to women who would be performing the hands-on practices of prolapse repair, fistula treatment, or assistance in difficult birth. In other words, no 'textual community' ever seems to have formed around the one text that most immediately reflected the Salernitan female tradition of medical practice. True, this failure may be due to the poor circulation of *Treatments for Women* in France: only eight copies of the independent Latin text are now extant and of these, only two possibly come from France.[35] One, possibly two fourteenth- or fifteenth-century French translators rendered the ensemble text in its entirety, but, as we saw, in the only one that is extant in full, the Latin's *obstetrices* have been eliminated, 'Trotula' reduced to the name of a disease, and the entire body of knowledge of women's medicine—gynaecological, obstetric, and cosmetic—has been assumed to be the male practitioner's preserve. In the French tradition, therefore, the unique achievement of Salerno—the capturing of women's medical practices in a written text—was lost. *Conditions of Women*, that bookish compilation of Arabic and Hippocratic lore, did succeed in generating female textual communities (if we can believe that the hopes of the *Quant Dex nostre Seignor* and *Si com Aristocele* were met in the actual audience the texts received, something for which we as yet have no manuscript evidence). But French male practitioners seem to have been as willing to ignore the practical complications of the gendered notions of shame as had all the male users of the Latin texts. Perhaps it was only his realization of the continuing authority of women in courtly circles that prompted the thirteenth-century French verse author of *Bien sachiés femmes* to open his text with a flimsy apostrophe to women to 'know well' that the following text assembled learning on 'their' diseases. His

---

[35] See Green, 'Development', pp. 135–48. Of the two copies of *Treatments for Women* possibly produced in France (BLL, MSS Sloane 434 and 1615), the former has excerpts only. Both copies migrated to England by the later Middle Ages and so may never have had much of an impact on French knowledge of Trota's practices.

scenario of how that learning will be *used*, however, is clearly focused on the masculine traditions of masters and their students. By the time the fourteenth- or early fifteenth-century translation *Regimen of Ladies* was composed, there was no longer any need to even pretend to address an imagined audience of women.[36]

'SO THAT MANY WOMEN THEREBY MAY BE COMFORTED IN ALL THEIR INFIRMITIES': JOHANNES HARTLIEB'S GERMAN TRANSLATION

The German tradition of gynaecological writing and translation is uniformly male-oriented though it is less easy to characterize along strict professional vs. lay divisions, perhaps because the practice of medicine was itself less confined to a corps of specialists defined by education or licensing as was the case in France. Only two translations of the *Trotula* are known, which is itself surprising given the sizable number of other German gynaecological texts in circulation by the fifteenth century.[37] The first German *Trotula*, from the early or mid fifteenth century, is situated in the one extant copy amid German and Latin recipes, medical texts, and astrological notes. An early owner (and perhaps the commissioner) of the manuscript was a male physician, Hermann Bach, who also owned (and helped write) a small collection of notes on urines, including women's, and a larger collection of German recipes and notes.[38] The second German translation, on the other hand, does show considerable novelty. It was made between 1460 and 1465 by a Munich physician, Johannes Hartlieb (d. 1468), who dedicated this quite creatively modified version of the *Trotula* not to another physician or surgeon, but to Siegmund, Duke of Bavaria-Munich, Count-palatine of the Rhine. Another copy was prepared soon after for Emperor Frederick III.[39] Hartlieb translated the *Trotula* as a companion volume to

---

[36] There is also another late medieval French gynaecological treatise addressed to male practitioners that I discuss in Chapter 6 below.

[37] Britta-Juliane Kruse, *Verborgene Heilkünste: Geschichte der Frauenmedizin im Spätmittelalter*, Quellen und Forschungen zur Literatur- und Kulturgeschichte, 5 (Berlin: Walter de Gruyter, 1996), who has made a comprehensive survey of late medieval German gynaecological literature, characterizes a 15th-century text she calls *Traktat über die Menstruation* as an excerpt from the *Trotula*. However, I find the correspondences very slight and have not included this text in my assessment of the German *Trotula* here. I have also realized that what I listed in 'Handlist II' as a third German translation (of the cosmetics only) is in fact an excerpt from the second translation, that by Hartlieb.

[38] On the *Flos mulierum/Blume der Frawen*, see Green, 'Handlist II', p. 95. Bach's books have, remarkably, stayed together to the present day. They are now MSS Benjamin 5, 9, and 11 at the University of California at Los Angeles.

[39] One copy of each version made during Hartlieb's lifetime is still extant; both were made by the same scribe. Hartlieb's *Buch Trotula* is currently being edited by Kristian Bosselmann-Cyran. For general information on *Das Buch Trotula* and the paired translation of the pseudo-Albertus Magnus, see Kristian Bosselmann-Cyran (ed.), *'Secreta mulierum' mit Glosse in der deutschen Bearbeitung*

his German rendition of the pseudo-Albertus Magnus *Secrets of Women*. He acknowledged that the *Secrets* offered little by way of advice that could be given to women for 'their secret diseases' (*irren gehaymen prechenn*); by appending a translation of the *Trotula*, Hartlieb seems, at least by implication, to be directing the latter text to a female audience. Echoing directly the sentiments of the *Conditions of Women* preface, he points out that he himself has seen women brought to the brink of death by their refusal to show their infirmities to men:

> Therefore it is indeed reasonable that the book *Trotula* be rendered into German so that many women thereby may be comforted in all their infirmities of whatever type they may be; and whatever diseases women might have, against these they will be forewarned with the teaching of Trotula as hereafter will be clearly and openly reported and written.[40]

But how women were supposed to actually get access to this source of aid and comfort is not clear: Duke Siegmund was not, in fact, married at the time Hartlieb wrote the book, and the continued pairing of the *Trotula* with the *Secreta*, to which other texts on generation would soon be added, suggests the distinct interests of male readers in women's nature and reproduction (a topic to which we shall return in the next chapter).

Hartlieb's decision to translate these two texts on 'woman's nature' for a male reader is all the more remarkable in that he himself recognized women as suitable patrons and/or dedicatees of his work. Two, perhaps three of his dozen earlier works were written for Anna of Braunschweig, the wife of his previous patron, Siegmund's father Duke Albrecht III of Bavaria-Munich. Though widowed and advanced in years, Anna was still alive in 1460 and may still have been alive when Hartlieb translated the *Trotula* for her son.[41] Moreover, right within the

---

von Johann Hartlieb, Würzburger medizinhistorische Forschungen, Band 36 (Pattensen/Hannover: Horst Wellm, 1985); *idem*, 'Ein weiterer Textzeuge von Johann Hartliebs '*Secreta mulierum*'- und '*Buch Trotula*'-Bearbeitung: Der Mailänder Kodex AE.IX.34 aus der Privatbibliothek des Arztes und Literaten Albrecht von Haller', *Würzburger medizinhistorische Mitteilungen* 13 (1995), 209–15; Green, 'Handlist. Part II', pp. 95–7; and Karin Zimmermann, 'Ein unbekannter Textzeuge der *Secreta mulierum* und *Trotula*-Übersetzung des Johannes Hartlieb in Cod. Pal. germ. 280', *Zeitschrift für deutsches Altertum* 131 (2002), 343–5.

[40] See Henry E. Sigerist, 'Johannes Hartlieb's Gynaecological Collection and the Johns Hopkins Manuscript 3 (38066)', in *Science, Medicine and History: Essays on the Evolution of Scientific Thought and Medical Practice in Honor of Charles Singer*, ed. E. A. Underwood, 2 vols. (London and New York: Oxford University Press, 1953), 1:231–46, at p. 245, for the preface of the Herzog-Version (my translation).

[41] Hartlieb's works for Anna (whose exact date of death I have been unable to determine) were a translation of the romantic epic, *Alexander*, one of the voyage of St Brendan and (of disputed authenticity) a book on chiromancy. See Klaus Grubmüller, 'Hartlieb, Johannes', in *Die deutsche Literatur des Mittelalters: Verfasserlexikon*, rev. ed., ed. Kurt Ruh *et al.*, 10 vols. (Berlin: De Gruyter, 1978–1999), Bd. 3, coll. 480–96. Obviously, Anna's advanced age in the 1460s may have made her an unlikely dedicatee of a work that incorporated obstetrics and cosmetics. Nevertheless, while it is possible that Hartlieb had discovered Muscio's text only recently before he translated the *Secreta* and the *Trotula* translations (he mentions Muscio's work in both texts and had had plans to translate it, too), it seems unlikely that the widely circulating *Trotula* was not known to him earlier in his career as a physician. One of Hartlieb's friends, Siegmund Gotzkircher (*c.*1410–75), owned his

prologue to his *Secrets of Women* translation, Hartlieb mentioned Muscio's late antique gynaecological text (which he considered to be a fairly recent discovery) and wondered why no German translation had yet been made of this book since it would be 'such a treasure *to midwives*'.[42] Hartlieb, apparently the first northern European writer since Thomas of Cantimpré to envisage an audience of midwives, did not, however, carry out his plan to translate Muscio; he abandoned the project, he says, because of the text's length. Midwives were certainly not his intended audience for the *Trotula*. Translating from a complete copy of the standardized ensemble, he omitted all of the *Treatments for Women* material aside from the instructions for restoring virginity. He translated the *Conditions of Women*'s chapters on menstrual irregularities, uterine dislocation, pregnancy tests, management of birth, and care of the newborn, but he omitted the sections on lesions and ulcers. It is generation, not women's diseases broadly conceived, that interests Hartlieb. He even includes the cosmetics, which other translators often ignored, in order to make women more attractive to their husbands.[43] Hartlieb's intent was to provide aristocratic male readers with a guide to understanding sexuality; the cosmetics were included to facilitate sexual coupling, apparently with the thought that male heads of households would convey the information to their wives (or lovers). His intent was to facilitate reproduction; addressing women was irrelevant.

The irony that Hartlieb could write two 'typically feminine' works for a female patron but dedicate his gynaecological work to males, that he could recognize the utility of translating a work on obstetrics for midwives but then not direct his gynaecological work to them, is striking but not surprising. Aside from a womb exorcism found in a thirteenth-century psalter owned by some German Dominican nuns and a brief charm to facilitate birth embedded within a larger medical collection owned by Barbara Holländersche in the late fifteenth century, we have as yet no evidence that the quite rich corpus of German gynaecological texts and recipe collections either was intended directly for or circulated among women prior to the sixteenth century.[44] At about the same time Barbara's book was being prepared, two texts focusing on regimen for pregnancy, childbirth,

own copy of the *Trotula* (see Appendix 1, item 68), though this was not the copy Hartlieb used for his translation.

[42] I discuss Hartlieb's understanding of Muscio's text in a forthcoming essay, 'The Sources of Eucharius Rösslin's *Rosegarden for Pregnant Women and Midwives* (1513)'. As was typical of the period, Hartlieb only recognizes Muscio's utility as a resource on obstetrics; the work's gynaecological content is never mentioned.

[43] See Chapter 5 below.

[44] German women who owned medical books (but not anything specifically gynaecological) include *Juncfrow* Guoteline von Eßlignen of Speyer, who in 1321 compiled or had compiled for her a diverse collection of medical texts written in Alsacian dialect; Elisabeth von Volkensdorf, an as yet unidentified Austrian woman from the first half of the 15th century who had six medical books among her collection of forty-eight volumes (some of which were on law); and Kunigunde Gross Schreiberin (d. 1470), a patrician widow turned Dominican nun, who brought a collection of medical recipes into the nunnery of St Katharina's in Nuremberg. See Green, 'Possibilities', p. 53–4.

and postnatal care were produced. Although both would go on to have fortunes as print texts, each in its earlier manuscript form survives in a single copy that gives no evidence of female use.[45] The former is found amid German texts on urines, astrology, questions and answers about the art of medicine, some of the pseudo-Aristotle *Problems*, and even excerpts from a formal commentary of Rhazes's *Liber Almansoris*. In other words, this looks very much like a compilation for a professional healer. The latter text, a more lengthy work that fills up the bulk of its small codex, actually addresses 'the common man' (*gemeinen man*), who should consult learned doctors or apothecaries if 'he' does not understand the technical terms in the text. Like most other vernacular traditions, German gynaecological texts are frequently found in codices that also incorporate Latin texts or recipes, and like the other vernacular traditions, these texts (some of which are just strings of gynaecological and obstetrical recipes) are found amid medical or surgical collections that have nothing to suggest female engagement either as owners or readers.[46]

'FOR TO DRAW OUT OF LATIN': ENGLISH LAYWOMEN AND DOCTORS, GENTLEMEN AND MERCHANTS

Whereas the German tradition of gynaecological writing seems to have been entirely male-oriented, as one moves further west across northern Europe the gendering of the vernacular becomes ambiguous again. There were three Dutch translations of the *Trotula*. One of the two fourteenth-century translations selects a few chapters of the *Conditions of Women* and embeds them in a larger medical compendium. Another, which employs a modified version of the proto-ensemble, uses the *Trotula* as the core of a long rhymed text on generation. Neither version has any address to a female audience, and the codicological contexts suggest ownership and use by male practitioners or clergy.[47] A third Dutch translation, however, departs radically from these earlier two and claims women as (or at least among) its audience and envisages them as both reading *and* listening.

---

[45] On the *Frauenbüchlein* (printed in 1495) and the *Rosegarden for Pregnant Women and Midwives* (printed in 1513), see Chapter 6 and the Conclusion below.

[46] In her book, *Verborgene Heilkunste*, Kruse continually referred to *Leseren/innen* ('male and female readers'), and even *Verfasseren/innen* ('male and female authors'), yet she never offered any evidence that women made up any significant portion of the audience of these texts. Kruse's own research turned up male owners for twenty-three of the fifty-one manuscripts she surveyed, a fact whose significance she does not address. One might add, too, that the circulation of Latin gynaecological texts remained just as vigorous for just as long in German-speaking territories as in other parts of western Europe.

[47] See Green, 'Handlist II', pp. 81–3. Since publishing my initial handlist, I have identified four additional copies of the first text, bringing the total to six. While I think the 14th- and 15th-century users were male, see Conclusion below for evidence that at least two copies were used by laywomen in the 16th century.

Making no mention of women's shame, it opens with a straightforward address to 'all women who will see this or hear it read'.[48] All three manuscripts bear a characteristic of possible use by women that, as we will see, distinguishes the three fifteenth-century English texts addressed to women: they all were produced as independent pamphlets rather than as elements of larger medical or surgical compendia. The two later copies, moreover, incorporate additional obstetrical material to supplement that of the original *Trotula*, a feature that likewise would characterize two of the contemporary texts addressed to women in England. Finally, all three copies of this Dutch translation are distinctive within the *Trotula* tradition, whether Latin or vernacular, in adding illustrations of various medical devices (pessaries, fumigation pots, etc.) that must have aided greatly in making the text comprehensible to readers not already familiar with common gynaecological practices.[49] But this Dutch translation also presents inherent contradictions, for the third copy, although keeping the nominal address to women, in fact presents a very male-oriented text. Produced around the middle of the fifteenth century, this copy adds material on surgical interventions in obstructed birth drawn from the Arabic authority Albucasis (including his images of surgical instruments) as well as material from the pseudo-Albertan *Secrets of Women* that described planetary influences on the unborn foetus or those of the twelve zodiacal houses. These changes would not, in themselves, work to exclude a female audience, but in fact this redactor makes other changes that may have had (or been intended to have) that effect. He interposes the midwife (*die hoeftmoeder*) back into all situations that involve actual manual manipulation of the female genitalia, exactly the same referencing of a subordinate assistant that we find in other gynaecological works meant for men.[50] And whereas the other two copies of this Dutch *Liber Trotula* acknowledged 'Trotula' as an authority on women's matters, this redactor suppressed all references to her and instead ascribed the entire work to 'Albertus', undoubtedly meaning the great Dominican authority Albertus Magnus.[51] Although created as an independent

---

[48] Brugge, Openbare Bibliotheek, MS 593, s. xv (western Flanders), ff. 1r–18r. The text was edited (poorly) by Delva, *Vrouwengeneeskunde*. This *Liber Trotula* is the only content of the manuscript, save for three added recipes on menstrual retention at the end.

[49] Reproductions of some of the images from Copenhagen, Det Kongelige Bibliotek, MS GKS 1657 can be found in Green, *Trotula*, pp. 32–33. The third copy, Hamburg, Staats- und Universitätsbibliothek, Cod. med. 798, s. xv med., pp. 85–256, also adds sections from Albucasis's surgical text along with accompanying images of surgical instruments.

[50] For example, in rendering the obstetrical sections of Albucasis' *Surgery*, the Dutch redactor retains all five references to the *obstetrix* in the Latin, and adds four additional references to the *hoeftmoeder* to clarify that it is this female attendant, and not the male addressee, that performs the manual tasks. See Brigitte Kusche, 'Laatmiddelnederlandse Fragmenten uit de *Chirurgie* van Albucasis', *Verslagen en mededelingen*, Koninklijke Academie voor Nederlandse Taal- en Letterkunde (Gent, 1980), pp. 370–420.

[51] The text opens (Hamburg, cod. med. 798, p. 85) with the rubric: *Hic incipit Alberti liber de secretis mulierum*. References to 'Albertus seit' (Albertus says) and 'Ic Albertus' (I, Albertus) litter the text. See Chapter 5 below for Albert's role in this story.

pamphlet, it was soon bound with a Latin copy of the pseudo-Albertus *Secrets of Women* as well as the Latin *Trotula* ensemble. The address to 'all women who will see this or hear it read' now is buried far below lengthy appeals to authorities such as Avicenna, Hippocrates, and Boethius.[52] At best, the address to women has become a flimsy concession to the unlikely possibility that any woman would ever come close to this text with its Latin headings, scholastic digressions, and clerical tone; at worst, it reflects the oversight of a hasty redactor who failed to suppress this now extraneous passage.

It would be interesting to think that whoever was responsible for the first two redactions of the Dutch *Liber Trotula*—the ones that seem authentically meant for women—was aware of the contemporary English tradition, for the parallels in gendered rhetoric and textual form are astoundingly similar.[53] Building on the earlier Anglo-Norman tradition, where, as we saw, three texts at least nominally claimed a female audience, so in English three different texts would be addressed to women in the late fourteenth and fifteenth centuries. But just as the French and the Dutch translations for women ended up sooner or later back in the hands of men, so, too, the English texts show a contest between men and women over their possession. In fact, the earliest English gynaecological text was neither a translation of the *Trotula* nor a text meant for women, but rather a translation of a Latin adaptation of Muscio (which had itself probably originated in the university context of Paris) meant to instruct its male readers on the basics of female physiology and obstetrics. In the sole extant copy, *Nature of Women* is found among astrological and other natural philosophical texts in English and Latin, a context suggestive of non-therapeutic uses.[54] As we will see, English was never a 'women-only' language in medicine. The English tradition is unique, however, in that it was the first to articulate a female perspective on the problematic male uses of gynaecological literature.

The earliest of the five English translations of the *Trotula, The Knowing of Woman's Kind in Childing*, taps not simply into textual traditions but also social

---

[52] The phrase, 'Ic bidde alle vrouwen . . .', appears on p. 89, well after the main prefatory material describing this redactor's purpose and authorities on pp. 85–8.

[53] On political and cultural ties between England and the Low Countries in this period, see Erik Kooper (ed.), *Medieval Dutch Literature in its European Context* (Cambridge: Cambridge University Press, 1994). Jacqueline of Hainault's (d. 1436/7) transference of English medical books to Flanders upon her marriage to her fourth husband is a singular instance of such interconnections (Green, 'Possibilities', p. 55), but her story also shows that English books had no audience there. Other evidence for transmission across the Channel, perhaps in the other direction, includes a Latin abbreviation of the *Trotula* ensemble, currently known only in a copy made in late 15th-century Flanders but obviously originating earlier, which served as the basis for the third Middle English translation of the *Trotula*, the ambiguously entitled *Secreta mulierum*. See also Chapter 5 below on Chaucer's Dutch connections.

[54] Monica H. Green, 'Obstetrical and Gynecological Texts in Middle English', *Studies in the Age of Chaucer* 14 (1992), 53–88; repr. in Green, *Women's Healthcare*, Essay IV, at pp. 84–8.

traditions already ensconced in England.[55] It draws not on the Latin *Trotula* but an early version of the Old French prose translation, *Quant Dex nostre Seignor*, which had been circulating in England since at least the middle of the thirteenth century and had already given rise to the Anglo-Norman verse text discussed above. It is from his French source that this Middle English translator gets his initial authorization to address women, although he articulates much more forcefully the 'women only' character of his text. He now finally makes explicit the potential for a written text to liberate women from male scrutiny:

And because women of our tongue know better [how] to read and understand this language than any other, and [so that] every literate woman may read it to others who are unlettered and help them and counsel them in their maladies *without having to show their disease to man*, I have drawn this [out of the treatises of diverse masters] and written it in English.[56]

Interestingly, this English text makes no direct appeal to women's shame as an argument for women's use of the text, even though that topos had figured prominently in its French source. Nevertheless, the *Knowing of Woman's Kind*, even more than its French source, is a real 'woman's text': the grammatical addresses, the topical content, and the codicological context (of at least of three of the five extant copies) all point to a female audience, both intended and real. The author does not presume a great deal of prior knowledge of anatomy or basic physiology, though he does assume the reader will be able to absorb such information when it is presented in a straightforward way. One of the most striking features of the text is the entirely novel material the author introduces on male/female differences and the physiology of menstruation and uterine suffocation. The author usually retains a coolly descriptive third-person mode for accounts of symptomatology and etiology, but therapeutic instructions are almost always couched in direct second-person addresses to the (female) reader—except, that is, for a few chapters describing how the midwife (referred to in the third-person and so not the immediate addressee) should handle difficulties in birth.[57] The text, therefore, seems to be addressed not to professional practitioners but to knowledgeable laywomen concerned to help themselves and their neighbours. The

---

[55] Although Alexandra Barratt (ed.), *The Knowing of Woman's Kind in Childing: A Middle English Version of Material Derived from the 'Trotula' and Other Sources*, Medieval Women: Texts and Contexts, 4 (Turnhout: Brepols, 2001), suggests that *Knowing* was composed in the early 15th century, this is simply the date of the earliest extant manuscript and does not rule out a late 14th-century composition. In fact, *Knowing* has distinct correspondences with the 14th-century Muscian text *The Nature of Women*.

[56] Barratt, *Knowing*, lines 18–22, my emphasis. Barratt edits the two main versions of this text in facing-page format. My quotations come from the earlier, Douce version, based on OBL, MS Douce 37 (SC 21611), s. xv in., ff. 1r–37v.

[57] There is only one instance where the 'you' receiving instructions is clearly contrasted with (and is assumed not to be identical with) the woman to be treated; cf. Barratt, *Knowing*, MS D, lines 941–2: 'and yf ye thyrst [thrust] hit [*sc.*, a uterine tumour] hard þe pacient schall suffyre gret grevans . . .'.

special needs of a female audience are further reflected by the addition (from the Muscio adaptation *Non omnes quidem*) of new material on how to handle both normal and malpresented births—a medical function that remained decidedly in the hands of women.

We know nothing, unfortunately, about the translator of *Knowing of Woman's Kind*. There are no therapeutic additions to the text to indicate his direct experience as a practitioner,[58] but his mastery of general medical theory (as well as his obvious competence in Latin) suggests that he may well have been a cleric who considered translation work an act of charity.[59] All the more striking, then, is his awareness of and even downright hostility to current masculine uses (and misuses) of gynaecological texts, which (as we will see in more detail later) he attempts to forestall. His desire to reach a female audience does seem to have been at least partially fulfilled. No owner's marks can confirm this, but the codicological context of three of the five extant copies of *Knowing* suggests that at least on occasion it was owned by women: *Knowing* either appears as an independent pamphlet (which, as we have seen, the Latin *Trotula* almost never did), or with a few additional English recipes on gynaecological and other matters (to be bound later with another woman-directed gynaecological text), or with a devotional text of the kind we would expect to be owned by women.[60] In this last copy, the scribe has even added the claim that *Knowing* was written 'at the pleasure of my lady', perhaps in reference to the woman who commissioned the manuscript.[61] The small format of these three copies of *Knowing* is reminiscent of the Books of Hours and prayerbooks that many women of the period owned;[62] these are not workbooks of an active physician but private possessions, perhaps to be pondered

---

[58] The one extended section that does not come from his French or Latin sources is a series of recipes, prayers, and charms to aid childbirth (Barratt, *Knowing*, lines 359–76). These can, however, be documented from other English sources and do not reflect the compiler's own unique practices. A section at the end of the text on apostemes (tumours) comes from an as yet unidentified source.

[59] The two Latin sources, the pseudo-Cleopatran *Gynecology* and the Muscian adaptation *Non omnes quidem* often circulated together as parts I and III, respectively, of a three-text compendium. (The middle text was the *De passionibus mulierum A*.) Two extant copies of the group are known from England, and catalogue references show the group was or may have been available at both Christ Church and St Augustine's, Canterbury, and at the Priory of St John the Baptist in Launde (Leicestershire), where John Leland found a copy of *Gemissae [sic] libellus ad Cleopatram de menstruis et matrice* when he was searching for materials to support Henry VIII's divorce from his wife Katherine. On translation as an act of charity, see Faye Marie Getz, 'Charity, Translation, and Language of Medical Learning in Medieval England', *Bulletin of the History of Medicine* 64 (1990), 1–17.

[60] These are, respectively, OBL, MS Douce 37 (SC 21611), s. xv in., ff. 1r–37v, the earliest extant copy; Cambridge, University Library, MS Ii.VI.33, s. xv, ff. 33r–68r; and BLL, MS Sloane 421A, *ante* 1530, ff. 2r–25v, where *Knowing* appears with a brief English 'regiment of helthe' for body and soul, followed by two English recipes for delivering a woman of a dead foetus. On all the Middle English texts, see Green, 'Obstetrical and Gynecological Texts'.

[61] Barratt, *Knowing*, pp. 4 and 32.

[62] Barratt, *Knowing*, gives their dimensions as $5^3/_8 \times 3^7/_8$ inches (Douce 37); 6×4 (Cambridge University Library Ii.VI.33); and $8^1/_4 \times 6$ (Sloane 421A).

over slowly for general edification or communal discussion, perhaps to be carried to the bedsides of kinswomen and neighbours for emergency consultation.

The two other extant copies of *Knowing of Woman's Kind*, however, are harder to connect with 'typically feminine' patterns of reading. One situates a somewhat abbreviated copy of *Knowing* amid English works on astronomy, astrology, fishing, bookmaking, and magic. Astronomy and astrology seem to have been, like medicine, a 'borderline' area where only a handful of women of the upper classes treaded; for fishing, bookmaking, and magic, we thus far have no evidence of female textual involvement at all.[63] The other dubiously gendered copy locates *Knowing* next to an anonymous Middle English andrological and gynaecological text that speaks not to women but to a professional (apparently male) practitioner; the other contents are an English receptary, several English herbals, and miscellaneous recipes in English and Latin. Written in the middle of the fifteenth century for an unknown reader, by the end of the century it was in the possession of one Jhon [*sic*] Barke.[64]

The differing interests of male and female audiences in vernacular gynaeco- logical texts continue to be seen in the seven other English gynaecological texts composed in the following century. Four of these were translations of the *Trotula*, each done, apparently, in ignorance of the existence of its predecessors. As on the Continent, *Condition of Women*'s articulation of the problem of women's shame seems not at all to have been taken as a disqualification of male gynaecological practice. The Middle English *Liber Trotuli* ('The Book of Trotulus', the only medieval case where the authoress 'Trotula' has been masculinized) was produced sometime in the first half of the fifteenth century from the intermediate version of the *Trotula* ensemble.[65] It dutifully translates the shame claim,[66] yet there is nothing in the text itself to suggest that a direct female audience was intended. The translator has, for example, suppressed the instructions in ¶149 of the

---

[63] BLL, MS Additional 12195, s. xv². Upper-class women's rare involvement in astrology and other divinatory sciences in addressed in Monica H. Green, 'Gendering the Audiences of Medieval Scientific Texts: The Case of Chiromancy' (presented at the 38th International Medieval Congress, Kalamazoo, Michigan, May 2003). Given the poor quality of this particular manuscript, it seems unlikely to have been made for an upper-class recipient. I therefore find it difficult to accept Barratt's arguments (*Knowing*, p. 37) that this manuscript could have been made by or for a woman, especially since there is evidence to connect it with the house of Augustinian canons in North Creake, Norfolk.

[64] OBL, MS Bodley 483 (SC 2062), s. xv med. On the andrological text, see Green, 'Obstetrical and Gynaecological Texts', pp. 83–4. The manuscript was probably owned in the mid 16th century by John Twynne of Canterbury (d. 1581).

[65] Grammatically, the genitive *Trotuli* could be either masculine or neuter, yet the latter makes no sense as a possessive form.

[66] BLL, MS Additional 34111, s. xv med., f. 197r: 'for woman is more febil than man be way of kynd and hathe grete greuaunce be fele tymes in beryng of children, and hathe mo diuers sekenes than the man and nameliche a boute the membres that bien in the most priue place of alle the body and wil noght telle to the leche for shame the sekenes that be falleth be cause that she dar noght suffreth more greuaunce'. This translator omits the original author's claim to have drawn on other books; instead, Galen and Hippocrates are directly acknowledged as authorities.

Treatments for Women in which Trota (or her representative) had given detailed, hands-on instructions on repairing a prolapsed uterus with ano-vaginal fistula. The translator omits the instructions to massage the uterus with warm wine and butter and restore it to its place, omits the directions on how to sew up the fistula, and omits the injunctions to keep the woman in bed, abstaining from both baths and foods that might induce coughing. Rather, all he includes is the single recipe to powder consound and sprinkle it, together with anise and cinnamon, on the lesion.[67] This translation is, in fact, notable for its paucity of obstetrical material; neither midwives nor any hands-on treatments (save one) are ever mentioned.[68] In the single known manuscript the text is found amid a massive collection of *experimenta* of various medical authorities, all clearly intended for professional medical practice.[69] There is nothing about this 'Book of Trotulus', then, to suggest that it was meant for the use of either female patients or female healers.

The translator of the so-called Middle English *Secreta mulierum* ('The Secrets of Women'), made perhaps around the middle of the century, even while still asserting (in the authorial voice) that he was motivated by 'the love of women', stresses the masculine origin of the work by emphasizing that it was composed with 'the fatherly help of Hippocrates and Galen, the philosophers and fathers of physic'. 'Trotula' as author makes no appearance here.[70] The text is marked

---

[67] BLL, MS Additional 34111, f. 206v.

[68] The exception is the instruction from ¶56 of the Latin *Conditions of Women*, where it was couched in the passive, to manually reposition a prolapsed uterus (f. 202r: 'and than lege to honde to the marice and do it in his stede'). This translator (or perhaps the scribe of this particular manuscript) is often inattentive to keeping his grammatical forms consistent; in this same paragraph, the same (implied) 'you' of the imperatives not only replaces the uterus and prepares certain remedies, but also drinks one of them! It is not clear whether the absence of all the obstetrical material from *Conditions of Women* is a deliberate omission or the result of what appears to be a lacuna between ff. 203v and 204r. Notably, however, of the thirteen *Treatments for Women* obstetrical chapters, the only ones that appear here are recipes for three postpartum conditions (¶¶149 on ano-vaginal fistula, much abbreviated as just noted; 229 on postpartum pain, and 230 on haemorrhoids due to childbirth).

[69] In addition to the description of Additional 34111 in Green, 'Obstetrical and Gynecological Texts', see Hunt, *Anglo-Norman Medicine*, 2: 10–11. The longest text in the manuscript, a 300-page Middle English translation of the Latin *Speculum medicorum*, is introduced as a 'litel boke' that doctors have assembled so 'þat seke men shal noght long perish and þat leches unconyng may be holpyn of many þenges' (Hunt, 2:10).

[70] Cambridge, Jesus College, MS 43 (Q.D.1), s. xv, f. 70r: 'Be cawse that woman bene febeler of nature, and for ther bene often tymes greuyd in chyld berthe therfor be diuerse tymes they habundaunt sekenes and most abowte the preuy membris that bene ordrynyd in the offyse of nature and they thorowgh schame and rednesse of face helyn and wolle nowt be aknow ne they durnowt schewe ne sey to leches half the party of here sykenes weche ffallen abowte here secrete partyes'; f. 70v: 'the fadyrly help of epocras and Galyene the fylosofers and ffaderrs of fysek'. The omission of 'Trotula's' name as author may well have been a deliberate decision of the translator, since we do find her name attached to the single extant copy of the Latin version that served as the translator's source: LWL, MS 517, Miscellanea Alchemica XII (*olim* Phillipps 2946), s. xv ex. (probably Flanders), ff. 129v–134r. The anecdote about Trota/'Trotula' in ¶151 is not included in this version.

by extensive omissions: included are only selected chapters from *Conditions of Women* on retained menses (believed to be the chief impediment to conception), excessive menstruation, problems of fertility, and difficult birth. From *Treatments for Women*, there are only a few passages on excessive bloodflow after birth, certain urogenital disorders, and mechanisms to 'restore' virginity. None of the more 'hands-on' remedies are included. These omissions are the work not of the English translator but an earlier Latin abbreviator, whose condensed version of the *Trotula* ensemble was still circulating in Flanders at the end of the fifteenth century. Just as this later Flemish copy is found incorporated into a volume of Latin and Dutch alchemical and magical texts, so we find two copies of the English translation amid collections of Latin and English medical and other scientific texts. Once again, translation into the vernacular seems to have altered the character of the text's audience very little. In the third extant manuscript, this 'Secrets of Women' was originally part of a small pamphlet containing uroscopy texts and miscellaneous medical recipes. It was soon bound, however, into a personal collection of poetry and legal texts compiled by a Cheshire gentleman, Humphrey Newton (1466–1536), whose domestic interests in the text we will return to shortly.

The fourth English translation of the *Trotula*, entitled both *The Book called 'Trotela'* and *Secreta mulierum*, shows a more interventionist approach to the text. This version seems to have started off as a fairly literal translation of *Conditions of Women* in the first half of the fifteenth century,[71] although in the only complete copy we have of it (which dates from the latter half of the sixteenth century) it has been modified to stand at an intermediate point between the 'self-help' versions addressed to women and those oriented toward professional or learned lay male audiences.[72] New material has been added. For example, a Plinian account of the noxious properties of the menses is inserted: contact with menses kills crops, rusts iron, and turns dogs rabid. Yet instead of directing the 'moral' of these observations to men (that they should flee menstruous women), we instead find the admonition that 'Therefore good women shall not meddle with men in that time of that sickness unless it were a wife that cannot by any excuse or

---

[71] BLL, MS Sloane 121, s. xv med., ff. 106r–107v. This is only extant in a single bifolium (comprising ¶¶91–116, the obstetrical portions of the text) inserted into a compilation of several other volumes (one of which includes the third Middle English translation, *Secreta mulierum*). It is therefore impossible to know in what codicological context the original version circulated or whether the additional material found in the second copy, from more than a century later, reflects the original translator's work.

[72] Although this second, complete copy of the text (Longleat House [Warminster, Wiltshire], MS Longleat 333, ff. 33r–43v) dates from the second half of the 16th century, a number of features suggest that this scribe is copying a much earlier text. First, several Latin phrases (which this copyist often mangles badly) must have been added to the text at an earlier stage. Second, the presence of a version of the *peperit* charm (fol. 40v: 'Sancta Maria peperit et matrix eius non doluit: Christum genuit qui suo sanguine nos recttinit [*sic*]') suggests composition of this version prior to the suppression of Mariology in the 1540s. I therefore find nothing in this expanded version of the text that would contradict a 15th- or early 16th-century date of composition.

entreaty defend [against] her husband'.[73] Male aphrodisiacs intended as aids to conception are added, though these are phrased in such a way that it is not clear whether the man himself is preparing these remedies or they are being prepared for him (perhaps by his wife). There are also extensive obstetrical instructions that provide more clinical detail than any other medieval text known in England. For example, in the section, 'Means to help and to provoke the birth and to make the labour easier and without great pain', the compiler adds these instructions: 'First, the woman that labours must either sit grovelling or else upright leaning backward according as it shall seem most commodious and necessary to the party or as she is accustomed'.[74] The text closes with the thoughtful suggestion that if the reader finds the medicaments described therein too technical, s/he can copy down the prescription and send it off to a professional apothecary for preparation.[75] The text seems, then, to have been intended for a domestic context, reflecting both the concerns for progeny common to males and the concern with the very real hazards of childbirth more directly threatening women. In fact, despite the ascription of this text to a male author, 'Iohn of Burgwen' ('Trotela' here being understood as a title), this text seems the closest we have seen yet to a 'neutral' text, one that could serve the needs and concerns of both the men and the women in a domestic setting, a setting in which the other contents of the manuscript (short tracts on herbs; medical and culinary recipes as well as ones for making ink, dyeing clothes, distilling, etc.; and works on prognostication) would have had an equally utilitarian value. Discerning *usage* in a domestic setting is difficult (a topic to which we will return below), but the *Book called 'Trotela'* is nonetheless an intriguing exception to the gender-segregated patterns we have seen thus far.

The last medieval English translation of the *Trotula*, in contrast, the *Book Made [by] a Woman Named Rota*, instead of combining men's and women's interests, presents them as if they are fundamentally opposed. In this case, the two extant manuscripts present us with a 'woman's version' and a 'man's version' of the same vernacular translation. The *Book*, made perhaps as late as the turn of the sixteenth century, is a free rendition of a few select chapters of *Conditions of Women* and *Treatments for Women* along with other material. It is focused primarily on the 'many maladise and disseases' that afflict the uterus and has only minimal obstetrical material.[76] Although there is no direct address to women in

---

[73] *Boke called Trotela*, MS Longleat 333, f. 33r.   [74] *Ibid.*, f. 42r.

[75] *Ibid.*, f. 43v: 'And if thow be noght so conyng to wirk by your medicyns as ther names is wrytten her for strangnes, maik thy bylles in forme as it is her wrytten and send them to the ypoticaries and that may be sone sped.'

[76] Whether the translator had access to only a fragmentary copy of the ensemble or chose not to translate the more detailed prescriptions of *Treatments for Women* is unclear. The text overall is very abbreviated and contains material not original to the *Trotula*; it seems unlikely to have functioned well as a handbook specifically for midwives. Nevertheless, midwives may have been part of the intended audience, for the suggestion that the 'good midwife' will have a certain oil with her at all times could be read as professional counsel.

the preface, in one copy the text is clearly intended for the use of the patient who will be treating herself or for the use of her female attendant. The text is often quite explicit in detailing what different practitioners—barber, apothecary, and midwife—should do or provide.[77] More frequently, self-treatments are described; only if a woman cannot perform certain procedures by herself should she then have another woman help her. In one case the text insists, using the direct second-person, that the woman must anoint herself internally, no matter how embarrassed she is; in another, an impersonal third-person prescription for an emmenagogue suddenly shifts to the second person: 'and within an hour and a half you shall feel your flowers [menses] begin to break and come forth'—hardly an appropriate comment to make to a male physician. In the other copy of *The Book of Rota*, however, which the physician and alchemist Robert Green of Welby made for his own use in 1544, all the self-treating references (except for one final slip) appear in the third-person. It is probably no coincidence that the attribution to 'a woman named Rota' is also missing in Green's copy.[78]

Robert Green's appropriation of the *Book of Rota* demonstrates, once again, that there was no way to guarantee that texts intended for women would stay in their hands. Indeed, long before Green was active in the 1540s there was a whole corpus of vernacular gynaecological literature circulating in England, most of which gave no indication at all that women, whether lay or professional, were the intended audience. I will have more to say about male physicians' practice of gynaecology in fifteenth-century England in Chapter 6, but here one further Middle English text merits analysis since, like the *Book of Rota*, it has both a men's and a women's version.

The most widely circulating Middle English gynaecological text, *The Sickness of Women*, was not a translation of the *Trotula* but of the gynaecological chapters of Gilbert the Englishman's *Compendium of Medicine*. The earlier of its two different versions (often found as part of the full translation of Gilbert's *Compendium*) bears no statement of intended audience, while the later adaptation is intended (or so the added preface claims) for women.[79] Like many of the *Trotula* translators, the

[77] Midwives are referred to three times in Cambridge University Library, MS Ii.VII.33 once as the attendant who should replace the prolapsed uterus; once as the birth supervisor; and in one case describing how to stretch out the vagina during birth, with the statement that 'a good mydwyfe shuld euer haue thys oyle with her when she goth to thys secret occupacion' (i.e., childbirth). A barber is to be called when there is need to let blood, and certain items are said to be obtainable from apothecaries—in one case the price is even given.

[78] Glasgow, Glasgow University Library, MS Hunter 403 (V.3.1), an. 1544, pp. 347–63. Because it retains the material on contraceptives (which clearly derives from the original Latin *Trotula*) which the Cambridge copy lacks, Green's copy cannot be a copy of the latter, which may in turn suggest that the female address was not original. Nevertheless, I am inclined to believe that the female address was original, as Green's inadvertent slip into a nonsensical second-person address at the very end of his text suggests that he himself had been transposing second-person addresses into third-person forms as he transcribed his text.

[79] *Sickness of Women 1* seems to have originated as part of a complete translation of Gilbertus's *Compendium*, but was then split off to circulate independently. It is extant in twelve copies (vs. the

author of *Sickness of Women 1* probably did not feel it necessary to explicitly claim a particular audience because he expected the text's readers to be the same sorts of people who read medical texts in general: professional (and normatively male) practitioners and interested laymen. In most of the twelve extant manuscripts, *Sickness 1*'s codicological context suggests that it was used by surgeons or general practitioners—the one known owner is a certain Richard Dod of London, barber-surgeon—and most of the other copies of the text have a similar technical, often surgical, focus suggesting use by practitioners. Richard Dod's copy, as well as two others, clarified that male readers had 'permission' to read this text by opening with the direct address, 'Sirs'. It was probably a merchant, however, who commissioned the compilation of one of these 'male' copies of the text, for we find here, alongside astrological material and in the same hand as the gynaecological text, some notes for merchants on spices, cloth, wine, and weights and measures.[80]

As for the second, 'female' version of *Sickness of Women*, its address to a female audience is problematic as it conflicts with certain other elements of the text. Not only does *Sickness 2* have only third-person references to the female patient and the midwife (meaning that neither party is addressed directly), but despite its inclusion—as in its *Trotula* counterpart, *The Knowing of Woman's Kind*—of a substantial amount of obstetrical material (here including the foetus-in-utero figures drawn from Muscio's *Gynaecia*), its equally substantial amount of Latin (some of it addressed directly to men!) undermines the compiler's own prefatory claim to be writing a text that women can use themselves 'so that one woman may help another in her sickness'.[81] Read closely, in fact, this preface never asserts that men should *not* read the text; rather, those men who do read it are simply warned that they should not misuse it.

Sickness of Women 2's codicological context in two of the four extant manuscripts parallels that of the English and Dutch *Trotulas* addressed to women: they are independent fascicles where the gynaecological text appears

English *Trotulas* which are extant in one to five copies each), and was adapted in the mid 15th century into a second version that was ostensibly intended for female use though, in two of its four copies, actually appears in male-owned codices. The latter text is edited, with extensive commentary, in Monica H. Green and Linne R. Mooney, 'The *Sickness of Women*', in *Sex, Aging, and Death in a Medieval Medical Compendium: Trinity College Cambridge MS R.14.52, Its Texts, Language, and Scribe*, ed. M. Teresa Tavormina, Medieval and Renaissance Texts and Studies, 292, 2 vols. (Tempe, AZ: Arizona Center for Medieval and Renaissance Studies, 2006), vol. 2, pp. 455–568.

[80] Longleat House (Warminster, Wiltshire), MS Longleat 174, s. xv²; other sections contain calendrical material, a uroscopy text, and a synonymy of herbs in Latin and English. My thanks to Kate Harris, librarian to the Marquess of Bath, for sharing with me her draft description of this manuscript.

[81] Green and Mooney, *Sickness*, lines 17–18: 'that oo womman may help another in hir sikenes and nat discure hir privitees to suche vncurteys men'. We argue there that a variety of features in this peculiar text suggest its composition by a male author familiar with such university texts as Avicenna's *Canon* even though there is nothing about the work that could be called 'scholastic'.

as the main work and the other contents (a brief devotional 'regimen' in one copy, a recipe for *aqua vitae* in the other) would fit well with 'typically feminine' interests we have documented from other sources.[82] It is the other two manuscripts, however, that show the tension over use of the text for, again like the *Trotula*, *Sickness of Women 2* was also pulled into compendia used by men. In one manuscript, compiled just after the middle of the fifteenth century, this supposedly woman-oriented text was drawn back into the same codicological context in which the earlier, 'men's' version of *Sickness of Women* had already circulated: that is, into a collection of technical works meant for use by surgeons. Whether the surgeon who originally commissioned this rather elegant (and therefore, expensive) manuscript was male cannot be known for certain, but the codex is certainly 'masculine' in its professional character.[83] In the other instance, a manuscript copied in London in the 1460s (probably directly from the surgeon's copy), *Sickness 2* was assimilated into a massive collection of Middle English tracts on medicine, astrology and astronomy, mathematics, and the seven liberal arts. The manuscript was commissioned, apparently, by the merchant Thomas Cook, who served as mayor of London in 1462–63, and it later passed into the hands of his secretary, John de Vale. The codex as a whole shows an aspiration to acquire knowledge on longevity, generation, and other scientific topics that normally circulated within university settings. In fact, Cook seems to have commissioned from this same scribe a veritable 'Everyman's Library', consisting not only of this massive medical and scientific compendium, but also matching volumes that contained London city, guild, and legal affairs; apocryphal and authentic books of scripture and devotional, didactic, and contemplative treatises; and treatises on state ceremony, heraldry, and chivalry.[84]

The Cook/de Vale manuscript raises an important question: for those vernacular texts that circulated within the lay realm, is not the distinction between 'men's texts' and 'women's texts' too hard and fast? Wouldn't women have had access to books in their husbands' libraries, and might not 'household books' have been a venue in which men and women might equally share access to medical knowledge? Defining what 'household books' actually were has been a point of contention among scholars; one reasonable formula is 'a repository of practical information of more or less domestic kinds—recipes and remedies and instructions on matters such as dyeing, fishing, arboriculture, and book

[82] In addition to Green and Mooney, *Sickness*, see also Monica H. Green, 'Masses in Remembrance of 'Seynt Susanne': A Fifteenth-Century Spiritual Regimen', *Notes and Queries* n. s. 50, no. 4 (December 2003), 380–4.

[83] BLL, MS Sloane 2463, s. xv². See Chapter 6 below on this manuscript's 16th-century owners.

[84] See Linne R. Mooney, 'The Scribe', in *Sex, Aging, and Death in a Medieval Medical Compendium: Trinity College Cambridge MS R.14.52, Its Texts, Language, and Scribe*, ed. M. Teresa Tavormina, Medieval and Renaissance Texts and Studies, 292, 2 vols. (Tempe, AZ: Arizona Center for Medieval and Renaissance Studies, 2006), vol. 1, pp. 55–64.

production—which various members of a household may have wished to consult'.[85] But did those 'various members of a household' always include the women?

It is hard to know, of course, what went on inside the confines of the domestic setting, and we still have much to learn about the use of the vast numbers of gynaecological and obstetrical remedies we find scattered throughout later medieval manuscripts.[86] If one starts by looking at an English treatise on a topic of fundamentally domestic interest, tree grafting, for example, and then explores various codices that contain the work, one finds an array of volumes that seem to fit this general description of 'household book'. 'Medicine' figures as a common element, with every one of the manuscripts (save a single-leaf fragment) having some sort of medical texts or recipes.[87] Women would presumably have been members of most if not all of these 'households', yet only four of the eighteen codices contain material specifically on women's medicine and in only one case does it seem plausible that the women of the house would have been the principal users of the codex.[88] In two of the other cases, the gynaecological material is wholly or partly in Latin, while in the fourth copy three brief gynaecological

[85] Julia Boffey, 'Bodleian Library, MS Arch. Selden.B.24 and Definitions of the 'Household Book'', in *The English Medieval Book: Studies in Memory of Jeremy Griffiths*, ed. A. S. G. Edwards, Vincent Gillespie, and Ralph Hanna (London: The British Library, 2000), pp. 125–34, at p. 125. Boffey's main argument is to suggest that the term 'household book' might also be used to describe books (sometimes of primarily literary character) created within the context of the household rather than by professional scribes.

[86] One of the largest categories of recipes that Linda Ehrsam Voigts and Patricia Deery Kurtz found in compiling their survey of Middle English scientific and medical texts was gynaecology and obstetrics. See Linda Ehrsam Voigts, 'Multitudes of Middle English Medical Manuscripts, or the Englishing of Science and Medicine', in *Manuscript Sources of Medieval Medicine: A Book of Essays*, ed. Margaret R. Schleissner, Garland Medieval Casebooks, 8 (New York: Garland, 1995), pp. 183–95.

[87] One of the seventeen manuscripts with Nicholas Bollard's treatise on arboriculture studied by Boffey, Private Collection MS 45, has only veterinary medical texts. I have expanded Boffey's analysis to include an additional copy listed in Linda Ehrsam Voigts and Patricia Deery Kurtz, eds., *Scientific and Medical Writings in Old and Middle English: An Electronic Reference*, The Society for Early English and Norse Electronic Texts, CD-ROM (Ann Arbor: University of Michigan Press, 2000).

[88] This exception is Aberystwyth, National Library of Wales, MS Brogynton II.1 (*olim* Porkington 10), which has been suspected to have been composed for the women and children, as well as the men, of a gentry family near the Welsh borderlands; besides its medical and scientific content, it includes considerable amounts of devotional, educational, and recreational material. Even in this case, however, it is clear that the pamphlet containing the scientific and medical material originated independently and may have little relation to the rest of the codex's contents. See Auvo Kurvinen, 'MS Porkington 10: Description with Extracts', *Neuphilologische Mitteilungen* 54 (1953), 33–67 (rept. Modern Language Society, Helsinki. Amsterdam: Swets and Zeitlinger, 1968); Daniel Huws, 'MS Porkington 10 and its Scribes', in Jennifer Fellows, *et al.*, eds., *Romance Reading on the Book: Essays on Medieval Narrative presented to Maldwyn Mills* (Cardiff, 1996), pp. 208–20; and Katherine J. Lewis, 'Model Girls? Virgin-Martyrs and the Training of Young Women in Late Medieval England', in *Young Medieval Women*, ed. Katherine J. Lewis, Noël James Menuge, and Kim M. Phillips (Phoenix Mill: Sutton, 1999), pp. 25–46, where she examines the Aberystwyth ms in the context of seven household books that were likely used by women.

recipes (along with others on treating lice, worms, snakebites and so forth) are added by a later hand to a collection of medical and alchemical texts.[89] While compilations intended specifically for female domestic use continue to be identified, thus far these codices have given no evidence of a particular feminine interest in medicine.[90]

Indeed, it seems that book ownership and book use within the heterosexual domestic context could be just as segregated by gender as elsewhere. One manuscript long recognized as a perfect example of a 'household book' is also one of the few where we have an identifiable owner of an English *Trotula*. As noted above, Humphrey Newton of Pownall, Cheshire, owned a copy of the translation that bears, in the two other extant copies, the Latin title *Secreta mulierum*. We will return to the significance of this particular form of the text in the next chapter. Here, what interests us is how Newton might have used this copy of the *Trotula*, which is abbreviated to stress generational issues rather than women's diseases more broadly. The quire in which this English *Trotula* appears was probably written in the 1470s (when Newton would have still been a child) and so could not have been assembled for his own specific tastes. Nor do we know exactly when Newton acquired it—whether, for example, it was before or after his marriage in 1490 (at the age of 24) or around 1497 when he became the head of the Newton family and so the full bearer of responsibility for carrying on the line. Newton made no annotations to the *Trotula* that would give us direct evidence of how he was reading the text. (Perhaps unfortunately for him, this version of the *Trotula* lacked the chapters on regimen for the wet-nurse, which would have proved useful since we know he employed at least one.)[91] Nevertheless, Newton's addition (in his own hand) of a variety of Latin and English medical recipes, including one 'Ffor to make a woman to conseyue child', and perhaps his insertion of a loose leaf with two Latin paragraphs on uterine mole and (quoting Avicenna) the signs of

[89] These manuscripts are OBL, MS Rawlinson C.506, which contains the opening chapters of the Latin *Practica* of Trota; MS Bodley 591, which contains a Latin adaptation of Muscio's *Gynaecia* meant to be used to instruct midwives (see Chapter 3 above); and Cambridge, University Library, MS Ee.1.13, where three English gynaecological recipes are added on f. 130r–v.

[90] For example, in Lewis's sample of seven codices containing saints' lives probably intended for female use, only one, the Aberystwyth ms, has any gynaecological material. The absence from all six other codices of any medical material save some veterinary recipes in one volume and a brief verse regimen in another is telling evidence that there seems to have been no particularly gendered association of women with medical writings. Medical texts are likewise absent from the manuscripts examined by Mary C. Erler, *Women, Reading, and Piety in Late Medieval England* (Cambridge: Cambridge University Press, 2002); and Carole M. Meale and Julia Boffey, 'Gentlewomen's Reading', in *The Cambridge History of the Book in Britain, vol. III: 1400–1557*, ed. Lotte Helinga and J. B. Trapp (Cambridge: Cambridge University Press, 1999), pp. 526–40.

[91] On Newton's employment of a wet-nurse named Katherine, see Deborah Youngs, 'Servants and Labourers on a Late Medieval Demesne: The Case of Newton, Cheshire, 1498–1520', *Agricultural History Review* 47 (2000), 145–60, at pp. 151 and 154.

pregnancy, suggests his particular interest in discerning viable from non-viable pregnancies.[92] Such a concern for progeny would certainly fit in with other elements of Newton's personality, for although he seems to have spent the bulk of his career on his estates in Cheshire, he expended extraordinary effort, both bureaucratic and cultural, in 'family investment'. A micromanaging landlord who kept a firm hand over his labourers, he also dabbled in literary culture, collecting excerpts from the likes of Chaucer and the *Gawain* poet and composing his own verses.[93] He assembled instructions on the proper elements of courteous deportment, how to carve fowl, and how to orchestrate a bridal feast. Newton looked after his afterlife as much as his earthly one, collecting visions of purgatory as well as indulgences. Humphrey Newton's household book was, therefore, very much a product of Newton's own self-fashioning and intimately reflects his ambitions. As Ralph Hanna reminds us, 'Newton shows that a household is constituted . . . by an estate and a patrimony.'[94] Newton's efforts to maintain and enlarge that patrimony would have been in vain had he been unable to secure heirs, in which task he did in fact prove successful: his wife bore him four sons and six daughters.[95] Yet there is nothing in his book to indicate that he shared directly with his wife the literate tasks connected with his role of head of household.[96]

Through extensive studies of the phenomenon of vernacularization in the later Middle Ages, it has become clear that the main clientele for both commissioned and 'speculative' medical manuscripts (manuscripts prepared by a stationer's shop without a particular purchaser in mind) was, in addition to the medical practitioners we have already encountered, a bourgeois class, both urban and on landed estates, who had acquired some basic Latin and, along the way, some rudimentary rhetoric and logic as well.[97] This kind of often bilingual, or in England, trilingual, literacy would have been acquired primarily for business

---

[92] OBL, MS Lat. misc. c. 66, s. xv ex, ff. 90r and 87b, respectively.

[93] Ralph Hanna, 'Humphrey Newton and Bodleian Library, MS Lat. Misc. C.66', *Medium Aevum* 69 (2000), 279–91, finds that 'such [literary] fragments testify to Newton's access to a substantial library of Middle English' (p. 285). On Newton's characteristics as a landlord, see Youngs, 'Servants and Labourers'.

[94] Hanna, 'Humphrey Newton', pp. 288–9. On Newton's business affairs and concern with not only his own lineage but that of his neighbours, see Deborah Marsh, '"I see by sizt of evidence": Information Gathering in Late Medieval Cheshire', in *Courts, Counties and the Capital in the Late Middle Ages*, ed. Diana E. S. Dunn (New York: St Martin's, 1996), pp. 71–92.

[95] Rossell Hope Robbins, 'The Poems of Humfrey Newton, Esquire, 1466–1536', *Publications of the Modern Languages Association of America* 65 (1950), 249–81, at p. 250.

[96] The only other contemporary hand in the book that has thus far been recognized is that of one of Humphrey's sons, who was adding to the collection some years after Humphrey died (Robbins, 'Poems', p. 255).

[97] Linda Ehrsam Voigts, 'What's the Word? Bilingualism in Late-Medieval England', *Speculum* 1:4, (1996), 813–826; and Bernhard Schnell, 'Die volkssprachliche Medizinliteratur des Mittelalters—Wissen für wen?', in *Laienlektüre und Buchmarkt im späten Mittelalter*, ed. Thomas Kock and Rita Schlusemann (Frankfurt am Main: Peter Lang, 1997), pp. 129–45.

and administrative purposes,[98] though, as with Humphrey Newton, aspirations toward a more refined way of living may have been cultivated as well. Though not holding degrees from the university, men of these up-and-coming classes nevertheless sometimes aspired toward the kind of knowledge cultivated at the universities, knowledge that could aid them in controlling both the natural and the social world around them: not simply agriculture, therefore, but also prognostic arts (whether by thunder, names, handreading, etc.), astrology, and alchemy. Among these concerns was interest in, perhaps even anxiety over, generation and the ability to produce heirs who could inherit the patrimony that these men of substance had so laboriously built up. It is for this reason, apparently, that we find men like Thomas Cook and Humphrey Newton incorporating gynaecological material into their household compendia.

The vernacularization of the *Trotula*, and the creation of other vernacular texts on women's medicine in the later Middle Ages, bears both marked similarities to and differences from other areas of medicine affected by the shift to the vernacular. Gynaecological texts seem to have been chosen for vernacularization no more or less often than other kinds of medical texts that addressed the practical rather than theoretical aspects of medicine. For example, all the major surgical writers of the thirteenth and fourteenth centuries—Bruno, Theoderic, William of Saliceto, Lanfranc, Henri de Mondeville, Guy de Chauliac—were rendered into various vernaculars, often multiple times. Rarely do the translators articulate a theory of translation or an explicit claim to a hoped-for audience. Often, the only reference is to 'simple people' or 'those who are not great clerics [but nevertheless] wish to exercise the practice of surgery'.[99] In no case have I found a medical translator expressing fear that use of the vernacular might increase access to women, nor is there any active prohibition against women reading.[100] On the other hand, aside from a dozen or so herbals or general regimens commissioned by or addressed to specific noble women,[101] I have as yet found no vernacular medical text beyond certain cosmetic works and the gynaecological writings examined here that claims women as, or among, its intended audience. In other words, women are envisaged as audiences of medical works only when a specific woman is involved as patron or dedicatee, or when the topic of the text connects generically with the female body or feminine roles. In fact, even though gynaecology was more inherently tied to the physical, sexed body of women than the superficially gendered habits of cosmetics, gynaecological texts—and so the assembly of knowledge that they embodied—were less closely tied to female readers. A fourteenth-century Catalan

---

[98] W. Rothwell, 'Anglo-French and Middle English Vocabulary in *Femina nova*', *Medium Aevum* 69 (2000), 34–58.

[99] Bazin-Tacchella, 'Adaptations françaises', at p. 173.

[100] We will, however, find such active prohibition against women's reading in the case of another (not strictly medical) text, to be discussed in Chapter 5.

[101] See Green, 'Possibilities', Tables 2 and 3.

author, Johan Reimbamaco, included near the end of a work he actually titled *The Book Called Trotula* some gynaecological material as well as a brief general health regimen; he even claimed that his text would free its female reader from reliance on physicians for all except the most serious conditions. Yet he sees *cosmetics* as the central concern of 'women's medicine'; it is that topic, not gynaecological disorders, that makes up the bulk of his text.[102] If, as in Johan Reimbamaco's text, 'women's medicine' is taken to revolve specifically around cosmetics (even Johan's gynaecological material is more focused on vaginal hygiene and remedies for stretch marks than serious uterine conditions), then such texts did indeed liberate women from the need to submit to a physician's authority. But for gynaecological disease and more serious obstetrical threats, male practitioners were the prime creators and clinical deliverers of knowledge.

The effect of vernacularization of the *Trotula* on men seems to have been that the audience was not so much changed (the association with high learned medicine can still be found in some cases) as broadened beyond a narrow elite. Most of the identifiable male owners of the vernacular *Trotula* and other vernacular texts on women's medicine were professional practitioners—men like Master Pierre the French surgeon, Hermann Bach the German physician, or Richard Dod the English barber-surgeon—many of whom had some competence in Latin. Yet equally significant is the passage of the texts into the hands of lay males, like the king of France, a duke and emperor in Germany, or simply an aspiring country gentleman in England like Humphrey Newton. This appetite among male readers for works that explained the female body was such that even the texts addressed to women were not off limits: the French *Quant Dex nostre Seignor*, the Dutch *Liber Trotula*, and the English *Knowing of Woman's Kind* and *Sicknesses of Women 2* all sooner or later fell back into the hands of men. Nor was there any way that women could have prevented this relapse. While translation into the vernacular may have increased women's access to the texts, it also increased men's.

But not, it seems, without a fight. We find a hint of this gendered struggle in *The Knowing of Woman's Kind*, the earlier of the two English translations of the *Trotula* written for women. As we saw, the assertion that the book should be shared among women derives from the French and suggests a continuity in usage among upper-class French- and English-speaking women in England. Yet there is also something completely new here. Omitting the list of medical writers that had assured the antiquity and authority of the original text, the English translator substituted instead an entirely different perspective on proper male involvement with the text:

---

[102] Madrid, Biblioteca Nacional, MS 3356, f. 22va–b: 'E sapiatz que en aquest libre no dic totes les malaties de la mare ni totes les medicines sino aqueles que son per aiensar, e ja ho he a vos dit en altre loch, que aquest libre no parla sino de embeliment'. On this text more generally, see Montserrat Cabré i Pairet, 'From a Master to a Laywoman: A Feminine Manual of Self-Help', *Dynamis: Acta Hispanica ad Medicinae Scientiarumque Historiam Illustrandam* 20 (2000), 371–93.

And if it should happen that any man read this, I beg and charge him on Our Lady's behalf that he read it neither in spite nor in order to slander any woman nor for any other reason than to heal or help them, dreading that vengeance might befall him as has happened to others who have exposed [women's] private matters in order to slander them. And let him understand that women who are alive now have no more evils than those women who are now saints in heaven.[103]

Spite? Slander? Vengeance? These are indeed fighting words. But what is the 'fight' about?

'AND IF IT SHOULD HAPPEN THAT ANY MAN READ THIS': A TUG-OF-WAR

Prior to the fourteenth century, 'slander' had never appeared in the vocabulary of western gynaecological literature. 'Shame', 'reluctance', 'embarrassment'—all these sentiments had figured as rhetorical topoi in gynaecological literature since Antiquity to justify women's medical practice or, at the very least, the assembling of knowledge on women's diseases and the recording of it in writing.[104] It is conceivable that this new concern was simply about the perceived impropriety of discussing women's 'private matters' publicly, even when motivated by the best therapeutic intentions. Yet the English author of *The Knowing of Woman's Kind*, as we noted before, had *deleted* the reference to women's shame that the French translator, from whom he was drawing, had faithfully preserved from the Latin *Conditions of Women*. Something very different is going on here and while it clearly connects with the issues of women's shame we have encountered before, the stakes have gotten much higher.

Reticence simply to talk about the reproductive organs or their functions is surely one element of the problem. How women talked about such issues among themselves is one of the many aspects of medieval women's lives virtually inaccessible to us. What is better documented (if only by the silences that surround it) was the problematic nature of talking about such issues in mixed-sex company. Writers of French Romance literature, for example, no matter how detailed they may have been on matters of love or sex, never explicitly utter the word 'menses' (*menstrué*) or any of its euphemisms, and are generally reticent to discuss other, more specific aspects of female physiology.[105] Even writers of fabliaux, that raunchy genre of humorous tales, may be willing to use various vulgarities for the sexual organs themselves, but shy away from discussing their

---

[103] Barratt, *Knowing*, lines 24–31.   [104] See Chapter 1 above.

[105] In French gynaecological texts, terms used for menstruation include *menstrués* or *mestrués* ('menses'); *les fleurs* ('the flowers'), the most common term; *les maladies secrettes* ('the secret maladies'); and *le sang mestruel* ('menstrual blood'). For discussion of menstruation and the lochia in French literature, see Peggy McCracken, *The Curse of Eve, the Wound of the Hero: Blood, Gender, and Medieval Literature* (Philadelphia: University of Pennsylvania Press, 2003).

functions or their diseases. Christine de Pizan's famous controversy over the *Romance of the Rose* at the turn of the fifteenth century hinged, in part, on her accusation against Jean de Meun for using obscene language. (He had referred to the male genitalia by their common name, *coilles*.) The cultural obsession with female sexual purity rendered problematic any public discussion, no matter how well-intentioned, of diseases of the female genitalia; the potential for scandal, as we saw in previous chapters, was always there.

But as the male author of the Hippocratic *Diseases of Women* had already recognized in the fifth or fourth century BC, it was impossible to *treat* women's diseases unless they were named and discussed. Medieval male practitioners, in expanding their practice to include not simply women's general medical conditions, but their gynaecological ones as well, were faced with the same problem. As we have seen, most of the editors, copyists and, apparently, readers of the *Trotula*, whether in Latin or the vernacular, blithely ignored the problematic questions of male practice on female patients, apparently because they had simply not yet formulated any formal rationale for their practice. The off-hand dismissal in 1322 of Jacoba Felicie's arguments for the need for women to treat women is typical of this failure to engage in a rational justification of male gynaecological practice.[106] It was only the rare medical writer who at least articulated the need for techniques such as 'the leech's subtle asking'. All the more surprising, therefore, is a uniquely explicit confrontation of this problem in a French translation of the *Trotula* mentioned earlier, the *Treatise on the Many Maladies Which Can Happen to Women and on Their Secret Maladies*, which elaborates on the shame topos of the *Conditions of Women* preface in a novel way:

And first, because women are ashamed to confide in and reveal themselves to men and physicians concerning their secret diseases, and because in the past many have allowed themselves to be grievously harmed rather [than disclose their illness to men], we have fully translated the conditions from which their diseases arise and all the organs of their secret natures. All these things are ordered one after the other. However, because women are ashamed to name these things in the manner in which we are accustomed to name them in French, we will name each organ by another name which they do not customarily have. Thus, women will name them more readily without being ashamed.[107]

---

[106] See Chapter 3 above.
[107] *Un Traictié de plusieurs maladies qui peuent avenir aux femmes, et de leurs maladies secretes*, partially transcribed in Jules Camus, 'La Seconde Traduction de la Chirurgie de Mondeville (Turin, Bibl. nat. L.IV.17)', *Bulletin de la Société des Anciens textes français* 28 (1902), 100–19, at p. 109: 'Et premier, pour ce que lez femmez sont honteuses de prendre conseil et ellez descouvrir as hommes et as phisicienz de leurs maladies secrettes, et que moult de dames se lairoient ainchois grever durement, avons plainement translaté lez causes desquellez les maladies viennent et tous lez instrumens de leurs secrettes natures. Toutes sont ordonnéez l'une après l'autre; mais, pour ce qu'ellez ne soient honteuses de nommer en telle maniere que nous lez nommons communement en romant, nous nommerons cascun instrument par aultre non que a coustume n'ont; si les nommeront plus habondament sans estre honteuses.'

The translator (who is now functioning as an author in his own right) goes on to list his new terms: 'the first gate' (*le premiere porte*) for the vagina, 'the tongue' (*le langue*) for the clitoris, 'the seed' (*le semence*) for the sperm (male or female).[108]

In laying out these euphemisms one by one, the translator is clearly not writing a text for women's own use, offering women a vocabulary they can use *among themselves* to talk about their diseases. While we know nothing about the audience claims of this text (the bulk of the manuscript, including the *Trotula*, was unfortunately destroyed in a fire in 1904),[109] the rearranged structure of the text as well as the specialized content of the codex (a massive 539-leaf compendium of medical and surgical texts) suggest that the volume as a whole was intended for professional use by a surgeon. The euphemisms are provided, therefore, in order to give male practitioners—the 'we' who are not ashamed to use the normative French vocabulary for the reproductive organs—a language to offer women, so that women, in turn, will speak to men. What this text shows, then, is the need for tact and delicacy when men are discussing women's diseases with their patients. Women's shame was merely an unfortunate obstacle to male medical practice, not an absolute impediment to it.

Still, the problem did not go away. And as with the problem of shame as it effected medical practice (discussed in Chapter 2), it is important again to stress that this was *men's* problem as well as women's. The fifteenth-century Dutch translator of the *Trotula* who was addressing women seems particularly reluctant to discuss sexual matters or anatomical details, and when he does, it is in an apologetic mode. He begins the description of the anatomy of the womb with the plea 'Now you women, do not take offense, what is said here is natural and also useful.' He abbreviates, 'for fear that one might curse me', the discussion of the etiology of uterine suffocation (which is caused by either retained menses or the female semen retained in women who are not sexually active). In a chapter on excessive heat in the womb, the translator breaks off a description of how a pessary should be inserted 'on account of criticism by women'.[110] The strongest statement comes in the opening lines of the text: 'I ask all women who will see

---

[108] Jules Camus, 'Premier, nous nommerons le premiere porte, qui est menbre de generacion, alias, *volve*. Item appellerons le langue qui est enmy, *pignon*. Item appellerons le semence, *esperme*'. Camus cuts off his transcription here, though when portions of the text were embedded into a French natural historical encyclopedia (BNF, MS fr. 212, s. xv ex.), the list (which is slightly different here, omitting *le langue*, which is an extremely rare acknowledgement of the existence of the clitoris) continues on with terms for the uterus, the menses, and the afterbirth. See Chapter 5 below.

[109] One hundred leaves of the manuscript survived the fire of 1904 that engulfed the Turin library, but these contain only the surgical text of Mondeville. From the excerpts transcribed by Camus, it is obvious that *Conditions of Women* has been adapted into a form more closely resembling the 'secrets of women' tradition than the therapeutically oriented *Trotula*. The text was rearranged, apparently, to focus attention on generation more than women's diseases *per se*. Some later, modified excerpts are also directed to a male audience. See Chapter 5 below.

[110] *Liber Trotula*, ed. Delva, pp. 160, 179–80, 182.

this or hear [it] read, I ask them not to curse me, because I have not written this to injure them but [only] for their profit.'[111]

Some of the new prefatory sentiments we find in late medieval gynaecological texts are not apologia directed to women, however, but admonitions to potential male readers of the texts. When this Dutch translator apologizes to his female audience, for example, he may be doing so on the assumption that he is speaking only to women. But he may also be apologizing to whatever women happen to be in the *mixed* audience he assumes his text will find. As we have seen, his book did come into the hands of a Latinate, surgically oriented, scholastically minded editor who quite decidedly changed the character of the text even while retaining the nominal address to female readers. The original Dutch author's attempts to reassure women that he does not wish to harm them suggest that in the late medieval period gynaecological texts sometimes were—or could be conceived to be—intended to harm or offend women.

But still, the question is *how*? How could gynaecological texts—these works so fundamentally focused on describing women's diseases and detailing their cures—be used to *harm* women? The answer, in short, is that some men using these texts were motivated by something other than the desire to gain therapeutic knowledge. What is at issue is not so much what the texts contain as *how* they are read. Returning to the English context, we find the compiler of the mid fifteenth-century text, *Sickness of Women 2*, laying out an unflattering depiction of what men do with the knowledge they obtain of women's diseases:

[A]lthough women have various maladies and many terrible sicknesses more than any man knows, as I said, they are ashamed for fear of reproof in times to come and of exposure by discourteous men who love women only because of their lusts and unsavory desires. And if women become sick, such men despise them and fail to realize how much sickness women have before they bring them into this world. And therefore, in order to help women, I will write of how to help women's secret maladies so that one woman may aid another in her illness and not disclose her secrets to such discourteous men.[112]

Here, the initial issue of men's misuse of gynaecological knowledge seems to lie in men's ridiculing of women for their diseases. Yet there is an implied suggestion that if women turn to men for help, they will be not only ridiculed but may actually be sexually exploited by men 'who love women only because of their lusts and unsavory desires'. Still, there is no prohibition of male reading here, nor even any suggestion of what a man might do with this text were he to read it. In fact, it seems likely that this author, who was apparently himself an active practitioner of women's healthcare, *expected* men to be involved in women's care.[113] Thus,

---

[111] Brugge, Openbare Bibliotheek, MS 593, f. 1r: 'Ic bidde alle vrouwen die dit sullen sien ofte horen lesen, hem biddic dat si my niet ne vloucken, want ic ne hebbe hem dit niet ghescreven te scaeden maer te haren profite' (Delva, *Vrouwengeneeskunde*, p. 160). This passage is nearly identical in the Copenhagen and Hamburg manuscripts.

[112] Green and Mooney, *Sickness*, lines 8–18.   [113] Green and Mooney, *Sickness*.

this disparagement of 'discourteous men'—with its implied suggestion that their interests in women's bodies are ultimately sexual—may have simply served both to warn male readers of the text to behave themselves and to reaffirm this author's own beneficent intentions in compiling the book.[114] A quite sizable portion of the corpus of both Latin and English gynaecological texts circulating in fifteenth-century England clearly was in men's hands, a fact that usually needed neither apology nor explanation. Yet, there was some discomfort. As already noted, the direct address 'Sirs' was added at the beginning of several manuscripts of *Sickness of Women 1*, which otherwise has no explicit statement of intended audience. Apparently, this rare usage of the masculine address (rare because it would normally have been gratuitous) was meant to reassure male readers that they did indeed have 'permission' to read the text.[115]

Recognition of alternate, ill-intentioned readings of gynaecology was not confined to medical texts intended for a female audience. In the *Arzneibuch* ('Book of Medicine') that he compiled sometime around 1400, a Dutch surgeon named Albrecht van Borgunnien introduced the section on gynaecology with the warning 'This book is not suitable for all men to read, rather [it is] only for those who are honest and understand the best way, for we all have come from women.'[116] Albrecht's warning points to the heart of his concern: *dis*honest men might misuse his book, forgetting the respect they owe to women who have borne them. Later in the century, a German surgeon, Hans Seyff von Göppingen, expressed a nearly identical sentiment when he copied a German tract on female physiology and anatomy into his own medical handbook:

This book is called the Secrets of Women. This book should be neither read nor listened to by anyone unless he be reasonable. For God has created in womankind many secrets of nature, and it would not be good if anyone who is not reasonable should know it, and that is why this book should be guarded.[117]

---

[114] I discuss this author's active engagement in gynaecological and obstetrical practice in Chapter 6 below.

[115] Only one other scientific or medical text in Middle English has thus far been identified beginning with the generic plural 'Sirs' to address a male audience: it is 'a gentlemanly treatise' on fishing and fowling (cf. OBL, MS Add. A. 60, ff. 1–17, a s. xix transcription of a now lost medieval ms from CTC); my thanks to Linda Voigts for this reference. In checking the *Index of Printed Middle English Prose* and the *Index of Middle English Prose: Handlists* (nos. 1–17), I find the generic plural address 'Sirs' used as an opening address in only three other texts: two of the sermons in John Mirk's cycle of sermons known as the *Festial* and a treatise on confession.

[116] As cited in Gundolf Keil, 'Die Frau als Ärztin und Patientin in der medizinischen Fachprosa des deutschen Mittelalters', in *Frau und spätmittelalterlicher Alltag: Internationaler Kongress, Krems an der Donau, 2. bis 5. Oktober 1984* (Vienna: Österreichischen Akademie der Wissenschaften, 1986), pp. 157–211, p. 211: 'Dyt bok temet alle man nicht to lesen sunder de erbar syn vnde alle dink to den besten vorstaᵉn, wente wi sint alle van vrouwen gekomen.' My thanks to Margaret Schleissner for translating this passage for me.

[117] Preface to a work that Kruse entitles *Sieben Erklärungen zur weiblichen Sexualität und zur Reproduktion*, in Kruse, *Verborgene Heilkünste*, p. 265; my thanks to Ann Marie Rasmussen for assistance with this translation. Another copy of the same work, which may have been owned by the male Franciscans of Munich, opens similarly.

Men themselves recognized that prurient readings of material on women's bodies by males, particularly adolescents, needed to be forestalled by warnings and injunctions. For example, in the margin at the beginning of some Latin excerpts from Muscio's *Gynaecology* in a fifteenth-century manuscript, a later commentator added the warning: 'Not to be read by a pure and innocent eye. Avert your eyes lest they see vanity.'[118] However intriguing this self-policing among men themselves may be, what is most striking about the Dutch and English gynaecological texts addressed to women is that these authors (who I assume to have all been male) believe that women *already know* that men use gynaecological texts to disparage them. The reading of texts on women's medicine was thus about more than the practice of women's medicine. It was also about women's honour—and the potential threat of slander.

[118] Berlin, Staatsbibliothek Preussischer Kulturbesitz, MS lat. qu. 373, *c*.1470 (S. Germany), ff. 156r ('Non legatur ab oculo puro et simplici. Averte oculos ne videant vanitatem') and 159v. Although conceivably the commentator may be expressing sincere concern for the moral well-being of young monks, the text that follows is entitled *Secreta secretorum mulierum*, 'the secrets of the secrets of women', a title which would surely attract more attention than it would avert. The manuscript was owned by Master Hildebrandus Brandenburg, who then donated it to the Carthusian house of Buxheim.

5

Slander and the Secrets of Women

He hadde a book that gladly, nyght and day,
For his desport he wolde rede alway;
He cleped it Valerie and Theofraste,
At which book he lough alwey ful faste.
And eek ther was somtyme a clerk at Rome,
A cardinal, that highte Seint Jerome,
That made a book agayn Jovinian;
In which book eek ther was Tertulan,
Crisippus, Trotula, and Helowys,
That was abbesse nat fer fro Parys,
And eek the Parables of Salomon,
Ovides Art, and bookes many on,
And alle thise were bounden in o volume.

Geoffrey Chaucer, *The Canterbury Tales*
(before 1400)

'I have seen another small book in Latin, my lady, called *The Secrets of Women*, which discusses the constitution of their natural bodies and especially their great defects'. [Lady Reason] replied, 'You can see for yourself without further proof, this book was written carelessly and colored by hypocrisy, for if you have looked at it, you know that it is obviously a treatise composed of lies.'

Christine de Pizan, *Book of the City of Ladies* (1405)

In the Prologue to her *Tale*, Chaucer's Wife of Bath describes a 'book of wikked wyves' that her fifth husband, the clerk Jankyn, liked to read from 'every nyght and day... / Whan he hadde leyser and vacacioun / From oother worldly occupacioun'.[1] Chaucer's Wife, Dame Alice, speaks with repugnance of this book recounting women's many wiles and relates how it gave occasion to an extraordinary row between husband and wife. Christine de Pizan, writing her

---

[1] Geoffrey Chaucer, *The Canterbury Tales, The Wife of Bath's Prologue* III (D), 669–85, in *The Riverside Chaucer*, ed. Larry D. Benson, 3rd edn (Boston: Houghton Mifflin, 1987), p. 114.

great defence of women in France just a few years after Chaucer's death, speaks with equal distaste of another book that disparaged women, the so-called *Secrets of Women*, a book we might best characterize as a 'natural history' of women.[2] Chaucer's and Christine's citations of books offensive to women have more than just chronological similarity. They both reflect a convergence of medical and natural philosophical interests in women that would profoundly affect the way gynaecological literature was read in the later Middle Ages, particularly in northern Europe.

In previous chapters, we have already seen not only ample evidence for the growing interest of male physicians in fertility, but also the interests of laymen ranging from country gentlemen and urban merchants to noblemen, who were reading vernacular gynaecological texts out of their interests in understanding generation. They were continuing the pursuit that natural philosophers and clerics in the twelfth and thirteenth centuries had already started of questions like how the seed (in both men and women) is produced and how the foetus develops, being distinguished now by a more active desire to *use* that knowledge to influence fertility. Much of this interest narrowed into questions about women's physical nature or women's 'secrets', which in turn produced two parallel phenomena. On the one hand, gynaecological texts (particularly the *Trotula*) were adapted to make them focus less on women's diseases in their entirety and more on making the female body a properly functioning locus of reproduction. Both within the universities and outside them, both in Latin and in the vernaculars, gynaecological texts were excerpted, rearranged, abbreviated and in other ways manipulated to serve new purposes.[3] The second phenomenon was the creation of a distinct natural-philosophical tradition of the 'secrets of women', most prominently represented by a late thirteenth-century work of that title commonly, if falsely, attributed to the Dominican preacher Albertus Magnus (d. 1280). Although the therapeutic character of gynaecological texts was very different from the speculative character of the pseudo-Albertan text, their common focus on issues of generation allowed them to be seen as virtually interchangeable, sometimes being paired with one another, sometimes circulating in identical codicological contexts as if it didn't matter which particular text was included. Some of these new readings of gynaecological literature were more localized, some more peculiar than others. But all reflect new habits of thinking about the female body.

---

[2] Christine de Pizan, *The Book of the City of Ladies*, trans. Earl Jeffrey Richards (New York: Persea, 1982), I.9.2, p. 22. I have modified Richards' translation slightly, omitting the Latin title he inserted. As I argue in Green, 'Traittié', it seems clear that even though de Pizan knew that the *Secrets of Women* had been composed in Latin, she was citing from the French translation of the text.

[3] I discuss these developments at greater length in Green, 'From "Diseases of Women" to "Secrets of Women": The Transformation of Gynecological Literature in the Later Middle Ages', *Journal of Medieval and Early Modern Studies* 30 (2000), 5–39.

The *Trotula* was, ironically, fundamentally inadequate for answering many of the questions being asked of it, for it had almost nothing detailed to say of women's anatomy, sexual physiology, or many other matters. It could, however, claim an importance that all the gynaecological chapters of learned medical compendia could not: it could claim authorship by a female authority who revealed 'women's secrets' to men. The fact that 'Trotula' could serve as a mouthpiece for views on women (some of which were nowhere to be found within the *Trotula* texts themselves) heightened another dimension of the new natural-philosophical and medical readings of gynaecological literature: their connections with clerical misogyny, a tradition of compiling litanies of the alleged evils and deceits of women often as a means to dissuade celibate priests and monks from engagement with the opposite sex. German- and Dutch-speaking areas formed a distinct epicentre from which the pseudo-Albertan text spread its influence, although even in places like England where the pseudo-Albertan text had almost no impact, the discourse of the 'secrets of women' could be found coupled with misogynous discourse across a wide range of male literates who had been imbued with such rhetoric from their school days on. This is the contemporary discourse on women that Chaucer captured in his caricature of the clerk Jankyn. In France, Christine de Pizan recognized the misogynous intent of much of the discourse about the female body in the early fifteenth century when she denounced the *Secrets of Women* as 'a treatise composed of lies'. De Pizan never mentions 'Trotula', though had she done so it is likely she would have denounced her as well. We have no direct evidence of how other women reacted either to the author-figure 'Trotula' or to the new ways gynaecological literature was being read by men. But the rhetorical 'policing' around gynaecological texts that we saw in the previous chapter, together with other evidence, suggests that this double manipulation of the authoress 'Trotula' and the body of literature meant to help rather than harm women did not go unnoticed.

FROM 'WOMEN'S DISEASES' TO 'WOMEN'S SECRETS': ATTITUDES TOWARD GENERATION

Around 1435, a manuscript was prepared in Germany that contained, as its only illustration, a 'disease woman' drawn rather clumsily onto the opening flyleaf. A formalized depiction of the afflictions to which the female body was subject (cf. Fig. 3.6 above), the 'disease woman' was followed by Bernard of Gordon's long Latin encyclopedia, the *Lily of Medicine*, which was in turn followed by the *Trotula* and then short works on *materia medica*, urines, and recipes in Latin and German.[4] The earliest known owner of the manuscript may also have

---

[4] See Chapter 3 above.

commissioned it: Martin von Geismar (d. 1450), whom we've met before, a master of arts, licentiate in canon law, head of the cathedral chapter of St-Peters in Fritzlar (diocese of Mainz) and later a canon in Worms. Von Geismar owned nearly five dozen books but only two were on medicine.[5] Why would such a cleric need a diagram of a 'disease woman' (with uterus opened, as in most copies of the image, to display a tiny foetus) and a copy of the *Trotula*? Earlier, I raised the question whether von Geismar and other clerics who owned gynaecological or obstetrical materials had been involved in instructing midwives by showing them such images or reading to them (in simultaneous translation) from their Latin books.[6] We know too little about von Geismar's pastoral duties to conclude with any certainty that he was not engaged in such instruction, but other evidence suggests that he had rather different objectives in owning this manuscript. First, it also includes, just a few leaves after the end of the *Trotula*, the short *Interrogations on the Treatment of Sterility*, that fourteenth-century Montpellierain work with forty-one questions that need to be asked of the woman to determine a couple's fitness for procreation. The second hint comes in von Geismar's inventory of his books, where he describes the *Trotula* not as 'The Book on the Sufferings of Women According to Trotula' (which is how the text is headed in the manuscript itself), but as *dicta super secreta mulierum*, 'Sayings on the Secrets of Women'.[7]

The Latin term *secreta* ('secrets' or, literally, 'things set apart or hidden') is of classical origin and might have been used by any author or scribe to refer to texts on women's diseases throughout late Antiquity and the early Middle Ages. Nevertheless, although, as we have seen, the idea that shame about gynaecological disease was an inhibiting factor in the proper provision of care for women was very old, the heading 'women's secrets' was in fact never used as a title for gynaecological writings prior to the thirteenth century.[8] Even then, the term was not used as a simple equivalent for 'lore on women's diseases' but rather implied something more specific: it was that *part* of the lore on women's conditions that related most immediately to generation.[9]

Despite theological suspicions about sexuality as a dangerous and disruptive force, medical and natural philosophical writers proved themselves quite willing to discuss freely the nature of coitus (at least from the male perspective) and

[5] The other, now Kassel, Stadt- und Landesbibliothek, 4° Ms. med. 21, *c*.1380, contains Gerard de Solo's commentary on the ninth book of Rhazes's *Liber ad Almansorem* (a general medical textbook), other works on practical medicine, and various recipes.

[6] See Chapter 3 above.

[7] Ludwig Denecke, 'Die Bibliothek des Fritzlarer Stiftsherrn Martin von Geismar († 1450)', *Hessisches Jahrbuch für Landesgeschichte* 28 (1978), 80–109, at p. 93.

[8] Green, 'From "Diseases of Women"'.

[9] On the *Secrés de femmes*, the first French translation of the *Trotula*, see Chapter 4 above. On the very different uses of the term 'secrets of women' and its variants in the Hebrew tradition, see Carmen Caballero Navas, 'Secrets of Women: Naming Female Sexual Difference in Medieval Hebrew Medical Literature,' *Nashim: A Journal of Jewish Women's Studies and Gender* 12 (2006), 39–56.

to prescribe remedies to assuage or stimulate sexual desire.[10] Beyond concern with the sexual act *per se*, already in the twelfth century a tradition of question-and-answer works now known as the Salernitan Questions devoted considerable attention to such issues as the cause and physiology of menstruation, why prostitutes conceive so rarely, and why women seem to infect men with leprosy (which was thought to be sexually transmitted) but are not afflicted themselves. From the cathedral schools, this natural philosophical interest moved in the thirteenth century to the universities where, bolstered by the newly available Aristotelian texts and Arabic commentaries, long disquisitions on generation were composed like Albertus Magnus's works on animals and on generation in the 1250s and 1260s and Giles of Rome's (d. 1316) *On the Formation of the Human Body in the Uterus*.[11] Among physicians, general medical texts addressed such issues as why (as it was supposed) women take greater pleasure in sex than men.[12]

One result of this intensified interest was the convergence of medical and natural philosophical interests in the reproductive and sexual capacities of the female body. Up until the thirteenth century, gynaecological literature had existed largely in isolation from these discourses on generation and sexuality. Neither the *Trotula* nor most of the gynaecological texts that preceded it were much concerned with questions like how the embryo develops, how female reproductive anatomy compares or contrasts with that of the male, whether or not the female produces seed, what the mechanisms of intercourse are. Gynaecological texts were fundamentally practical, insistently therapeutic, and a measure of this gap is the simple fact that speculative texts on reproductive anatomy or generation almost never circulated in the same codicological contexts as gynaecology.[13] Yet the natural philosophical speculations of the cathedral schools and later the

---

[10] On theological views, see James A. Brundage, *Law, Sex, and Christian Society in Medieval Europe* (Chicago: University of Chicago Press, 1987); and Pierre J. Payer, *The Bridling of Desire: Ideas of Sex in the Later Middle Ages* (Toronto: University of Toronto Press, 1993). On medical and scientific views, see Danielle Jacquart and Claude Thomasset, *Sexuality and Medical Knowledge in the Middle Ages*, trans. Matthew Adamson (Oxford: Polity Press; Princeton: Princeton University Press, 1988); Mary F. Wack, *Lovesickness in the Middle Ages: The 'Viaticum' and its Commentaries* (Philadelphia: University of Pennsylvania Press, 1990); Joan Cadden, *Meanings of Sex Difference in the Middle Ages: Medicine, Science and Culture* (Cambridge: Cambridge University Press, 1993). Peter Biller, *The Measure of Multitude: Population in Medieval Thought* (Oxford: Oxford University Press, 2000), offers a definitive analysis of broader interests in generation and population.

[11] See M. Anthony Hewson, *Giles of Rome and the Medieval Theory of Conception: A Study of the 'De formatione corporis humani in utero'*, University of London Historical Studies, 38 (London: Athelone Press, University of London, 1975); James A. Weisheipl (ed.), *Albertus Magnus and the Sciences: Commemorative Essays, 1980*, Studies and Texts 49 (Toronto: Pontifical Institute of Mediaeval Studies, 1980); Danielle Jacquart and Claude Thomasset, 'Albert le Grand et les problèmes de la sexualité', *History and Philosophy of the Life Sciences* 3 (1981), 73–93; and Cadden, *Meanings*.

[12] Mary F. Wack, 'The Measure of Pleasure: Peter of Spain on Men, Women, and Lovesickness', *Viator* 17 (1986), 173–96; Jacquart and Thomasset, *Sexuality*; and Cadden, *Meanings*.

[13] Green, 'From "Diseases of Women"'.

universities did ultimately have an impact on gynaecological literature, manifested particularly in texts and vernacular traditions on the margins of university culture itself. Out of the general interest in sexuality and generation there gradually grew a specialized literature that fused natural philosophical concerns to understand generation with medical concerns to control it.

It is thus no accident that the most important work in this new genre of the 'secrets of women'—indeed, the text that has come to define the field of inquiry—should have drawn directly on the *Trotula* for some of its material.[14] The Latin *Secrets of Women*, composed probably in the late 1200s, was attributed as early as the fourteenth century to the great Dominican theologian of Cologne, Albertus Magnus. This attribution, while apocryphal, reflects the text's more or less direct connection with Albertus's circle and perhaps even its composition by one of his students. Albertus had devoted considerable energy to making the scientific works of Aristotle comprehensible within a Christian framework, and he focused intensely on the Greek philosopher's biological writings. The *Secrets of Women* is in a way a continuation of Aristotle's discussions of generation, here with a particular emphasis on explaining how the female menses act as both a purgative process in the cold female body and as a seminal fluid.[15] Beginning with the generation of the embryo out of the male's semen and the female's menstrual blood, the text then recounts the development of the foetus and how the different planets affect it while it grows, how certain animals are generated spontaneously, disorders in fetal development and birth, signs of conception and the foetus's sex, signs of virginity or unchastity in a woman, uterine suffocation (which is included here because it is the product of disordered menstruation), and impediments to conception. Particularly surprising, giving the title, is what is *not* here: there is no general description of female reproductive anatomy nor any extended explanation of female sexual response. Commentary traditions that developed in the fourteenth and fifteenth centuries to a certain extent filled these gaps.[16]

Clearly, the pseudo-Albertan *Secrets of Women* only partially fulfilled the growing curiosity about this subject, for in the two centuries following its composition we find various examples of the co-optation of the *Trotula* into

---

[14] I document this reliance in an as yet unpublished essay, 'Slander and the Secrets of Women: The *Meretrices* Version of the *Trotula* Ensemble'.

[15] Unlike most medical writings, the *Secrets of Women* follows the Aristotelian line in denying the existence of a female seed independent of the menses. This issue of whether or not women produced semen (from their 'testicles') as well as menstrual blood, or only the latter, was a key point of argument between natural philosophers (who largely followed Aristotle) and physicians (who followed Galen's belief that women did indeed produce seed). Indeed, in one of the early manuscripts of the pseudo-Albertan *Secrets of Women* (Munich, Bayerische Staatsbibliothek, Clm 22300, an. 1320, Erfurt), the text is actually called *The Book on Generation and Corruption*, a deliberate echo of the title of one of the Aristotelian texts on which it was loosely based.

[16] There are at least seven distinct commentary traditions, none of which have been studied in detail.

the 'secrets of women' tradition in German- and Dutch-speaking regions. The *Trotula* was manipulated in various ways: its title was often changed from 'The Diseases of Women' to 'The Secrets of Women', and it was amended and abbreviated to suit a narrower focus on sexuality and reproduction. It was also directly paired with the pseudo-Albertan text. In all, of some two dozen copies of the Latin *Trotula* gynaecological treatises made in Germany and the Low Countries in the fourteenth and fifteenth centuries, sixteen in some way manipulate or situate the texts to draw them into alliance with the 'secrets' tradition. The *Trotula* could 'pass' for the *Secrets of Women*, serving the same functions as a resource for 'the natural history of women'.

To return, then, to Martin von Geismar's volume, we can see that his interests fit more with the 'secrets of women' traditions—the concern to understand and attempt to control the female body as a site of generation—than a concern to instruct midwives. To judge from the large number of Aristotelian texts and commentaries that he owned, von Geismar had broad interests in natural philosophy.[17] Just as von Geismar could reduce 'the sufferings of women' to the narrower category of 'the secrets of women' (under which title it was well paired with the work on infertility and the visual guide to the interior of the female body), so we see similar collections turning up in the hands of clerics as well as physicians, laymen, and university-trained scholars with interests in natural philosophy.

After von Geismar's death, his books were returned to the Collegiate church of St Peter in Fritzlar, which, a few decades earlier, had already inherited a copy of the pseudo-Albertan *Secrets of Women* from a rector and canon in Thuringia named Johannes Rymph.[18] Similar interests can be found among von Geismar's contemporaries. In Salzburg, either Erhard Manseer himself or the canons of the Archabbey of St Peter added a list of twenty-five impediments to conception in a manuscript of the *Trotula* that Manseer had copied out while in Leipzig.[19] In Nuremberg, the male Dominicans had both a gynaecological text (possibly the *Trotula*) and the pseudo-Albert, *Secrets of Women*, as did the physicians, Herman Schedel and his cousin Hartman.[20] In Munich, Siegmund Gotzkircher, the

---

[17] Interestingly, although von Geismar had a copy of some questions on Aristotle's general theoretical work of generation, *De generatione et corruptione*, he didn't have a copy of Aristotle's more detailed work, *De generatione animalium*.

[18] Kassel, Stadt- und Landesbibliothek, 8° Ms. med. 10, an. 1360 (or 1368?). Rymph was also a canon at the cathedral of St Martin in Kassel.

[19] Salzburg, Erzabtei St Peter, MS b V 22, *c.* 1456 (ff. 149r–162v, with the *Trotula*, were copied in Leipzig).

[20] For the Nuremberg Dominicans' copy of the *Secreta mulierum*, and what may have been a copy of the *Trotula*, see Bayerische Akademie der Wissenschaften, *Mittelalterliche Bibliothekskataloge Deutschlands und der Schweiz* (Munich: Beck, 1969–83), vol. 3, pt. 3, pp. 495–6, see Appendix 1, n. 1. The copy of the pseudo-Albertan text is still extant: Erlangen, Universitätsbibliothek, MS 673 (Irm. 917). The Schedels owned between them one copy of the *Secreta mulierum* (Munich, Bayerische Staatsbibliothek, Clm 444, s. 14 ex., S. Germany, which also included the Salernitan *Women's Cosmetics*) plus three copies of the *Trotula* gynaecological treatises. See Appendix 1, items 64 and 67.

court physician and friend of the German translator Johannes Hartlieb, owned a copy of each text.[21] In Bohemia, the physician Johannes Rudolt not only copied out the *Trotula* with his own hand, but he also rearranged it (deleting all the now extraneous cosmetics), added both the title 'Secrets of Women' and an attribution to 'Master Albertus', and then paired it with the pseudo-Albertan *Secrets of Women* and a brief text on the signs of conception.[22] Once translated into the vernacular, the *Secrets of Women* and the *Trotula* shifted to lay audiences. As we have already seen, Johannes Hartlieb made his paired translations of the *Secrets of Women* and the *Trotula* for his patron, Siegmund, Duke of Bavaria-Munich (with a special version prepared soon after for the Emperor Frederic III).[23] A southern Tyrolean nobleman, Anton von Annenberg (1426/30–83) apparently purchased a copy of the earlier, anonymous southern German translation of the *Secrets of Women* in the early 1470s, adding it to his collection of legal, religious, and humanistic texts.[24]

Beside these identifiable owners of 'secrets of women' literature (all of whom date from the fifteenth century), we can infer similar interests among the as yet unidentified owners of dozens of other copies of the pseudo-Albertan text and other works labelled 'the secrets of women' in the fourteenth and fifteenth centuries. The pseudo-Albertan text often circulated in natural philosophical contexts, appearing with Aristotle's series of works on sensation, sleep, etc. (the so-called *Parva naturalia*), Albertus Magnus's works on astronomical phenomena or the properties of stones, tracts on astronomy, and so forth. We find the *Trotula* absorbed, in precisely the same way, into exclusively or predominantly natural philosophical compendia.[25] Even alchemists were interested in the texts.[26]

[21] Margaret R. Schleissner, 'A Fifteenth-Century Physician's Attitude Toward Sexuality: Dr. Johann Hartlieb's *Secreta mulierum* Translation', in Joyce A. Salisbury, ed., *Sex in the Middle Ages* (New York: Garland, 1991), pp. 110–25, confirms Gotzkircher's ownership of *Trotula* Wolfenbüttel 784 (see Appendix 1, item 68) and of Graz, Universitätsbibliothek, MS 594, s. xv med., where the *Secreta* appears at the end of a large collection of medical texts.

[22] Appendix 1, item 69.   [23] See Chapter 4 above.

[24] Frank Fürbeth, 'Die spätmittelalterliche Adelsbibliothek des Anton von Annenberg: ihr Signaturensystem als Rekonstruktionshilfe', in *Sources for the History of Medieval Books and Libraries*, ed. Rita Schlusemann, Jos. M. M. Hermans, and Margriet Hoogvliet (Groningen: Egbert Forstern, 1999), pp. 61–78. The manuscript von Annenberg owned had been made in 1439 (Vienna, Österreichische Nationalbibliothek, MS 12490). On this early translation, see Margaret R. Schleissner, 'Pseudo-Albertus Magnus: *Secreta mulierum cum commento*, Deutsch: Critical text and commentary', PhD dissertation (Princeton University, 1987).

[25] With the exception of two copies in the Sorbonne where small pamphlets or loose gatherings were later bound into volumes with natural philosophical texts (see Appendix 1, items 39 and 40), all copies of the *Trotula* with predominantly natural philosophical content come from Germanic areas.

[26] Manuscripts with the *Trotula* amidst alchemy are LWL, MS 517 (*olim* Phillipps 2946), s. xv ex. (probably Flanders); and Kremsmünster, Stiftsbibliothek, MS 72, s. xv med. (Austria). Manuscripts of the *Secreta* that include alchemy are New Haven (Connecticut), Yale University, Beinecke Library, MS Mellon 9, *c.* 1440 (probably Prague), with medical and alchemical texts in Latin, Czech, German, transliterated Arabic, and Polish (Constantinus Africanus's *De coitu* immediately follows the *Secreta mulierum*); and OBL, MS Bodley 484 (SC 2063), s. xv med. (England), which includes medical and alchemical texts, plus a tract on confession.

Clearly, then, we can see how widespread this interest in 'women's secrets' was. But what were such readers *doing* with these texts? Were they being used to inform confessors how they ought to interrogate their flock?[27] To help canon lawyers understand the nature of generation when they had to assess consanguinity?[28] To instruct preachers how to censure women for their 'wiles'[29] or to aid witch-hunters in their tasks?[30] Clearly, it will take a full-fledged cultural history of the *Secrets of Women* in late medieval German society to determine why so many fourteenth- and fifteenth-century clerics, physicians, and laymen shared an interest in 'women's secrets'.[31] The more limited question that concerns us here is what effect this very broad interest in generation had on the way gynaecological literature was read. Examination of three cases of the pairing of the *Trotula* and the pseudo-Albertan text can help us understand how the two texts functioned as a complementary pair.

One of the later manifestations of this pairing are the German translations made by the Munich physician Johannes Hartlieb just after the middle of the fifteenth century, whose reasons for seeing the texts as complementary we have already examined.[32] I have also argued that, whatever his claims to sympathize

[27] Manuscripts of the *Secreta mulierum* with confessors' manuals include: Saint-Gall, Stiftsbibliothek, MS 828 an. 1402–49, which includes Johannes Nider's *Manuale confessorum*; BAV, MS Pal. lat. 310, s. xiv, which includes Anselm's *De passione domini*, sermons, an explanation of symbols, the *Scala fidei*, a tract on the ten commandments, sentences from the Bible, more sermons, a tract on confession, and yet more sermons; and Wolfenbüttel, Herzog-August-Bibliothek, MS 648 Helmst. (von Heinemann 698), an. 1382, 1391, which includes what is perhaps an excerpt from the *Secreta* alongside the so-called *Labryrinthus*, a tract on Latinity, an admonition to priests, a list of authoritative statements of the church fathers, and hymns.

[28] Manuscripts of the *Secreta* that include texts on consanguinity include Erfurt, Wissenschaftliche Bibliothek, MS Q. 157 (to which Amplonius latter added a commentary); and Freiburg im Breisgau, Universitätsbibliothek, MS 168, an. 1481 (upper Rhine area) which places the *Secreta* next to the pseudo-Aristotelian *Problemata*, texts on succession, excerpts on succession from Justinian's *Novellae*, tables and notes on consanguinity, tracts by the theologian Jean Gerson, more notes on consanguinity, an *Ars memorandi*, and a text on spheres.

[29] E.g., New Haven, Connecticut, Yale University, Beinecke Library, MS Beinecke 462, s. xv[2] (Austria), where the *Secreta* is found with a heavily annotated copy of the *Doligamus* of Adolfus of Vienna, a series of fables on the deceitful conduct of women; and Philadelphia, University of Pennsylvania, MS lat. 180, s. xv (Germany?) where the *Secreta* is preceded by (1) a brief tract on the art of coitus (for purposes of reproduction only, of course), (2) the proverbs of Secundus, (3) signs by which to determine if a woman is bearing a male or a female child, (4) punning *artes mulierum*, and (5) an extended definition of *meretrix*.

[30] The same hand that wrote the copy of the *Secreta* in Klagenfurt, Studienbibliothek, MS cart. 113 (an. 1431) prefaced it with a text on the witches' sabbath. The codex also contains (in different hands) the *Problemata Aristotelis; Auctoritates philosophiae naturalis* and Isidore, *Sententiae aliquot*; and some Latin sermons.

[31] As of this writing, I have identified 105 extant copies of the Latin *Secreta mulierum*, three-fourths of which were made in the 15th century. Since the *Secreta* began to appear in print by 1475 (at least fifty editions would appear by 1500), the availability of this text must have been extraordinary.

[32] Chapter 4 above. Schleissner, 'Fifteenth-Century Physician's Attitude', p. 117, has usefully suggested that the one embodied the theory (*wort*), the other the practice (*werck*) of the science of generation.

with women's sufferings, Hartlieb intended both texts to meet the interests of his *male* readers. By the time he got to the *Secrets* and the *Trotula* between the early and mid-1460s, Hartlieb had already translated that famous instruction booklet on courtly love, Andreas Capellanus's *Tractatus amoris*, which may indicate his desire to entertain rather than merely educate his lay patrons.[33] As with his translation of the *Trotula*, Hartlieb's *Secrets* is more a novel interweaving of a variety of sources than a straightforward translation. He drew, of course, upon the original *Secrets*, but also, he says, from Macrobius, 'Trotula', Muscio, Gilbert the Englishman and other natural-philosophical writers to produce a book 'on the nature of women and what is peculiar to them in all matters. Also how a man shall live and deal with women so that true love and friendship may not be destroyed between married people.' Indeed, Hartlieb's pride in his craftsmanship bordered on immodesty: 'I do not think that any book has ever been written in the world that could be more useful and more amusing for all married people.'[34] Hartlieb included repeated warnings that the work not be used 'for lust' (*zupulerey*), apparently implying that this knowledge on women should not be used to seduce women (or as erotica?).[35] In a work addressed to the bachelor Siegmund, these claims seem disingenuous, suggesting that Hartlieb had always had a wider audience in mind.

The *Trotula* forms a suitable complement to the *Secrets* because, Hartlieb informs his reader,

[it] tells about many secret matters of women, namely, how they may become pregnant and how they shall behave during pregnancy; also how they shall purify themselves in childbed. The book also tells of all infirmities of women which cause displeasure to men, be they infirmities of the vagina, of the hands, mouth, teeth, or skin. It gives such great remedies that it seems a real miracle that a woman can acquire so much beauty.[36]

---

[33] Klaus Grubmüller, 'Hartlieb, Johannes', in *Die deutsche Literatur des Mittelalters: Verfasserlexikon*, rev. edn, ed. Kurt Ruh *et al.*, 10 vols. (Berlin: De Gruyter, 1978–99), Bd. 3, coll. 480–96.

[34] Partial English translation in Henry E. Sigerist, 'Johannes Hartlieb's Gynaecological Collection and the Johns Hopkins Manuscript 3 (38066)', in *Science, Medicine and History: Essays on the Evolution of Scientific Thought and Medical Practice in Honor of Charles Singer*, ed. E. A. Underwood, 2 vols. (London and New York: Oxford University Press, 1953), 1:231–46, pp. 235–6; cf. Kristian Bosselman-Cyran (ed.), '*Secreta mulierum*' mit Glosse in der deutschen Bearbeitung von *Johann Hartlieb*, Würzburger medizinhistorische Forschungen, 36 (Pattensen/Hannover: Horst Wellm, 1985), pp. 91 and 111–13. Interestingly, although Hartlieb claimed in the *Secreta* to be incorporating material by the 'queen' Trotula, aside from a handful of references to her I have found nothing that actually draws on the original Latin *Trotula* texts.

[35] Bosselman-Cyran, '*Secreta mulierum*'. My thanks to Margaret Schleissner for bringing Hartlieb's admonitions to my attention. Sigerist, 'Johannes Hartlieb's Gynaecological Collection', pp. 233–4, sees Hartlieb's claims as a deliberate disguise for what he describes as an *ars amatoria*. Schleissner, 'Fifteenth-Century Physician's Attitude', on the other hand, finds Hartlieb's concerns more sincere.

[36] As translated by Sigerist, 'Johannes Hartlieb's Gynaecological Collection', p. 236; cf. Bosselmann-Cyran, *Secreta mulierum*, p. 109. Hartlieb's characterization of *Das Buch Trotula* appears in the introduction to his translation of the pseudo-Albertus Magnus *Secreta mulierum*, with which the *Trotula* was paired.

Ensuring women's fertility and making women sexually attractive to men: these are the main features of the *Buch Trotula* in Hartlieb's eyes, not the care of women's diseases because they are distressing or dangerous to women. As we have seen, Hartlieb's translation presents only those chapters that conform to his idea of what the text *should* be about: by eliminating all of the *Treatments for Women* material aside from the instructions for restoring virginity as well as the *Conditions of Women* chapters that did not immediately pertain to generation, Hartlieb did indeed make the *Trotula* into a perfect complement to the *Secrets of Women*.

What is striking about Hartlieb's project is how directly he takes the learning of Latinate scholars and replicates it for a lay, vernacular audience. The collection of the Erfurt bibliophile, Amplonius Ratinck (d. 1435), active a few decades before Hartlieb, demonstrates what interests a physician/natural philosopher might have had in these texts. Amplonius, a master of arts and doctor of medicine who had studied at the universities of Cologne and Paris, later serving as rector of the former university and personal physician to Archbishop Frederick III of Cologne, catalogued his massive library of 635 volumes between 1410 and 1412, dividing it into several distinct classifications. Besides theology and canon and civil law, he grouped his books under the headings of mathematics, alchemy, natural philosophy, and medicine. Amplonius owned four copies of the *Trotula*, five of the *Secrets of Women*.[37] Although he no doubt had multiple copies simply because they appeared in pre-made volumes he had acquired for other reasons, there is no doubt that he did have specific interests in the texts. His method of cataloguing says a great deal about how he placed these works in his categories of knowledge.

Two of the *Trotula* copies (both still extant) were found in strictly medical collections and Amplonius duly classified them among his medical books.[38] One was a collection of mostly Salernitan texts, the other a miscellany of later medical texts that was bound with a copy of the *Articella*. Amplonius catalogued his other two volumes with the *Trotula* under natural philosophy. One volume (no longer extant) contained perhaps two versions of the pseudo-Aristotelian *Secretum secretorum*, the sayings of Secundus (a collection of notoriously misogynistic jibes as well as other pithy sayings),[39] a pseudo-Boethian tract on the discipline of scholars, Seneca's tract on the remedies of fortune, sayings of both theologians and philosophers, the book of Petrus Alfonsus on clerical discipline, and finally the *Trotula*.[40] (This manuscript is, in fact, strikingly similar in content to the one from Jena described in Chapter 2 above, which had belonged to the monks

[37] Amplonius may have also owned a copy of *Women's Cosmetics 3*; see Appendix 1, item 56.

[38] Pommersfelden, Bibliothek der Grafen von Schönborn, HS 178 (2642) (*olim* LXII/178), s. xiii ex./xiv in. (Italy); and *ibid.*, HS 197 (2815) (*olim* LXII/197), s. xiv² (Germany), the latter with the *meretrices* version.

[39] See Alcuin Blamires (ed.), *Woman Defamed and Woman Defended: An Anthology of Medieval Texts* (Oxford: Clarendon, 1992), pp. 99–100. ('What is a woman? The confusion of man, an insatiable beast, continual nagging . . .').

[40] Ms Phil. nat. 46; see Wilhelm Schum, *Beschreibendes Verzeichniss der amplonianischen Handschriften-Sammlung zu Erfurt* (Berlin: Weidmann, 1887), p. 814.

Heinrich and Friedrich of the monastery of Mildenfurth at just this same time.) The other copy of the *Trotula* in Amplonius's natural philosophical section combined a handful of surgical and anatomical texts with several of the same natural philosophical texts in the manuscript just mentioned, plus texts on such topics as the inundation of the Nile, the distinction of forms, and works of Aquinas and Albertus Magnus. Notably, the *Trotula* appears in this last copy paired with the *Secrets of Women*.[41] All of Amplonius's other copies of the *Secrets of Women* appear in the natural philosophy section amid works on philosophy, astronomy, physiognomy, meteorology, etc.[42] Amplonius also owned a fifth copy of the *Secrets* which, though not listed in his catalogue, is the most direct evidence of his interest in the text: found with texts on civil and canon law, the *Secrets* is here supplemented by a commentary that Amplonius copied out in his own hand.[43] Amplonius's unusual interest in these two texts was very probably stimulated during his student days in Paris. There, it seems, he copied from an error-ridden transcript the otherwise unattested lectures of the Parisian philosopher Jean Buridan (d. *c*.1360) on 'the secrets of women'.[44]

Amplonius Ratinck, as the sheer size of his library indicates, was ordinary neither as a physician nor a university scholar. But in pulling the therapeutic text of the *Trotula* so intimately into a context of natural philosophical speculation about generation, to the point where gynaecology and the 'secrets of women' were virtually indistinguishable, he was completely typical. A manuscript from Brabant from *c*.1300 shows just how difficult it is to draw a clear line between medical and natural philosophical uses of gynaecological and 'secrets of women' texts.[45] Containing one of the (if not the) oldest extant copies of the pseudo-Albertan text as well as a particularly peculiar adaptation of the *Trotula* (about which, more in a moment),[46] the codex as a whole comprises Latin and Dutch medical recipes, a tract on urines, medical excerpts from the pseudo-Aristotelian

[41] Erfurt, Wissenschaftliche Bibliothek, MS Amplonian Q 15, *c*.1352–54 (Cremona and Erfurt by German scribe). The *Secreta* is here called *Mistica herarum, id est occulta dominarum.*

[42] These are Erfurt, Wissenschaftliche Bibliothek, MS Amplonian O 79, an. 1341, listed in Amplonius' 1412 cat. as MS phil. natur. 53; MS Amplonian Q 234, an. 1352 (Liège), listed as Phil. nat. 59; and MS Amplonian Q 342, s. xiv, listed as Phil. nat. 29.

[43] Erfurt, Wissenschaftliche Bibliothek, MS Amplonian Q 157; see Schum, *op. cit.*, p. 420. The part of the codex with the *Secrets* had previously belonged to one Johannes Sosati of Göttingen. Unfortunately, I have not been able to obtain a microfilm of this manuscript to determine whether the commentary is Amplonius's own composition or not. He similarly inserted pamphlets written in his own hand into thirteen other codices in the collection.

[44] Erfurt, Wissenschaftliche Bibliothek, MS Amplonian Q 299, s. xiv, ff. 167r–175v: Jean Buridan, *Questiones de secretis mulierum, inc.*: Utrum generatio animalium sit perpetua; *expl.*: Explicit questiones bone a reverendo mag. Buridano pertractate ab Amplonio Rensie in Gallia super secreta mulierum notate difficulter, quoniam exemplar studencium erat incorrectum.

[45] Paris, privately owned ms, *c*.1300 (Brabant). See Green, 'Handlist I'.

[46] The three earliest mss are Paris, Private Collection, *c*.1300 (Brabant); Munich, Bayerische Staatsbibliothek, Clm 22297 (Windberg 97), an. 1320 (Erfurt); and Clm 22300 (Windberg 100), s. xiv in. Clm 22297 situates the *Secreta* amid natural philosophical texts, while Clm 22300 places it amid medical texts, excerpts from Seneca, and formulae for writing letters. A fourth manuscript,

Secret of Secrets, two tracts on physiognomy attributed to Albertus Magnus, a life of Aristotle, the misogynous sayings of Secundus, a table of vices and virtues, the *Trotula* followed immediately by the *Secrets of Women*, excerpts from the Gospels, Christian healing charms in Dutch and Latin, a tract on how the king of the Persians tried to woo a queen he loved, a work on the properties of stones, trees and herbs, two tracts attributed to Hermes, works on astrology, a table to calculate whether a patient will live or die based on the letters of his/her name, a brief text on the medicinal properties of animals, Petrus Hispanus's compendium of therapies called the *Thesaurus pauperum* (in which 'Trotula' had been frequently cited as an authority), a multiplication table, and a tract on dream interpretation attributed to the prophet Daniel. Various notes in Latin and Dutch fill the margins throughout. The overall concern of the volume is medical, but there is a clear overlay of scholastic and clerical interests: philosophy, physiognomy, biblical texts are present here, as well as religious charms and various works reflecting a keen desire to comprehend the world in its many aspects. To judge from the many *notas* added in its margins, the *Secrets of Women* was read closely,[47] while the therapies of the *Trotula* were supplemented by additional gynaecological recipes scribbled elsewhere in the margins. Who compiled this manuscript? Who used it? Should we classify him as a physician? a natural philosopher? a cleric? In a sense it hardly matters. Although a notable increase in *Secrets* ownership by clerics is discernible in the fifteenth century, overall what is striking is how easily the *Secrets* and allied gynaecological texts seem to have travelled across several different classes of Latin and vernacular readers—physicians, religious men, natural philosophers, and elite laymen—who all participated in a shared discourse on women in the fourteenth and fifteenth centuries. And that discourse had one profoundly distinctive feature: a tendency toward misogyny.

'MORE EVIL AND DANGEROUS THAN THE VENOM OF A SERPENT': WOMEN'S SECRETS AND MISOGYNY

In 1458, the pseudo-Albertan *Secrets of Women* was incorporated as the opening text into a manuscript that included Latin treatises on viniculture attributed to Arnau of Villanova and Albertus Magnus; a work of 'subtle observations on the maintenance and order of a household' (mostly a collection of cooking recipes); and some miscellaneous notes on proper eating habits and other matters, some of

---

Admont, Stiftsbibliothek MS 635, a medical compendium, has been described as 13th century, but I have not yet been able to examine the manuscript myself to confirm the date.

[47] For example, the annotator (who may have been the original scribe) adds a *nota* alongside a passage in Chap. V describing a vein that links the uterus and breasts (f. 54ra) and another one alongside an interpolated section citing Avicenna for a test to see if the woman is bearing a male child (f. 56va).

which were added by a later owner of the manuscript, the Heidelberg humanist, historian, and court chaplain to Elector Frederick I of Pfalz, Matthias Kemnat (d. 1476).[48] Kemnat's small codex seems intended to serve as a guide to the management of his household. All the more striking, then, that the *Secrets of Women* text should open with a boldly coloured initial of a male figure sticking his tongue out at the woman who stands beside him (Fig. 5.1).

A peculiarity of the 'secrets of women' tradition is the failure not only by the author of the pseudo-Albertan text but also of his commentators and the many compilers and copyists of other texts entitled 'secrets of women' actually to define what they meant by the term. The closest pseudo-Albertus came was to open the text with the claim that he had been asked to 'make manifest the nature and hidden conditions and secrets *in women*'.[49] Given that men and even the planets are as much involved in generation as women, the title 'secrets of *women*' doesn't really make sense.[50] Why and for whom are these secrets 'secret'?

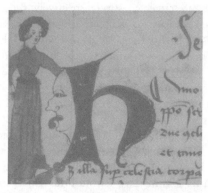

FIG. 5.1 Opening initial of a mid fifteenth-century copy of pseudo-Albertus, *Secrets of Women*; the male figure sticking his tongue out at the woman is suggestive of the text's attitude toward women.

---

[48] BAV, MS Pal. lat. 1382, part VI, an. 1458; the *Secreta* appears on ff. 117r–168v. Kemnat's pamphlet would later be bound together with six other manuscripts, including a copy of the *Trotula* by Martinus Rentz (d. 1503), Professor of Medicine at the University of Heidelberg.

[49] Paris, Private Collection, f. 46ra: 'Cum uestra fauorabilitas ac gratuita societas me rogauerit ut quedam vobis de hiis que *apud mulierem* naturam et conditiones occultas et secreta sunt manifestarem, visa petitione nulla pigricia. A compilatione breuis et compendiosi tractatuli de impetrata me retraxit. Sed pusilla et iuuenalis mea mens secundum eius possibilitatem et temporis oportunitatem quia ad aliena retrahantur, vestro cupiens appetitui satisfacere habeat presentem epistolam'. For a slightly different reading in one of the other early manuscripts, see Green, 'From "Diseases of Women"'. I also discuss the terminology of 'secrecy' at further length there.

[50] Lynn Thorndike, 'Further Consideration of the *Experimenta, Speculum astronomiae*, and *De secretis mulierum* Ascribed to Albertus Magnus', *Speculum* 30 (1955), 413–43, p. 430, notes that the words *et virorum* ('and of men') are included in the earliest copy of the 'Scribit philosophus' commentary. Be that as it may, most manuscripts, even the earliest, concur in labelling the work simply *Secreta mulierum*.

'Secret' can, of course, mean 'hidden away' and that would certainly describe much of the processes involved in generation: they are 'hidden away' inside the female body. Such 'hiddenness' was no less true of the heart, lungs, or other viscera, yet to my knowledge there are no traditions of speaking about the 'secrets' of those organs or the processes they perform. Rather, the 'secrets of generation' become the 'secrets of women' because the 'hidden' processes of generation primarily go on inside the recesses of the female body. They are, in other words, *hidden from men*.

Now, for men to talk about women among themselves is not necessarily misogynous. All intellectual discourse about women, or any other matter, that went on inside the universities, *studia*, cathedral, or monastic walls in the Middle Ages necessarily occurred outside the earshot of women. Rather, what pushes the *Secrets of Women* into the territory of misogyny is the attitude of *suspicion* it projects toward women. In the eyes of the author of the pseudo-Albertan text, the hiddenness of 'women's secrets' is not simply biological. In the chapters on the signs of foetal sex and female chastity, respectively, the author mentions that there are some women who are 'so astute' that they know how to lie in order to invalidate pregnancy or chastity tests.[51] For such women, the interrogator needs to employ alternate methods—in other words, knowledge about generation is to be *extracted* from women. Little wonder, then, that the *Secrets of Women* is structured as a male-to-male conversation.[52]

The commentaries which soon began to accrete around the texts in the mid fourteenth century play out the misogynous possibilities of this closed male conversation even further. Here we find the standard Aristotelian view of women as failed males; here the Plinian account of the poisonous properties of the menstrual blood in *all* women, not just old ones. Indeed, one commentator, after having repeated three times how harmful the female's menses are, wonders why women don't poison themselves with their own lethal blood.[53] These views

---

[51] In the Paris manuscript, these are cap. VIII, *De signis vtrum sit vir uel mulier*, and cap. IX, *De signis castitatis et corruptionis*; in Helen Lemay (trans.), *Women's Secrets: A Translation of Pseudo-Albertus Magnus' 'De secretis mulierum' with Commentaries* (Albany: State University of New York Press, 1992), pp. 126–31, the latter chapter is divided in two. In Paris, Private Collection, the passages read as follows: 'quia quedam mulieres sunt tam astute quod illud considerantes semper opposito modo dicent quam sit rei ueritatis' (f. 56va-b); and 'Tamen quedam mulieres tam astute inueniuntur. quod omnibus istis optime sciunt obuiare' (f. 57rb).

[52] Schleissner, 'Pseudo-Albertus Magnus'. Even within an all-male community, this treatise should not be shown to those who are 'boys whether in age or in morals' (Paris, Private Collection, f. 46ra: 'Rogansque vestram instanciam ut in hoc opere et negotio constans et celans satis ne alicui paruo tam in etate quam in moribus ad presentiam veniat promitteris'). Indeed, the Brabant manuscript, our earliest witness to the text, reinforces this concern in its opening heading: 'Here begins the book or treatise on the Secrets of Women which by law ought not be divulged among little boys and youths' (*ibid.*: 'Incipit liber seu tractatus de secretis mulierum qui non debet de iure inter paruos et iuuenes diulgari').

[53] The oldest copy of the commentary beginning 'Scribit philosophus decimo ethycorum' seems to be Utrecht, Universiteitsbibliotheek, MS 723, an. 1353, ff. 46r–77r. This is what Lemay terms 'Commentary A' in her translation (Lemay, *Women's Secrets*).

were not original to the commentators, of course, and the reader determined to find such negative views of women could have readily located them in a number of other writings. But just as the pithy sayings of the philosopher Secundus could serve as a touchstone for such clerics as Amplonius or the compiler of the Brabant manuscript, so the *Secrets of Women* and its commentaries functioned as a summary of how the female body functioned as a necessary but also dangerous aspect of generation. 'Women's secrets' are not simply inaccessible to men; they are also potentially dangerous to them. Men have no means of control over them *except* by attempting to know and understand them.

If the *Secrets* tradition embodies so much misogyny and has so much potential to generate further misogyny, would not its affiliation with medical traditions, and more particularly with gynaecology, make the latter seem intentionally disparaging, too? The ease with which misogynous rhetoric could fuse onto gynaecological knowledge once the latter had been expropriated for 'secrets of women' purposes is exemplified by a lengthy insert, attributed to a certain Albert de Trapesonde, found in a fifteenth-century copy of a French encyclopedic work, the *Placides and Timeus*, made for Louis de Bruges, seigneur de Gruthuyse.[54] Drawn in part from the *Trotula* treatises as well as other medical and natural philosophical works, this additional section discusses a variety of embryological, obstetrical, and gynaecological issues with many standard questions about the 'nature of women' such as why (as it was believed) prostitutes conceive so rarely or how women who have been raped could conceive at all. Just prior to the gynaecological section, there comes a chapter explaining 'How Galen, the great philosopher and physician, speaks of the natural secret of women':

Galen, a great philosopher of old, says that the maladies of women ought to be concealed from men and especially those which have to do with childbearing. He doesn't speak at all of the flowers [menses], for men ought to hear nothing of them in order that they never copulate with women while they have their flowers, for, if a woman conceives during [her period], the infant will be stinking, red, tainted and mischievous. And the flowers are a venom more evil and dangerous than the venom of a serpent, for if one throws some of them on a green herb, it will dry up, and if a dog eats some, it will be seized by madness, and if someone should lay some in the notch of a tree, never again will it bear good fruit. But the other diseases ought equally to be concealed, except from physicians, for from their ancient books they know these diseases better than women. And because such maladies are subtle and because it is difficult to know whence they arise and where they proceed, it is expedient that women know the causes, reasons and manners of their diseases, and which and of what sort are the instruments of their natural secrets.[55]

---

54 BNF, MS fr. 212, s. xv ex. This copy was prepared for the bibliophile Louis de Bruges by one of his more skilled calligraphers.

55 Claude Thomasset (ed.), *Placides et Timéo ou Li secrés as philosophes: Edition critique avec introduction et notes* (Geneva: Droz, 1980), pp. 264–5. This depiction of Galen's theories is, of course, completely spurious.

Although the author mentions that 'it is expedient that *women* know the causes, reasons and manners of their diseases', ensuring women's ability to cure those diseases by themselves is clearly not his intent: women must turn to male physicians for that knowledge. Rather, his greatest concern is for the potential threat *to men* of their knowledge about women's 'secrets', the most dangerous of which is menstruation. Amazingly, this author introduces an excerpt from the French version of the *Trotula* that had laid out a vocabulary for women to use so that they could speak without shame to a male practitioner.[56] Here, however, it is the *author's* shame, not women's, that constrains his discussion. He claims he will 'speak under cover' and he lays out the terms he will use to designate the vagina, the hymen, the seed, the womb, 'les maladies secrettes' (which he subsumes under the single rubric, 'les fleurs', which usually refers only to menstruation) and the afterbirth.[57] Despite this cover of modesty, the author in fact does freely and fully discuss the 'secrets' of women for the benefit of his male audience. And what constitutes 'women's secrets' for him are solely matters of generation, not women's diseases more broadly.

'TROTULA... WHO TEACHES THE NATURE OF WOMEN'

As we saw in Chapters 1 and 2, the author-figure 'Trotula' was generated out of a misreading of the title *Trotula*, which itself was a positive acknowledgement of Trota's authoritative relationship to the text(s). Whether attributed to Trota or 'Trotula', the assumption of female authorship 'made sense' in the gendered structures of medical practice in the twelfth and thirteenth centuries.[58] But 'Trotula' also came to be seen as an authority whose name could be invoked for a variety of views on women, whether or not they could actually be found in any of the *Trotula* texts. This habit of appropriation of 'Trotula's' authority goes back to the first half of the thirteenth century. The commentary to a Middle French translation of Ovid's *Art of Love* (written *c.*1215–35) cites 'Trotula' 'who teaches the nature of women' (*qui enseigna la nature des femmes*). What is surprising is the subject on which she is supposedly an authority: women's immodesty in going to public games in order to see and be seen, a topic found nowhere in

---

[56] See Chapter 4 above.

[57] Thomasset, *Placides et Timéo*, p. 265: 'Mais pour tant que je me vergongne dire, je voeul en parler en couvert et, a une chascune equalité, je changeray le nom des natures et tout premierement le premier porte, je l'appelleray le sain, et ce qui est au my lieu, je l'appelleray 'pignonus'; et ce que se dit 'sperma', je l'appelleray semence et le lieu ou quel la semence de homme est rechupte et assemblee, je l'appelleray matrice; les maladies secrettes, je les appelleray les fleurs; et les choses qui sieuvent l'enfant, je les appelleray secondines'.

[58] See Chapter 3 above.

the *Trotula* texts.⁵⁹ On the contrary, it is a deliberate perversion of the sincere assertion of women's shame before male doctors in the preface to *Conditions of Women*. In a more learned setting, the thirteenth-century Portuguese physician Petrus Hispanus addresses in his commentary on the *Articella* text, the *Isagoge* of Johannitius, the question of whether women delight in intercourse more than men. In typical scholastic fashion, he weighs the arguments for and against the opinion. One of the authorities he cites is 'Trotula', whom he credits with the opinion that women desire sex more than men. Curiously, Petrus says that 'Trotula has damned woman' (*dempnavit mulierem*) in putting forward this opinion.⁶⁰

This habit of expanding 'Trotula's' authority beyond the scope of the original Salernitan texts even came back to affect the *Trotula* texts themselves. The so-called *meretrices* version of the *Trotula* ensemble remarkably attributes *Conditions of Women* and *Treatments for Women*, respectively, to two prostitutes, mother and daughter, confusing 'Trotula' as title with 'Trotula' as author's name.⁶¹ The ascription is first found in a Brabant manuscript of *c*.1300, the earliest pairing of the *Trotula* with the *Secrets of Women*; a second copy comes from the late fourteenth century and was owned by Amplonius Ratinck; and a third is found in a later fifteenth-century manuscript written in northern Italy apparently for a German student.⁶² The *meretrices* group presents several unusual features beyond the attribution. Although the text of *Conditions of Women* and *Treatments for Women* is in most respects normal (only one chapter of *Women's Cosmetics* is included here), the editor has emended what he apparently saw as deficiencies in the information provided by adding two lengthy inserts, one on the anatomy of the uterus from 'the *summa* of king Alexander' and another on sterility and

⁵⁹ Ovid, *L'Art d'amours: Traduction et commentaire de l'Ars amatoria d'Ovide*, ed. Bruno Roy (Leiden: E. J. Brill, 1974), p. 81; Lawrence B. Blonquist, trans., *L'Art d'amours (The Art of Love)* (New York: Garland, 1987), p. 79.

⁶⁰ My deepest thanks to Miguel de Asua of the Universidad Nacional de San Martín in Argentina, for sharing with me his transcription of Peter's commentary in Madrid, Biblioteca Nacional, MS 1877, f. 42rb. Another possible expansion of the abbreviation here might be *de[s]pernavit* ('she disparaged woman'); unfortunately, none of the other three extant copies of Petrus's commentary is complete so we have no further witness to this particular passage.

⁶¹ Aside from a passing reference to *meretrices-obstetrices* in ¶193 of BLL, MS Harley 3407, s. xiv ex./xv in. (a copy produced in France during the Hundred Years War though reflecting an English textual tradition), I have found no other linking of 'Trotula' or the *Trotula* texts to prostitution. Ruth Mazo Karras has informed me (personal communication) that she likewise found no association of midwifery and prostitution in her researches on the latter institution in later medieval England.

⁶² Paris, Private Collection; Pommersfelden 197; and Berlin, Deutsche Staatsbibliothek, MS Hamilton 433, s. xv² (N. Italy). The attribution alone was later copied into the margin of a manuscript owned by the Nuremberg physician Hermann Schedel (Munich, Bayerische Staatsbibliothek, Clm 660, s. xv¹, Germany?); the text in this copy is not, however, related to the *meretrices* group.

the generation of the seed, including astrological influences. He also added one additional remedy to the section on 'restoratives' of virginity, several more remedies for breast pain and swelling, a new contraceptive recipe (with the proviso that it ought not be told to all women), and instructions for making a sort of harness for an excessively large penis so that it not injure a woman with a small vagina during intercourse.

Why attribute the text to prostitutes? 'Trotula', in both the gynaecological and even the literary traditions, had always been considered learned, but the compiler of this revised version was apparently looking for a different kind of authority than the medical expertise traditionally accorded to the Salernitan healer. A hint of his reasoning comes from the pseudo-Albertan *Secrets of Women*. Beside the 'astute' women who deflected inquiries about their pregnancy or chastity, the *Secrets* author also referred to 'learned women' (*mulieres docte*). These are no great philosophers like Aristotle or physicians like Galen. These are prostitutes. For example, in the chapter on the formation of the foetus (including astral influences on it), he recounts that although women do not know the reason why certain members of the body are more likely to be severely injured if the affliction occurs when the moon is in the sign that dominates that member, they nevertheless know the effect. To illustrate, he mentions a method women use to wound the penis of their male partner by putting a piece of iron in their vagina: 'certain prostitutes are learned in these and other similar [practices]'.[63] Similarly, he attributes a method for inducing abortion to 'prostitutes and other women learned in this wickedness'.[64] It is sexual experience, then, and not medical, that the two authors of the *Trotula mulierum* seem to be credited with: 'two prostitutes, mother and daughter, who travelled through many lands in order to gain experience'. The fiction that they should be mother and daughter undoubtedly further enhanced the feminine 'secrecy' of the texts by stressing the intimate relation between parent and child.[65]

---

[63] Pseudo-Albertus Magnus, *De secretis mulierum*, in Paris, Private Collection, f. 50ra: 'Et sciatis socii mei quod quamuis causam huius rei quedam mulieres occultant et occulta ignorant, tamen quedam effectum cognoscunt et plura mala ex isto operantur. Cum vir cum eis in coitu est, accidit quandoque viris lesio magna et grauis et ex imperfectione [Clm 22297 has *infectione*] membri virilis per eas et per ferrum appositionem prout quedam *meretrices docte sunt in istis et in aliis consimilibus*' (my emphasis).

[64] *Ibid.*, f. 53ra: 'Et ideo meretrices et alie mulieres docte in ista nequitia'. There is a third reference to prostitutes in the Paris manuscript, not duplicated in either Clm 22297 or 22300, that explains why prostitutes' semen is not retained because of frequent intercourse (f. 59ra). Although in later versions of the text, midwives (referred to three times in chap. 5, *De exitu fetus de utero*) would be called *discrete* (used twice) and *expertes*, here in the Paris manuscript they have no qualifiers at all (f. 54ra–b).

[65] As we have seen, the mother–daughter tie was also stressed by Thomas of Cantimpré when he attributed the obstetrical selections from Muscio to Cleopatra and her daughter; see Chapter 3 above. The Hebrew *Sefer ha-Toledet*, a translation of Muscio's *Gynaecia*, is, in contrast, set in the form of a dialogue between the tragic biblical heroine Dinah and her father; the choice of a masculine source is in this case meant to suggest scientific understanding, of which women are incapable; cf. Ron Barkaï, *Les Infortunes de Dinah: le livre de la génération. La gynécologie juive au*

Presented as the work of two truly 'learned' women, then, and enhanced with the kind of information that a 'secrets' reader was really interested in, it is not at all surprising to find that in two of the three *meretrices* manuscripts the *Trotula* should be seen as the perfect complement to the pseudo-Albertan *Secrets of Women*.

Equally specious in its appeals to 'Trotula's' authority is the *Placides and Timeus*, a later thirteenth-century French natural philosophical encyclopedia, whose author articulates most clearly the attractions of being able to claim that his source is written 'from a woman's point of view'. Cast in the form of a dialogue between the master Timeus and his young princely pupil, the *Placides and Timeus, or the Secrets of the Philosophers* draws on a variety of encyclopedic and scientific works to cover four areas of knowledge necessary to a philosopher-prince: God and his creation, human reproduction, meteorology, and finally the history of the transmission of laws and the birth of feudal civilization. Three references to 'Trotula' are found in the long section on reproduction. Calling 'Trotula' a philosopher and stressing her experience and her beauty, the author says that 'physicians who know something derive great authority and much solid information' from 'Trotula' because she could both speak of what she 'felt in herself, since she was a woman', and, also because she was a woman, 'all women revealed their inner thoughts more readily to her than to any man and told her their natures'. As with the French translator of Ovid, however, the actual content of the *Trotula* seems to have been irrelevant: none of the subsequent discussion of 'women's natures' in the *Placides and Timeus* derives from the Salernitan texts.[66] After his lavish praise of 'Trotula's' special attributes, the author of the *Placides and Timeus* goes on to use her authority to support a statement that women desire intercourse more when they are pregnant than at other times.[67] 'Trotula' is also cited as an authority for the term *molla*; although *Treatments for Women* makes mention of a certain growth in the uterus, it is not clear that the mole is being referred to and in any case the term itself is never used.[68] When the author of the *Placides and Timeus* wished to speak of women's nature he called not only upon 'Trotula' 'to whom all women disclosed their thoughts more willingly than to a man', but also 'Hermafrodites', a man who dressed in women's clothing and passed amid the company of women and learned their 'private natures'. He also referred to Sirenis, 'another

---

Moyen-Age, trans. Jacqueline Barnavi and Michel Garel (Paris: Cerf, 1991), pp. 131–2. A German poem from this period, 'How the Wife Taught Her Daughter Whoring', likewise exploits the idea of how women pass on their 'secrets' from one generation to the next; see Ann Marie Rasmussen, *Mothers and Daughters in Medieval German Literature* (Syracuse: Syracuse University Press, 1997).

[66] Thomasset, *Placides et Timéo*, pp. 133–4; see also *idem, Une vision du monde à la fin du XIIIe siècle: Commentaire du Dialogue de 'Placides et Timéo'* (Geneva: Droz, 1982), pp. 160–61.

[67] Thomasset, *Placides et Timéo*, pp. 135–6.

[68] Thomasset, *Placides et Timéo*, p. 148. On the reference to growths in the womb in *Treatments for Women*, see Green, *Trotula*, ¶111. What is now called the hydatidiform (or hydatid) mole is an abnormal placental growth, sometimes with, sometimes without the presence of foetal tissue.

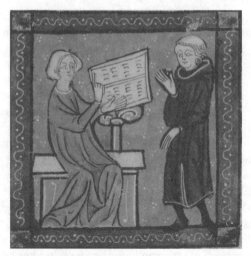

Fig. 5.2 'Trotula' expounding on the nature of women in a copy of the *Placides et Timéo*, which may have been owned by Clemence of Hungary; the rubric reads 'How the woman reads to the clerk the secrets of nature' ('Comme la fame lit as clers les secrés de nature').

sage femme'. In other words, even though male authorities such as Aristotle and Galen may be cited on aspects of generation, there is something about women's nature that remains thoroughly hidden from men, something that can only be learned from a woman—or from a man who has lived as if he were a woman.

The earliest extant copy of the *Placides and Timeus* (written in 1304) shows this strikingly. In an image bearing the rubric 'How the woman reads to the clerk the secrets of nature' (Fig. 5.2),[69] a woman is seated on a bench in front of a book perched on a lectern. She holds up her right finger in a gesture of teaching to the tonsured clerk who stands in front of her. The image is a depiction of 'Trotula' who, the text tells us, 'looked in her books and found confirmation of all which nature revealed to her and, from that, she knew most of the nature of women'.[70] Thus, both text and image support the fiction that 'Trotula' is an extraordinarily learned woman who was acknowledged even by male clerks as a great authority on 'woman's nature'. But it was an ambivalent authority, one that could be co-opted as easily to condemn women as to aid them.

'Trotula' was not the only female authority so used. The names of Cleopatra, the emperor Constantine's mother Helen, and a certain queen Aelis were also

---

[69] Rennes, Bibliothèque Municipale, MS 593, f. 532r: 'Comme la fame lit as clers les secrés de nature'. The image falls between ¶¶291 and 292 of Thomasset's edition.

[70] *Placides et Timéo* ¶291 (p. 134): 'et celle regardoit en ses livres et trouvoit concordance en ce que nature lui en devisoit et, par ce, elle savoit grant partie des natures as femmes'.

occasionally invoked for authority on women's secrets.[71] For example, in a later medieval adaptation of the French *Quant Dex nostre Seignor* translation (which, like most independent translations of the Salernitan *Conditions of Women*, had no attribution to 'Trotula'), we find the heading: 'Here begins the book of the secrets of ladies which Constantine, Galen and Hippocrates made. And it was made, too, by Helen, the mother of Constantine, who knew all of nature and understood all the properties of herbs.' Later, Helen's expertise is reaffirmed: 'Helen, the mother of Constantine, who knew the ways of women'.[72] But 'Trotula', perhaps simply by virtue of the broad circulation of the *Trotula* texts, was by far the best known feminine figure. As late as the 1460s, while conceding that Galen, Rhazes, and Avicenna had also written on gynaecology, Johannes Hartlieb claimed 'but all that is tiny compared to what Trotula wrote and learned'.[73] He even elevated her stature to that of a queen of Greece! As we have seen, there was no necessary reason to keep the figure 'Trotula' tied to the actual content of the *Trotula* texts. Any sort of theory about women could be pinned to her name. But the fact that authoress, text, and *topic* of the text were so intimately linked was more than convenient. The existence of the secrets of women texts—the existence of a whole mindset of pursuing these secrets—was furthered and enabled by having those 'secrets' come out of the mouth of a woman.

READING LIKE JANKYN: FROM SECRETS TO SLANDER

Jankyn's 'book of wikked wyves' might well be the most thoroughly studied book that never existed.[74] No manuscripts have ever been found with the entire combination of treatises that Chaucer listed as its contents, and it has been argued that Chaucer was simply drawing from a collection of anti-matrimonial 'classics' gathered in his own library, to which he added other 'titles which give Jankyn's book a distinctive individuality well adapted to its dramatic role in the Wife of Bath's Prologue'.[75] From the context of his citation, it is clear that Chaucer thought 'Trotula' to be an author's name, not (or not simply) the title of a book.[76] Chaucer gives no biographical identification for her—as he does for the

---

71 Green, 'Traittié'. On the ascription of obstetrical instructions to Cleopatra, see Chapter 3 above.

72 Green, 'Traittié'.   73 Bosselman-Cyran, 'Secreta mulierum', p. 110.

74 Ralph Hanna III and Traugott Lawler (eds.), *Jankyn's Book of Wikked Wyves*, using materials collected by Karl Young and Robert A. Pratt (Athens: University of Georgia Press, 1997-).

75 Robert A. Pratt, 'Jankyn's Book of Wikked Wyves: Medieval Antimatrimonial Propaganda in the Universities', *Annuale mediaevale* 3 (1962), 5–27, at p. 6.

76 What Chaucer meant by the reference to 'Trotula' cannot be determined by the manuscripts of the *Tales* themselves. John M. Manly and Edith Rickert (eds.), *The Text of the Canterbury Tales, Studied on the Basis of All Known Manuscripts*, 8 vols. (Chicago: University of Chicago Press, 1940), 5:70, find only one insignificant variant form, 'Trocula', and this in only two of several dozen

only other female authority in the list, Heloise[77]—and he makes no mention of her writings. He assumes, in other words, that mere mention of her name would be enough to bring to the reader's mind an association that made her function in Jankyn's book obvious. So why did he cite her? Most scholars have followed a suggestion made a century ago that 'Trotula' was included because her writing was pornographic.[78] This line of argument assumes that Chaucer viewed the texts as a source of information on female sexuality, hinting at the lustiness of the oft-married Wife of Bath herself. Yet I think our modern reductionist focus on sexuality falsely induces us to assume that anything that talks about the genitalia is *only* about sex. Aside from the chapters in *Treatments for Women* and *Women's Cosmetics* prescribing means to make a sexually experienced woman appear like a virgin again (¶¶190–5, 231, and 307–9) or the chapter found at the end of many copies of *Women's Cosmetics* and earlier forms of the ensemble instructing the woman on precoital hygiene (¶305f), little in any of the three *Trotula* texts would by modern standards—or, I believe, medieval ones—be considered blatantly erotic. There is very little discussion of female sexual physiology and (except for the *meretrices* version, which did not circulate in England) virtually no description of female anatomy that might be used to inform the sexually curious. No instructions are given on how to copulate well, either with the intention of

---

manuscripts of the *Tales*. Furthermore, Professors Susan Schibanoff and Stephen B. Partridge have informed me that the reference to 'Trotula' (and all the other authorities in Jankyn's book) is never annotated by the major glossators of the *Tales*; my thanks to them both for advice on this matter.

[77] Heloise and 'Trotula' are also the only 'modern' authorities in the list. Although Chaucer is clearly drawing on Walter Map's (1140-*c*.1209) *Letter of Valerius to Ruffinus* as well as ancient authorities that only resurfaced in the 12th century, he does not refer to Map or any other medieval male author by name.

[78] George L. Hamilton, 'Trotula', *Modern Philology* 4 (1906), 377–80, at p. 379. Charles and Dorothea Singer, 'The Origin of the Medical School of Salerno, the First University: An Attempted Reconstruction', in *Essays on the History of Medicine Presented to Karl Sudhoff on the Occasion of His Seventieth Birthday November 26th 1923*, ed. Charles Singer and Henry E. Sigerist (London: Oxford University Press, 1924; repr. Freeport, NY: Books for Libraries Press, 1968), pp. 121–38, describe the *Trotula* texts as having 'something of the 'Peeping Tom' about them' (p. 129). This assumption continues to the present day; see Michael Uebel, 'Pornography', in *Dictionary of the Middle Ages. Supplement I*, William C. Jordan, editor-in-chief (New York: Charles Scribner's Sons, 2004), pp. 490–93. In a slightly different vein, some scholars have suggested that Chaucer is playing on 'Trotula's' name, implying that she 'trots around' (in the sense of pandering) or that the French form of Trota's name (Trote) evokes the word for 'turd' (*crote*); see Eric W. Naylor, 'Nunca le digas trotera' (*Libro de buen amor*, 926c)', in *Homenaje al Profesor Antonio Vilanova*, ed. Adolfo Sotelo Vázquez and Marta Cristina Carbonell (Barcelona: Universidad de Barcelona, 1989), pp. 461–74. Perhaps in medieval France and England (and even Spain) people snickered over the verbal coincidences, but no such associations are ever made by the scribes or annotators of the *Trotula* manuscripts themselves. Blamires, *Woman Defamed*, follows Pratt in suggesting that the citation of 'Trotula' is 'mere name-dropping' (p. 218), though this still begs the question of why hers is a name worth dropping. As I have explained elsewhere ('Traittié'), I believe the wicked portrait of 'Dame Trote' by the 13th-century poet Rutebeuf refers to the historic Salernitan healer Trota and not the gynaecological author-figure 'Trotula'.

reproducing or of simply seeking pleasure.[79] The reader turning to the *Trotula* treatises as a source of explicit erotica would surely have come away disappointed.

Actually, Chaucer need never have cracked open any of the dozens of copies of the *Trotula* texts in England nor heard 'Trotula' directly mentioned to have decided that her name belonged in Jankyn's book. Known for his exceptionally broad range of French reading, Chaucer may have included 'Trotula's' name simply because he had found it in the early Ovid translation cited above or the *Placides and Timeus*.[80] Chaucer's reference may, therefore, be nothing more than a literary allusion to show off his learning.

Or perhaps Chaucer's reference to 'Trotula' was merely an inside joke. One manuscript of the *Trotula* had been donated to Merton College, Oxford, probably by the physician and mathematician Simon Bredon in 1368. Perhaps Chaucer, who had connections with Merton, looked at this 'book made by a Salernitan woman who is called Trotula' (*liber factus a muliere Salernitana que Trotula uocatur*), noticed that the only marginal annotations in the *Trotula* were an odd form drawn beside ¶¶190–5 on 'repairing' virginity and an additional *nota* beside ¶231 on the same topic, and then deemed these few recipes sufficient grounds for including her in Jankyn's book.[81] Yet Chaucer clearly expected that his readers (who consisted of much wider group than the fellows at Merton) would readily recognize the joke.

It seems to me unlikely that Chaucer—though no physician, still obviously well-versed in the major medical authorities[82]—could have been unaware that 'Trotula' was the principal name associated with gynaecological literature. After all, England was more heavily supplied with copies of the texts than anywhere else

---

[79] Such information could readily be found elsewhere, for example in Constantine the African's *On Sexual Intercourse* which was readily available in England; see Lister Matheson, 'Constantinus Africanus: *Liber de coitu* (*Liber creatoris*)', in *Sex, Aging, and Death in a Medieval Medical Compendium: Trinity College Cambridge MS R.14.52, Its Texts, Language, and Scribe*, ed. M. Teresa Tavormina, Medieval and Renaissance Texts and Studies, 292, 2 vols. (Tempe, AZ: Arizona Center for Medieval and Renaissance Studies, 2006), vol. 1, pp. 287–326; or in works that derived from Avicenna's *Canon*. See also Helen Lemay, 'William of Saliceto on Human Sexuality', *Viator* 12 (1981), 167–81.

[80] Although not rare, the Old French Ovid seems to have had no more than a modest circulation before the 15th century, the date of all five extant manuscripts. The *Placides et Timéo* enjoyed a better circulation throughout the later Middle Ages. It now exists in eight manuscripts ranging in date from 1304 to the end of the 15th century; to the seven manuscripts listed by Thomasset, add Glasgow, University Library, MS Ferguson 241, s. xv ex., ff. 1r–65r. It was printed numerous times in the 16th century. On the pervasive influence of French literature on Chaucer's writings, see Haldeen Braddy, 'The French Influence on Chaucer', in *Companion to Chaucer Studies*, ed. Beryl Rowland, rev. ed. (New York and Oxford: Oxford University Press, 1979), pp. 143–59.

[81] On Oxford, Merton College, MS 230 (N.1.3), s. xiv in. (England, probably Oxford), see Appendix 1, items 6 and 7.

[82] And perhaps acquainted with several physicians; see Huling E. Ussery, *Chaucer's Physician: Medicine and Literature in Fourteenth-Century England*, Tulane Studies in English 19 (New Orleans: Tulane University, Department of English, 1971).

in Europe. Notably, Chaucer's inclusion of 'Trotula' amidst Jankyn's catalogue of misogynistic writers is nearly contemporaneous with the Middle English translation of the _Trotula_ that warns against men's slanderous readings of gynaecological texts. That is, even as Chaucer is describing a fictive tome that could be used as a weapon against women, the English translator is issuing a veritable threat of divine vengeance against male slanderers who would use a gynaecological text not to help women, but to disparage them. Both works may, in different ways and for different purposes, be exaggerating the tug-of-war over gynaecological literature. Yet both, I believe, reflect attitudes toward and uses of gynaecological literature that were in fact becoming increasingly common throughout Europe in the later medieval period.

In England as on the Continent, the misogynous potential of the _Trotula_ lay in their utility in answering 'secrets of women' questions. The pseudo-Albertan _Secrets of Women_ never circulated well in England: only one extant Latin manuscript was produced in Britain (and that not until the mid fifteenth century) and only one of some fifty printed editions prior to 1500 came from an English press.[83] There is no evidence that a Middle English translation of the text was ever made. Nevertheless, it is striking how many other parallels there are with the Continental patterns, both in the interest in generation and in the use of the terminology of 'women's secrets'. The earliest known use of the term 'secrets of women' as a title, as we have already seen, is the inscription _Les Secres de femmes_ in the thirteenth-century French adaptation of the _Conditions of Women_'s chapters on generation, which was copied in England perhaps as early as the third quarter of that century. A brief Latin dialogue on questions relating to sex and generation, which in another form had circulated in England since at least the turn of the thirteenth century, is found in a fourteenth-century English manuscript under the title _The Greater Treatise on the Secrets of Women._ The epithet 'the greater' contrasts it, in turn, with another text in the same manuscript (this one more similar to the pseudo-Albertan text) entitled _The Little Treatise on the Secrets of Women._[84] Also in the fourteenth century we find a Middle English translation of an adaptation of Muscio—entitled _On_

---

[83] OBL, MS Bodley 484 (SC 2063), s. xv med. (England), ff. 1r–33r. The two other copies now in British collections were produced in the Low Countries (Glasgow, University Library, MS Hunter 414, ff. 86v–96v, an. 1414) and Germany (LWL, MS 11, an. 1374). The work was printed in London in 1485, ten years after editions had begun appearing on the Continent.

[84] CTC, MS O.2.5 (1109), s. xiv, ff. 75ra–85vb (_maior_) and ff. 130va–132va (_parvus_). There is also an additional section on ff. 206rb–207rb, _quare mulieres communiter sunt minores hominibus, pallidiores et lenitiores et frequenter menstruant_ ('why women commonly are smaller, paler, and smoother than men, and why they menstruate frequently'); a later hand calls this a _Secretorum mulierum appendix_. On the first text (for which she adopts the standardized title _On Human Generation_), see Cadden, _Meanings of Sex Difference_, pp. 89–103. The earliest known copy from England of this series of questions is OBL, MS Auct. F.3.10, _c._ 1200, ff. 118r–153r, where the dialogue appears at the beginning of a longer series of questions; this text is edited in Brian Lawn, _The Prose Salernitan Questions_ (London: British Academy/Oxford University Press, 1979), pp. 1–155. The _Parvus tractatus_ is also found (untitled) in CTC, MS R.14.45 (916), s. xv, ff. 24r–27r.

the Secrets (or Nature) of Women—that, in its original Latin version, had sat in the libraries of the Sorbonne and St Victor in Paris since at least the early 1300s.[85] Beside the two copies of the *Trotula* which he donated to the library of St Augustine's in Canterbury, the astronomer John of London (fl. 1310) gave a volume with an unidentified 'practical text of gynaecology on the secrets of women'.[86] John Erghome (d. *c*.1385), master of theology and prior of the convent of Augustinian friars at York, owned a copy of the *Trotula maior* which he referred to as 'on the secrets of women' in a collection of mostly Salernitan medical tracts. The Augustinian friars at Leicester had a copy with exactly the same title, here embedded (as was common in German circulation) in an extraordinary collection of astronomical and natural philosophical texts. This trend would continue well into the fifteenth century.[87] Texts entitled 'secrets of women' (whatever their actual content may have been) were considered appropriate reading for cultivated gentlemen with natural philosophical and/or medical interests: although Humphrey Newton's copy of that abridged Middle English translation of the *Trotula* did not bear the title *Secretum mulierum* (as it did in the other two extant copies), his interests may have been the same as those of Thomas Stotevyle (*c*.1408–*c*.1466), a prominent Suffolk lawyer who, earlier in the century, owned among his forty books on law, theology, history, medicine, and literature (including the *Canterbury Tales*) 'a small book on the secrets of women'.[88]

---

[85] See Chapter 4 above.

[86] Montague Rhodes James, *The Ancient Libraries of Canterbury and Dover: The Catalogues of the Libraries of Christ Church Priory and St Augustine's Abbey at Canterbury and of St Martin's Priory at Dover* (Cambridge: Cambridge University Press, 1903), p. 346, item 1262: *Practica Genescie de secretis mulierum*. In between the gynaecological text and the pseudo-Boethius treatise on the discipline of scholars were three other practical medical texts.

[87] On the copy at Leicester, see Appendix 1, item 27. The title 'secrets' even appears in the 15th-century Oxford copy of the *Practica secundum Trotam*. Examples of incorporation of gynaecological texts into natural philosophical collections include a copy of the English Gilbertus Anglicus *Sickness of Women 1* (the 'men's version') which was originally copied with a Middle English translation of the popular natural philosophical *Secreta secretorum*, traditionally attributed to Aristotle and was later bound with several Latin scientific texts (OBL, MS Lyell 36). Even when remaining in medical contexts, gynaecology might be accompanied by 'nature of women' concerns as when another copy of *Sickness of Women 1* was incorporated into an array of Latin and English medical texts; later in the volume we find a series of questions (in Latin) on why women desire intercourse more than men, why when women are pregnant they desire sex more while animals do not desire it at all, why women menstruate but men do not, why menstruation is monthly, why women and eunuchs have soft voices, why women do not have beards but men do (BLL, MS Harley 2375, s. xv; *Sickness of Women 1* appears on ff. 19r–29v, the questions on women on f. 54v).

[88] See D. H. Turner, 'The Eric Millar Bequest to the Department of Manuscripts. I. The Medieval and Renaissance Manuscripts', *British Museum Quarterly* 33 (1968–69), 16–37 and pl. 8, for a brief description of London, British Library, MS Additional 54233; the list of Stotevyle's books, made in 1459–60, is on f. 3r (reproduced as Turner's plate 8). Item 9 on the list is a *paruus liber de secreta* [*sic*] *mulierum*. Stotevyle was a member (from 1424) and later governor of Lincoln's Inn, one of four training schools for barristers in 15th-century England; see W. P. Bailbon, *Records of the Honorable Society of Lincoln's Inn: The Black Books*, 5 vols. (London: Lincoln's Inn, 1897–1968), vol. 1, *passim* (s.n. Stuteville).

These English interests in women's secrets also paralleled those on the Continent by developing alongside clerical misogynous literary traditions, which were alive and well and even flourishing in English learned circles, particularly at Oxford.[89] Already in the early fourteenth century, teachings similar to those contained in the 'secrets of women' tradition were given to English boys in grammar school: discourses on the nature of the menses and the development of the foetus are all bracketed by the standard vituperations (drawn from the philosopher Secundus and others) of women in general and of prostitutes and postmenopausal old women in particular. 'Place a restraint on yourself', the boys are warned, 'beware woman's poison: the vessel which you feel is delightful is full of diseased blood.'[90] These warnings came in the course of a commentary on the *Discipline of Scholars* falsely attributed to Boethius. The same pseudo-Boethian text was found at the end of John of London's volume containing 'A Practical Gynecological Text on the Secrets of Women'. Indeed, it has been suggested that those extant collections of misogynistic lore that are most similar to Jankyn's 'book of wykked wyves' 'seem designed to indoctrinate young men in Latin grammar and antifeminism simultaneously'.[91] English clerics would have thus had exposure to both natural philosophical and medical ideas akin to continental traditions on the 'secrets of women', and they would have been well-versed in attitudes toward women that hardened as traditional clerical misogamy veered into misogyny.

It is just such a university cleric that Chaucer, writing in the 1390s, satirizes in his depiction of Jankyn. If Jankyn had indeed had a copy of the *Trotula*, how would he have read it? A manuscript of the ensemble now at Winchester College suggests how a reading of the *Trotula*, informed by the 'secrets' traditions, might veer into blatant misogyny.[92] The manuscript's contents are mostly medical and thoroughly typical of the practical, therapeutic concerns of the majority of *Trotula* manuscripts: texts on surgery, anatomy, and *materia medica*, plus general texts on medical praxis and prognosis. Only slightly unusual are a tract on the

[89] Pratt, 'Jankyn's Book'.

[90] Cf. the lectures of William Wheatley (fl. 1305–17, headmaster of the grammar school at Stamford in Lincolnshire in the early 14th century and later of that at Lincoln cathedral), as described in Michael Johnson, 'Science and Discipline: The Ethos of Sex Education in a Fourteenth-Century Classroom', in Helen Rodnite Lemay, ed., *Homo Carnalis: The Carnal Aspect of Medieval Human Life*, Acta XIV, Center for Medieval and Early Renaissance Studies (Binghampton: SUNY Center for Medieval and Renaissance Studies, 1990), pp. 157–72 (quote from p. 164). Wheatley is also credited with authorship of a tract entitled *De signis prognosticis futurae sterilitatis* (Oxford, New College, MS 264, s. xiv, ff. 253ra–264rb), a treatise on the famines of the mid-1310s though this has only passing discussion of issues of human generation.

[91] Ralph Hanna III, '*Compilatio* and the Wife of Bath: Latin Backgrounds, Ricardian Texts', in *Latin and Vernacular: Studies in Late-Medieval Texts and Manuscripts*, ed. Alistair Minnis (Woodbridge: D. S. Brewer, 1989), pp. 1–11, at p. 2.

[92] Winchester, Winchester College, Warden and Fellows Library, MS 26, s. xiii ex./xiv in. (England). My thanks to Roger Custance, Librarian at Winchester College, for permission to consult this manuscript *in situ*. Nothing is known, unfortunately, about the manuscript's medieval provenance; it first appears in the College's catalogue in 1634.

medicinal properties of various animals (including camels, elephants, gazelles, and leopards) and an incomplete Anglo-Norman verse tract on the diseases of hunting birds. What makes the manuscript thoroughly distinctive are readers' marks added by several fourteenth- or fifteenth-century readers, at least four of whom can be distinguished by their hands, inks, and characteristic marks (or, as we will see, cuts).[93] None of them wrote any substantive textual commentaries on the *Trotula*. Rather, they marked the text with simple marks, *notas*, or, most interestingly, marginal sketches that give an often visceral sense of their reactions to the text. Such marginalia, which we might otherwise be inclined to dismiss as doodlings, are in no sense uncommon in medieval manuscripts. They served as a mechanism to spark recollection, to retrain the eye on passages that the reader thought most worthy of note.[94] But precisely because they were *selective*, the marginalia in this Winchester manuscript show us what elements of the *Trotula* a small group of readers in England were most interested in.

The first annotator is one of these 'doodlers', preferring visual mnemonics to words as he marked the text. He confines his 'comments' to the *Trotula*, showing no interest in any of the dozen other texts in the manuscript. Even in the *Trotula* he remains silent for quite some time, skipping over the extensive discussions of menstruation, uterine suffocation, uterine prolapse, cancers, lesions, etc. in *Conditions of Women*. Only when he comes to the chapter on sterility (¶75, f. 45r, Fig. 5.3) does he become engaged.[95] Here he adds the head of a bearded man at the beginning of the chapter. Beside a recipe below for aiding conception, he draws a hedgehog, the symbol of self-preservation (¶77). He became particularly excited on the next page (¶¶82–86, f. 45v, Fig. 5.4), adding three pointing hands alongside the final remedy to promote conception and the following contraceptives that come with the justification that some women need to avoid pregnancy lest they die. He then adds a capped and bearded male head, who gazes at the text below, another contraceptive recipe (¶87). This same annotator probably also added some particularly vivid illustration alongside the closing

[93] Because some marks are clearly written around and/or in reaction to others, it is possible to date the relative order of the different hands. For all the reasons examined in Chapters 2 and 4, I assume that all of these 'commentators' were male.

[94] Mary Carruthers, *The Book of Memory* (Cambridge: Cambridge University Press, 1990) argues that vulgar marginalia are merely mnemonics, the point of the vulgarity being to shock and therefore stimulate recollection. Michael Camille, *Image on the Edge: The Margins of Medieval Art* (Cambridge, MA: Harvard University Press, 1992), critiques common assumptions of the irrelevance of marginalia, gargoyles, and other 'monkey business' (his term) on the edges of medieval art. The marginalia in Winchester 26 differ from the kinds of marginal 'commentaries' Camille discusses, however, in that they are clearly the additions of later hands, not those of the original scribe or illuminator.

[95] The paragraph numbers refer to numeration in my edition of the *Trotula* standardized ensemble (Green, *Trotula*). Since the Winchester manuscript contains an earlier, fuller version of the ensemble (what I have called the intermediate ensemble), it contains some additional chapters not found in the modern edition. For the numeration of these, see the full concordance to all the versions of the *Trotula* in Green, 'Development'.

passages of *Conditions of Women* where additional aids to conception had been discussed (¶¶129–31, f. 46*v). Apparently, these 'comments' were too vivid, for a later reader cut out the whole upper quarter of that page—text, margin, and all.[96] The nature of this offending illustration may be gauged from the following page, where *Treatments for Women* begins. Here, our annotator first added a stork beside a remedy, new here in this copy of the text, that will either provoke the menses or expel the dead foetus.[97] That illustration was placid enough. More unsettling for the late medieval exciser, apparently, was a sketch just below of a duck with, as its head and neck, a skeletal face and vertebrae. This bizarre hybrid illustrates a passage likening the prolapsed womb to 'a wild beast of the forest, that wanders this way and that' (¶140, f. 47r, Fig. 5.5). Our knife-wielding exciser attempted to remove this disturbing image, too: a slash cuts right through it, though it seems he gave up as it was too hard to cut out a section from the inner (bound) margin.[98]

Moving along, our annotator adds a penis and scrotum dressed up as a fish next to the chapter on swelling of the penis (¶154, f. 48r, Fig. 5.6). Next to an unguent, said to be used by Salernitan women for sunburn, lesions caused by the sun or wind, and facial excoriations made in mourning for the dead, the annotator adds a suitably mournful face (¶167, f. 48v, Fig. 5.7). On the next page, a fang-baring wild man's head is drawn opposite the chapter on teeth loosened by cold (¶187, f. 49r top). Further down the page beside the chapter on swelling of the vagina caused by coitus, a 'Nota' is about to be eaten by a hideous man (¶196, f. 49r bottom, Fig. 5.8). Finally, as the twelfth of his 'comments', our annotator sketches in a monkey, symbol of uncontrolled sexuality and filth, pointing to the chapter on women who suffer from excessive odour or sweat (¶205, f. 49v, Fig. 5.9). The end of the text is missing, though again it is conceivable that its loss was not accidental: it would have contained the original closing chapter of *Women's Cosmetics* (¶305f), a detailed account of sexual hygiene that counselled how to prepare a scented water and powder for anointing the genitalia. Although this chapter would later be deleted from a version of *Women's Cosmetics* that promised to help women preserve themselves 'decently' and from the revised version of the full ensemble, in all manuscripts where it remains, whether Latin or vernacular, it is never singled out for comment by scribes or annotators.[99]

---

[96] This exciser cannot be dated precisely, but because a 16th-century annotator (who was adding headings to several of the texts in the upper margins) wrote *around* the excision of f. 46bis, the exciser must be late medieval or early 16th-century at the latest. (My thanks to Dr Richard Gameson for his assistance in dating this later hand.) That the exciser was reacting to something on the *verso* of f. 46bis can be determined by impressions of the knife cut left on the verso of the preceding leaf.

[97] It appears in the position of what should have been ¶136, which was instead a remedy for excessive menstruation.

[98] Again, a cut in the leaf underneath (f. 48) confirms the direction and force of the attempted excision.

[99] The passage appears in both of the two vernacular renditions of the intermediate ensemble: the 14th-century Italian *Segrete cose delle donne*, and the 15th-century English *Liber Trotuli*.

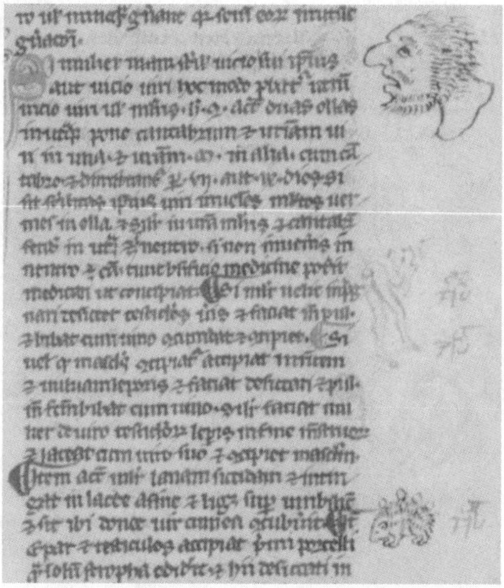

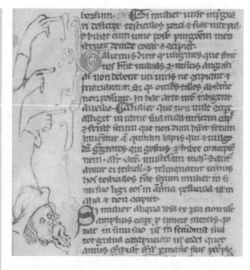

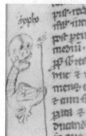

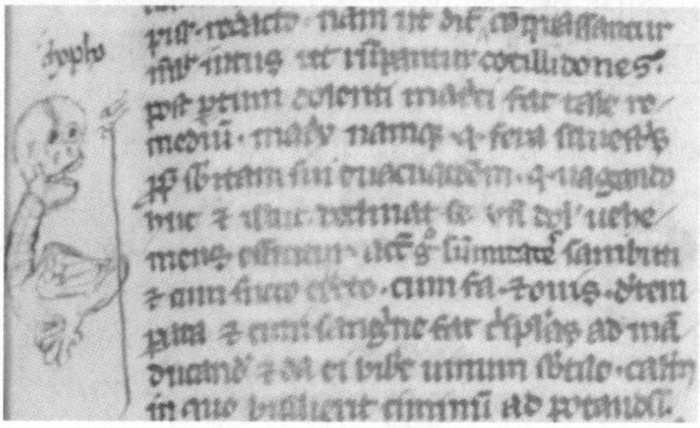

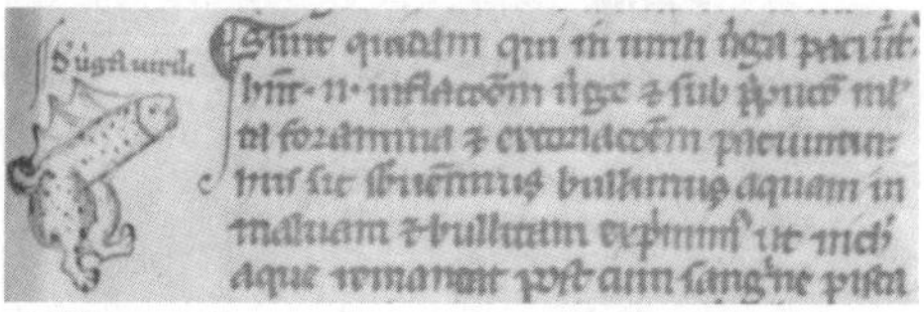

Left to right:

FIG. 5.3 From the Winchester manuscript 45r.
FIG. 5.4 From the Winchester manuscript 45v.
FIG. 5.5 From the Winchester manuscript 47r.
FIG. 5.6 From the Winchester manuscript 48r.

In the Winchester manuscript, however, given the pattern we have seen thus far, this chapter would have likely elicited both an extreme flourish from the annotator and an equally extreme reaction from his later medieval exciser.

What was perhaps the second annotator of the manuscript had more limited interests, which seem to have been medical.[100] He confined himself to the occasional *nota* symbol alongside passages of interest to him. His markings start in Bruno's *Surgery* and run through the manual of medical ethics and diagnostic procedures attributed to the Salernitan physician Archimattheus, where he adds six *notas*. Two fall beside simple problems of diagnosis, but the

---

[100] The relative order of the first and second annotators is not completely clear. The only point at which their annotations overlap is on f. 47r in the *Trotula*. While it is possible that the *Nota* annotator marked those passages first, the narrowness and crampedness of his marks here (in contrast to the thicker marks he makes elsewhere) lead me to believe that he was writing after the 'doodler'.

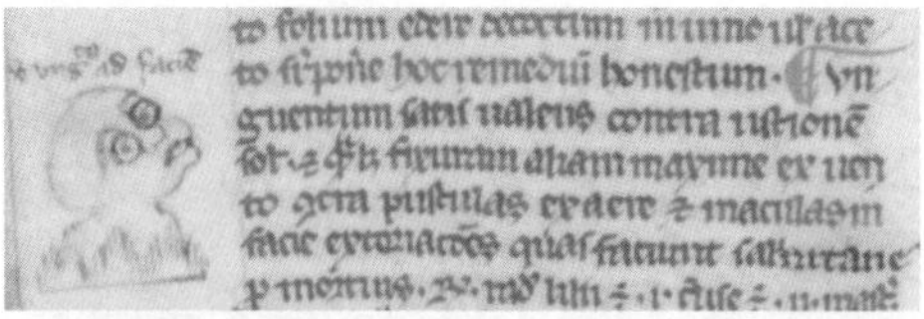

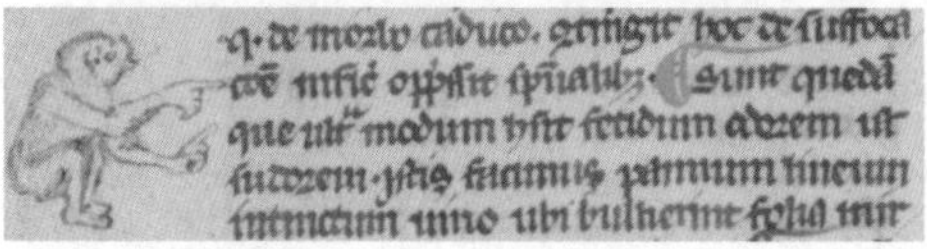

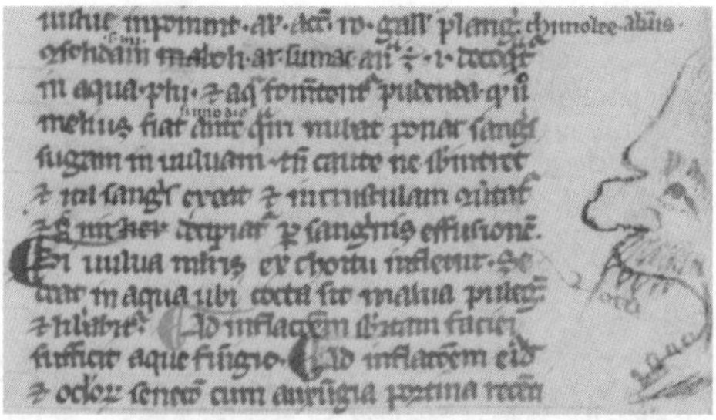

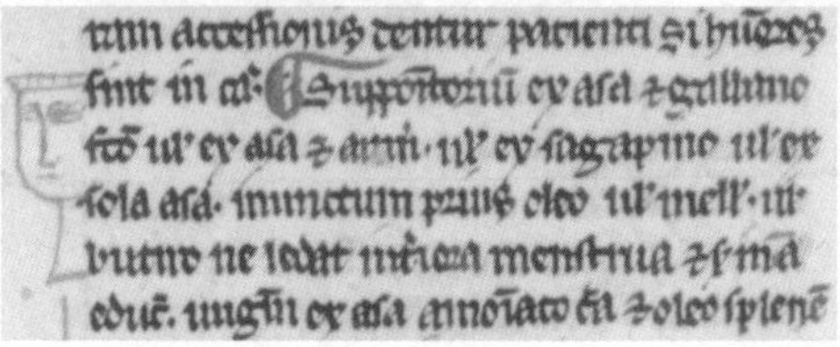

Left to right:

Fig. 5.7 From the Winchester manuscript 48v.
Fig. 5.8 From the Winchester manuscript 49r.
Fig. 5.9 From the Winchester manuscript 49v.
Fig. 5.10 From the Winchester manuscript 74v.

other four mark passages warning of particular problems of patient–physician interactions, one of them being the warning to the physician to avoid compromising conduct with female members of the (male) patient's household.[101] No more of this annotator's *notas* appear until more than halfway into the *Trotula* where he re-marks the passages on the emmenagogue/foetal expulsive and uterine wandering that the first annotator had already highlighted so vividly.

The third annotator, who like the first has a penchant for visual annotations, also has very special interests, chief among them women and generation, though he also seems to have some personal concerns. He begins in Bruno of Longobucco's *Surgery* where we find a fanged boar's head in the margin beside a cure for tooth pain.[102] No more 'commentary' comes again until five leaves later when he adds a face next to a recipe for exfoliating the skin.[103] In Archimattheus's treatise on physician decorum, this third annotator highlights the *notas* that his predecessor had already made. He duly marks the passage on avoiding inappropriate conduct with the women of the house with a gendered marker: a cloven-hoofed figure with a woman's head and a dog's rear-end.

In the *Trotula*, our third annotator (like the first two) remains silent for quite some time, skipping over all the general gynaecological topics. Between the head of a bearded man at the beginning of the chapter on fertility and

101 *Trotula.*, f. 36v. See Chapter 1 above.

102 Winchester MS 26, f. 19v. The dog in the bottom margin below a cure for lesions under the tongue is in a different ink and perhaps a different hand.

103 *Ibid.*, f. 26v.

the hedgehog below (Fig. 5.3 above), the annotator draws a figure defecating beside a passage describing a recipe of powdered testicles of a boar to be taken in wine by the woman (¶75a).[104] Beside both this recipe and the one following (¶76, for conceiving a male child) he adds a written *nota*. The following pages have similar marks flagging passages on pregnancy and care of the infant. In the third, cosmetic part of the *Trotula* (which the first two annotators had left untouched, with the possible exception of the lost end of the text), the third annotator adds *notas* and sometimes figures beside recipes for the hair (including one for hair loss),[105] while simple crosses mark the chapters on signs of the dead foetus, bad breath, body odour, two vaginal constrictives (all three annotators having skipped the earlier recipes on this topic in *Treatments for Women* with no comment whatsoever),[106] and finally two remedies for whitening the face. Our third annotator's interest in generation did not stop with the *Trotula*. In a subsequent text, on the medicinal properties of animals, he marked with crosses all allusions to generation, whether they be contraceptives, abortifacients, aids to produce a male child, aphrodisiacs, or anaphrodisiacs. We also begin to see signs of another topic of interest: he marks with a cross the statement that the tooth of a leopard, when suspended from the neck, aids against forgetfulness. Finally, this third annotator's interest in generation spills over into yet another text, the alphabetized herbal *Circa instans*, where he begins to mark every recipe relating to women with a woman's head: the suppository with asafetida to bring out the menses or the afterbirth (f. 74v, Fig. 5.10); the emmenagogues made of aloe, chaste tree (*agnus castus*), lovage (*apium rifus*), ammoniac gum, and mugwort (*artemisia*); anise for uterine distress; amber and asphalt for uterine suffocation; and dill (*anetum*) for uterine pain.[107] By the following page, however, our annotator finally seems to have had his fill of women's reproductive issues: he notes, by sketching a penis and scrotum in the margin, how garlic (*allium*) can be used for opening the hepatic and urinary vessels, yet he 'says' nothing about its uses for provoking the menses. Our annotator has, in fact, lost interest altogether, for after the A's no more gendered markings appear.

The marginalia in the Winchester manuscript are in no way random or thoughtless. After the *Trotula* and the gendered 'comments' at the opening of the *Circa instans*, only four marginal figures appear in the remaining 150 leaves of the manuscript: in the *Circa instans*, a little hybrid stands opposite the remedy for restoring the memory, a dragon appears opposite the remedy for tooth pain, a man's stubby head by the recipe for ringing in the ears, and a

---

[104] The designation '¶75a' refers to the recipe that, in the standardized ensemble, was repositioned as ¶82; see Green, *Trotula*.

[105] This recipe (¶261) was altered in the revised ensemble because of a scribal error: for the original *Ad capillos cadentes* (for hair loss), it read *Ad capillos candendos* (for whitening the hair). See Green, *Trotula*, p. 172.

[106] ¶¶190–5 and 231.   [107] Winchester MS 26, ff. 74v–78r.

stag's head next to a recipe for arthritis in the general medical compendium by Roger de Barone.[108] Aside from women's sexuality and capacity to reproduce (especially male children), the only subjects our third annotator seems interested in are tooth pain, loss of both hair and memory, and other irritations of old age. The first and third annotators have no fundamental disagreements about what is most interesting—or most deserving of comment—in the *Trotula* texts. Neither annotator is interested in the sufferings, the *passiones*, of women in their broadest sense. Menstrual difficulties, uterine prolapse, cancers and lesions all are passed over. Rather, these readers are interested in issues surrounding generation: infertility, contraception, production of male offspring.

Are the 'annotators' of the Winchester manuscript just silly old men, giggling over a text on women's diseases even as they extract from it recipes useful for controlling the fertility of their paramours or their own problems of tooth pain or baldness? Are they examples of the 'uncourteous', spiteful, and slanderous men the Middle English gynaecological prefaces referred to? Are they Jankyn grown old, deaf, and mean? Whether this copy of the *Trotula* had actually been called 'women's secrets' or been acknowledged as the work of a female author, we don't know: if the text had an author's name or title, it probably would have been found at the (now lost) end of the text.[109] Yet in their manner of annotating, these commentators have reduced this expansive collection of remedies for women's various ills to a bare sexual and generational minimum: these readers have clearly turned to the *Trotula as if* it were 'secrets' literature. No other copy of the *Trotula* has anything like the marginalia of the Winchester manuscript, which clearly reflects a quite specific context of reading.[110] Whether the manuscript had previously been housed in a university library or some other institution we do not know nor, obviously, can we know whether Chaucer knew anything about such habits of annotation. Nevertheless, it exists. And as with Matthias von Kemnat's copy of the *Secrets of Women* with its crude gesture towards women, the Winchester manuscript shows how marginalia that might initially be taken as whimsical or playful appear, on closer analysis, rather more vulgar and threatening. When these readers turn to women, their jokes become cruel.

In England, as on the Continent, the *Trotula* texts have *become* 'the secrets of women': even if they still had little of the more blatantly misogynistic 'secrets'

---

[108] There are also a handful of marginal *notas* marking individual recipes. The loss of least four original quires and the two leaves concluding the *Trotula* raises the possibility that the codex originally had more marginalia.

[109] In all other texts written by this hand, the title appears in the explicit. In most copies of this version of the ensemble (which was the fullest form of the text), if the text is complete the attribution to 'Trotula' is found.

[110] In all other cases where there are annotations in the *Trotula* manuscripts, whether they are in Latin or the vernacular, the comments are strictly medical.

of women's physiology (the horrors of menstruation) or female sexuality (their lusts and deceits) as found in the pseudo-Albertan *Secrets of Women* and its commentaries, the *Placides and Timeus*, and similar works, through a radically reductive reading of their content and original intent the *Trotula* treatises came to be perceived as a principal source of the 'secrets' of female fecundity—how to insure conception, successful birth, and a renewed cycle of fertility. The Chaucer scholar, Robert Pratt, concluded that Jankyn's 'book of wikked wyves' was just a literary conceit, that no real manuscripts ever existed that brought together all the authorities Chaucer lists. That may well be true, but the Winchester manuscript shows how the *Trotula* might have been read in a spirit similar to that epitomized by Jankyn's book. As both the Continental and the English developments demonstrate, such readings—whether by physicians or clerics, natural philosophers reading in Latin or laymen reading in the vernacular—were dictated not so much by what was in the texts as by what the reader expected to find there.

'TROTULA, MISTRESS OF WOMEN'?

But what if that reader were a woman? With few exceptions, the epithet 'secrets' was not used when authors or translators strove to address or create textual communities among women. Nor was 'Trotula' paraded prominently as an authority that women, recognizing her (like Agnodice) as another woman, could automatically trust. Viewing the 'secrets of women' tradition and the uses of female authorities from a female perspective produces a much different image of 'Trotula's' and the *Trotula*'s fame and leads us closer to understanding the very real effects of the gendered inequalities of literacy and the impact of clerical misogyny.[111]

Already in the thirteenth century, both Trota and 'Trotula' had been honoured with the epithet 'lady' (*domina*).[112] An image of 'Trotula' in a copy of the *Trotula* ensemble from early fourteenth-century France conveys her stature over women: she stands holding an orb in her raised hand, as if showing her dominion over

---

[111] For a particularly thoughtful exposition of the problems of documenting the historical effects of misogyny, see Judith M. Bennett, 'Misogyny, Popular Culture, and Women's Work', *History Workshop* issue 31 (Spring 1991), 166–88.

[112] A 13th-century Anglo-Norman cosmetic text refers to 'Dame Trote' twelve times. The epithet *domina* was added to Trota/'Trotula's' name in the anecdote of her cure in several 13th- through 15th-century copies of the text: Leipzig, Universitätsbibliothek, MS 1215, *c.*1225–50; BLL, MS Sloane 783 B, s. xv; Munich, Bayerische Staatsbibliothek, Clm 8742, s. xiii ex./xiv in.; and BNF, MS lat. 7056, s. xiii med. She was likewise elevated to *domina* in the opening rubric of BNF, MS lat. 16191, s. xiv in., a copy eventually held by the Sorbonne library (see Appendix 1, item 41), and in the 14th-century Irish translation. She was also called *domina* in a late 14th- or early 15th-century gynaecological compilation made in England, *Signa retencionis menstruorum*, in Oxford, Magdalen College, MS 164, s. xv in. (England), ff. 247r–259v.

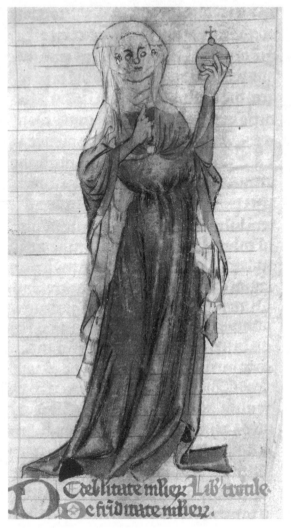

Fig. 5.11 A portrait of 'Trotula' holding an orb, perhaps to suggest (as other manuscripts describe her) that she is *domina mulierum*, 'mistress of all women'.

the world (Fig. 5.11). And in the copy of the Latin *Trotula* that lay on the shelves of Charles V's library in Paris, her more elevated status was confirmed. She was now *Trotula, domina mulierum*: 'Trotula, mistress of women'.[113] These were, of course, Latin copies of the texts and so probably circulated in the hands of male readers. They give us no hint of how *women* reacted to the female

---

[113] On Charles's copy, see the Introduction above.

figure of 'Trotula'. Did they even know of this legendary *mulier Salernitana*? The collective *mulieres Salernitane* may have been encountered in other reading. Isabelle of Portugal (1397–1471), for example, a queen of France famous for her medical ministrations to the poor, owned a copy of a French adaptation of the Salernitan *Circa instans*, which included over a dozen references to the *femmes Salernitaines*.[114] But there is little evidence that 'Trotula' herself was widely known, let alone admired, by female readers. As we have seen, the late fourteenth- or early fifteenth-century English *Knowing of Woman's Kind* and its mid fifteenth century imitator, *Sickness of Women 2*, as well as the contemporary Dutch *Liber Trotula*, all invited women's use at the same time as they 'policed' the texts to defend against inappropriate use by men. Yet only the last of these makes any claim to be the work of a female author.[115] In fact, in all the vernacular translations of the *Trotula* addressed to women, 'Trotula' was either never mentioned as authoress or, if she was, little elaboration of her identity was offered.[116] Only the late fifteenth-century English *Book Made by a Woman Named Rota* celebrates the female author's name without irony or artifice, but this in a form that harkens back, not to the personified title of a book that had been the object of so much manipulation, but to the real given name of the woman from Salerno.

Nor did women (or those authors who claimed to speak on their behalf) often attempt to use the concept of 'women's secrets' as a barrier to keep men out of their affairs. The only two female-addressed versions of the *Trotula* that employed the epithet 'secrets of women'—the thirteenth-century French 'sermon' on generation and the Latin verse rendition—were both meant to be conveyed *to* women by male interlocutors.[117] Here we begin to see the powerfully divisive potential of the idea of 'women's secrets', for the term means

[114] BNF, MS fr. 12321, s. xv¹. As the most widely circulating of all the texts that referred to the *mulieres Salernitane* (it was used by apothecaries and doctors throughout Europe), the *Circa instans* was probably the chief vehicle for the *mulieres'* continuing fame in the late Middle Ages. See Chapter 6 below.

[115] The closing rubric *Liber Trotularis* in one of the four copies of *Sickness of Women 2* is the product of a misunderstanding by a single scribe; no other copy of the text bears that attribution. See Monica H. Green and Linne Mooney, 'The *Sickness of Women*', in *Sex, Aging, and Death in a Medieval Medical Compendium: Trinity College Cambridge MS R.14.52, Its Texts, Language, and Scribe*, ed. M. Teresa Tavormina, Medieval and Renaissance Texts and Studies, 292, 2 vols. (Tempe, AZ: Arizona Center for Medieval and Renaissance Studies, 2006), vol. 2, pp. 455–568, at p. 568.

[116] In the English *Knowing of Woman's Kind*, with its poignant address to women, we do hear of an *unnamed* lady of Salerno (Barratt, *Knowing*, p. 86, line 685) as well as Cleopatra and her daughter and even 'Dame Fabina Prycyll'. The French *Conditions of Women* (*Quant Dex nostre Seignor*, one of the sources for the English text) never bears 'Trotula's' name, which is in fact true of most copies of *Conditions of Women* when it circulated independently. Yet given 'Trotula's' popularity in England it is notable that neither the translator nor any copyist connected the text to her. The Dutch *Liber Trotula*, as we have seen, initially confuses the author's name and the title, and when it does present 'Trotula' as an author, it depicts her as 'a woman very wise and knowledgeable about the secrets of women and their secret defects'.

[117] See Chapter 4.

one thing when used by women themselves, another when used by men. When the author(s) of the original twelfth-century Salernitan *Treatments for Women* spoke of letting midwives' incompetence remain 'our secret among women', and when Jacoba Felicie, in claiming her duty to provide care for women at her trial in 1322, spoke of 'the secrets and concealed matters of [woman's] nature' and 'the secrets of women and their secret associations', both were being deliberately defensive, saying, in effect, 'this is a women's affair and it should *stay* a women's affair'. 'Women's secrets' for them, as for men, meant lore about the female body or practices surrounding it that are not simply hidden (i.e., interior) but hidden from men. But the *desire* to pull a curtain of secrecy around women's affairs has a very different motive when the term is used by women themselves: it *protects* women from the threat to their honour that men represent.

Wouldn't a female authority have been attractive to women, a reassurance that the knowledge she disseminated was authentic and well-intentioned? Or, to use the Wife of Bath's metaphor, wouldn't the lion's story look different if the lion were the painter?[118] In fact it need not, as the inclusion of 'Trotula' and Heloise in Jankyn's book shows. Use of a female authority by men in fact increased men's ability to claim the truth of their views, since they were supported by the authority of a woman herself.[119] Men could both boast of their knowledge about women to female listeners and continue to draw boundaries around that knowledge so that it would not be compromised or challenged by women. Latin was masculinized enough by the thirteenth century that even the possibility of a female reading audience of 'secrets of women' literature was never articulated. There might be concern about keeping material out of the hands of boys, but no prohibition of female reading was needed as it was too unlikely. With the vernacular, however, there is not so much of a tug-of-war, as we saw with gynaecological texts, as simply an awareness that once women knew the things men were saying about them, there would likely be a reaction. Yet there were also reasons why men might *want* to share secrets literature with women.

A remarkable family of vernacular translations of the pseudo-Albertan *Secrets of Women* has as its framing device a male lover's appeal to his female beloved. In French, Dutch, Lower Rhenish, and Italian versions, the authorial voice claims that a woman—'the most worthy and perfect woman in the world'—has *asked* him to write 'something profitable' on the nature of women. He begs her that she not then be offended by its contents, for not only is what he is going to say true, but he has written it out of love for her.[120] The Rhenish copy (which dates from

---

[118] Chaucer, *Wife of Bath's Prologue*, line 698.

[119] For a wonderful analysis of this point from the perspective of women's writing, see Jennifer Summit, *Lost Property: The Woman Writer and English Literary History, 1380–1589* (Chicago: University of Chicago Press, 2000), p. 27.

[120] On this text and its various versions, see Green, 'Traittié'. Ongoing research by Orlanda Lie at the University of Utrecht promises to further disentangle the complicated evolution of this text. For the current whereabouts of the French copy owned in the nineteenth century by Alexandre Colson

the mid fourteenth century) and the Dutch one (which dates from 1405) both appear in small pamphlets, similar in format to the woman-addressed versions of vernacular gynaecological texts in English and Dutch. The Dutch copy (which has further interpolations begging the addressee to grant this redactor 'her favours') actually has the name of its possible recipient, one Margareta Godevartse of Udim, embedded in the text as an acrostic. The French version (which may have been the progenitor of all the others) survives today only in fifteenth-century copies, in one case accompanied by the French encyclopedic work, *Placides and Timeus*, and in all the other copies by surgical texts. The remarkable claim that a work full of detailed accounts of menstrual blood, difficulties in childbirth, and monstrous births should function as a love trinket is yet another aspect of the *Secrets of Women* tradition that demands teasing out to discover the full range of discursive meaning that must have been at play here. Yet the existence of these texts does suggest how the *Secrets of Women* could function as a device for engaging in 'sex talk' between the sexes. At some point in the French tradition, someone created the fiction of a papal bull that served to keep the text out of the hands of women: 'And it is forbidden in the decretal *Ad meam doctrinam* by our Holy Father the pope on pain of excommunication to reveal [this book] to a woman'.¹²¹ But was this fictitious decretal meant to avert 'sex talk', or something else?

A rather different, more malicious reason for a man to selectively share 'women's secrets' with a woman is exemplified by Jankyn's use of his 'book of wikked wyves'. He not only read it for his own pleasure, but he would also occasionally read it to his wife Alice. The book serves not only as a source of private edification for Jankyn, but also as a weapon with which to humiliate and subjugate his unruly wife. In this instance, the effect of silencing was not achieved: Dame Alice, enraged one night while Jankyn was reading, ripped out three pages of the book. The ensuing quarrel resulted in the burning of the book and a restoration of domestic harmony.¹²² Part of Chaucer's fiction, therefore, is not only to have captured the contemporary uses that were made of the *Trotula*, but also to depict women's hostility toward female authorities like Heloise and 'Trotula' who give clerks ammunition for their assaults on women. Like *Knowing of Woman's Kind* and the Dutch *Liber Trotula*, Chaucer's

---

and previously believed to be lost, see now Anna Viganò, Patrizia Tomba, and Luciano Merlini, 'A Manuscript Worth a Villa: Vittorio Putti's Acquisition of the Guy de Chauliac Manuscript', *Acta orthopaedica Scandinavica* 70, no. 6 (December 1999), 531–5. There was also a second independent French translation of the *Secrets of Women* made probably in the 15th century directly from the Latin; it has no prohibition against female reading.

¹²¹ Green, 'Traittié', p. 153. Interestingly, this injunction was altered slightly in the Italian translation, which no longer specified *women* as the excluded audience: 'Quin a presso sono iscritti i segreti delle femine, traslatato di latino in uolgare. E sono uietati per la sancta madre ecclesia che non si lascino leggiere a omgni maniera di gente'.

¹²² *Wife of Bath's Prologue*, lines 701–812.

conceit assumes that women *did* know something about the ways men talked about them.

Some women (like Chaucer's Dame Alice or the Dutch woman Margareta Godevartse) may have learned about 'secrets' discourse through their husbands or lovers, some through the sermons of their parish priests. Some may even have engaged with the texts directly. The oldest extant copy of the *Placides and Timeus*, and the one from which the image of 'Trotula' in Figure 5.2 comes, was written in 1304 as part of a huge compendium of French natural philosophical and devotional works produced, perhaps, for Queen Jeanne of Navarre (d. 1305). It was probably owned soon after by Clemence of Hungary (d. 1328), Jeanne's daughter-in-law.[123] The figure of 'Trotula' presented here as a learned woman who 'reads to the clerk the secrets of nature', holding up her right hand in a gesture of instruction, may have been not simply plausible but attractive and inspiring to the manuscript's female readers.[124] We don't know how Jeanne, Clemence, or any other women who may have seen this book or the other tracts that spoke of the 'secrets of women' reacted, either to the content of the 'secrets' or to the fact that they were being conveyed by a female interlocutor to men. In fact, to date not a single female-authored reference to 'Trotula' or any gynaecological text has been found. Yet there was one woman who both recognized the 'secrets' tradition and challenged its misogyny. That she was simultaneously silent on 'Trotula' may not have been a coincidence.

In 1405, Christine de Pizan singled out the French translation of the pseudo-Albertan *Secrets of Women* for especially harsh criticism in her great catalogue of ancient and medieval women worthies, the *City of Ladies*. In this extended counter-attack on anti-feminism, Christine astutely recognized the spuriousness of the papal decretal, arguing that it had been added 'because the man who wrote it knew that if women read it or heard it read aloud, they would know it was lies, would contradict it, and make fun of it'.[125] Christine de Pizan is an extraordinary figure on a number of levels (and so to that degree atypical), but she may give evidence that other medieval women did not so easily internalize

---

[123] Rennes, Bibliothèque Municipale, MS 593, an. 1304. This 539-leaf volume comprises an astronomical work translated for Queen Jeanne de Navarre by its author William of Saint Cloud and encyclopedic works on history and natural and political philosophy like Gossuin de Metz's *Image of the World*, Pierre de Beauvais's *Mappemonde*, Brunetto Latini's *Treasure*, and works of Marian devotion. Unusually, we know quite a bit about the genesis of this massive manuscript. Its principal scribe was the Parisian Robin Boutemont, whose mother was probably Erembourc, a manuscript illuminator still alive in 1299. The illuminations in the manuscript were an early work of the so-called Master of Thomas de Maubeuge illuminator, who would go on to a distinguished career illustrating histories, romances, and other luxurious manuscripts; among the Master's collaborators were the scribe and illuminator couple, Robert and Jeanne Montbaston. See Richard H. Rouse and Mary A. Rouse, *Manuscripts and their Makers: Commercial Book Producers in Medieval Paris, 1200–1500*, 2 vols. (Turnhout: Harvey Miller, 2000), vol. 2, pp. 26, 128, 178–9.

[124] On the symbolism of the raised hand, see Helen Solterer, *The Master and Minerva: Disputing Women in French Medieval Culture* (Berkeley: University of California Press, 1995).

[125] De Pizan, *City of Ladies*, Book I, cap. 9, pp. 22–3. See also Green, 'Traittié'.

the misogynistic views being propagated about them in clerical culture. As we have seen, already in the thirteenth century the fictional Queen Ginover was being depicted as sceptical of 'that which I have often heard read' about women's nature in medical books,[126] and perhaps some of the few highly educated women who owned medical books were able to form their own opinions about female nature.

But perhaps women were not always able to distinguish the messenger from the message. The literary scholar Barbara Newman has noted how Heloise, the learned abbess and passionate lover of Peter Abelard, was appropriated as a misogynistic authority in later medieval literary traditions because of her critiques of marriage and its incompatibility with the philosophical life. This appropriation may explain, Newman suggests, why Heloise is included in Jankyn's 'book of wikked wyves' but excluded from Christine de Pizan's *City*.[127] 'Trotula', too, finds no place in the *City*, yet fits as comfortably in Jankyn's book as does Heloise. Whether Christine, a physician's daughter, ever directly encountered the *Trotula* we do not know. Her father, trained in Italy where the *Trotula* faded from importance earlier than in northern Europe, is unlikely to have still considered 'Trotula' a relevant authority on women's medicine.[128] But if Christine, who had been raised and educated primarily in France, had looked among the medical books in Charles V's library—that magnificent collection up in the tower of the Louvre where in the 1390s and early 1400s she seems to have spent many an hour perusing the works of philosophers and poets—she would have found the royal library's Latin copy of *Trotula, domina mulierum*. Knowing Latin and intrigued to find a work by a female author (one of only two represented in the whole royal library, the other being the ethereal Sybil), Christine might have taken it down from the shelf to examine it.

Why shouldn't she have found the work of this 'mistress of women' admirable, appealing as it did in sympathetic terms to the sufferings of women and the need to aid them in their distress? True, she may have doubted the *Conditions of Women*'s opening claims of women's universal physical frailty, but there was no assault here on women's moral character, no morbid litany of the evil properties of menstrual blood, no salacious recounting of women's insatiable sexual desires. But had Christine also looked on these same shelves among the works of scientists and philosophers whose works she so admired, she would have found Charles's three copies of the *Placides and Timeus*, where 'Trotula' is seen revealing women's secrets to men. She may even have seen an image similar to Figure 5.2 of 'Trotula' lecturing from her books to a male cleric. Christine no

[126] See Chapter 3 above.

[127] Barbara Newman, 'Authority, Authenticity, and the Repression of Heloise', *Journal of Medieval and Renaissance Studies* 22 (1992), 121–57. De Pizan clearly knew about Heloise, whose story she refers to in another of her writings.

[128] See Chapter 6 below.

doubt would have assumed, rightly, that 'Trotula' was being granted authority specifically because, as a woman, she could speak on the 'secrets' of women. And, as we have seen, Christine would have been right to assume that the *Trotula* texts themselves—in the new, modified form in which they were circulating in the fourteenth and fifteenth centuries—had become interchangeable with texts properly belonging to the *Secrets of Women* tradition.[129] She would have had every reason, in other words, to assume that the French *Secrés des dames* was gynaecology and that the *Trotula* was 'secrets' literature. It would only be natural, then, that Christine should form a thoroughly negative image of gynaecological literature and, consequently, of 'Trotula'.

By holding up a female authority against women and by reading gynaecological texts (to which women had so little access and even less control) as if they were 'secrets' literature, medieval male intellectuals and physicians may well have made the *Trotula* and other gynaecological texts seem to be sources of pernicious information that women—excluded from the production of this knowledge—had good reason to resent and fear. We cannot know if the warning in *Knowing of Woman's Kind*'s preface that men read the text 'neither in spite nor in order to slander any woman' represents an echoed *cri de coeur* of a woman who had herself been maligned or humiliated by male misuses of gynaecological literature. But we do know that it can be no coincidence that that poignant rhetoric was composed at virtually the same moment that various clerks were annotating the Winchester manuscript with their selective 'comments' on generation and female sexuality, and when Chaucer was imagining Jankyn's fictive book wherein 'Trotula' figured as an authority on 'wikked wyves'.

By the middle of the fifteenth century, in the Low Countries, in France, in England, and especially in Italy, while laymen and clerics continued to read the 'secrets of women', male physicians and surgeons would become confident enough in their own understanding of 'women's secrets' that such female authorities as 'Trotula' could be ignored. The gynaecological traditions in fact parted ways with the pseudo-Albertan work by the end of the century: with but one exception, the *Secrets of Women* never appeared with gynaecological texts after the transition to print and hardly any newly composed gynaecological texts of the fifteenth or sixteenth century would use the term 'secrets of women' in their titles.[130] Nevertheless, the effect of medieval habits of reading about women's secrets was permanent: the misogynous potential of male-controlled intellectual

---

[129] Evidence for the whole phenomenon of the 'secrets of women' tradition in France, including the circulation of the *Trotula* there, can be found in Green, 'Traittié'.

[130] The Latin pseudo-Albertan text was first printed in 1475, with at least fifty editions by 1500. The exception to the trend to segregate the pseudo-Albertan text from gynaecological literature was a German compilation that first appeared in 1526 called *Ehstand Arzneybuch*, 'Medicine for Married Life'; see Appendix 2, item 14. For 16th-century printed gynaecological texts that use the term 'secrets of women' (all of which are in the vernacular), see Appendix 2, items 5, 16, 57, 59, and 62 (note).

traditions on the female body had been realized and concerns about male misuses of gynaecological texts would extend well into the sixteenth century, with prefaces that continued to warn male readers not to abuse the information contained therein. As the editor of the most widely circulated text on women's medicine in sixteenth-century England observed, 'every boy and knave [has access to] these books, reading them as openly as the tales as Robin Hood'.[131]

[131] Thomas Raynalde, ed. and trans., *The Byrth of Mankynde, Otherwyse Named the Womans Booke. Newly set furth, corrected and augmented* (London: Thomas Raynalde, 1545), f. D verso. On continued concerns about male misuse of gynaecological texts and other writings on generation, see the Conclusion below.

6

The Masculine Birth of Gynaecology

I leave such treatment to male physicians, for it is not the work of women.

Michele Savonarola, *Regimen for the Women of Ferrara* (*c*.1460)[1]

By the time Michele Savonarola (d. 1466) was writing his *Regimen for the Women of Ferrara* in the middle of the fifteenth century, 'Trotula' had long since disappeared from the pantheon of gynaecological authorities acknowledged by northern Italian physicians. The last Italian medical writer who made direct use of the *Trotula* was Niccolò Falcucci (d. 1412) and even he made only vague allusions to the text, never mentioning 'Trotula's' name or acknowledging that he drew on the work of an alleged female authority.[2] For Savonarola and his peers in the mid fifteenth century, gynaecology was a field where masculine authorities reigned supreme: Galen, Rhazes, Avicenna, and, in Savonarola's humanistic worldview, even such ancients as Ovid and Augustine. Nor was masculine authority limited to the written page or the role of distant advisor. When he wrote his vernacular regimen to aid Ferrarese women in conception, birth, and child care, Savonarola repeatedly advised his female audience, both laywomen and midwives, to leave certain tasks to the male physician or surgeon: the prescribing of medicines, surgical intervention in obstructed birth, treatment of postpartum fever.[3] This vernacular work reinforced his vision of the proper gender division of medical labour, for some twenty years earlier he had put the

---

[1] Michele Savonarola, *Il trattato ginecologico-pediatrico in volgare 'Ad mulieres ferrarienses de regimine pregnantium et noviter natorum usque ad septennium'*, ed. Luigi Belloni (Milan: Società Italiana di ostetricia e ginecologia, 1952), p. 127: 'lasso tal cura a medici, che non è opera da donne'.

[2] Falcucci twice draws some incidental material directly from the *Trotula*: he refers to the striking flower analogy from the *Conditions of Women* (¶3) when discussing the nature of menstruation, and later includes the contraceptive employing barley (¶87). I have found no Italian copies of the *Trotula* after the beginning of the 14th century with the exception of two 15th-century collections of random excerpts (Basel, Öffentliche Universitätsbibliothek, MS D.III.1, *c*.1420, ff. 115ra–116ra; and Seville, Biblioteca Capitular y Colombina, MS 7–4–25, s. xv[1], f. 128ra–b), and a copy of the *meretrices* version of the ensemble made, apparently, for a German student from a German exemplar but written by an Italian scribe (Berlin, Deutsche Staatsbibliothek, MS Hamilton 433, s. xv[2], ff. 51ra–71ra).

[3] See, for example, Savonarola, *Ad mulieres ferrarienses*, pp. 87–8, 117, 125, 127, and 130.

bulk of what he knew about gynaecological and obstetrical conditions into his Latin *Greater Practica*, which was meant for other Latinate male physicians like himself.

Physicians and surgeons north of the Alps were not quite so confident as their Italian confrères of either their knowledge or their social authority in the field of women's medicine, but they, too, grew bolder. They began, for the first time since Antiquity and the anomaly of the twelfth-century *Conditions of Women*, to compose new texts. Not just strings of recipes or isolated *consilia*, or even, as had the Montpellierain physicians in the fourteenth century, small specialized tracts on fertility, but whole texts devoted to women's conditions. As with the vernacular translations of the *Trotula* we surveyed in Chapter 4, these new Latin and vernacular texts found an audience not simply among professional male practitioners, but also among elite laymen anxious to have knowledge, maybe even control, over their own and their wives' reproductive capacities. As a group, these fifteenth-century productions would be rendered obsolete within a century, but they had served their purpose: they had established the competence of book-learned men to oversee virtually all aspects of women's health, even to the point of supervising the midwife in her tasks.

It is against this background of slow but steady fifteenth-century expansion of the intellectual and social competence of men in the field of gynaecology that we must understand the revolution of the sixteenth century. Or perhaps 'intensification' would be a better word, for while the traditional defining features of the transition to early modernity in intellectual culture—humanism and the printing press—did have their effect, it was more to reinforce and intensify the gendered divisions already established in the fifteenth century than to challenge or change them.

The first development was the creation of obstetrical literature, works focusing on childbirth. Aside from a few random excerpts, there was no prior genre of such specialized writing. The two texts that had had the most detailed obstetrical information—Muscio's late antique *Gynaecology* and Albucasis's *Surgery*—were meant, respectively, for midwives who *combined* obstetrical and gynaecological expertise, and for male surgeons who would instruct midwives on what they needed to do in case of difficulties. Savonarola, by directing his mid fifteenth century *Regimen for the Women of Ferrara* to midwives as well as the elite women of the city, became the first author expressly to address midwives since late Antiquity. Savonarola's Italian *Regimen* seems to have had no impact outside northern Italy. But unbeknownst to him, his more technical Latin *Practica* found an extraordinarily wide audience: the obstetrical portions were translated into German and, combined with the technology of the printing press, were used to create the anonymous German *Frauenbüchlein* ('Women's Handbook', *c.*1495) and the phenomenally popular *Rosegarden for Pregnant Women and Midwives* of Eucharius Rösslin (1513). Between 1516 and 1580, the latter would be translated into most of the western and central European languages and become *the* text for midwives throughout all of Europe. At the same time, however, male surgeons were expanding their expertise in obstetrical emergencies, and by mid century the first obstetrical work written for surgeons' use had appeared.

Gynaecology, the province of physicians, took a different course. Already around the turn of the century, humanist physicians had rediscovered the ancient medical heritage of Celsus and Pliny and begun to move away from the traditional medieval authorities. Then, in the second quarter of the sixteenth century, the rediscovery of the ancient Hippocratic gynaecological corpus brought the imprimatur of the Father of Medicine to this 'new' field, *gynaikeia*, which could now legitimately claim its importance as a distinct subdiscipline of medicine. As Hippocrates (or the voice they imagined to be Hippocrates) said, 'The healing of women's diseases differs from the healing of men's diseases'—in one phrase both establishing the ontological distinction of 'women's diseases' and demanding a separate system of therapy.[4] In the act of creating or re-creating these ancient roots of gynaecology, sixteenth-century physicians were able not simply to sever themselves from the more embarrassing aspects of their scholastic medieval past (including all association with the 'secrets of women' traditions), they were able to secure this ancient field's respectability as a masculine endeavour. As with obstetrics, the printing press certainly facilitated the dissemination of both the Hippocratic gynaecology and the explosion of new gynaecological writings in the latter half of the century, but aside from its role in standardizing anatomical images, it was in no sense a causative factor.

The sixteenth century thus witnessed two developments: the creation of the literate midwife—the creation, that is, of an *expectation* that midwives would ideally avail themselves of written texts just as physicians, surgeons, and apothecaries had done for 200 years or more—and the creation both of male midwives *avant la lettre* and of gynaecology as a field of intellectual specialization. What the sixteenth century did *not* create, however, was any new sense that women had authoritative knowledge in women's medicine beyond their skill in attending uncomplicated births. In one of the great ironies of medical history, the archetypal medieval gynaecological text, the *Trotula*, was revived on the belief that it reflected *ancient* medical learning. 'Trotula' as an authoress momentarily received new life, too, but within twenty years she was erased again, the victim of a philologist's creative emendation. With not a single medieval or 'modern' woman credited as an authority, the recovery of the Father of Medicine together with these other sixteenth-century developments would reinforce the message that, childbirth aside, women's medicine was 'not the work of women'.

---

[4] *Diseases of Women* 1.62, in Ann Ellis Hanson, 'Hippocrates: *Diseases of Women* 1', *Signs: Journal of Women in Culture and Society* 1 (1975), 567–84.

FROM FERTILITY TO GYNAECOLOGY: THE FIFTEENTH CENTURY

When he ascended the throne in 1364, the French dauphin (now King Charles V) had been unable to produce a living heir after fourteen years of marriage. This led him to make changes in the coronation ceremony for his wife, Jeanne de Bourbon, in order to heighten the traditional aspects of the queen's unction as a fertility ritual. Not simply was she anointed on her head and breast but special, newly composed prayers were recited over her: 'And together with Sarah and Rebecca and Leah and Rachel, all blessed and revered women, may she be worthy of being made fruitful and rejoice in the fruit of her womb'.[5] Whether Charles's acquisition of Latin and French copies of the *Trotula* coincided with this period of reproductive insecurity we don't know,[6] but in any event they were the only texts on gynaecology or fertility he had on his library shelves. Eighty years later, the young Count of Foix, Gaston IV (r. 1436–72), no doubt aware how devastating the lack of male heirs had been to his county in recent years and anxious to insure his own reproductive success,[7] instead placed his faith in the 'new' medical science: he commissioned a novel tract on generation and childbirth from Pierre Andrieu, a physician at the University of Toulouse. As we have seen, small specialized tracts on infertility had begun to be composed already *c.*1300, well before the devastation of the Black Death could even be imagined.[8] While these Montpellierain texts would continue to circulate in the fifteenth century (as the *Trotula* did, too, though more in translation than in Latin), the fifteenth century witnessed a surge of new activity that moved the physician as well as the surgeon beyond the role of the 'hands-off' counsellor who diagnosed and prescribed from a distance, into roles that brought them more immediately into contact with the bodies of their female patients. Whether in Italy, France, or northern Europe, we see a new empiricism, an increasing approach near the female genitalia. My concern in the following survey of fifteenth-century gynaecological writings, therefore, is not simply to document the regularity of men's involvement with women's medicine (which, as we saw in Chapter 2, was

---

[5] Claire Richter Sherman, 'The Queen in Charles V's "Coronation Book": Jeanne de Bourbon and the "Ordo ad reginam benedicendam"', *Viator* 8 (1977), 255–99 and plates, at p. 292.

[6] We only know that the books were in his library when it was first inventoried in 1373.

[7] On the problems of succession in the reigns of Gaston's two predecessors, see William Henry York, 'Experience and Theory in Medical Practice during the Later Middle Ages: Valesco de Tarenta (fl. 1382–1426) at the Court of Foix (France)', PhD dissertation, The Johns Hopkins University, 2003, pp. 180–1.

[8] Although the first waves of the Black Death in the 14th century had hit all classes equally hard, noble families in particular seem to have developed new anxieties about preserving their lineages. Joel Rosenthal, 'Mediaeval Longevity and the Secular Peerage, 1350–1400', *Population Studies* 27 (1973), 287–93, documents the failure of a direct male line in one-fourth of English noble families every twenty-five years in the fourteenth and fifteenth centuries.

already substantial in the thirteenth and fourteenth centuries), but also to assess, in their subtle asides as well as their sometimes boastful claims, the breaching of the taboo against male sight, and even touch, of the female genitalia. I will argue that these passing comments, oblique though they sometimes are, are the manifestations of a widespread re-gendering of gynaecological practice that occurred at the bedsides and in the corridors of the houses of female patients.

Italy

Prior to the fifteenth century, the 'hands-off' nature of male gynaecological practice was rarely discussed directly but was reflected in the subtle grammatical choices that authors made in their writings: the use of passive injunctions—'let this be done', 'have this applied'—together with a corresponding absence of first-person accounts. Aside from the remarkable frankness of one of the later medieval French translators of the *Trotula* who provided an alternative vocabulary that women could use to explain their problems to male physicians,[9] fifteenth-century texts are characterized as much as earlier ones by an absence of *explicit* discussion of how the male physician was supposed to manoeuvre the delicate negotiations of cross-sex practice. Nevertheless, close reading of the new fifteenth-century writings shows a pronounced increase in first-person accounts. These, together with other indicators, suggest not simply an increase in male practitioners' advisory roles, but, I will argue, an actual increase in their access to the female patient's body. The taboos against male sight and touch of the female genitalia did not disappear entirely, but they were relaxed considerably.

Take, for example, a fifteenth-century copy of the Montpellierain *Treatise on Sterility*, where the text has been substantially amplified by a redactor's own first-person accounts of his successes in treating women. He attests that one method is particularly well proven to aid in the conception of boys instead of girls, 'as I have seen this tried through true, unquestionable experience by many women who went without offspring for a long time, one for 22 years, another for 15, another for 13, another for 11, and another for 9. And for all of these I proved this and found it to be true.'[10] He then goes on to the detailed case of a woman who was about forty years old who had never borne a child or even shown any signs of having conceived. She was very fat and of a phlegmatic constitution, yet despite the poor prognosis, our author did succeed in getting her to bear a child. We need not take all these success stories to be true or even credit our author for the efficacy of his remedies in order to gather the more important historical fact: he believed he was competent to treat infertility in women and that it was

---

[9] On the *Treatise on the Many Maladies Which Can Happen to Women and on Their Secret Maladies*, see Chapter 4 above.

[10] BLL, MS Sloane 3124, s. xv (Italy), ff. 331v–354v, at f. 352v. In the manuscript, the text is attributed to Maurus of Salerno, though this cannot be the famous Maurus who wrote and practised there in the late 12th century.

appropriate that his advice be sought out for such treatment. Any gynaecological intervention that he made was considered completely within the bounds of his normal practice. Similarly, a fifteenth-century Italian owner of Bernard of Gordon's *Lily of Medicine* annotated his copy with his own clinical commentary. He notes treatments or observations he has made of female patients suffering from *reuma*, intestinal flux, excessive menstruation, and uterine suffocation. He adds additional remedies alongside the chapters on obstetrics; to be sure, these consist of only fumigations, plasters, potions, and amulets (that is, there is nothing more 'hands-on' to his practice than that of earlier male practitioners), but his role as an *adviser* in such situations is apparent.[11]

Other, more substantial writings show an even greater move beyond the distant advisory role of earlier male involvement with female patients. Niccolò Falcucci, a Florentine physician who around 1400 composed seven massive *Sermons* on medicine, dedicated the sixth of his 'sermons' to the anatomy, physiology, and diseases of the reproductive organs, both male and female; this section alone runs to over 300 pages in extant manuscript copies. In his gynaecological chapters, we find the same reliance on learned, written authorities that characterized all of Niccolò's work; Niccolò's work is, in this sense, very much the product of traditional scholastic synthesis. Yet we also find here an extraordinary number of personal attestations: 'I saw two aborted foetuses in the wife of Jacobus Dinus del Pecora'; 'I saw a woman from among the general masses who after birth was so tightly constricted by the midwife that she remained closed so that her husband was never able to insert his penis nor was any medicine capable of opening her up, and thus was she rendered sterile.'[12] These attestations are no more common in the gynaecological chapters than elsewhere in his sprawling work, but that is precisely what is notable: he has as much personal *observational* experience with gynaecological conditions as with any other aspect of medical practice.

Whether that observation was accompanied by any direct 'hands-on' involvement in the care of his patients is harder to determine. His chapters on uterine mole, obstruction of the womb, and uterine prolapse—which to varying degrees require visual inspection and manual manipulation for their diagnosis and treatment—show him simply mouthing the treatment recommendations of his learned (written) authorities. In the chapter on the mole, although he gives two personal attestations of cases he has seen (one of the wife of Franciscus Gabrielis, one again of the wife of Jacobus Dinus), he gives no indication that he has *treated* either woman.[13] In the chapter on obstruction of the womb (or rather,

---

11 LWL, MS 130, an. 1330 (Montpellier); the later annotations are on ff. 67v, 109r, 135r–v.

12 I have examined Niccolò Falcucci, *Sermonum liber scientie medicine, Sermo sextus: De membris genitalibus* in several manuscript copies as well as the 1507 Venice printed edition. My citations here come from Utrecht, Universiteitbibliotheek, MS 692, s. xv, where the sixth *sermo* appears as an independent codex. The passages come from Tract I, cap. 6: *De anothomia matricis* (Utrecht 692, f. 10r); and Tract III, cap. 24 (correctly, 25): *De opilatione matricis* (f. 134rb).

13 Falcucci, Tract III, cap. 20: *De mola matricis* (Utrecht 692, f. 115va).

the vagina), in addition to the woman whom the midwife had closed up too tightly, Niccolò asserts that, 'just as I have seen', the opening of the vagina can be so small as to inhibit the menstrual flow as well as entry of the penis during intercourse. Did Niccolò himself actually examine such women's genitals? The narrative frame 'I saw' may simply mean that 'he heard' of a case, or perhaps that he saw the woman as a patient but never made the physical examination. Again, later in this same chapter when he describes how the exterior orifice is able to be known 'by sense for it is able to be seen and touched', whereas the interior orifice 'is able to be known by the midwife when she inserts her anointed finger' into the vagina, he is simply echoing his source Avicenna.[14]

In the chapter on uterine prolapse, however, we actually find evidence of Niccolò's practice. Niccolò says he has seen a woman who suffered from a swelling that tipped to one side, and he has seen the wife of one Andreas Salsitie whose uterus ruptured and extruded entirely outside, but who was nevertheless able to conduct her domestic affairs for many years. In neither case does Niccolò say that he has treated these women. Yet elsewhere he proudly recounts his own experience (*ego expertus sum*) in applying a rotten hen's egg to a woman's prolapsed uterus: 'and I marveled at its immediate reduction'. He tried it again on an old woman, with similar results. True, he admits, the stench is so awful as to be nearly intolerable, but that can be taken care of by covering up the woman so the smell does not reach her nose.[15] Although, following his sources, throughout the chapter he has the midwife do all the manual work of restoring the uterus to its place and applying various unguents, he notes that often, after a woman has suffered uterine suffocation, 'the physician *or* the midwife can feel a sort of round mass in the place immediately above the navel'.[16] The male physician, therefore, is clearly authorized to touch the belly of his female patients and he is obviously intimately involved in the diagnosis and prescription of treatment for the full range of gynaecological diseases. As for obstetrics, Niccolò's personal attestations all but disappear in the chapters on childbirth: 'I myself have seen' cases where women suffer terribly when the afterbirth is not removed, 'especially in Lady Bartholomea, the wife of Falco de Peris'. This, and a statement where he remarks on whether phlebotomy is harmful to pregnant women, suggest his involvement in care for women before and after birth, but not during.[17]

In the next half century, northern Italian writers move beyond Falcucci and his dependence on previous writers. Their works, ever longer in size and more

[14] Falcucci, Tract III. cap. 24 (correctly, 25): *De opilatione matricis* (Utrecht 692, f. 134ra–b).

[15] *Ibid.*, Tract III, cap. 26: *De precipitatione matricis et remotione eius a suo loco naturali* (Utrecht 692, f. 138rb).

[16] *Ibid.*, f. 136vb: 'Et quandoque sentit post suffocatione medicus vel obstetrix quasi aliquid rotundatum esse in loco quo immediate est supra vmbilicum'.

[17] *Ibid.*, Tract III, cap. 9: *De partu in generali* (Utrecht 692, f. 99rb); Tract III, cap. 16: *De aborsu in generali* (f. 109rb). Although he mentions both Caesarean section (here quoting Bernard de Gordon) and surgical removal of the dead foetus, he does not elaborate on *who* is to perform those procedures.

extensive in detail, show less and less verbatim dependence on Avicenna or other Arabic or Latin authorities. They also, to some extent, start to move the topic of women's diseases outside the traditional framework of the *a capite ad calcem* order of the medical encyclopedia where gynaecological diseases were always paired with andrological conditions. In 1440 the Pavian physician Antonius Guainerius dedicated his *Treatise on the Womb* (*Tractatus de matrice*) to Filippo Maria Visconti, the Duke of Milan, with florid appeals to the Duke's desire for progeny. Guainerius intended the *Treatise* to serve as just one part of an encyclopedic *Practica* that he had planned, but he says he wanted to publish his work on the female generative organs now, independently, lest he fail to complete the whole work. Similar evidence of involvement in gynaecological care can be found in the individualized *consilia* of various elite northern Italian physicians from this period: Antonio da Scarperia (1350/2–1433), Antonio Cermisone (d. 1441), Bartholomeus de Montagnana (d. *c.*1451), Giovanni Matteo Ferrari da Grado (d. 1472), and Alessandro Sermoneta (d. after 1492) all wrote *consilia* on gynaecological and obstetrical conditions that show their involvement in a variety of routine and complicated cases.

By the time we reach Michele Savonarola, writing in the 1440s and 1460s, therefore, there is nothing unusual at all about his extreme confidence in proclaiming that major aspects of women's healthcare are the province of male physicians and surgeons and 'not the work of women'. Savonarola had taught and practised medicine in Padua before being called to the court of Ferrara in 1440; soon thereafter, he composed his magnum opus, the *Practica maior*. Savonarola devoted his two longest chapters in the whole book to generation (which in itself is unsurprising since intervention in fertility remained the most important element of male gynaecological practice), yet his other gynaecological chapters are distinctive both in their level of detail and the frequency of his personal attestations of cases he has seen. To be sure, Savonarola is nearly as textually dependent as Falcucci was before him: he, too, relies heavily on Avicenna and (without acknowledgement) on a work composed in southern Italy in the early fourteenth century, Francesco da Piedemonte's *Supplementum*.[18] Nevertheless, Savonarola added enough novel and personalized elements that we can glimpse his image of the ideal male practitioner.

Although this practitioner defers to the midwife whenever there is need to insert a hand into the female patient (to feel for hardness obstructing the vagina, to report whether the veins of a prolapsed uterus are replete, to masturbate a woman suffering from uterine suffocation, to assess pregnancy or blockage of the vagina, to feel for the mole),[19] in almost all other respects he relies on his own assessments. When, for example, Savonarola referred to the use of a mirror below

[18] See Chapter 2 above.
[19] Michele Savonarola, *Practica maior* (Venice: Vincentius Valgrisium, 1561); all subsequent citations refer to Tractatus VI, cap. XXI. References to the midwife's manual assessments occur on ff. 250va, 257vb, 258ra, 258va, 258vb, 259ra, 260va, 262vb, 264vb, 265va, 268vb, 270rb.

the genitals to determine whether a woman was suffering from lacerations of the vagina, he was simply following Avicenna (and perhaps also Francesco, who was using the same source).[20] Yet neither Avicenna nor Francesco had specified that it was *the physician* who was to do this inspection. Like William of Saliceto before him, Savonarola implies that there is no difficulty with a male practitioner using instruments to examine a female's genitalia.[21] He also relies on his interrogation of the patient: he cites the report of one woman who told him she never felt herself being impregnated even though she conceived ten times; eliciting the woman's report on the regularity of her menstruation is crucial to the physician's ability to assess pregnancy.[22] Aside from a woman from Filtri who suffered a menstrual flux continuously for fourteen months but whom he was nevertheless able to cure,[23] Savonarola's anecdotes are less about his own clinical experiences than extreme cases that help him make a point. Thus, when discussing a question debated since the time of Hippocrates—whether phlebotomy could be recommended for a pregnant woman—Savonarola mentions that he saw the niece of Lord Prosdocimus lose more than sixteen pounds of blood through a nosebleed that lasted twelve days, yet she was able nevertheless to give birth to a healthy child who was then twenty years old.[24]

Another sign of Savonarola's confidence in his role as physician to women is that he voluntarily brings up the subject of shame. Having already addressed the general anatomy and complexional dispositions of the uterus in his first chapter, he then returns to the signs of the different complexions in the second chapter. It is important, he explains, to be very clear about these signs 'both because the organ is well hidden and because of their embarrassment, women do not reveal conditions that harm it'.[25] Here, at last, we have an articulated response to the vagueness that had troubled literate traditions of gynaecology ever since the Salernitan *Conditions of Women* was composed in the twelfth century. The more women are embarrassed, the more deeply their conditions are hidden; the more they are hidden, the more informed and solicitous the male physician needs to be.

---

[20] Michele Savonarola, rubr. 16: *de rhagadijs matricis* (f. 257ra): 'deinde manifestantur tactu, aut uisu: tactu digitis, ut dicetur item quia apud coitum sentitur dolor non consuetus; ut in positione cannae clysteris in ano: uisu; quia uirga exit sanguinolenta. *item quia medicus per impositionem speculi ea comprehendit*' (my emphasis). I believe Avicenna, and Savonarola following him, were indeed referring to a simple mirror. See nn. 49 and 62 below, however, for the possibility that a speculum in the modern sense—that is, a special tool for viewing the vagina—is in use in 15th-century southern France and Spain.

[21] On William of Saliceto, see Chapter 2 above.

[22] Savonarola, *Practica maior*, rubr. 24, *de sterilitate et causis impraegnationem difficultantibus* (ff. 262ra and 264rb).

[23] *Ibid.*, rubr. 7: *de fluxu menstruorum non naturali* (f. 254rb): 'in ultimis habui experientiam in domina quadam filtrina, quae passa erat fluxum menstruorum. xiiii. mensibus . . . et sunt expertae'.

[24] *Ibid.*, rubr. 31, *De aborsu, et causis eius* (f. 267rb).

[25] *Ibid.*, rubr. 2, *De signis complexionis matricis* (f. 250ra): 'haec non fecerim tibi ex secundo techni magis notis; quoniam de cura eius, ut dixi, plus quam sollicitus esse uolo, etiam quia membrum est occultum ualde, et propter uerecundiam mulieres non ita eius nocumenta detegunt'.

There is no argument here for providing women with learned *female* practitioners so the problem of shame might be avoided. On the contrary, Savonarola insists how much the physician must instruct the midwife to gather the information *he* needs to do his work of diagnosis. Later, Savonarola returns to problems caused by women's reluctance to reveal their afflictions: because 'ladies' (*dominae*) are reluctant to disclose their problems with excessive menstrual flux, this condition is usually only brought to the attention of physicians when it is well established and, unfortunately, difficult to cure. 'Rarely', therefore, 'does treatment of this bring honour to the physician . . . Consider this well!'[26]

In laying out the proper roles of physician, midwife, and female patient, Savonarola also indicated a fourth figure now even more regularly involved in women's healthcare: the surgeon. Savonarola did not automatically concede every aspect of surgery to surgeons. In his chapter on apostemes (tumours or lesions) in the uterus, he readily described what he calls *il schizarolo*, a special instrument used to administer medicines into the uterus. And he retains and modifies Avicenna's description of an operation to open up tissues that are blocking the vagina, recommending to the physician that he use his discretion in deciding whether he should incise little by little over the course of several days or do it all at once. Yet overall he seems to prefer to leave surgical interventions to surgeons. Indeed, at one point he suggests that surgical interventions on the vagina have become frequent enough that *unnecessary* surgeries are the cause of apostemes.[27] Also among the duties of surgeons he includes removal of the dead foetus.[28]

There are few surgical writings from fifteenth-century Italy so it is difficult to confirm how commonly surgeons could be found who were capable of performing an embryotomy. Described by Albucasis and Avicenna, the operation had failed to receive discussion among the surgical writers prior to Guy de Chauliac, who himself, writing in the 1360s, spoke only vaguely of using the hands, hooks, and grippers to extract the foetus 'whole or in pieces'.[29] The Bolognese surgeon Pietro d'Argellata (d. 1423), however, speaks of it as if it were a regular part of his practice. This is especially striking since Pietro was extremely derivative in his surgical writing, relying heavily on authorities such as Galen, Lanfranc, Dioscorides, Serapion, Avicenna, and Albucasis. He seems uninterested in causes of diseases, symptomatology, etc. (he is, in fact, quite willing to defer to 'our Lords, the physicians' on many subjects). His frequent assertions that whatever cures the testicles or penis is good for the breasts or vagina, which are derivative

---

[26] *Ibid.*, f. 253va: 'postremo scito, quod raro medici consequuntur honorem de cura eius; quia dominae uerecundantur detegere hanc passionem; et ideo vt plurimum non nisi inueterata ad manus peruenti medicorum. et ideo considera'.

[27] Savonarola, *Practica major*, rubr. 10, *De apostemate matricis*: 'Causa apostematis matricis est primitiua . . . aut disruptio facta ab obstetrice, cum foetus recipit: aut incisio non debite facta'.

[28] *Ibid.*, ff. 250va-b, 252rb, 254vb, 255ra, 256vb, 257ra, 263va, and 270rb.

[29] Guy de Chauliac, *Inventarium sive Chirurgia magna*, ed. Michael R. McVaugh, with Margaret S. Ogden, Studies in Ancient Medicine, vol. 14, I and II (Leiden: Brill, 1997), 1:388.

of Guy de Chauliac's homology, do not lend confidence that he has much personal experience in gynaecological practice. Be that as it may, there are also some notable instances where he switches from recounting the opinions of his predecessors to offering his own observations and experiences. In the chapters on breast diseases, for example, he refers repeatedly to his own experiences with cures of hot apostemes of the breasts and coagulation of the milk. In the chapter on scrofula of the breasts, he asserts both that in some cases it is better to simply alleviate pain than attempt a cure, and, in others, that it is better to leave the condition incompletely healed than to attempt an overly aggressive cure which might end up killing the patient.[30] He also describes both embryotomy and Caesarean section, in both cases implying that he has performed these procedures on several occasions. Writing in mid century, the Pavian physician Giovanni Matteo Ferrari da Grado (*c.*1400–72) could unproblematically counsel that 'if [the foetus] has died, a surgical operation is necessary and for this a diligent and experienced surgeon should be chosen'.[31] Thus when we find Jacopo Berengario da Carpi's account at the end of the century of a vaginal hysterectomy performed for uterine prolapse by his surgeon father, we should see this in line not only with the advancing anatomical knowledge of late medieval Italian practitioners, but with their increasing practical experience as well.[32]

If all of these accounts of male gynaecological and even obstetrical practice in fifteenth-century northern Italy are true, then a change must have occurred not simply in how male physicians and surgeons practised, but in how their female patients *let* them practise. Boccaccio's claims about the 'liberating' effects of the plague in the mid fourteenth century notwithstanding, there is nothing to suggest that sexual modesty was any less important for women of the fifteenth century than before.[33] At least some of the increased knowledge that Italian practitioners had was due to the simple fact that the women they observed were dead. Katharine Park has shown that a driving force behind the increase

[30] Pietro d'Argellata, *Chirurgia* (Venice: Benedictus Senuensis, 1480), p. 140a–b: 'Et ego dico quod in hoc casu melius est paliare quam curare et infamiam incurrere ut faciunt emperici qui omnem egritudinem curare uolunt . . . Dico ego quod melius est dimittere aliqualiter egrum quam totaliter egrum quod uidi semel. Ita una domina prope burgum galerie cui superuenti empericus: quidam et uoluit ipsam curare et cum corruptorio uoluit apostemationem remouere et finaliter eam interfecit et in ista uene erant magne in loco uel circa locum.'

[31] Giovanni Matteo Ferrari da Grado, *Practica* (Venice, 1521), p. 341: 'Quod si [foetus] fuisset mortuus operatio chirurgica erit necessaria et in hoc eligatur diligens et expertus chirurgicus', as cited by Carl Oskar Rosenthal, 'Zur geburtshilflich-gynaekologischen Betätigung des Mannes bis zum Ausgange des 16. Jahrhunderts', *Janus* 27 (1923), 117–48 and 192–212.

[32] Jacopo Berengario da Carpi, *Commentaria cum amplissimis additionibus super anatomia Mundini* (Bologna: Girolamo Benedetti, 1521), f. CCXXV. On developments in anatomy, see Katharine Park, *Secrets of Women: Gender, Generation, and the Origins of Human Dissection* (New York: Zone Books, 2006).

[33] Sharon Strocchia, 'Gender and the Rites of Honour in Italian Renaissance Cities', in *Gender and Society in Renaissance Italy*, ed. Judith C. Brown and Robert C. Davis, Women and Men in History Series (London and New York: Longman, 1998), pp. 39–60; and Trevor Dean, 'Gender and Insult in an Italian City: Bologna in the Later Middle Ages', *Social History* 29 (2004), 217–31.

in anatomical activity in fifteenth- and sixteenth-century Italy was the desire to 'penetrate' the 'secrets' of women's bodies. Already in the fourteenth century, the availability of a female cadaver at a medical school autopsy was cause for excitement (and an enlarged number of permitted spectators), and in the fifteenth century postmortems became even more common.[34] Nor should we discount the possibility that male practitioners may have learned something of gynaecological conditions, and developed their practical expertise, by observing prostitutes and domestic servants, whose bodies were more readily available to them. Savonarola tells the following story: 'I knew of a young woman having a skin thus covering [her vaginal opening] with whom young men were unable to have intercourse, even when she was willing; a certain experienced surgeon named Novellus, learning of this, cut the skin obstructing the vagina . . . and more than one hundred students were thus able to enter her.'[35] Similarly, when he explains what signs the physician should look for to detect impending miscarriage, he gives the example of the physician recognizing it in a woman of his household, whose normal complexion he would know well; he even gives a recipe for an aperitif used *in casu nostro*.[36]

The relatively rare opportunities to conduct autopsies or examine prostitutes clearly do not account for the many personal observations and case histories that characterize fifteenth-century writings, however. Bartholomeus and other writers of *consilia* often name their upper-class female patients, a practice that would have been unthinkable had any impropriety been attached to male gynaecological practice. Savonarola was as highly attuned as anyone to the need for both practitioner and patient to maintain respectability: he called women 'the trumpet of physicians', the creators and sustainers of a physician's good reputation, and he seems to have taken great care to turn that power to

[34] Park, *Secrets of Women.*

[35] Savonarola, *Practica major*, rubr. 5, *De mala compositione matricis, et de eius oppilatione*, f. 250rb-va: 'et ego cognoui iuuenem habentem sic pellem cooperientem eam, et cum qua iuuenes coire non poterant ipsa uolente, et quidam chirurgicus et expertus nomine Nouellus hoc sciens ei scindit pellem ante uuluam stantem et magnam fecit aperturam ita, ut ingressi sint plures quam centum socii'. Bernard de Chaussade, to be discussed below, includes the story of a Parisian medical licentiate, Johannes Cortui, perhaps to be identified with the Jean Courtin, licensed in 1466, discussed by Ernst Wickersheimer, *Dictionnaire biographique des médecins en France au Moyen Age*, 2 vols. (1936; repr. Geneva: Librairie Droz, 1979), 1:388, and Danielle Jacquart, ed., *Supplément* to Ernest Wickersheimer, *Dictionnaire biographique des médecins en France au Moyen Age* (Geneva: Librairie Droz, 1979), 152. Bernard explains how he died during intercourse with a prostitute in 1472. Although nothing in Bernard's account indicates that the prostitute (identified by her *nom d'emprunt*, 'La Belle Cypriane') was physically examined, it is stated that she was interrogated about the death. On prostitutes in Bologna and their student clientele, see Carol Lansing, 'Concubines, Lovers, Prostitutes: Infamy and Female Identity in Medieval Bologna', in *Beyond Florence: The Contours of Medieval and Early Modern Italy* (Stanford, CA: Stanford University Press, 2003), pp. 85–100 and 256–8.

[36] Savonarola, *Practica maior*, rubr. 30: *De conseruatione embrionis et cautela aborsus*, f. 267ra: 'Sexto, quando medicus timet aborsum, et praecipue in muliere sibi domestica: quia cognoscit matricis eius dispositionem'.

his best advantage.[37] As we have already seen, the scenario he envisioned of gynaecological treatment had the physician and midwife working in tandem; apparently, as long as female attendants were present to 'chaperone' the encounter, attendance by a male physician or surgeon was not problematic.[38] Rather than reflecting a decline in moral standards, the rise in male gynaecological practice in fifteenth-century Italy rather seems to confirm the rising status of learned medicine. Patrician and bourgeois men wanted the best care for their wives and daughters, and women, apparently, often concurred that the 'best care' was to be had from male practitioners. By the late fifteenth century, upper-class women themselves were requesting that autopsies be performed on their bodies after death so that the cause of their sickness (and the implications for their children) might be known.[39] Given the extraordinary material and social investments in reproduction that were made by the upper classes of northern Italy in the fifteenth century, it would have been more surprising if male practitioners had *not* been involved in gynaecological and some aspects of obstetrical practice.[40]

France

No comparably intense tradition of anatomical practice seems to have developed north of the Alps in the fifteenth century.[41] Nevertheless, both gynaecological and, to a lesser extent, obstetrical practice by men was expanding. As in previous centuries, ownership of texts on gynaecology lay in men's hands: aside from

[37] Savonarola, *Practica maior*, rubr. 1, *De descriptione, anatomia, et complexione matricis, ac de eius colligantia cum reliquis membris*, f. 249va: 'ut omnino dominabus succurramus, quae sunt medicorum tubae'. In the section on medical ethics in what was perhaps his earliest writing, Savonarola insisted that the two most important elements of a physician's comportment were handsome physical appearance and the avoidance of an over-easy presumption of knowledge; see Tiziana Pesenti Marangon, 'Michele Savonarola a Padova: L'ambiente, le opere, la cultura medica', *Quaderni per la Storia dell'Università di Padova* 9–10 (1976–7), 45–102, plus genealogical tables, at p. 89. In other words, he was very conscious of the need to impress his patients.

[38] In the images of gynaecological or obstetrical encounters I have reviewed, a female patient will be alone with men only in cases of autopsy or Caesarean section (in which case she was already dead or dying). Living patients (e.g., in childbirth scenes) will always have female attendants if a male physician or surgeon is present. See, for example, Jacqueline Musacchio, *The Art and Ritual of Childbirth in Renaissance Italy* (New Haven and London: Yale University Press, 1999), pp. 116–18, 128; and Renate Blumenfeld-Kosinski, *Not of Woman Born: Representations of Caesarean Birth in Medieval and Renaissance Culture* (Ithaca, NY: Cornell University Press, 1990), *passim*.

[39] Park, *Secrets of Women*.

[40] On the intense culture of reproduction in late medieval and Renaissance northern Italy, see Musacchio, *Art and Ritual*.

[41] Though see now Vivian and Christine Nutton, 'The Archer of Meudon: A Curious Absence of Continuity in the History of Medicine', *Journal of the History of Medicine and Allied Sciences* 58, no. 4 (October 2003), 401–27, for indirect evidence for regularized anatomical practices in late 15th-century Paris. Montpellier had instituted annual anatomies for instructional purposes in the early 15th century if not earlier. In neither city, however, is there evidence of regularized forensic or diagnostic anatomy.

Anne de Beaujeu, the dedicatee of a Latin text on fertility at the end of the century (about whom more later), not a single fifteenth-century French woman has been documented as the owner of a gynaecological text.[42] The Latin *Trotula* dropped off in popularity in the fifteenth century and was rarely copied in France, but it could still serve as the focal point of a veritable *summa* on fertility that was compiled in the middle of the century in eastern France; Johannes de Bursalia (fl. 1433–55), a physician trained at Paris and Montpellier, was interested enough in some sections of the *Trotula* on fertility, uterine prolapse, and uterine distemper to copy them into his own miscellany.[43] In French translation, as we saw in Chapter 4, the *Trotula* retained its popularity well into the fifteenth century, being incorporated into collections of surgical and other practical medical texts. Also in French, surgical collections often contained a translation of the pseudo-Albertus Magnus *Secrets of Women* (here expanded with Thomas of Cantimpré's instructions for midwives) as well as two other brief gynaecological works.[44] Likewise, the Latin Montpellierain treatises on fertility maintained their popularity in the fifteenth century while the newer Italian treatises by Falcucci and Guainerius began to make headway into France as well.

The real evidence for male gynaecological and obstetrical *practice*, however, comes not from the passive circulation of texts but from hints, asides, and sometimes even straightout assertions that show how a variety of French male practitioners were carving out increasingly large areas of gynaecological expertise and negotiating these changes with both their female patients and their female colleagues, the midwives. Guillaume de Naste (fl. 1466–70), for example, doctor of medicine and counsellor to the Duke of Burgundy, owned an unusual copy of Niccolò Falcucci's *Sermon* on gynaecology: what had been four separate tractates on the generative organs in Falcucci's original—one on generation in general, one on the male organs, one on the female organs, and one on enhancing the sexual experience—were here rearranged. Women's diseases were placed first and several of the andrological conditions were dropped. As with most of the books that he owned, Guillaume annotated this one with observations of cases he

---

[42] French noblewomen of the 15th- and early 16th-century were, nevertheless, notable for their high rates of ownership of herbals and other small practical medical texts. See Green, 'Possibilities'.

[43] The *summa* on fertility, BNF, MS lat. 7066, s. xv med., is a codex written by many hands, among them a member of the Faculty of Medicine at Paris, Pierre Pilatre. It had an unprecedented thirteen texts and excerpts exclusively on gynaecology and generation, including two different versions of the *Trotula*. Judging from the number of different hands that later added recipes, the codex was well used. Johannes de Bursalia's compendium is now Seville, Biblioteca Capitolar y Colombina, MS 5–1–45, an. 1452–3. Most of the other 15th-century French owners of the *Trotula* seem to have been simply passing around old copies; see Appendix 1, items 43–50.

[44] On the French *Secrets des dames*, see Green, 'Traittié'. The two other small French texts were Bernard de Gordon's (?) *Dix règles pour quoi l'on peut entendre pourquoy les femmes ont chascun mois leurs fleurs* and Jean de Trabarmaco's (?) *Des aydes de la mayre des dames et de leurs medecines*; see Monica H. Green, 'Medieval Gynecological Texts: A Handlist', in *Women's Healthcare*, Appendix, pp. 1–36, pp. 7 and 16.

had seen among his own clientele in Lille.[45] For example, at the bottom of one of the pages describing childbirth, Guillaume writes 'Note that it is a great and sovereign good when a woman is quiet and obedient in her labour.' Niccolò's text had said nothing about the benefits of women's subdued behaviour in birth nor was it a common topos in gynaecological literature; however Guillaume came to this opinion, it was not through his written authorities. Guillaume also shows his awareness of male surgical interventions when he notes, alongside the chapter on obstruction of the vagina, that he himself saw, while visiting Montpellier, a woman who was 'unveiled' by a barber-surgeon's tool. Alongside the chapter on uterine prolapse, he notes that 'it is known from the woman [herself] whether her uterus is inverted or not, as I have seen'. He then notes, alongside Niccolò's indications of the appearance of the urine in women with a prolapsed uterus, that he has seen the same thing in the wife of Jean le Saumir, the lady of Barbenson, and the wife of the Lombard.[46] At no point does Guillaume encounter one of Niccolò's frequent statements 'I saw' with any hint of scepticism or opprobrium that a male practitioner should have such access to female patients.

Fifteenth-century France also saw the composition of new material on gynaecology, all of it showing the increasing hands-on involvement of male practitioners. Valesco of Tarenta (d. after 1426), court physician to the famous Gaston Phoebus, count of Foix (d. 1391), and his successors, embedded his gynaecological material in a general medical encyclopedia where, like those of Niccolò Falcucci and Michele Savonarola, it is replete with anecdotes and observations culled from personal experience.[47] Valesco is surprisingly detailed in his accounts of some diseases, especially uterine lesions. He laments the cases when women's slowness to seek counsel with physicians results in conditions difficult or impossible of cure,[48] and he sees one of the physician's tasks as differentiating morbid conditions from pregnancy, which would involve him quite regularly in women's care. Twice he mentions instruments to inspect or apply treatment to the uterus, and the midwife is nowhere to be found.[49] In

---

[45] Lille, Bibliothèque Municipale, MS 334, s. xv, here entitled *Nicholus, De passionibus mulierum.* On Guillaume de Naste, see Wickersheimer, *Dictionnaire,* 1:257 and Jacquart, *Supplément,* 109.

[46] Lille, Bibliothèque municipale, MS 334, ff. 72v, 164r and 171r.

[47] Valesco de Taranta, *Philonium* (Lyons: Scipio de Gabiano, 1535); all quotations are from Book VI. For Valesco's biography and analysis of his practice, see York, 'Experience and Theory'.

[48] For example, in discussing windiness and inflation of the belly after birth, Valesco assures his reader that any postpartum woman who immediately employs the medicines he has described will be cured; those who don't suffer from swollen bellies for the rest of their lives. Later, he notes that women, thinking themselves pregnant (due to swelling of the belly and absence of menstruation), 'do not right from the start show themselves to physicians' (*a principio non se ostendunt medicis*), hence further aggravating the condition; *Philonium,* cap. 16, f. 350rb-vb). Likewise he notes women who mistake the pains and swelling of their belly due to apostemes for pregnancy and so do not seek out the counsel of a physician; they end up becoming dropsical and dying (cap. 17, f. 352vb).

[49] Valesco, *Philonium,* cap. 12 (on excess menstruation), f. 342rb: 'necesse est argaliam [a catheter] vel siringam vel aliud instrumentum inuenire ad immittendum medicinam in matricem'; cap. 20

his chapter on birth in particular, we sense a closer approach to the birthing room than we have seen in earlier writers. For example, he is far more specific in detailing how the midwife should anoint the pudenda and the vagina prior to birth; how, if four hours of labour have passed and the patient has not eaten, she should be given certain restoratives; how the midwife, having had the woman lie supine with her legs spread open, should then cover them with a cloth lest cold air come in; and how she should then have her breathe with short, strong breaths. No such detail could be found in Valesco's sources, suggesting that, like his Italian brethren, he had crossed the threshold into the birthing room.

Several decades after Valesco had served at the court of Foix, the new count, Gaston IV, commissioned a treatise on fertility and birth from Pierre Andrieu, a master of medicine at the University of Toulouse.[50] Pierre's work, *The Golden Apple* (*Pomum aureum*), written in 1444, treated both the theory and the practice of generation: the theory explained the process of generation, the determinants of the sex of the foetus, the factors that affected whether the child resembled one or another of his parents (or even others), and the signs of pregnancy. The practice addressed miscarriage and ways to avoid it, the process of birth and how it should be managed, care of the woman after birth, and care of the child through infancy. Unlike Avicenna or any of his other sources, Pierre provides detailed instructions on how the parturient should be positioned so that the mouth of the womb can better be viewed during birth. He explains how the water in which the just-birthed woman washes should be used by no other woman, but immediately be disposed where no one else will find it as should the afterbirth itself. He even refers to a remedy for tightening up the belly after birth that he had used successfully on Gaston's own mother.[51] All this suggests Pierre's own experience in (or just outside) the birthing room.

A third new gynaecological composition from this period, a French treatise entitled *On the Diseases Which Can Occur in the Generative Organs of Women*,

---

(on difficult birth), f. 359vb: 'Si foetus est mortuus extrahatur et dilatetur vulua cum instrumento chirurgico quod dilatat orificium matricis et membratum expellatur'. Valesco's reference to a 'surgical instrument which dilates the orifice of womb' is one of the first clear medieval references to the vaginal speculum that I have found. Described in three different forms by Albucasis (whose descriptions in turn differ from instruments known in Antiquity), it is unlikely, given the severe distortions in the depictions of the instruments in the Latin Albucasis, that any functional instrument was ever reconstructed on the basis of that text. Valesco's first patron, Gaston Phoebus, had owned an illustrated copy of Albucasis's *Surgery*, so it remains possible that he was referring to an idealized instrument rather than anything commonly in use. But see below.

[50] Pierre Andrieu, *Pomum aureum*, BNF, MS lat. 6992, s. xv med., ff. 79r–90v; my deepest thanks to Michael McVaugh for providing me with a printout from his film of this manuscript. For further information on the biography of Pierre (fl. *c.*1430–59, also called Pierre Andree de Pulcro Visu), see Wickersheimer, *Dictionnaire*, 2:612, and Jacquart, *Supplément*, 226–27.

[51] Since Jeanne d'Albret died in 1436 before Gaston himself ascended the throne, this indicates that Pierre was practising in the court of Gaston's father, Jean I (r. 1412–36), as well.

shows the kind of care urban women might receive from male practitioners.[52]
Writing probably in Picardy around 1440 or 1450, this anonymous male author
covers such topics as generation of the child, the nature of the menses, specific
gynaecological conditions such as menstrual problems and uterine displacement,
as well as the signs of pregnancy and management of birth. There are several
levels on which the author gives evidence of his own gynaecological practice
and of his assumption that his readers (presumably other male practitioners
like himself) will relate to their female patients in much the same manner. The
author recounts, first of all, his own success in curing certain diseases. He says
that with a certain remedy 'many women were cured by me at Paris as well as
Rouen and Amiens in Picardy of their "white flowers" '.[53] He also claims to have
cured a young bourgeoise in Paris when she suffered uterine prolapse and severe
haemorrhage in the middle of the night. As with the other fifteenth-century
writers, the midwife is still present. But it is very much the male physician who
is in control. In cases of a malpresented foetus it is the *physician* who must see to
it that the child is pushed back into the womb and turned, and it is the *physician*
who, if there are twins or triplets, must see to it that they are brought forth one
after the other.[54] In the case of the young bourgeoise whose uterus prolapsed,
although the uterus was actually manually repositioned by a midwife, it was our
male author who was sought out by the woman's husband in the middle of the
night and he that diagnosed the condition and prescribed treatment.[55]

   That these three gynaecological writers were not social innovators in mas-
culinizing gynaecological practice is suggested by the trial of a male practitioner,
Jean Domrémi, who was prosecuted by the Faculty of Medicine in Paris between

---

[52] Anonymous, *Des maladies qui peuuent souruenir es membres generatifz de la femme*, found
uniquely in BNF, MS fr. 2043, s. xv med., ff. 77r–99v. While the author's gender is not confirmed
by any grammatical indications (none of the few first-person statements employ gendered verbal
forms), I take his engagement with university medicine (Hippocrates, Aristotle, and Avicenna), his
quotations from Latin, his consistent identification with the male *médecin*, and his distancing from
the female *sage-femme* as evidence of his masculinity. On the date of composition of this text (which
must postdate 1429), see Ernest Wickersheimer, 'La descente de matrice d'une bourgeoise de Paris
et la monstre bicéphale d'Aubervilliers. Deux observations du XV siècle', *Progrès Médical* no. 47
(Nov. 17, 1931), p. 2099.

[53] BNF, MS fr. 2043, f. 85v. By 'white flowers' (*de fleurs blanches*), the author is referring
to some kind of vaginal discharge. The 'flowers' was a common term in many of the European
vernaculars for menstrual blood. See Green, *Trotula*, pp. 21–22; and Green, 'Flowers, Poisons, and
Men: Menstruation in Medieval Western Europe', in *Menstruation: A Cultural History*, ed. Andrew
Shail and Gillian Howie (New York: Palgrave, 2005), pp. 51–64.

[54] BNF, MS fr. 2043, s. xv, f. 99r: 'le medecin doit faire remectre l'enfant'; f. 99v: 'Et se la mere
auoit deux ou troys enfants ensemble en son ventre le medecin doit faire que l'ung viengne apres
l'autre'.

[55] BNF, MS fr. 2043, f. 92r: 'et elle apperceut sa marris hors de son corps auec tres grant
habundance de sang et lors commenca a appeller son mary. Et luy failly la parole et me vint
querir son mary pour mectre remede a la jeune. Et lors feis asseoir vne ventouse sur le ventre de la
bourgeoyse et fy remectre la marris en son lieu par la matrone durant tous jours la grant ventouse
auec les remedes dessusdits, par quoy fut parfaictement guerie ladite jeune bourgeoyse ne oncques
puys ne luy aduint tel accident en sa marris.'

1423 and 1427. Jean's trial is similar in many ways to that of Jacoba Felicie a century earlier.[56] Although Jean had been practising for many years in Paris, the case that seems to have initially elicited the Faculty's wrath was one of a pregnant woman whom he had cured. She had been attended by certain male physicians who, despairing of her life, renounced her case as hopeless, saying that the only thing they could do was to have her opened up (*fère ouvrir ladite femme*) in order to save the child. Jean, however, gave her some kind of medicine and, at the time of the trial, reported that she was not only still alive but in good health (*en bonne santé*); her child was apparently born without incident since Jean could now report that it, too, was alive. The Faculty of Medicine (who were joined in their suit by the whole University of Paris) credited Jean's cure to sheer luck. The University physicians who were pursuing him did not, however, prosecute him because he was a man caring for a pregnant woman, but rather because he was a man practising medicine without a licence. Later, in January 1424, the case turned from a civil procedure to a criminal trial when Jean was accused of *crimes horribles*, that is, infanticide, because of at least two miscarriages he caused by his inexpert use of scammony, a powerful expulsive. Apparently, therefore, Jean was regularly treating pregnant women.[57]

Jean, like Perretta Petone a decade before him, protested in his defense not simply that he was a highly experienced practitioner (he vacillated in his story whether he was a surgeon or a physician), but that he did, in fact, own a medical book despite the Faculty's claims that he was illiterate. (Unlike Perretta, Jean admits that he has to have his son, an apothecary, read it to him.) And he also similarly protested that there were lots of other unlicensed practitioners in Paris, including women assisting in birth, whom the Faculty never prosecuted. This was true, the Faculty's representatives replied, but in practising obstetrics such women were simply following the normative principles of *de ventre inspiciendo* (literally, 'on inspecting the belly'). This was an ancient Roman legal concept stipulating that, if a wife or recent widow was suspected of being pregnant with a presumptive heir, a group of women and midwives was to be gathered to examine her and confirm the pregnancy.[58] Clearly, the phrase was being used here in Jean's trial as shorthand

---

[56] Laurent Garrigues, 'Les Professions médicales à Paris au début du XVe siècle: Praticiens en procès au parlement', *Bibliothèque de l'École des Chartes* 156 (1998), 317–67. The significance of Jean Domrémi's trial for the history of women's medicine has been discussed by Susan Broomhall, *Women's Medical Work in Early Modern France* (Manchester: University of Manchester Press, 2004), pp. 54–55, who, however, misinterprets two key elements of the account: *venterie* (which she interprets as evidence that Jean practised 'obstetrics') should instead be translated as 'longwindedness' (the physicians are complaining of his pompous self-defense), while the reference to *abortivorum* is not a claim that he practises abortions but rather that he has caused accidental miscarriages by the remedies he prescribed. Geneviève Dumas and Faith Wallis, 'Theory and Practice in the Trial of Jean Domrémi, 1423–1427', *Journal of the History of Medicine and Allied Sciences*, 54, no. 1 (Jan. 1999), 55–87, present an English translation of the appeal case (from 1423–7) before the royal court though this, too, is marred by several transcriptional errors.

[57] Unfortunately, we don't know the outcome of this latter accusation.

[58] Justinian, *Digest*, 25.4: *De inspiciendo ventre custodiendoque partu.*

to refer to women's traditional practices of attending childbirth. Such women, the physicians imply, were not practising *medicine*, or if they were it was only minimally. All others who practised medicine were rightfully subject to prosecution. What the Faculty is saying, in effect, is that when a *man* attempts to care for a pregnant woman, that work is necessarily medical, an understanding that accords with everything we have seen about developing male physician competencies in gynaecology over the previous three centuries. What is striking here—precisely because it goes unstated—is that nobody is contesting the prerogative of male practitioners to attend to pregnant women. The initial attendance of the male physicians on the pregnant woman, the threat of surgical intervention (the alleged plan to open the woman and cut the baby out), even the woman's acceptance of Jean's ministrations after the learned physicians abandoned her—all these are treated in the narrative as if they were common occurrences. Jean is being prosecuted for his care of pregnant women only because he does it badly: without Latin, without learning, without books, and without a licence.

From Valesco de Tarenta and Pierre Andrieu practising in the south of France, to our anonymous Picard author in Paris and Normandy and Guillaume de Naste in Lille, to Jean Domrémi in Paris itself, we find a new confidence among male medical writers and practitioners in their claims to authoritative knowledge on women's medicine. Near the end of the century, in 1488, the royal physician Bernard Chaussade completed his *Treatise on Conception and Generation, Especially of Male Children* for his patroness and patient, Anne de Beaujeu, former regent of France and current Duchess of Bourbon, who though married for fourteen years had yet to produce an heir.[59] Aside from the gender of his dedicatee, Bernard and his text were typical of the state of women's medicine in fifteenth-century France. Still untouched by the humanistic influences of later fifteenth-century Italian medicine,[60] Bernard did little more than build on the tradition of the earlier Montpellierain fertility treatises in co-opting gynaecological disease categories into his framework for explaining the causes of infertility. Bernard does not venture into obstetrical territory in the text itself (given Anne's sterility, it is hardly yet relevant), yet his service as personal physician not simply to Anne but also her mother, Charlotte of Savoy (wife of Louis XI), her sister-in-law, Anne of Brittany (wife of Charles VIII, whose marriage Anne had herself arranged), and even to Anne of Brittany's mother, Margaret of Foix, makes it highly unlikely that he would have stayed very far from the door of their lying-in rooms. Bernard's treatise did not prove as effective as Pierre Andrieu's earlier in the century—Anne would end up only bearing a single child, a daughter Suzanne—but it is Bernard's very mediocrity that shows how normative male expertise in women's medicine had become.

---

[59] Bernardus Chaussade, *Tractatus de conceptione et generatione praecipue filiorum*, BNF, MS lat. 7064 (28 Dec. 1488), ff. 1r–82v.
[60] The most recent Italian author Bernard cites is Niccolò Falcucci.

Active involvement of both physicians and surgeons in the diagnosis and care of women's gynaecological and obstetrical conditions can be documented all across western Europe in the fifteenth century. Tentative steps were taken in England to rework older material into new forms.[61] In Germany (as we will see in more detail in a moment) interests in generation and childbirth became increasingly concentrated in the latter half of the century. While evidence for male gynaecological practice has yet to be gathered for Spain, the casual presence of a *speculum matricis* ('a speculum for the uterus') among the surgical belongings of a mid fifteenth-century barber-surgeon in Barcelona suggests that it was common.[62] All the writers whom we can identify are male, and all the anonymous texts display clear signs of masculine genesis, such as competence with Latin, familiarity with learned university discourse, and deferral to a third-person midwife who is specifically (and sometimes solely) charged with assistance at birth and manipulations that involve the vagina. And most of these writers direct themselves to audiences of other males. Indeed, one of the most striking things about fifteenth-century gynaecological writers, even those north of the Alps, is their confidence in moving beyond their earlier textual authorities and expanding their command over women's medicine.

ANCIENT MODELS AND MODEL ANCIENTS: THE SIXTEENTH CENTURY

At this point, therefore, it should be clear that the masculine birth of gynae-cology was not a phenomenon of the sixteenth century but of the century preceding it, when physicians and surgeons moved well beyond their earlier 'hands-off' advisory role to a more active engagement both intellectually and clinically with the diseases of women. It is all the more surprising, then, that the achievements of the fifteenth century seem at first glance to have been ephemeral, for in the sixteenth century the landscape of gynaecological knowledge was transformed yet again. The works of the Italian authors mentioned above enjoyed healthy afterlives in print for several decades, yet with but two exceptions, none of the new specialized gynaecological compositions of the fifteenth century, whether intended for men or women, whether composed in Latin or a vernacular, would make the transition into print. How viable could this new area of male medical engagement be if its works were so easily eliminated?

---

[61] See Chapters 4 and 5 above.

[62] Lluís Cifuentes, 'La Promoció intellectual i social dels barbers-cirurgians a la Barcelona medieval: L'obrador, la biblioteca i els béns de Joan Vicenç (*fl.* 1421–64)', *Arxiu de Textos Catalans Antics* 19 (2000), 429–79, at pp. 439 and 472. The 15th-century Valencian physician-surgeon Bartolomé Martí had 'una siringa dargent pera siringar homens e altra siringa pera siringar dones'; Luís García-Ballester, 'Tres bibliotecas médicas en la Valencia del siglo XV', *Asclepio* 18–19 (1966–67), 383–405, at p. 385.

Viable enough, apparently, to remake itself despite the technological revolution brought on by the printing press and the intellectual revolution occasioned by the spread of humanism to medicine. It was able to do so, I will argue, precisely because the *social* foundations of masculine gynaecology were already so deeply laid.

Medical writings were as quick to be represented in the new technology of printing as any other field but, as was common, printers initially tended to favour not novel compositions, but works of already recognized popularity that they knew would sell. Most of the gynaecological works that appeared in the first few decades of print were either attached to the *oeuvres* of famous men—Galen, Arnau de Vilanova, Bernard of Gordon, and Constantine the African—or they were the gynaecological sections of larger *summae* of the great Italian encyclopedists of the fifteenth century. Aside from the extraordinary popularity of the pseudo-Albertus Magnus *Secrets of Women* (which was published over fifty times prior to 1500, and many more times thereafter), there is no evidence of a special interest in women's medicine. Ludovico Bonaccioli's Latin *Enneas muliebris* ('Nine Books on Women'), published in Ferrara *c*.1502–3 and dedicated to Lucrezia Borgia, was an oddity: an entirely new composition, it was unusual not so much in being dedicated to a woman (Bernard Chaussade, as we have seen, had already recognized the value of noble female patronage) but in eschewing a therapeutic focus for a more discursive, compendious survey of scientific opinion on generation.[63] This and two other exceptional German works aside (about which, more in a moment), the printing press initially had a negative effect on the field of women's medicine, narrowing the variety of texts being produced for public consumption.[64] This was hardly an auspicious beginning, yet within a hundred years the field had replaced several times over everything that was lost, producing well over six dozen printed texts, many of which went through multiple editions.[65]

---

[63] Ludovico Bonaccioli, *Enneas muliebris* (Ferrara: Laurentius de Rubies?, *c*.1502–3?). There is some confusion about whether this dates from 1502–3 or 1505 (the printed text itself bears no date). See G. Stabile, 'Bonaccioli, Ludovico', *Dizionario biografico degli Italiani*, vol. 11 (1969), pp. 456–8.

[64] In Germany and the Low Countries, manuscript production of certain medieval texts continued well into the 16th century; in England, there seems to have been an earlier disruption in manuscript usage, with few new manuscripts of medieval texts being copied after *c*.1530. In southern Europe, the impact of print occurred even earlier.

[65] See Appendix 2. In compiling this list, I have included all specialized texts that addressed the anatomy, physiology, or pathology of the female body with, at least potentially, a therapeutic goal. Thus, for example, I have included Gabriele Zerbi's 1502 study on uterine anatomy, while omitting such texts as the multiple reprints of the pseudo-Albertus *Secreta mulierum* and works that only addressed foetal development, such as the 1515 edition of Giles of Rome's tract on the formation of the foetus. Nor have I attempted to assess the continuing presence of gynaecological material within medical encyclopedias more generally, such as the extraordinarily influential Book VII of Aetius of Amida's *Tetrabiblos*, which Janus Cornarius translated into Latin in 1542. Finally, this list does not even begin to reflect the masses of manuscript and other archival materials (university lecture notes, new texts circulating only in manuscript, and bodies of correspondence) that will no doubt

For the history of women's medicine, the sixteenth century can be divided into two halves. The first is dominated by the birth of specialized obstetrical writing, usually in the vernacular, and the creation of a completely new audience, midwives, who now for the first time since late Antiquity could claim to have 'professional books' of their own. As I will show, this development came directly out of later medieval interests and concerns and owed nothing to 'the Renaissance' other than its savvy exploitation of the possibilities of print. The second half of the century presents a much more typical Renaissance story: the rediscovery of the Hippocratic gynaecological texts (the bulk of which had been unavailable to the West for over 1500 years) offered a major ancient authority for the field of gynaecology—indeed, the highest authority possible. This corpus, in turn, spawned the creation of new specialized texts in Latin of unprecedented length and detail which proliferated from the middle of the century on; many of these were reprinted in the three increasingly large editions of the *Gynaeciorum libri*, 'The Books of Gynaecology', which served not simply as a textbook but also as a physical monument to the stature of the field. Because of these two parallel developments, by the end of the sixteenth century books existed in a variety of languages around which both male 'gynaecologists' and female midwives could create professional identities. But those identities were as gendered as ever: the authoritative stature of men in both gynaecology and obstetrics had never been higher, while that of women, who remained confined to the role of midwife, was only slightly elevated by their entry into the realm of literate medicine. The fundamental character of sixteenth century gynaecology was defined not by intellectual breaks from its medieval past (considerable though they were) but by continuity with the social structures that male and female practitioners of the sixteenth century had inherited from the late Middle Ages.

The birth of obstetrics

As I have argued throughout the previous chapters, the one group left out of the rise of literate medicine in the later Middle Ages was also the group that could in theory have made most use of the obstetrical aspects of gynaecological writings: the midwives. The creation of texts specifically on the subject of childbirth assistance, directed ostensibly to midwives as well as parturient women, began as we have seen with Michele Savonarola's *Regimen for the Women of Ferrara*, written *c*.1460. Savonarola's *Regimen*, composed in the local Ferrarese dialect, had a limited circulation and spawned no direct imitators in Italy, where texts for midwives would not be written again for another hundred years.[66] Nevertheless,

---

be unearthed once scholars begin to look for them. On the development of anatomy as it relates to women, see Park, *Secrets of Women*.

[66] Aside from the 1538 Italian translation of Rösslin (see Appendix 2, item 21), the first newly composed Italian texts for midwives date from 1563 and 1595 by Marinelli and Mercurio, respectively (see Appendix 2, items 44 and 77).

Savonarola's teachings on certain aspects of women's medicine were to have more influence than he—or any medieval author, for that matter—could ever have imagined possible.

At first glance, the German-speaking territories of the late fifteenth century would hardly seem likely to produce what would become the most influential texts on obstetrics of the early modern period since they had no prior tradition of addressing texts on women's medicine to female audiences. This was not for lack of interest in the *topic* of women's medicine. As in England, the *Trotula* was still the most widely circulating text on women's medicine in fifteenth-century Germany, being reworked into new forms and, as we saw in Chapter 4, twice translated into German. The Latin Montpellierain fertility treatises were also readily available as were, from the mid fifteenth century on, the writings of the great north Italian physicians, whose works were being brought to Germany by students returning from their medical studies in Padua, Bologna, and Ferrara. These Latin writings were supplemented by a fair number of German texts on women's medicine, which tended more toward recipe collections and general descriptions of basic physiological processes. Moreover, as we saw in Chapter 5, German-speaking territories were distinguished by their extraordinary appetite for knowledge of the 'secrets of women', an appetite that not only led monks, priests, and laymen to read gynaecological texts and the pseudo-Albertan *Secrets of Women* indiscriminately, as if both of these very different textual genres provided the same kind of information, but also to the proliferation of the 'disease woman' figures and the foetus-in-utero figures derived from Muscio's late antique *Gynaecology*. Johannes Hartlieb's paired *Secrets of Women* and *Trotula* translations, which we examined in previous chapters, would be amplified early in the sixteenth century by the addition of the gynaecological sections from one of the most popular medical texts of the day, the so-called *Medical Pamphlet* (*Fasciculus medicine*) attributed to 'Johannes Ketham', together with a German rendering of selections on sexuality and reproduction from a pseudo-Aristotelian series of natural philosophical questions.[67] Most strikingly, the fifteenth and sixteenth centuries saw the introduction of the licensing of midwives in southern German cities.[68] Unlike France, where such licensing seems to have been exclusively an ecclesiastical affair, in German territories midwives were licensed by the individual municipalities, with doctors of medicine often being asked to verify the women's capabilities.

[67] These latter two texts are edited in Britta-Juliane Kruse, *Verborgene Heilkünste: Geschichte der Frauenmedizin im Spätmittelalter*, Quellen und Forschungen zur Literatur- und Kulturgeschichte, 5 (Berlin: Walter de Gruyter, 1996), pp. 337–69. On the significance of the pseudo-Ketham *Fasciculus medicine* for female anatomy, see Park, *Secrets of Women*.

[68] Sibylla Flügge, *Hebammen und heilkundige Frauen: Recht und Rechtswirklichkeit im 15. und 16. Jahrhundert*, 2nd ed. (Frankfurt am Main: Stroenfeld, 2000), finds evidence for midwives' oaths in southern Germany from as early as 1417; the earliest extant regulation comes from Regensburg in 1452. Whether there were any direct links between the German trend toward licensing and that documented earlier in France and Brussels (see Chapter 3 above) is unclear.

In short, there was an extraordinary amount of interest in matters of generation at all levels of literate society in fifteenth-century Germany reflecting, I would suggest, concern among learned men—be they medical masters, priests and preachers, or male heads of households—to monitor the knowledge that wives and midwives had about the processes of generation and birth. The early fifteenth-century Latin and German Apocalypse manuscript, for example, that we examined in Chapter 3 for its use of the Muscian foetus-in-utero figures and other material on women (Figs. 3.5 and 3.6 above), reflects the interests of clerics in managing the processes of birth: after noting the importance of having 'good and experienced midwives' when the foetus malpresents, the obstetrical section not only includes an image of a male practitioner performing a Caesarean section (with the heading 'let the learned doctor incise [the woman]') but goes on to advise 'Let the male physician (*medicus*) avoid there being shouts and lamentations [at the parturient's bedside] such as women are accustomed to make'.[69] As we have seen, Johannes Hartlieb had praised Muscio's late antique gynaecological text (which he considered a fairly recent discovery) and wondered why no German translation had yet been made of this book since it would be 'such a treasure to midwives'.[70] Hartlieb, like his predecessors in the twelfth and thirteenth centuries, was ultimately defeated by Muscio's *Gynaecology*, abandoning his plan to translate it probably because it trafficked too heavily in the outmoded and incomprehensible theories of the ancient Methodists. His assessment of the value of the work does, however, indicate that the *sentiment* that midwives might benefit from having their own 'professional books' (a view which, of course, had been Muscio's own motivation for writing) was attractive in later fifteenth-century southern Germany.

It is in this general context, therefore, that we must view the genesis of the two earliest printed obstetrical texts, the *Frauenbüchlein* ('Women's Little Book' or 'Women's Manual') from around 1495 and the *Rosegarden for Pregnant Women and Midwives* by Eucharius Rösslin in 1513.[71] The *Frauenbüchlein* is indeed a 'little book' in three chapters: one on the regimen and other preparations that should be made prior to birth, one on the regimen after birth, and one listing the various complications that can arise in the postpartum period. It is not a midwives' text since it offers little information on conducting a birth. Nor can

---

[69] LWL, MS 49, *c*.1420 (Germany), f. 38v: 'Et sic bone obstetrices et experte in hoc opere debent haberi . . . doctus medicus incidatur . . . Caueat ibi medicus ne ibi sint clamores et luccus ut solent mulieres'.

[70] On knowledge of Muscio's text in southern Germany in this period, see Monica H. Green, 'The Sources of Eucharius Rösslin's *Rosegarden for Pregnant Women and Midwives* (1513)' (forthcoming). As was typical of the period, Hartlieb only recognizes Muscio's utility as a resource on obstetrics; the work's gynaecological content is never mentioned.

[71] Both the *Women's Manual* and the *Rosegarden* are known (from the single manuscript copy of each that now survives) to have had an earlier existence. Neither one, in its manuscript form, is explicitly addressed to a female audience, a characteristic they share with all other currently known gynaecological texts in German. See Green, 'Sources'.

it quite be called a 'self-help' manual, since the third chapter lists the disease headings but does not explain what one should do about them other than to take one's concerns to a doctor. In other words, it is a guide for *lay*women to help them conduct their pregnancies and lyings-in productively.

The *Rosegarden*, in contrast, very much constitutes a midwives' handbook, giving the most detailed obstetrical and pediatric instructions of any independent text since Muscio's *Gynaecology*. Indeed, on many levels, it surpasses Muscio's work in descriptive detail. Dedicated to Katharine, Duchess of Brunswick-Lüneburg (in northern Germany), whom the Frankfurt-based author, Eucharius Rösslin, had served five years prior to publishing the work, the *Rosegarden* lays out in its first nine chapters basic information on the development of the foetus, a regimen to be followed prior to birth, and full descriptions of how childbirth itself, whether normal or abnormal, ought to be managed. The final three chapters cover care of the newborn.[72]

Rösslin employed the excerpts from Muscio's *Gynaecology* that had accompanied the images of various possible malpresentations at birth. Rösslin's main textual source, however, was not ancient at all but almost modern: Rösslin (or rather, an earlier German translator from whom Rösslin himself was borrowing) lifted most of his material directly from Savonarola's Latin *Practica*.[73] Thus, when Rösslin recommends that the parturient have any potentially complicating genital boils, ulcers, or warts attended to by a surgeon prior to birth, he is following Savonarola's own recommendation that women rely on male surgeons for such prenatal gynaecological care. When he is describing the birthing chair 'that women of southern Germany and Romance-speaking lands are accustomed to use', he is echoing Savonarola's claim that this is a chair women 'in diverse regions' use. When Rösslin explains how the midwives attending a birth should encourage the labouring woman through her pains by telling her she will give birth to a son, he is echoing Savonarola's same assessment of the relative value of males versus females in fifteenth-century Italian culture. Perhaps most importantly to the future professional capacity of German midwives, when Rösslin explains that for any *serious* obstetrical or postpartum condition, the midwives or attendant women were to call on surgeons or physicians, he is mirroring exactly Savonarola's view that 'such treatment . . . is not the work of women'.

Through Rösslin's unacknowledged deployment of Savonarola's obstetrics, therefore, the northern Italian model of the midwife as a subordinate assistant to the male physician or surgeon was transmitted to German-speaking territories. Or rather, to all of western Europe, for not only would Rösslin's *Rosegarden* go

---

[72] Eucharius Rösslin, *Der Swangern Frauwen und hebammen Rosegarten*, facsimile reproduction of the 1513 Strasburg edition, ed. Huldrych M. Koelbing (Zürich: Verlag Bibliophile Drucke von J. Stocker, 1976).

[73] Savonarola, in turn, had lifted much of his material from the Neapolitan writer Francesco da Piedemonte; see Green, 'Sources'.

through over a hundred German editions in the course of the next two and a half centuries, but it was very quickly translated into Dutch, Latin, French, English, Czech, Spanish, and Danish.[74] I will return in the Conclusion to some specific features of the social impact of Rösslin's work. Here, it is important to note that, even with the unprecedented international impact of Rösslin's work, which for the first time gave midwives their own 'professional book' in their field, they could no more claim a *monopoly* on access to printed knowledge on obstetrics than medieval female readers could claim on manuscript gynaecological texts. As we have seen, already in the fifteenth century surgeons like Pietro d'Argellata made certain aspects of gynaecological and obstetrical surgery a regular part of their practice, and Savonarola certainly expected surgeons regularly to be on hand to deal with genital obstructions, fistulas, and growths, and to remove the dead foetus when necessary. By the mid sixteenth century male surgeons were not only incorporating obstetrical instructions into their treatises on anatomy, but they were writing independent obstetrical texts, sometimes for the instruction of midwives, sometimes for their own edification.[75]

The earliest example of the latter was a work first published by the French surgeon Ambroise Paré (*c*.1510–90) in 1549. Noting that he was drawing on the experiences of master barber-surgeons Thierry de Hery and Nicole Lambert, 'whom we have many times observed', Paré walks his reader through the normal length of gestation, the causes and symptoms of miscarriage, the signs by which to determine whether the infant was living or dead, and the method for extracting it in either case.[76] Once the surgeon has determined that the woman is not beyond hope (for if she is, he should commend her to God and retire), he can go about aiding her. Remarkably, the first interventions are not surgical: Paré begins by recommending potions, plasters, fumigations, sternutatives (substances that induce sneezing), etc., just what midwives or physicians would have used. If these do not work, however, one must have recourse to surgical interventions, which he then goes on to describe in detail. In contrast to the derivative work of Rösslin, Paré seems to be reflecting a tradition of empirically acquired knowledge by barber-surgeons. Hippocrates is the only authority whom Paré cites, and

---

[74] See Appendix 2 for information on these translations. The Danish text is found only in a manuscript copy.

[75] Space does not permit here analysis of the obstetrical writings of Jakob Ruf, Johannes Coninck, or François Rousset. For Ruf's and Rousset's work, see Appendix 2, items 33–4 and 58–9; and 60, 68, and 73, respectively. For Coninck's, which was never printed, see Willy Braekman, 'Johannes Conincks Instructies voor Vroedvrouwen uit de zestiende eeuw', in *Volkskunde* 88 (1987), 120–30. On the incorporation of obstetrical material into French anatomical and surgical writings from as early as 1545, see Valérie Worth-Stylianou, *Les Traités d'obstétrique en langue française au seuil de la modernité. Bibliographie critique des 'Divers Travaulx' d'Euchaire Rosslin (1536) à l' 'Apologie de Louyse Bourgeois sage-femme' (1627)* (Geneva: Droz, 2006), pp. 25 and *passim*.

[76] I have used the 1550 edition: Ambroise Paré, *Briefve collection de l'administration anatomique, avec la maniere de conjoindre les os: et d'extraire les enfans tant mors que vivans du ventre de la mere, lors que nature de soy ne peult venir a son effect . . .* (Paris: Guillaume Cavellat, 1550), quotation from f. 88r.

while he mentions at certain points how the surgeon ought to interrogate the mother (whether, for example, she has recently felt any movement of the foetus), at no point does he mention a midwife with whom he is collaborating. On the contrary, it is the surgeon himself who should apply ointments to the vulva to ease passage of the child, it is he who should remove the rings from his fingers, it is he who gently puts his hand 'without any violence' into the uterus to ascertain the position of the foetus. Midwives (*les obstetrices matrones, soy disans sages femmes*), who had previously been uniquely responsible for such internal examinations, only appear when Paré is criticizing them for their errors, when, for example, he was called in on a case where the midwives, by pulling too forcefully on an extruding arm, had caused it to become gangrenous.[77] The male surgeon has, in other words, now passed the last barrier to male practice of women's medicine: he can put his hand into the vagina. Paré's closing line is especially striking: after having explained in painful detail each step of extracting the foetus from its dead mother via Caesarean section, he says 'and for the rest, leave [the child] to God and to the women'.[78] It is with the tasks of mothering and nursing the newborn that Paré now recognizes 'women's work' to begin.

Paré, acknowledging that he has been trained in his obstetrical work by two other male practitioners, gives absolutely no hint that it is problematic for male surgeons to be attending birth. Although the fact that the surgeon has to assess immediately the life-or-death prospects of the labouring woman shows that he is not being called in early in labour (and hence is not the *routine* birth attendant),[79] once he is called in his authority not simply to direct the therapeutic protocol but to perform all necessary manual operations himself is unchallenged. We might be inclined to think that Paré (who was so unusual in a number of respects, including his rapid climb from humble social origins to the pinnacle of medical society) was merely a rare instance, were it not that, when the first ordinances for midwives were passed in Paris in 1560, it was stipulated that if the child presented 'other than head first, which is the normal delivery, or feet first, which is the next most normal delivery, the midwives should take advice from male physicians or surgeons'.[80] Whether Paré was himself involved in drafting these ordinances is not known (he did not become Surgeon-in-Ordinary to the French king until 1563), but he would be responsible for training subsequent

---

[77] I have used the 1550 edition: f. 93r. His only other reference to midwives is on f. 94v, when he notes that they call the umbilical cord 'the little entrail' (*le petit boyau*).

[78] *Ibid.*, f. 96r: 'et de la reste laisse l'enfant a Dieu et aux femmes'.

[79] Adrian Wilson, 'William Hunter and the Varieties of Man-Midwifery', in *William Hunter and the Eighteenth-Century Medical World*, ed. W. F. Bynum and Roy Porter (Cambridge: Cambridge University Press, 1985), pp. 343–69, examines in detail the importance of timing of the call for the male surgeon. As he notes, it is only when the male midwife was called in at the *beginning* of labour (or even booked for it in advance) that male midwifery finally moved beyond its lugubrious associations with the desperate scenarios of foetal or maternal death.

[80] Thomas G. Benedek, 'The Changing Relationship Between Midwives and Physicians During the Renaissance', *Bulletin of the History of Medicine* 51 (1977), 550–64, at p. 557.

generations of surgeons, including the husband of the early seventeenth-century midwife-author, Louise Bourgeois.[81] The fact that the second French translation of Rösslin's *Rosegarden*—that produced by Paul Bienassis in 1563—would be directed primarily to male surgeons rather than female midwives shows the comfortable position they had achieved in French obstetrics.[82]

Thus, despite the relatively early appearance of the French translation of Rösslin's *Rosegarden*, French midwives' late entry into the realm of literate medicine (if they did indeed enter, for no study has yet been done to prove they read either of the two French translations) did not preclude the further development of men's skills and expertise in obstetrics. In fact, all the midwives of sixteenth-century Europe would find that the boundaries of their profession had been set long before they themselves had the opportunity, as authors or self-regulating guildswomen, to define their own sphere of practice.

The father of medicine reclaims his paternity

The birth of obstetrics as a specialized field of medical writing for midwives and surgeons could, theoretically, have happened without any accompanying changes in the character of gynaecological writing or theorization. As we have just seen, the role of midwives did not expand in the sixteenth century beyond what it had already become in the late Middle Ages: attendance at normal birth with deferral to male physicians or surgeons when difficulties arose. Nor did the increasing involvement of male surgeons in difficult births alter the physician's role as the main consultant on women's internal gynaecological conditions. The defining tasks of the physician remained his involvement with regulating women's menstruation, ensuring fertility, and addressing other internal diseases of the female genitalia. At the end of the sixteenth century, the Venetian physician Scipione Mercurio would still be claiming that getting on with pharmacists and knowing how to make women fertile were the two most important factors in a physician's social success.[83] Ever since the twelfth century, 'the diseases of women' had established a niche for itself as a collection of subheadings in the larger category of 'diseases from head to toe', and even though it was clearly growing in scope and theoretical sophistication in the fifteenth century, it could conceivably have remained in that niche, comfortably within the purview of general (male) medical practitioners.

It is not surprising, therefore, that even when the fifteenth-century writers we have examined did compose new gynaecological works, no one articulated a reason *why* 'the diseases of women' should constitute its own separate field.

[81] On Bourgeois, see the Conclusion below.

[82] Worth-Stylianou, *Traités d'obstétrique*, p. 92.

[83] Richard Palmer, 'Pharmacy in the Republic of Venice in the Sixteenth Century', in *The Medical Renaissance of the Sixteenth Century*, ed. A. Wear, R. K. French, and I. M. Lonie (Cambridge: Cambridge University Press, 1985), 100–17, at p. 105.

As early as the first half of the fourteenth century, Italian and French authors began to speculate that Hippocrates had written a text specifically devoted to women's diseases,[84] but since no such text was known to them, they had no guidance in articulating what the specific rationale for this specialization might be. The writers who composed specialized texts on gynaecology seem to have been entirely unaware of each other's existence and there is no intertextuality among them—no references or subtle allusions to each other's works. Thus, none of these writers (or, apparently, their readers) had any explicit identity as collaborators in a shared enterprise.[85] An English author who pieced together a Latin gynaecological compendium out of other sources readily available in England provided neither title nor preface to his work, leaving his reader wondering what his intention was in synthesizing all these opinions on women's diseases.[86] The French author of the much more original *Diseases Which Can Occur in the Generative Organs of Women*, which moves well beyond the older French tradition of addressing simply sterility, offers no preface but simply jumps immediately into an Aristotelian explanation of how generation occurs as a joining of male and female.[87] For others, the specific topic of fertility was used to justify treating women's conditions separately from general medicine, though logically this focus demanded consideration of andrological conditions as well. Thus when Antonius Guainerius (who wrote with the ultimate intention of placing his *On the Womb* within an encyclopedia) 'pre-released' it with its own unique preface to his patron Philippo Maria, he gave as his rationale for writing specifically on women's (and men's) diseases the concern with progeny. Pierre Andrieu independently echoed this sentiment in his *Golden Apple*, though his greater focus on birth meant that both andrological and gynaecological diseases generally received less attention. The fifteenth-century translators or Latin adaptors of the *Trotula* could, of course, draw on *Conditions of Women's* justification of gynaecology as a separate concern because of women's greater suffering in reproduction. It was only, however, when gynaecological writers specifically addressed audiences of women—as did the authors of the English *Knowing of Woman's Kind in Childing*, the revised version of the English *Sickness of Women*, the Dutch *Liber Trotula*, and of course Savonarola in his *Regimen for the Women of Ferrara*—that we find substantive prefatory justifications for the creation of separate texts on women's conditions. And here, as we saw in

[84] Tiziana Pesenti, 'Le *Divisiones librorum Ypocratis* nei commenti all'*Articella*', *Medicina nei secoli* 14 (2002), 417–37, esp. pp. 426 and 428.

[85] The one exception I have found is the Middle English *Sickness of Women 2*, whose author seems to have been using the earlier *Knowing of Woman's Kind* as both model and foil to his own composition.

[86] This is what I have dubbed (from its incipit) Anonymous, *Signa retencionis menstruorum*. It appears in its unique manuscript copy alongside several early medieval gynaecological works. See Green, 'Medieval Gynecological Texts', pp. 31–2.

[87] BNF, MS fr. 2043, f. 77r: '[C]omme dit Aristote en son liure des bestes, la generation est fecte en la femme, et l'omme ne suffist pas a faire generation s'il na femme qui luy ayde'.

Chapter 4, the rationale was based on the distinct audience involved rather than the distinctive nature of the subject matter.

Yet as a glance at Appendix 2 will show, suddenly, in the middle of the sixteenth century, 'gynaecology' did indeed explode as its own distinct subdiscipline, with major works (some of them sizable monographs) appearing with ever increasing frequency. These were not isolated compositions, written for the eyes of a single patron faced with a personal crisis of infertility. As with the adaptors and imitators of Rösslin's *Rosegarden*, these gynaecological writers recognized the existence of a larger discourse on women's diseases and actively tried to contribute to it. While there is no indication that the explosion of new gynaecological literature in the latter half of the sixteenth century was accompanied by the birth of 'the gynaecologist' as a specialist (any more than writing a treatise on 'the French disease' would have made one a syphilologist), this period witnessed the creation of gynaecology as a legitimate, and legitimately distinct, field within medicine.

My interest here, of course, is not to chronicle this whole complicated development of sixteenth-century gynaecological writing, but rather to assess how this enterprise was gendered. Just as medieval authors of gynaecological texts could rarely articulate why gynaecology should be a specialized topic within medicine, so medieval practitioners were decidedly inarticulate on why men could claim expertise in women's medicine. Just as the Faculty of Medicine in Paris had no substantive reply to Jacoba Felicie's claim that women should be treated by other women, so a century later in the case of Jean Domrèmi they could offer no explanation for the continued dominance of women in obstetrics other than to claim lamely that, in accordance with Roman law, women were just 'inspecting' other women's bellies. No justification or rationale for male gynaecological authority was ever articulated, and perhaps none was needed since male practitioners of women's medicine did not yet comprise a distinct textual or social community. In the middle of the sixteenth century that changed. As the field was defined, so too was a sense of who had authoritative knowledge within it. Unsurprisingly, the official 'birth' of gynaecology served to confirm the masculine authority that had already been established in the late Middle Ages rather than to question it. Although the idea of feminine authority in this field was momentarily toyed with, it not simply soon disappeared but was soundly eradicated.

Unlike the birth of obstetrics, which involved a failed humanist revival of Muscio's *Gynaecology*, the birth of gynaecology as its own separate field was very much due to the successes of humanism: in this case, the recovery of the works of (or attributed to) the Father of Medicine, the ancient physician Hippocrates.[88] It

---

[88] The 'prince of physicians', Galen, never wrote any texts specifically on women's conditions other than a work on the anatomy of the uterus. The misascription of the Latin Metrodora translation, *Diseases of Women, Version A* to Galen originated in the 14th-century manuscript

is reflective of his historical moment that when Ludovico Bonacciuoli was writing his treatise on generation for Lucrezia Borgia at the beginning of the sixteenth century, he could only cite Hippocrates through the evidence of the *Aphorisms*, that rather disjointed collection of pithy truisms that taught the physician such things as 'Haemoptysis [coughing up blood] in a woman is removed by an eruption of the menses' (V, 32). In some respects, Bonacciuoli's printed text resembles Bernard Chaussade's manuscript book on fertility in addressing an essentially academic work to an aristocratic female patron. It differed drastically from Chaussade's work, however, in completely rejecting its medieval forebears. Bonacciuoli cites the leading Arabic medieval authors on occasion, but the text overall is a humanistic *tour de force*—literally a revival of the views of the ancients (everyone from Herodotus to Pliny) on the nature of generation and sexual reproduction.

The humanism that characterized Bonacciuoli's work had been spreading throughout medical writing since the 1460s. The most famous call to reject the alleged barbarisms and distortions of medieval Latin writers (and in his case, even Arabic authorities) came from Niccolò Leoniceno of Ferrara. He was only the most extreme of a number of medical writers who believed that the ancients, and particularly the Greeks, held a wisdom that had since been lost to the world.[89] Compare, for example, the early fifteenth-century encyclopedic work of Valesco of Tarenta with that of Alessandro Benedetti (*c*.1450–1513), a Venetian physician who wrote a similarly comprehensive work about a hundred years later. Valesco's *Philonium*, as we have seen, was typical in structure of the medieval medical encyclopedia, his sixth book being devoted to the diseases of the generative organs, both male and female. Valesco usually cited his authorities by name: Bernard of Gordon, Haly Abbas, Constantine, Avicenna. Benedetti, adhering to the same encyclopedic format but writing after the full impact of humanism on medicine, abandoned every one of these medieval authorities, citing instead the wisdom of Paul of Aegina, Galen, Aristotle, and, quite frequently, the naturalist Pliny, whose work he had himself commented on a few years earlier.[90]

With the publication of the complete Hippocratic Corpus in 1525 (and subsequent refinements of the texts in the following years), gynaecology solidified as a 'modern' discipline with its own set of authoritative and (more or less) authentically ancient texts. The rediscovery of the Hippocratic gynaecological

---

tradition and was thus carried over to the printed *Opera omnia* of 1490. Galen's authorship was finally rejected in the 1530s.

[89] Vivian Nutton, 'The Rise of Medical Humanism: Ferrara, 1464–1555', *Renaissance Studies* 11 (1997), 2–19.

[90] Alessandro Benedetti, *Collectiones medicinae*, originally published Venice, 1493; I have used the 1549 Basel edition, here entitled *De omnium a uertice ad plantam morborum signis, causis, differentijs, indicationibus et remedijs tam simplicibus quam compositis*, in Benedetti's collected works, *De re medica opus insigne* (Basel: Henricus Petrus, 1549).

corpus, which had been so poorly preserved in the early Middle Ages as to have no cohesive identity,[91] solidified the field of gynaecology not only as a masculine preserve but specifically as a legitimate area of *specialization of knowledge*. As the Hippocratic author of *Diseases of Women I* had stressed, 'The healing of women's diseases differs greatly from the healing of men's diseases', and this assertion became the mantra on which sixteenth-century gynaecological writers established the legitimacy of their field.[92] Obviously, the Hippocratic gynaecological texts did not effect a transformation overnight. Unaccompanied by any ancient commentary tradition and themselves quite inconsistent in the views of the female body that they proposed, the works were hardly transparent in meaning or significance. Yet whereas the Frenchman Nicholas de La Roche (fl. 1516–42) could, in 1542, still write a gynaecological treatise very similar to a late medieval one with citation piled on citation and no overarching *theory* of what made women's diseases distinct, Giovanni Battista da Monte's (1498–1551) *Brief Works on Uterine Affections*, first published posthumously in Venice in 1554, used the Hippocratic text *Diseases of Women 1* as the basis for his argument that a specific focus on the uterus was needed because it was itself one of the vital organs, tied to all the others and afflicted by its own diseases both frequent and difficult of cure.[93]

I am by no means arguing, of course, that this intense level of activity can be credited in its entirety to the rediscovery of a handful of ancient Greek texts. After all, there was more than a two-decade gap between Calvi's publication of Latin translations of the Hippocratic gynaecology and the publication of any of the 'new' gynaecology influenced by it.[94] Georg Kraut's initial publication of the *Trotula* in 1544, which he treated as a rare discovery of a 'very ancient' text, is itself witness to the slow realization of the possibilities for re-visioning the field of women's medicine that the Hippocratic texts held in store.[95] And

[91] Monica H. Green, 'The Transmission of Ancient Theories of Female Physiology and Disease Through the Early Middle Ages', PhD dissertation, Princeton University, 1985.

[92] For example, in his preface to the third and largest edition of the massive gynaecological compendium, *Gynaeciorum libri*, Israel Spach mimed exactly the arguments from the Hippocratic *Diseases of Women I* in claiming how great the multitude of women's diseases are; the difficulty of recognizing these diseases until they have become inveterate; the ignorance of physicians in diagnosing these diseases, which is compounded by women's reluctance to reveal them; and the problems caused by physicians' treatment of women's conditions as if they were men's diseases (*viriles*). Hence, 'women's and men's diseases differ very much in their treatment' (*Multum enim muliebres morbi et viriles curatione discrepant*). Israel Spach, ed., *Gynaeciorum sive de Mulierum tum communibus, tum gravidarum, parientium et puerperarum affectibus et morbis libri Graecorum, Arabum, Latinorum veterum et recentium quotquot extant, partim nunc primum editi, partim vero denuo recogniti, emendati* (Strasburg: Lazarus Zetzner, 1597), ff. [ii]r–[iii]r.

[93] See Appendix 2, items 24 and 32.

[94] A second translation of the Hippocratic corpus in fact seems to have become the more standard one.

[95] On the major 'emendations' that Kraut made in his edition of the *Trotula*, see Monica H. Green, 'In Search of an 'Authentic' Women's Medicine: The Strange Fates of Trota of

even once its potential was recognized, the Hippocratic gynaecology still posed major challenges of interpretation, for there was much in its conceptualization of the basic mechanics of physiology that did not gibe with the Galenic paradigm that had dominated western medicine for the past 500 years. Indeed, it has been argued that only when physicians learned how to read the Hippocratic gynaecology through Galenic eyes did it become a viable resource for commentary and elaboration.[96]

The ability to reframe gynaecology as a specialty, with its focus on the singular organ of the uterus, depended on other transformations in sixteenth-century medicine as well. The anatomical studies of the late fifteenth and first half of the sixteenth century had radically transformed what could be known about the uterus and its structure.[97] The medieval schematized images of the female genitalia, as well as the 'disease woman', were displaced first by a figure of a seated woman, 'drawn from life' with internal organs displayed, in the widely circulating *Medical Pamphlet* and then, after the publication of Vesalius's *Six [Anatomical] Tables* in 1538, by new images of the female body circulating as fugitive sheets with flaps that could be lifted to show the internal organs.[98] Debates about the nature and function of the clitoris began in the latter half of the century, and already by 1583 Felix Platter (1536–1614), professor of anatomy at Basel University, provided the first comprehensive and systematic account of the peculiar features of the female skeleton, including a detailed woodcut.[99] Ambroise Paré's innovation in publishing a specialized text on emergency obstetrics for

Salerno and Hildegard of Bingen', *Dynamis: Acta Hispanica ad Medicinae Scientiarumque Historiam Illustrandam* 19 (1999), 25–54; and Green, *Trotula*, pp. xi–xiii and 59–60.

[96] Helen King, *The Disease of Virgins: Green Sickness, Chlorosis, and the Problems of Puberty* (New York: Routledge, 2003).

[97] These anatomical developments are fully recounted in Park, *Secrets of Women*.

[98] The so-called pseudo-Ketham *Fasciculus medicinae* was originally published in 1491 with a simple reproduction of the 'disease woman'; by 1494, however, in an Italian edition from Venice, the internal organs were completely redrawn and the accompanying text rewritten to focus on the anatomy of the reproductive organs rather than diseases in general. See Park, *Secrets of Women*. On the fugitive sheets, see Andrea Carlino, *Paper Bodies: A Catalogue of Anatomical Fugitive Sheets*, trans. Noga Arika (London: Wellcome Institute for the History of Medicine, 1999); and Karen Rosoff Encarnación, 'The Proper Uses of Desire: Sex and Procreation in Reformation Anatomical Fugitive Sheets', in *The Material Culture of Sex, Procreation, and Marriage in Premodern Europe*, ed. Anne L. McClanan and Karen Rosoff Encarnación (New York: Palgrave, 2002), pp. 221–49. Already in 1540 the second English translator of Rösslin's *Rosegarden*, Thomas Raynalde (or the publisher of that same name who brought out the 1540 edition), owned a copy of 'an anatomical print graven in copper the one man the other woman with their Intrayles thereto belonging'; I. Gadd, 'Raynald, Thomas (fl. 1539–52?)', *Oxford Dictionary of National Biography* (Oxford: Oxford University Press, 2004), online edition, <http://www.oxforddnb.com.library.lib.asu.edu:80/view/article/23209> accessed 24 December 2004.

[99] Katharine Park, 'The Rediscovery of the Clitoris: French Medicine and the *Tribade*, 1570–1620', in *The Body in Parts: Fantasies of Corporeality in Early Modern Europe*, ed. David Hillman and Carla Mazzio (New York: Routledge, 1997), 171–93; and Michael Stolberg, 'A Woman Down to Her Bones: The Anatomy of Sexual Difference in Early Modern Europe', *Isis* 94 (2003), 274–99.

fellow male surgeons was followed in the 1580s by a controversy about whether Caesarean sections could be performed on living women, with good results for both mother and child.[100]

The rediscovery of the Greek Hippocratic gynaecological texts would be followed by reclamation of the Greek gynaecological works of Rufus of Ephesus, fragments of Soranus, and 'Moschion', that is, our old friend Muscio, whose Latin *Gynaecology* had been translated into Greek in the late medieval period and then 'rediscovered' as another witness to the greatness of Greek medicine. One final ancient author was admitted to this select company: the ancient male Latin author Eros, who through philological genius was reclaimed for the field of gynaecology in 1555. 'He' forms the end of our story, for with his addition to the pantheon of gynaecological authorities, the demise of women's authority was complete.

Georg Kraut's publication of the *Trotula* in 1544 was ironic not simply because the texts were no longer much used even in the fifteenth century except in England (where they had always been popular) and central Europe (where students and masters at newly founded universities seem to have welcomed having copies), but also because he deliberately altered the text to make it look more 'ancient' than it was by classicizing the language and removing the more obvious medieval references. It is no coincidence that its second appearance in print three years later was in a collection of *ancient* medical writings.[101] In both of his editions of the *Gynaeciorum* (1566 and 1586–88), Hans Caspar Wolf republished Kraut's revised text of the *Trotula* but added one important innovation. He changed the attribution from 'Trotula' to Eros, a freed male slave of the Roman empress Julia: 'The book of women's matters of Eros, physician [and] freedman of Julia, whom some have absurdly named 'Trotula'' (*Erotis medici liberti Iuliae, quem aliqui Trotulam inepte nominant, muliebrium liber*).[102] Wolf apparently borrowed this fantastic thesis from Hadrianus Junius (Aadrian DeJonghe, 1511–75), a Dutch physician who had asserted in 1556 that textual corruptions accounted for the false attribution of numerous texts, among them the work of

Eros Iuliae the physician, a freedman who took his name from Julia Augusta, his mistress, [who] by corrupted nomenclature is now called Trotula or Eroiulia, a phrasing less than latinate due to the fault of the barbarous age; this is the in no way idle judgement of the learned Morillonus.[103]

---

[100] On François Rousset, see Appendix 2, items 60, 68, and 73. Most recently on the controversy involving his claims about Caesarean section, see Nutton and Nutton, 'Archer of Meudun', pp. 415–18.

[101] See Green, 'In Search of an 'Authentic' Women's Medicine'.

[102] Caspar Wolf, ed., *Gynaeciorum, hoc est de Mulierum tum aliis, tum gravidarum, parientium et puerperarum affectibus et morbis libri veterum ac recentiorem aliquot, partim nunc primum editi, partim multo quam ante castigatiores . . . .* (Basel: Thomas Guarinus, 1566), coll. 215–16.

[103] Hadrianus Junius, *Animadversionum libri sex, omnigenae lectionis thesaurus, in quibus infiniti penè autorum loci corriguntur et declarantur, nunc primùm et nati, et in lucem aediti* (Basel: Isengrinus,

I have thus far been unable to find anything about this 'learned Morillonus', but I suspect he came to his conclusion through the inventive hypothesis that

TROTVLAE LIBER DE PASSIONIBVS MVLIERVM

was somehow a corruption of the abbreviation:

EROT. IVLIAE LIBERT. DE PASS. MVL.,

the initial capital 'E' having been misread as a 'T' with other misreadings following from there.

Not surprisingly, the assertion is contradicted by nearly every historical reference in the text. Even with all of Kraut's deletions of telltale signs of medievalness, Eros's alleged connection to the Empress Julia, daughter of Augustus Caesar, would place him in the first century CE, rendering somewhat problematic the numerous references to Galen (129–c.216/17 CE) and the one to Paul of Aegina (seventh century CE).[104] Even allowing for the humanists' still vague understanding of ancient medical chronology, the hypothesis suggests the power of romanticized humanistic views of Antiquity. Interestingly, Wolf did not delete or alter 'Trotula's' name in the anecdote of her famous cure within the text, and it is unclear how he explained to himself her continued presence. He did, nevertheless, have the circumspection to change the feminine participle in the prologue that referred to the authoress (*compulsa*, 'I was moved [to write]') to the masculine form *compulsus*.

It seems unlikely that this final suppression of 'Trotula's' existence was deliberately misogynistic for the simple reason that deliberate misogyny was unnecessary. Masculine authority in women's medicine—now both emergency obstetrics and gynaecology—seemed so normative by the mid sixteenth century that there was no question of 'suppressing' women's authority since no one imagined they had any authority to suppress. Despite the 'Debate over Women' (*Querelle des femmes*) that had been going on in intellectual circles throughout Europe since the late fourteenth century, I believe there was no 'gender question' on the topic of women's roles in medical practice. Morillonus, DeJonghe, and Wolf were simply delighting in their own philological cleverness, rewriting the history of gynaecology in the image that they had of it in their own time.

The irrelevance of women's authority can equally be seen in the otherwise surprising neglect of that 'very ancient book' that the humanist Francesco Filelfo had been begging to borrow from the Milanese physician Filippo Pelliccione in 1449.[105] Discovered in 1427, the Milanese manuscript passed through

---

1556), p. 250. For Junius's biography, see Rochus von Liliencron, *et al.* (eds.), *Allgemeine Deutsche Biographie*, 56 vols. (Leipzig: Duncker and Humblot, 1875–1912), 4:736–7.

[104] References to the 12th-century Salernitans Copho and Magister Ferrarius remained in the text, but given their relative obscurity the chronological difficulties they posed may have not been immediately perceptible.

[105] See the Preface above. This manuscript is now Florence, Biblioteca Laurenziana Medicea, MS Plut. 73.1, s. ix ex./x in. See Augusto Beccaria, *I codici di medicina del periodo presalernitano*

the hands of at least ten different philologists and physicians over the course of the fifteenth century and was used for the first edition of the Roman Celsus's *On Medicine* in 1478. Yet it was not until 1494 that anyone bothered to copy out the gynaecological texts that included the references to 'certain women' that Filelfo had noted.[106] Even then, it seems, it was copied more out of philological interest than medical. Neither the *Gynaecology of Cleopatra* nor the *Book of Soteris* (a probably apocryphal dialogue between Soranus and a female student) nor even Muscio's Latin *Gynaecology* was ever published in full in the Renaissance. Rather, the late antique legacy of midwifery literature was condensed into a brief *Harmony of Gynaecologies* that Caspar Wolf compiled for the first edition of his *Gynaeciorum libri* in 1566. Although Wolf included the prefaces of the works of Muscio, Theodorus Priscianus, and 'Cleopatra'—all of which had indicated that the texts were meant for female audiences—one could easily read Wolf's *Harmony* without ever grasping the fact that these works depicted a world of gendered medical practice completely at odds with that prevailing in early modern Europe.[107]

The irrelevance of female authority is registered, too, in the genealogies that later sixteenth-century physicians wrote of their profession. Conrad Gesner's *Bibliotheca Universalis* of 1545, a massive medical bibliography, initiated the genre, while Israel Spach's *Nomenclator scriptorum medicorum* of 1591 was organized by subject for the first time. He includes works of 1436 medical authors, eighteen of whom are said to have written *De morbis mulierum* ('On the diseases of women'). 'Trotula' is mentioned here only as the 'absurd' false attribution of the work of Eros; the only other women listed are Cleopatra and Soteris, both of whom are identified from the Milanese manuscript.[108] Fifteen

---

(secoli IX, X e XI) (Rome: Storia e Letteratura, 1956), pp. 277–79. The general medical textbook of the non-physician Celsus generated enormous excitement because his prose was considered almost the equal of Cicero's. The first copy of the gynaecological material was made in 1494 apparently by Poliziano and his associates (now BAV, MS Vat. lat. 6337). To this day the bulk of the gynaecological material in this manuscript has never been edited or subjected to rigorous analysis.

[106] The manuscript contains gynaecological texts attributed to, addressed to, or mentioning several women: the female physician Theodote, who is said to have served the Egyptian queen Cleopatra and her sister Arsinoë; a midwife Soteris, who engages, as the pupil, in a master–pupil dialogue with the great Greek physician Soranus; a queen Fabiana Priscilla, who is mentioned as the author of a particular remedy for uterine difficulties; and a *medica* (female healer) Victoria, to whom a male author, Theodorus Priscianus, dedicates his short tract on women's diseases. The six-part *Liber ad Soteris* is so textually complicated that it is not yet possible to untangle any clear authorial entity.

[107] Wolf's *Harmonia gynaeciorum* (see Appendix 2, item 48) is a badly confused text, largely because Wolf was unable to unravel the complicated textual traditions of the late antique and early medieval gynaecological corpus. The Byzantine Greek translation of Muscio was published in full (*ibid.*, item 46), but it lacked the preface to the Latin original which had explained that the work's intended audience was midwives. Caelius Aurelianus's text was never discovered in the Renaissance and even now is known only through a single copy where it was fused with Muscio's text.

[108] Israel Spach, *Nomenclator scriptorum medicorum. Hoc est: Elenchus eorum, qui artem medicam suis scriptis illustrarunt, secundum locos communes ipsius Medicinae; cum duplici Indice et rerum et authorum* (Frankfurt: Nicolaus Bassaeus and Lazarus Zetznerus, 1591), p. 130.

years later, in 1606, the German physician Johan Georg Schenk published the first extended list of gynaecological authors.[109] The list, which went on for a full twenty pages, included the names of several dozen Greek, Latin, Arab, medieval, and Renaissance authors. Together with the massive volumes of the *Books of Gynaecology* themselves, Schenk's list served as a manifesto that gynaecology had 'arrived' as its own special field. The female authors included here were Cleopatra, Satyra, and Sotira. Schenck claims that 'Satyra's' work was found in the famous Milanese codex (where her name is actually spelled 'Soteris'), and he suggests that she may be the same as the 'Sotira' mentioned by Pliny in his *Natural History*.[110] In other words, these two or three ancient female authorities in gynaecology are validated because there was considerable ancient testimony to confirm their existence. It was only because of his commitment to humanism and its valorization of ancient medicine, therefore, that Schenk did not erase female authority entirely from the record.

Identifying Cleopatra and Satyra/Sotira as gynaecological authorities was also unproblematic precisely because they were so far distant. Other names of female medical authorities would likewise be dredged from the ancient record: Medea, Circe, Anguitia, Ocyroe, Hepione, Aspasia, Agameda, and other women of ancient myth and legend would be enumerated in Schenk's list and others. Yet in only one of these lists have I found a contemporary name: in 1598, Fortunato Fidele (*c.*1550–1630) published a brief list of women of *clara fama* ('noble fame') known for their medical skill among whom he included Sentia Salernitana, 'of recent memory'.[111] The question is not, of course, whether women completely ceased medical practice in the sixteenth century; as I will clarify in the Conclusion, they clearly did not. Rather, the question is whether in their conception of their new specialized field of *gynaikeia*, learned male

[109] Johannes Schenck, *Elenchus auctorum in re medica cluentium, qui gynaecia scriptis clararunt et illustrarunt*, published in Joannes Andernacus Guinterius (1487–1574), *Gynaeciorum commentarius, de gravidarum, parturientium puerperarum et infantium, cura. Nunc primum a Schenkiana bibliotheca in lucem emissus.* (Strasburg: Lazar Zetzner, 1609), pp. 37–56.

[110] Since Pliny and other ancient writers in fact list some half dozen different female authorities—a fact Schenk must certainly have been familiar with—Schenk's decision to omit these other names can only be explained by his chosen emphasis on gynaecological *writers*. That is, Pliny's 'Sotira' could be conflated with the 'Soteris' of the Milan manuscript, whereas none of the other female authorities aside from Cleopatra could be connected with extant texts. For a comprehensive listing of female medical authorities and practitioners in Antiquity, see Rebecca Flemming, *Medicine and the Making of Roman Women: Gender, Nature, and Authority from Celsus to Galen* (Oxford: Oxford University Press, 2001).

[111] Fortunatus Fidelis, *Bissus, seu medicinae patrocinium quatuor libris distinctum* (Palermo, 1598), Book II, cap. 12, p. 116: 'Verum fuisse olim non paucas mulieres, artis medicae haud in celebres: ne hac in re fortasse ambigas: non solum amplissimum est Platonis testimonium, qui in sua republica nullo discrimine, et viros et feminas ad medendi usum admittit: sed etiam apud Iureconsultos medicina facere liceat: Clara etiam sunt medicarum mulierum nomina, Medea, Circe, Anguitia, Ocyroe, Hepione, Aspasia, Agameda, Cleopatra, et nostra memoria Sentia Salernitana; multaeque praeterea aliae, quas, ne longus sim, minime attengo.' My thanks to Patricia Skinner for checking Fidele's text in the British Library copy.

writers could acknowledge a woman as their equal. The suppression of 'Trotula's' authority, the neglect of the 'certain women' of the Milanese manuscript, and the creation of lists of gynaecological authorities that limited the female entries to a handful of ancient or even mythological women—all at the same time that the authority of the father of medicine, Hippocrates, was being elevated further and further—secured the position of gynaecology as a field of masculine expertise.

In 1551, a printer in Frankfurt produced an edition of the long popular *Regimen of the School of Salerno*, a verse regimen of health composed probably in the early thirteenth century and reprinted dozens of times in the Renaissance. In this particular case, he included a woodcut depicting a female student at the medical school of Salerno (Fig. 6.1).[112] Perhaps as much as 'Trotula', the undifferentiated 'women of Salerno' *(mulieres Salernitane)* were well known throughout medieval Europe, primarily because of the several references to them in the single most popular work on *materia medica*, the *Circa instans* often attributed to the Salernitan physician Mattheus Platearius.[113] As late as the middle of the sixteenth century, at least certain readers were still willing to entertain the idea not simply of female medical expertise, but of *learned* female expertise on a par with that of men. By the time the next edition of the *Regimen* appeared in 1555, however, the classroom scene had disappeared, to be replaced by one showing the male masters of Salerno presenting their book to the English

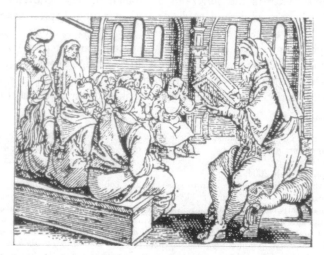

FIG. 6.1 A sixteenth-century woodcut depicting a female student at the medical school of Salerno.

---

[112] From Johannes Curion and Jacob Crell (eds.), *De conservanda bona valetudine opusculum scholae Salernitanae* (Frankfurt: Christian Egenolph, 1551).

[113] See Chapters 1 and 5 above. These references to the *mulieres* were usually included when the *Circa instans* was enlarged and/or translated into the vernacular, which happened numerous times.

king who had requested it. Even the fantasy of female medical authority conjured up by that single classroom scene was no longer tenable.

In March of 1578, the physician Corc Óg Ó Cadhla resided temporarily at the house of Brian Caomhánach in Kilkenny County, Ireland. He was there to treat Caomhánach's two daughters for menstrual disorders.[114] Corc Óg Ó Cadhla is no representative of a radical Renaissance transformation in medicine. A century after the printing press began to put medical texts into mass production, he is copying out an entire medical encyclopedia by hand, wishing he had proper vellum to write on instead of paper and apologizing that his handwriting is not better. A century after Niccolò Leoniceno had called for rejection of the corrupted texts and even more corrupted Latinity of medieval writers, he is copying, in Irish, Bernard of Gordon's early fourteenth-century text, the *Lily of Medicine*, which could hardly have been considered cutting edge even 200 years earlier. Yet in coming into the home of this mighty man, Brian Caomhánach, and treating his daughters for their gynaecological complaints, Corc Óg Ó Cadhla, off at the edges of Europe, shows the breadth of the successful masculinization of gynaecology.

Gynaecology was not uniformly incorporated into the practice of all fifteenth- and sixteenth-century physicians and surgeons, of course. There is no obstetrical material whatsoever in the *Surgery* of the Italian surgeon, Giovanni da Vigo (1450–1525), for example, and besides several substantive chapters on apostemes, indurations, and ulcers of the breasts, he limits his gynaecological material to the three perfunctory chapters on ulcers of the vagina and uterus.[115] Yet as with the exceptional cases we saw in the Middle Ages, da Vigo's context explains this lacuna: he spent the bulk of his career in service to a series of popes, in whose courts his interactions with female patients are likely to have been very limited.[116]

---

[114] Aoibheann Nic Dhonnchadha, 'Medical Writing in Irish, 1400–1700', in J. B. Lyons, ed., *Two Thousand Years of Irish Medicine* (Dublin, 1999); repr. *Irish Medical Journal of Medical Science* 169, no. 3 (July–Sept. 2000), 217–20; available at <http://www.celt.dias.ie/gaeilge/staff/rcsi1.html> accessed 13 July 2004.

[115] Giovanni da Vigo, *Practica in chirurgia* (Lyons: Jacob Myr, 1516); the chapters on the breasts appear on ff. 49va–52ra and f. 113ra–b, while those on the uterus and vagina appear on f. 121ra–vb. His chapters on conditions of the male genitalia, including hernia, run to at least ten times this length. Since the chapters on female conditions do contain a few references to personal practice or assertions of efficacy (e.g., *ista medella mamille imposita lactis exiccationem potenter effectum prestat* [50ra], *vidimus in tempestate nostra in nonnullis mulieribus tali apostemate laborantibus* [50rb], *vt plerumque vidimus euenire in tali dispositione* [f. 51va], *collirium, quod ego sepe numero expertus sum* [121vb]), I imagine da Vigo is reflecting practice he had among the wives of courtiers, household servants, and perhaps also visitors to the papal courts. Note that in the chapters on the genitalia, his analogous reasoning with conditions of the penis and anus is apparent.

[116] In her study of Avignon in the later 14th century (where the papal court was at the time ensconced), Joëlle Rollo-Koster found only five women in the employ of the pope: three washerwomen and two provisioners of textiles. See Rollo-Koster, 'The Women of Papal Avignon. A New Source: The *Liber Divisionis* of 1371', *The Journal of Women's History* 8 (Spring 1996): 36–59, at p. 45.

Nor was the geographic spread of this Renaissance 'revolution' uniform. Gynaecology in fifteenth-century England, although itself demonstrating signs of increased development, was largely unaffected by the new writing on the Continent.[117] In the sixteenth century, aside from Richard Jonas who translated Rösslin's *Rosegarden* into English in 1540 and Thomas Raynalde who revised it in 1545, none of the several dozen 'modern' authors on women's medicine hailed from England, and it would not be until well into the seventeenth century that England produced any gynaecological work of international prominence.[118] Nevertheless, even here there is evidence for the normativeness of male interest in and practice of gynaecology, as well as for the erasure of female authority. Robert Green of Welby, for example, while copying out a Middle English version of the *Trotula* in 1544, ascribed authorship not to 'a woman named Rota' (as had the other, earlier copy of this version) but to 'one expert in the anatomy and special [things] concerning the parts of a woman and the diseases often happening to them'. He does not explicitly say this was a man, but neither does he raise the possibility of female authorship. Later in the century, John Wotton, MD, bound a mid fifteenth-century copy of the Middle English *Sickness of Women 2*—a text explicitly addressed to women—in with his own handwritten, alphabetically arranged medical notes. The substantial sections of the latter devoted to gynaecology and obstetrics confirm his interest in women's diseases, while his references to Conrad Gesner (who had edited the Greek translation of Muscio's *Gynaecology* in 1565) show his engagement with gynaecological discourses on the Continent.[119] Another fifteenth-century copy of the *Sickness of Women* was owned by Richard Ferris, a master of the Barbers' and Surgeons' Company and sergeant surgeon to Queen Elizabeth; from him, the manuscript passed to John Felde (*c*.1520–87), an astrologer and associate of John Dee (1527–1609), who himself served the Queen as her philosopher. Dee, owner of a variety of manuscripts and printed texts on women's diseases and 'women's nature',[120] kept exhaustively detailed notes on his wife's menstrual cycles and

[117] The only sign that Italian or French developments reached England is the acquisition by the London physician, Roger Marchall (d. 1477), of a copy of Niccolò Falcucci's *Sermon* on the generative organs after mid century (Manchester, Chetham's Library, MS 27857 (Mun. A.3.134), s. xv², Flanders?).

[118] The national origins of the 16th-century writers represented in the 1597 edition of the *Gynaeciorum libri* were as follows: Germany and Switzerland (Platter, Ruf, Bauhin), France (de La Roche, du Bois, Le Bon, Paré, Rousset, de la Corde, Akakia, Jean d'Ailleboust), Italy (Bonacciuoli, Mercurialis, da Monte, Trincavelli, Bottoni), Spain (Mercato). England's late embrace of medical humanism was not distinct to gynaecology but a general characteristic; see Vivian Nutton, ' "A Diet for Barbarians": Introducing Renaissance Medicine to Tudor England', in *Natural Particulars: Nature and the Disciplines in Renaissance Europe*, ed. A. Grafton, N. G. Siraisi (Cambridge, MA: MIT Press, 2000), 275–94.

[119] For more on this manuscript, see Monica H. Green, 'Masses in Remembrance of "Seynt Susanne": A Fifteenth-Century Spiritual Regimen', *Notes and Queries* n. s. 50, no. 4 (December 2003), 380–4.

[120] The manuscript owned by Ferris and Felde is BLL, MS Sloane 2463, s. xv med. On Dee's selectivity in book buying, see Julian Roberts and Andrew Watson (eds.), *John Dee's Library*

recorded the astrological configurations at the times of their sexual couplings; he even examined a miscarried foetus early in their marriage, noting its indistinct form.[121] The unorthodox physician and occultist, Simon Forman (1552–1611), seems to have had a particularly successful gynaecological practice: 38 per cent of the female patients who consulted him came with gynaecological problems.[122] Mark Jameson (d. 1592), a clergyman and sometime medical practitioner in Glasgow, plotted out (at least on paper) a medicinal garden that contained a surprisingly high percentage of herbs with gynaecological and obstetrical properties. His annotations in his copy of Savonarola's *Practica* confirm his concern with menstrual difficulties.[123]

Gynaecology in sixteenth-century Europe was united neither by a single theoretical perspective nor a single group of authoritative texts that all practitioners would have acknowledged. Rather, the common element shared throughout Europe was the acceptability—and the *respectability*—of masculine interest in gynaecological and even obstetrical matters. Corc Óg Ó Cadhla could be called into the house of Brian Caomhánach to treat his daughters with no slur on the reputation of either the two men or the two women involved, in the same way that Michele Savonarola could involve himself in the medical care of the upper-class women of fifteenth-century Ferrara. When the Hippocratic gynaecological texts were rediscovered, there was no need to reconceive gynaecology or emergency obstetrics as a field where masculine involvement was appropriate. No *social* changes in medical practice (either in the relationship of physicians to midwives or male physicians to their female patients) were needed. Indeed, one might postulate that sixteenth-century gynaecology might have developed along much the same social path (if perhaps with somewhat less intellectual confidence) even if the Hippocratic gynaecology had never been rediscovered. The humanists never did find what was, in fact, the greatest ancient work in the field, Soranus's *Gynaecology*, and it seems likely that, had they done so, they would have been shocked by his assumption that the *midwife*, no less than male physicians or surgeons, was expected to be 'well versed in theory' and 'trained in all branches of therapy' (including diet, surgery, and drugs).[124]

Catalogue (London: Bibliographical Society, 1990), p. 14. For the *Trotula* manuscripts owned by Dee, see Appendix 1, item 33. Among his printed books we find a copy of Ruf's *De conceptu hominis* (item 401 in his catalogue), the two Italian treatises by Giovanni Marinelli, *Medicine partinenti alle infermità delle donne* and *Ornamenti delle donne* (items 857 and 858), and pseudo-Albertus Magnus, *De secretis mulierum* (item 2291).

121 Deborah E. Harkness, 'Managing an Experimental Household: The Dees of Mortlake and the Practice of Natural Philosophy', *Isis* 88 (1997), 247–62.

122 Barbara Traister, '"Matrix and the Pain Thereof": A Sixteenth-Century Gynaecological Essay', *Medical History* 35 (1991), 436–51.

123 J. H. Dickson and W. W. Gauld, 'Mark Jameson's Physic Plants: A Sixteenth Century Garden for Gynaecology in Glasgow?', *Scottish Medical Journal* 32 (1987), 60–2. My thanks to Karen Reeds for bringing this important study to my attention.

124 Soranus of Ephesus, *Soranus' Gynecology*, trans. Owsei Temkin (Baltimore: Johns Hopkins University Press, 1956; rept. 1991), p. 6. The only portion of Soranus's *Gynecology* known in the

Obviously, we do not yet know how far male gynaecological practice extended beyond social elites and major urban centres. Nor do we have much evidence whether female patients themselves offerred continuing resistance to the sight or touch of their genitalia by male practitioners. But some sense of the *normativeness* of male gynaecological and emergency obstetrical practice can be gleaned from sources far outside the learned and specialized medical treatises of physicians and surgeons themselves. Whereas male physicians and surgeons had only appeared in earlier hagiographic accounts long after the birth was over (as we saw in the cases of Flore Nicole and Dulceta of Marseille), by the later fifteenth century and even more so the sixteenth their presence at birth scenes is so routine as to be unworthy of special comment. In 1477, a Franciscan friar, Bartholomeus de Colle, brought up to date the collection of miracle stories connected with an early thirteenth-century secular Franciscan, Luchesius of Umbria. One was a story of how a woman labouring with a dead foetus was saved by a cloth that had been rubbed against the sainted man's relics. The woman, Bartholomeus tells us, had already 'tried the aid of physicians to no purpose, and had sought out in vain every remedy of old women and midwives'.[125] Bartholomeus's pairing of midwives *and* physicians as the normative authorities to summon in cases of difficult childbirth would be found in saints' lives throughout the sixteenth century. Ambrogio Taëgio, an early sixteenth-century Dominican writing some addenda to the miracles of a medieval inquisitor, Petrus Martyr, tells of a case where 'midwives and other women, *and physicians and surgeons, and many others*' were called in for a difficult labour.[126] The miracle is said to have taken place in 1307, before the involvement of male practitioners in birth would have been normative; I suspect, however, that this element of the story was Ambrogio's own sixteenth-century elaboration. Even the saints had to adjust their narratives to fit the times for much of women's medicine was, as Savonarola recognized, '[no longer] the work of women'.

16th century was a brief excerpt on the anatomy of the genitalia; see Appendix 2, item 37. The fuller text was not rediscovered until the nineteenth century, and even then with major sections missing. See Ann Ellis Hanson and Monica H. Green, 'Soranus of Ephesus: *Methodicorum princeps*', in Wolfgang Haase and Hildegard Temporini, eds., *Aufstieg und Niedergang der römischen Welt*, Teilband II, Band 37.2 (Berlin and New York: Walter de Gruyter, 1994), pp. 968–1075.

[125] *Acta Sanctorum*, 28 April, B. Lucensis seu Luchesius, cap. 4: 'frustra tentabat medicorum auxilium, et omne muliercularum et obstetricum remedium postulebat in vanum'.

[126] *Acta Sanctorum*, 29 April, S. Petrus Martyr, cap. XI: 'vocatisque obstetricibus et aliis feminis, medicisque ac chirurgicis, et aliis pluribus'. For other references to male practitioners at births, see *Acta Sanctorum*, 8 March, B. Ioannes de Deo (1588); 9 March, B. Catharina Bononiensis (1589); 18 March, B. Saluator de Horta (1600); 5 May, S. Angelus (1577); 17 May, B. Pasqualis Baylon (1595); and 18 June, B. Osanna Andreasia (*c*.1505).

Conclusion:
The Medieval Legacy:
Medicine of, for, and by Women

> Will there ever be a monument to the first woman physician . . . ? We
> need such landmarks of civilization not because those who died have lived
> for fame, no, but because the now-living, as well as those who will live
> long afterward, need encouragement for utilizing their capabilities, and
> monuments of this sort suggest to them the possibility of their so doing.
> The person who is covered by a monument is of no consequence, but the
> fact that a woman can work and make an impression upon civilization needs
> to be known to be remembered.[1]
>
> Marie E. Zakrzewska, MD (1881)

When she was twenty years old, a seventeenth-century German woman named
Justine Siegemund suffered from a morbid uterine growth and prolapse. Only
one of the midwives who attended her (in what they presumed was a regular
pregnancy) recognized the seriousness of her condition. A male physician was
eventually called in and it was to him and his medicines that Siegemund would
credit her cure. Probably because of this early reproductive tragedy, Siegemund
would remain childless the rest of her life. But it was also because of this tragedy
that she went on to study books of midwifery, trying to understand the causes of
obstetrical mishaps. She came to be recognized as an expert on difficult births,
eventually serving various members of the German nobility and producing in
1690 the first female-authored obstetrical text in the German language.[2]

[1] Marie E. Zakrzewska, letter of 28 May 1881, as cited in Agnes C. Vietor (ed.), *A Woman's
Quest: The Life of Marie E. Zakrzewska, M.D.* (New York: D. Appleton and Co., 1924; repr. New
York: Arno Press, 1972), pp. 404–5. On Zakrzewska's views on 'women's place' in medicine,
see Arleen Marcia Tuchman, 'Situating Gender: Marie E. Zakrzewska and the Place of Science in
Women's Medical Education', *Isis* 95 (2004), 34–57.

[2] Justine Siegemund, *The Court Midwife*, ed. and trans. Lynne Tatlock (University of Chicago
Press, 2005). My deepest thanks to Albert Rabil, editor of the Other Voice in Early Modern Europe
series, and Dr Tatlock for allowing me to consult the translation of Siegemund's treatise prior to
publication.

Siegemund was a direct inheritor of the transformations in women's medicine—medicine of, for, and by women—that we have chronicled in this book. The midwife's province as Siegemund depicts it in her book, *The Court Midwife*, is strictly limited to attendance at childbirth: the good midwife has knowledge to identify and then manually rectify malpresentations, but she should also turn to a male physician for advice when the gravity of the situation exceeds her skill.[3] The midwife of Siegemund's text performs some minor surgical procedures (such as using simple tools to extract uterine growths or dead foetuses), but she prescribes no medicines nor does she involve herself in any gynaecological conditions. Ironically, Siegemund was herself further weakening the very tenuous bond of gender—the linking of sexual identity so closely with notions of sexual modesty and the presumed 'natural' knowledge of women—that had kept routine childbirth attendance in women's hands throughout the medieval and early modern period. As a childless woman, she, like male physicians and surgeons, had to argue that *her learning* trumped the personal physical experience of motherhood and birth thought to qualify the traditional midwife. It is not merely fortuitous or coincidental, therefore, that the idealized midwife of Siegemund's text, whether student or teacher, is literate.

The nineteenth-century German midwife-turned-physician, Marie Zakrzewska, quoted above, can be placed in a direct line with the learned midwifery traditions that Siegemund represents. Where Zakrzewska differs radically from Siegemund, however, is that she, like hundreds of other women in her day, challenged the circumscription of women to the medical roles of midwife or nurse, claiming that women had the same rights and capabilities to practise learned medicine, in all its forms, as men did. The women of Zakrzewska's generation mounted a modern challenge to the gendering of learned medicine that had been established between the twelfth and sixteenth centuries, a challenge far more articulate and self-conscious (and perhaps, for that reason, more swift in its effects) than the slow masculinization of women's medicine in the later Middle Ages.

It is not my intent to chronicle these modern developments in this conclusion, though I would like briefly to ponder some morals that this story of medieval and early Renaissance women's medicine has for women's history more generally. There are many respects in which the masculine birth of gynaecology (and its parallel plot of women's exclusion from that birth) mirrors general narratives in European women's history that have developed over the last three decades. In terms of women's labour activities, for example, this story parallels quite closely what is now known about the increasing pressures pushing women out of the public labour force into a more domestic, economically dependent sphere. There are also some ways in which medicine's narrative differs from other areas of women's history: medieval women's multiple levels of engagement with both

---

[3] Siegemund's relations with male surgeons were much more contentious because they were more directly challenging midwives' monopoly over childbirth.

institutionalized and non-institutionalized religion, for example, were far more extensive than their presence in the field of medical practice, which was in turn a far more permeable field than law.

There are also certain morals of this story that tie the history of medicine to that of literacy. While the suppression of women's authority in the male spheres of literate, professionalized medicine was nearly absolute, women were never completely passive in the face of masculine dominance. Certain kinds of female medical practice never disappeared and, in a stunning turnabout, women in the sixteenth and seventeenth centuries, at least those of the upper classes, created an entirely new kind of women's medical authority in the domestic sphere: they created their own, largely feminine genre of medical writing, a new take on an old standard, the recipe collection. The seventeenth century also witnessed the appearance of the first women to write specifically on women's medicine since Trota. What even these women could not do, however, was reverse men's dominance over learned interpretations of women's medicine: if they moved beyond the field of childbirth assistance, these female midwifery writers did so in large part by relying on male authorities.[4]

What difference does it make whether women's medicine is constructed at its theoretical base, or practised in its clinical mode, by men rather than women? I have deliberately avoided throughout this book any discussion of the efficacy of the medicine theorized or practised by medieval men and women. As I will explain below, I don't believe there is any universal standard we can use to assess whether men's or women's medicine was 'better'. What we can do, however, is assess how far, how deeply, how profoundly, the medieval gender systems *made a difference* in how men vs. women theorized and practised 'women's medicine'. Gender, as modern theorists have come to understand it, is not simply a way of creating difference in a society. More importantly, it is a way of creating social inequality, differentials in power based on those (real or constructed) differences. Women may, at certain moments, have had separate traditions of medical knowledge-production and practice, but they never had equal ones, not even in Salerno. Thus, the issue is not 'what men did to women' as if in some grand conspiracy, but rather how much women, be they patients or practitioners, could or could not do for themselves.

It is this issue of women's ability to act as their own medical agents that leads me, finally, to ask how the *history* of women's agency in medicine itself functions

---

[4] Siegemund, whose work is strictly limited to difficult childbirth, cites by name only the Dutch anatomist Regnier de Graaf; her descriptions of the processes of labour (especially effacement) are strikingly original. Her predecessors Louise Bourgeois and Jane Sharp, who include more material on anatomy, infertility, and some other gynaecological conditions, are heavily dependent on prior textual authorities (all male-authored, of course), even if they remake them in novel ways; see Bridgette Ann Majella Sheridan, 'Childbirth, Midwifery, and Science: The Life and Work of the French Royal Midwife Louise Bourgeois (1563–1636)', PhD dissertation, Boston College, 2002; and Elaine Hobby, 'Gender, Science and Midwifery: Jane Sharp, *The Midwives Book* (1671)', in *The Arts of Seventeenth Century Science: Representations of the Natural World in European and North American Culture*, ed. Claire Jowitt and Diane Watt (Aldershot: Ashgate, 2002), pp. 146–59.

as a mechanism of stake-claiming, of carving out for women a place and a sense of legitimate ownership in the realm of healthcare. As the quotation from the nineteenth-century physician Marie Zakrzewska makes clear, history itself can function as a motivating force in women's engagements with medicine. Whereas Jacoba Felicie in the fourteenth century and even Perretta Petone in the early fifteenth century could readily identify with the female medical practitioners around them in Paris (even if only to argue 'If they can practise, why can't I?'), the late medieval/Renaissance erasure of female medical authority seems to have been quite effective: early modern women knew nothing of any female traditions of medical practice beyond midwifery and the domestic medicine they themselves practised in their homes. Although the present study is hardly the monument to female practitioners that Dr Zakrzewska envisioned, her acute observations on the historically contingent meanings of history do suggest why the laboured masculine birth of gynaecology over the course of the twelfth through sixteenth centuries remains relevant to us today.

'WHAT I HAVE LEARNED FROM MIDWIVES': THE MEDICAL AUTHORITY OF WOMEN

The maturing of gynaecology as an intellectually specialized discipline can be called a 'masculine birth' not only in the sense that it became a field dominated by (and in its literate aspects, solely populated by) men, but also in the more Baconian sense that it occurred largely without the input of women and, indeed, without any concern to involve them except in their roles as subordinate midwives or manual assistants and, of course, compliant patients.[5] Yet as this narrative has shown repeatedly, women were never completely passive in these developments. There was an active female subculture of women's medicine—medicine both by and for women—in twelfth-century Salerno, and the assumption that female practitioners would be caring in some manual capacity for childbirth and women's 'secret maladies' continued through the end of the period. Even with increasing legislation against them, female practitioners never disappeared entirely and, as we have seen, by the beginning of the sixteenth century midwifery actually caught up with the other medical professions in becoming a field with its own 'professional books'. The issue, therefore, is not women's universal exclusion from the production and delivery of women's medicine, but their exclusion from the production of *authoritative knowledge* in the field that was, in the most essential sense, their own.

It is clear that most male practitioners must have engaged at some level in dialogue with women, listening both to the complaints of their patients and the empirically acquired knowledge of midwives and other female practitioners.

---

[5] See the Preface above.

Valesco of Tarenta, the Portuguese physician practising at the court of Foix in the early fifteenth century, recounts a method women use themselves to treat uterine ulcers. He mentions a therapy that 'male and female physicians' use in Spain and a treatment for restoring milk that was used by 'a noble lady to whom women from all over used to flock as if pilgrimaging to Rome'.[6] Niccolò Falcucci, amidst all the remedies he gleaned from his written sources and all his personal attestations of efficacy, referred to an unguent for excessive menstrual flux 'which the Duchess of Austria used and which by some is called "the unguent of the Countess"'.[7] Michele Savonarola, despite his arrogation of major elements of gynaecological and obstetrical practice to the male physician and surgeon, recognized his fundamental reliance on midwives' cooperation for the successful treatment of his patients and his meriting of their 'trumpet' of fame. He could credit his own mother for certain information on the uterine mole just as much as his father.[8] And Giovanni Matteo Ferrari de Grado would admit that matrons and midwives were more expert in the application of therapies for uterine suffocation than physicians (_matronae et obstetrices sunt medicis peritiores_), though given that this therapy involved masturbation to expel the accumulated semen he was probably right to defer that task to women.[9]

Admittedly, this necessary reliance on female assistants was not always desired. A Parisian physician, Guillaume Boucher (d. 1410), refers to a case where the signs noted by the physicians were that the uterus had ascended, but they were deceived by the midwife who told them it was in its normal place.[10] Late in the sixteenth century, Girolamo Mercuriale (1530–1606) would refer to 'what I have learned from midwives' (_quod intellexi ab obstetricibus_) on the normal position of the foetus _in utero_, in effect ranking their opinion equal to the teachings of Hippocrates and Aristotle.[11] Yet on the very next page, he insists

---

[6] William Henry York, 'Experience and Theory in Medical Practice during the Later Middle Ages: Valesco de Tarenta (fl. 1382–1426) at the Court of Foix (France)', PhD dissertation, The Johns Hopkins University, 2003, pp. 132 and 190; the translation is my own.

[7] Falcucci, _De membris genitalibus_, in Manchester, Chetham's Library, MS 27857 (Mun. A.3.134), s. xv² (Flanders?), ff. 1r–285v, at f. 59r. The fact that this remedy already has a formal name suggests that Falcucci has not learned about it directly from this duchess, whoever she was. This same remedy was also mentioned in the 16th century by Jacques Dubois and Girolamo Mercuriale; see the 1597 edition of the _Gynaeciorum libri_, pp. 157 and 230.

[8] Michele Savonarola, _Practica maior_ (Venice: Vincentius Valgrisius, 1561), Tract. VI, cap. XXI, rubr. 17, _De mola_, f. 265rb.

[9] J. M. de Gradi, _Practica_, p. 350, as cited in Carl Oskar Rosenthal, 'Zur geburtshilflich-gynaekologischen Betätigung des Mannes bis zum Ausgange des 16. Jahrhunderts', _Janus_ 27 (1923), 117–48 and 192–212, at p. 143.

[10] Ernst Wickersheimer, 'Les secrets et conseils de maître Guillaume Boucher et de ses confrères: Contribution à l'histoire de la médecine à Paris vers 1400', _Bulletin de la Société Française d'Histoire de la Médecine_ 8 (1909), 199–305, at p. 279.

[11] Mercurialis, _De morbis muliebribus_, Bk II, chap. 2, _De partu vitioso_, in Israel Spach, ed. _Gynaeciorum sive de Mulierum tum communibus, tum gravidarum, parientium et puerperarum affectibus et morbis libri Graecorum, Arabum, Latinorum veterum et recentium quotquot extant, partim nunc primum editi, partim vero denuo recogniti, emendati_ (Strasburg: Lazarus Zetzner, 1597), p. 231.

that even though recognition of the signs of difficult birth is the business of midwives, these symptoms 'should also be known by the physician since often it happens that the midwives are stupid and ignorant and it becomes necessary for the physician to offer aid'.[12] Not simply should the physician be prepared to recommend baths to help dilate the uterine orifice or remedies to stimulate the expulsive faculty if the foetus has died, but just as much as the midwife he must have soft hands in order to aid delivery.

It has been argued recently that, after the devastations of the Black Death, many physicians began to turn away from strict adherence to theory and textual authority and to draw more heavily on their own empirical experiences and those of others.[13] But not all experience was equal. The fact that Valesco of Tarenta could make reference not only to his own experiences but also those of *indocti* surgeons (two of whom he even named), makes it all the more striking that he almost never accorded the same credence to female practitioners. True, he does not generalize from the lethal errors of two particular female practitioners to make sweeping condemnations of the medical capabilities of the whole sex,[14] but neither does he acknowledge that women's greater access to the bodies of their female patients might give them an authoritative knowledge he could never have. His contemporaries, moreover, were not always even as gracious as this. Valesco's successor as physician to the counts of Foix, Pierre Andrieu, on several occasions contrasts the practices of good, upright practitioners (*probos* and *probe mulieres et experte*) with 'old women and ignorant ones' (*vetulas et ignaras*) or even, more viciously, 'cursed old women' (*maledicte vetule*).[15] Midwives (*obstetrices*), in the two instances where they are mentioned, are treated neutrally, but it is clear that Pierre sees them neither as colleagues nor reliable sources of information.

Another example of how midwives could be written out of the creation of gynaecological and obstetrical knowledge comes from Alessandro Benedetti, the humanist Venetian physician and anatomist we met in the last chapter, who recounted in 1493 the following anecdote about a case of uterine mole:

We saw a woman [. . .] whom we immediately judged to have a mole in her uterus. The midwife announced that her vagina was shut. Three pessaries were made from galbanum, bdellium and oppopanax and inserted, and the mouths of the vagina were laid open by the wondrous work of nature. Then the midwife extracted the mole, torn into three pieces, which, when sewn back together, constituted the whole round mole [. . .] [A]nd it was found to be unformed, molded out of human skin, the matter inside without

[12] *Ibid.*, p. 232: 'Haec autem signa quanquam pertineant ad obstetrices, veruntamen sunt etiam Medico cognoscenda, eo quod saepe contingat obstetrices esse bardas, et ignaras, et necessarium sit Medici ministerium.'

[13] York, 'Experience and Theory'. [14] York, 'Experience and Theory', p. 123.

[15] Pierre Andrieu, *Pomum aureum*, BNF, MS lat. 6992: *per vetulas et ignaras ad dampnum quam plurimum pocius quam per probos exercetur* (f. 79rb); *istis maledictis vetulis* (f. 88va); and *alique maledicte vetule cum sujs pessimis artibus* (f. 89ra).

bones, without a heart, without a liver or intestines, but a kind of jumbled mass of flesh, with many veins dispersed through it, like a large round melon.[16]

Benedetti continues for two more long pages about the nature of the mole and its treatment. Yet he never mentions this midwife again or any others, either as sources of knowledge about the disorder or as therapists.

Indeed, what is surprising in the fifteenth and sixteenth centuries is that the disparagement of female practitioners seems to have *declined* from the rhetorical excesses of the thirteenth and fourteenth centuries. This was not because women had been completely eradicated as practitioners. Despite the prohibitive laws and trials of the fourteenth and early fifteenth centuries, women could still be found in medical practice throughout Europe at the end of the Middle Ages. Most of the spaces left open for female medical practice in the thirteenth and fourteenth centuries remained open in the fifteenth and sixteenth centuries to some degree. Cloistered religious women would presumably still have needed female phlebotomists and perhaps also *medice* to attend to certain of their gynaecological conditions,[17] midwives continued to attend normal childbirths, beguines and other religious women continued to serve as attendants at hospitals, while the spouses and daughters of male surgeons, barbers, and apothecaries often continued to contribute to the family business.

But for all of these groups their range of practice had shrunk to the same degree that male practitioners' professional identities had grown. Regulations in German-speaking areas established rules for licensing and even some medical training for midwives, but they also explicitly prevented them from making any surgical interventions in birth or engaging in anything that could be construed as medical practice (such as administering drugs). In France, while female surgeons were still to be found in provincial cities, after Perretta's trial in Paris in 1410 we find no further evidence of any female surgeon in the capital for the rest of the fifteenth century.[18] Likewise among barbers, we can

---

[16] Alessandro Benedetti, *Collectiones medicinae* (1493), as published in *Alexandri Benedicti veronensis, Medici ac Philosophi multis nominibus clarissimi, de re medica* (Basel: Henricus Petrus, 1549), p. 482.

[17] The presence of female medical practitioners within the cloister, even if only as phlebotomists, has not yet been explored for the early modern period, so we cannot know if there was a break in medieval traditions or not. Obviously, in Protestant parts of Europe, the Reformation would have eradicated this kind of female practice along with the institutions of nunneries.

[18] Laurent Garrigues, 'Les Professions médicales à Paris au début du XVe siècle: Praticiens en procès au parlement', *Bibliothèque de l'École des Chartes* 156 (1998), 317–67, p. 347. The only documented *chirurgienne* in Paris after Perretta seems to be one Guillemette Du Luys, who was in the service of Louis XI *c.*1479. She was identified as in charge of the 'lower stews' (*estuver . . . par dessoubs*); as such, she may have functioned strictly as a phlebotomist. See Ernest Wickersheimer, *Dictionnaire biographique des médecins en France au Moyen Age*, 2 vols. (1936; repr. Geneva: Librairie Droz, 1979), 1:267. Moreover, the only other female surgeon attested anywhere else in 15th-century France is one Martinette, to whom the mayor of Dijon grants special permission to hang a surgeon's sign on the understanding that she is only to treat the poor at a nearby hospital; Wickersheimer, *Dictionnaire*, 2:543. Susan Broomhall, *Women's Medical Work in Early Modern France* (Manchester,

see a decline in women's status over the course of the fifteenth century. In 1421, the Parisian female barber Emmelot was assessed the same tax by the occupying English forces as were two of her male colleagues and even a surgeon, suggesting that she was making a comfortable living off her work (or at least her workshop).[19] Yet Emmelot's success may have been becoming rarer. While it remained acceptable for the widows of barbers to continue shaving and hair-cutting, their practice of phlebotomy and minor surgical operations was strictly forbidden.

In fact, aside from midwifery and hospital-centred nursing, women's medical practice seems to have been entirely subsumed into the context of the patriarchal family, where it remained in a 'gray area' of both law and custom throughout the fifteenth century. The role of women in the transference of the material goods—and sometimes the skills—of medical practice was widely recognized. In 1484, the French regent Anne de Beaujeu (who would be the dedicatee of Bernard Chaussade's tract on fertility four years later) acted for her minor brother Charles VIII by issuing an ordinance that the apothecaries and spicers in Paris were now to be a regulated community, with a standardized four-year apprenticeship, oaths, and inspections to insure uniformity of practice and the product they sold. Among these detailed regulations were clear stipulations that the widows of apothecaries maintained the right to inherit and run their late husbands' workshops provided they did not remarry and provided they employed in their workshops a male colleague who had been properly accredited by the confraternity. Moreover, male heirs who had learned the craft under their mothers were just as entitled to exemption from guild entrance fees as those who had studied under their fathers or other male masters.[20] In other words, the woman as widow and mother could still serve as a conduit for the transference of goods and skills between generations of men. And if they were transferring *skills*, of course, then the women must have been practising at their husbands' sides

University of Manchester Press, 2004), p. 20 (following a 1906 unannotated study by Wicker-sheimer), claims that Charles VIII passed a law in 1484 formally denying women the right to practise surgery except when carrying on the workshop of their husbands. In fact, the 1484 law pertains to apothecaries (see below); indeed, there seems to be not a single law pertaining to women and surgery from this period, confirming that by this point the field had already become thoroughly masculinized. My thanks to Walton Schalick for his help on this point.

[19] Emmelot's tax of four ounces of silver was the same as that paid by a surgeon, Jean Dix Livres, and two barbers, Jean Lambert and Jean de Soulantes, and twice that paid by two other male barbers, Colin le Barbier and Nicolas Villart. See Danielle Jacquart, *Le milieu médical en France du XIIe au XVe siècle: En annexe 2e supplément au 'Dictionnaire' d'Ernest Wickersheimer* (Geneva: Librairie Droz, 1981), pp. 438, 440, 456–7, 460, and 465.

[20] *Ordonnances des rois de France de la troisième race, recueillies par ordre chronologique*, vol. 19, ed. M. le Marquis de Pastoret (Paris: Imprimerie Royale, 1835; repr. Farnborough: Gregg, 1968), pp. 415–17. These rights were maintained well into the eighteenth century; see Jean Flahaut, 'L'exercice de la pharmacie par les veuves d'apothicaires du XVe au XVIIIe siécles. 1ere partie: Aspects réglementaires', *Revue d'histoire de la pharmacie* 50, no. 335 (2002), 367–378; and *idem*, 'L'exercice de la pharmacie par les veuves d'apothicaires du XVᵉ au XVIIIᵉ siécles: 2ᵉ partie: Aspects humains', *Revue d'Histoire de la Pharmacie* 40, no. 336 (2002), 543–54.

while still alive, such as a husband and wife team of barbers we find in Bordeaux in 1415–24.[21]

Male practitioners (at least those at the craft level) therefore recognized that their own interests in establishing their profession as a transferable patrimony for their sons were positively served by allowing women to act as 'place holders' for deceased masters. But clearly there were limits. Between 1426 and 1428, yet another Parisian female practitioner, Jeanne la Poqueline, was claiming the right to practise barbery in the absence of her husband, Alain Poquelin, who had recently 'sold and given away her furniture and left without saying goodbye'. He was absent but not dead and that distinction was to prove her undoing. Initially, she was permitted to keep her shop open, but was prohibited from performing any barbering tasks (including phlebotomy) that involved surgical procedures. She seems to have persisted in her practice nevertheless, and was subsequently driven out of practice once and for all.[22] Other attempts to circumvent the normative exclusion of women could meet with similar opposition. In 1462, a seventy-year-old barber in Reims, Jean Estevent, essentially 'willed' his barbering business to his fifty-two-year-old wife, Isabelle, prior to his taking religious vows and abandoning his secular career. His fellow barbers were decidedly unhappy with this arrangement, and took action against Isabelle on the grounds that she had not been approved to practise. The case dragged on for three years (including Isabelle's direct appeal to the king); Isabelle won but the barbers of Reims took pains in 1473 when they revised their regulations to make sure no such incident would happen again.[23]

What is particularly striking about this increasing exclusion of 'the women of the house' from medical practice is that the practice of occupational endogamy—the marrying of daughters to other males in the trade—saw no signs of abating. In the later fifteenth century in Burgundy we find a high level of occupational endogamy among the surgeons and barbers in the moderate-sized town of Decize. Surgical tools are often included in the dowry when one barber marries his daughter off to another.[24] But we have no evidence that the women of these families were themselves recognized as medical practitioners. This pattern seems to have been replicated all over Europe.[25] Thus when, as we saw in

---

[21] Wickersheimer, *Dictionnaire*, v. 1, p. 224, s. n. Guillaume Abenant.

[22] Garrigues, 'Professions', pp. 344–49. Unlike Perretta, who really was the last documented female surgeon we can find in Paris in the 15th century, Jeanne la Poqueline was not the last of her kind: Perrette la Hance could still be found practising as a barber in the city at the end of the century; see Jacquart, *Milieu*, p. 467.

[23] Broomhall, *Women's Medical Work*, pp. 16–18 and 27.

[24] Christophe Giraudet, 'Le milieu médical à Decize à la fin du Moyen Âge', *Annales de Bourgogne* 72 (2000), 237–64.

[25] Annemarie Kinzelbach, '"wahnsinnige Weyber betriegen den unverstendigen Poeffel": Anerkennung und Diffamierung heilkundiger Frauen und Männer, 1450 bis 1700', *Medizin-historisches Journal* 32 (1997), 29–56, finds that aside from midwifery, women in Germany rarely practised medicine legally except as widows of deceased male practitioners. Doreen A. Evenden,

Chapter 3, a mid fifteenth-century Valencian apothecary willed all his movable goods to his wife *except* 'the things and tools that I have of my apothecary's art, and the books that I have of this art', he was acknowledging that his craft was a masculine art, one to be left preferentially to other males. This increasing sense not only that medicine was a profession but a *masculine* profession no doubt explains why laws regarding medical practice in the fifteenth century were not harsher against women: they didn't need to be. The medical professions had long since rebounded from whatever slight decline in prestige they suffered following the initial catastrophes of the Black Death in the mid fourteenth century,[26] and there were enough other elements of the social structure to ensure that male privilege would not be compromised by anomalous situations such as that of the abandoned wife Jeanne la Poqueline.

To be sure, there were other axes of power besides gender that differentiated medical practitioners from one another. Perretta Petone, the marginally literate Parisian surgeon, was marginal not simply as a woman or semi-literate, but also as a recent immigrant to the metropolis.[27] She shared this latter characteristic with Jean Domrémi, the male practitioner who, as we saw in the previous chapter, was prosecuted for his gynaecological and obstetrical practice in the 1420s. Outside the context of university towns and major metropolises, in situations where the men themselves were not fully professionalized, we find a broader range of practice by women. Women were still being licensed as surgeons in southern Italy in the early fifteenth century, just as they had been in the early fourteenth century.[28] In France, even without formal licensing, women could attain respect in their communities. A certain Isabelle practised as a 'physicienne' in Fécamp (on the Norman coast) in 1435; Jeanne de Chailly was a *médicine* in Lyons in 1493, as was a certain Louise in the village of Clermont in the mountains of central France in 1498.[29] Even the great university town of Montpellier had a *metgessa* in 1449.[30] The Spanish Cardinal Cisneros, while visiting Granada, could employ a Muslim woman to cure him in 1501 at the same time as he

'Gender Differences in the Licensing and Practice of Female and Male Surgeons in Early Modern England', *Medical History* 42 (1998), 194–216, finds that although widows of barbers could take over the shops and apprentices of their deceased husbands, widows of surgeons could not.

[26] Katharine Park, *Doctors and Medicine in Early Renaissance Florence* (Princeton: Princeton University Press, 1985), documented a temporary opening of the medical profession in Florence in first half century after plague, and it was in this period that she found four women practising as *medice*.

[27] In this respect, Perretta may have also been seen as one of many elements of disorder in a city then suffering from economic recession, decreased population, and a constant influx of immigrants from surrounding areas. See Claude Gauvard, Mary and Richard Rouse, and Alfred Soman, 'Le Châtelet de Paris au début du XVe siecle d'après les fragments d'un registre d'écrous de 1412', *Bibliothèque de l'École des Chartes* 157 (1999), 565–606, esp. p. 580.

[28] Francesco Pierro, 'Nuovi contributi alla conoscenza delle medichesse nel regno di Napoli negli ultimi tre secoli del medioevo', *Archivio Storico Pugliese* 17, fasc. 1–4 (1964), 231–41.

[29] Wickersheimer, *Dictionnaire*, 1:96 and 312; and Jacquart, *Supplément*, p. 201.

[30] Jacquart, *Supplément*, p. 48 on Biatris *la metgessa*.

was attempting to eradicate all last traces of Muslim civilization from the Iberian peninsula.[31] Anton Trutmann frequently cited the remedies of female healers in a medical compendium that he produced around the end of the fifteenth century in southwest Germany as did Count Palatine Ludwig V in his massive twelve-volume medical compendium composed in Heidelberg a few years later.[32] Indeed, Susan Broomhall opens her recent book on women's medical work in sixteenth-century France with the claim, 'For a majority of the French population during the period known as the Renaissance, most medical care would come at the hands of women.'[33] She then lists all the ways in which women would have been involved in the care of children, household members, the poor, the aged, and the dying. Why, then, if female medical practice was so pervasive, were women medical practitioners so ignorable by the male medical writers whose works we have chronicled here? The authors of the major fifteenth- and sixteenth-century gynaecological texts were, to the extent we can reconstruct their biographies, all university-educated, many holding professorships. Even as male practitioners, they could hardly be described as 'typical'. What relevance did the views of this elite group have for the broader spectrum of practitioners that made up the medical marketplace?

The answer, as I have argued throughout this book, is found in statements such as Broomhall herself cites. As the Parisian statutes for apothecaries asserted explicitly in 1514, any widow who takes over her late husband's workshop 'cannot take apprentices herself, *because she cannot call herself expert*'.[34] In 1580, the French writer André du Breil, in his aptly titled *Policing of the Art and Science of Medicine*, condemned the practice of widows taking over their husband's businesses, 'as if they were the inheritors of the knowledge of their husbands,

---

[31] L. P. Harvey, 'In Granada Under the Catholic Monarchs: A Call from a Doctor and Another from a *Curandera*', in *The Age of the Catholic Monarchs, 1474–1516: Literary Studies in Memory of Keith Whinnom*, ed. Alan Deyermond and Ian Macpherson (Liverpool: Liverpool University Press, 1989), pp. 71–5.

[32] Gundolf Keil, 'Der Hausvater als Arzt', in *Haushalt und Familie in Mittelalter und früher Neuzeit*, ed. Trude Ehlert *et al.* (Sigmaringen: Jan Thorbecke, 1991), pp. 219–243; and *idem*, 'Ludwig V', in *Die deutsche Literatur des Mittelalters: Verfasserlexikon*, rev. ed., ed. Kurt Ruh *et al.*, 10 vols. (Berlin: De Gruyter, 1978–99), vol. 5, coll. 1016–30, at col. 1025. At least two of these women appear quite extensively: Debra Stoudt counts approximately 400 entries for Anna Gremsin and more than 900 for Regina Hurleweg; Hurleweg, at least, seems to have authored a text and, given the corpus of her remedies, this seems likely for Gremsin as well. See Debra L. Stoudt, 'Medieval German Women and the Power of Healing', in *Women Healers and Physicians: Climbing a Long Hill*, ed. Lilian R. Furst (Lexington: University of Kentucky Press, 1997), pp. 13–42.

[33] Broomhall, *Women's Medical Work*, p. 1. For the continued presence of women in medical practice in other areas of early modern Europe, see, for example, Margaret Pelling, with Frances White, *Medical Conflicts in Early Modern London: Patronage, Physicians, and Irregular Practitioners, 1550–1640* (Oxford: Clarendon Press; New York: Oxford University Press, 2003); Gianna Pomata, *Contracting a Cure: Patients, Healers, and the Law in Early Modern Bologna*, translated by the author, with the assistance of Rosemarie Foy and Anna Taraboletti-Segre (Baltimore: Johns Hopkins University Press, 1998); and David Gentilcore, *Healers and Healing in Early Modern Italy* (Manchester: Manchester University Press, 1998).

[34] As cited in Broomhall, *Women's Medical Work*, p. 31; my emphasis.

like their goods'.[35] Like the physicians at the University of Paris in their trial of Jacoba Felicie, Du Breil makes the comparison with law:

[F]or it is no more acceptable that a widow of a physician, surgeon, apothecary, and barber practise medicine after the death of their husbands, than a widow of a judge, president, counsellor, lawyer, clerk, court usher or procurer, judge, plead, write or report causes and trials.[36]

Women, in other words, had no claim to the *authoritative knowledge* that distinguished the now professionalized, institutionally sanctioned practices of male physicians, surgeons, barbers, and apothecaries. Nor could midwives lay claim to a comparable authoritative knowledge for, even though they had their own 'professional books' by the early sixteenth century, these texts functioned (as I will explain in more detail below) quite differently for midwives than the esoteric books of learned physicians or surgeons did. There is little disparagement of female medical practitioners, therefore, among either fifteenth or sixteenth century male practitioners for the simple reason that the superior social standing of the book-learned physician or surgeon, long since gendered as male, was now unquestioned. Polemics against female practitioners appear only when male practitioners are moving into areas where they still feel somewhat insecure, such as the French practitioner Pierre Andrieu who in 1444 was writing the first text in France that specifically aimed to give instructions on birth and not just the prelude to it, fertility. Michele Savonarola, in contrast, writing in Italy where male involvement in birth was already common, attempted to elicit the cooperation of midwives; even when he identifies certain conditions as being caused by midwives' errors, he doesn't condemn them universally. For him, the superiority of learned male practitioners was already taken for granted.

Du Breil's choice of the law as the 'model' masculine profession was not inapt. Law, whether customary, Roman, or canon (ecclesiastical), had become book-dependent so early that practice by an illiterate was never a possibility. Although customary law continued to grant aristocratic women the right to administer justice in their own domains (and we do, in fact, find some women in possession of law books), the growing influence from the mid twelfth century on of Roman law—which included a legal dictate barring women from serving as magistrates—effectively disenfranchised women from any formal role in judicial proceedings in most aspects of both canon and civil law, whether as judge, advocate, or notary. Thus, there are no known cases of women being tried for illegally practising law in the Middle Ages for the simple reason that women got nowhere near the physical or intellectual spaces where law was practised other than as plaintiffs, petitioners, the accused, or witnesses.[37] Nor is there any

---

[35] Broomhall, p. 51.   [36] *Ibid.*, pp. 51–2.
[37] Elisabeth van Houts, 'Gender and Authority of Oral Witnesses in Europe (800–1300)', *Transactions of the Royal Historical Society*, Sixth Series 9 (1999), 201–20.

evidence women ever acted as notaries, perhaps the most common of literate professions in medieval Europe.[38]

Medicine differed from law in that, whatever the ambitions of learned physicians or surgeons to raise their field to a level of theory comparable to that of theology and law, it retained its necessarily empiric, hands-on character as a discipline of *practice*. Medicine was never as text-based as law, in the sense that one had to have one's books available at all times for consultation. Moreover, the practice of law was tied intimately with the dispensing of justice, which though contested between church and civil courts or feudal and royal ones, was confined to specified public venues. The practice of medicine, in contrast, was necessarily private, occurring in individual homes or at the apothecary's shop. Whereas the dispensing of justice could be deferred until an itinerant court came to the county or village or until the plaintiff took his or her complaint to the court, the dispensing of medicine often needed to be immediate and local, whenever or wherever the situation demanded. Aside from the lecture halls of the university, medieval medicine was never fully institutionalized in any settings outside the home; it thus remained incompletely professionalized, incompletely separated from the domestic sphere.[39] Books and book-learning added a very real patina of authority to medicine, but aside from the high learning of the universities, medicine remained porous, allowing women like Jacoba and Perretta, or men like Jean Domrémi, to enter. Its borders therefore demanded more active policing.

In several respects, therefore, the history of women's engagement with medicine as formal practitioners seems to follow the general trajectories of women's history in the transition from the late Middle Ages to the early modern period. Although the Middle Ages was never the 'golden age' that historians of more modern periods have sometimes imagined, it is possible to see a greater gender equity between men's and women's medical practices as late as the thirteenth and early fourteenth centuries than can be found in the fifteenth. Just as a microhistory of occupational categories in the northern city of Douai showed a general equity between the types of occupations in which men and women laboured in the thirteenth century, followed by an apparent closing off of many of those categories by the fifteenth, so on a larger scale historians of the early modern period have found that by the sixteenth century the exclusion of women from most occupational identities and their relegation to work of the household was well established. Just as women could be pushed out of the production of ale with the transition to the greater capital investment (and greater profit potential) of beer production, so with the increasing establishment of physic, surgery, and barbering as occupations in which one invested not only the time of

---

[38] My thanks to Timothy Strunk, Kathryn Reyerson, and Dan Smail for generously responding to my queries about women in legal and notarial culture. On notaries' literacy, see the Introduction above.

[39] Cf. Margaret Pelling, 'The Women of the Family? Speculations around Early Modern British Physicians', *Social History of Medicine* 8, no. 3 (Dec. 1995), 383–401.

education but also the material goods of tools and books was there an increasing masculinization.[40] Women could be avenues for the transfer of property and even sometimes of knowledge, but never of authority.

DID WOMEN HAVE A MEDICAL RENAISSANCE?

Ever since the historian Joan Kelly first asked 'Did women have a Renaissance?' in 1973,[41] it has been customary to question whether the great cultural turning points that affected men had an equal impact on women. The 'medical Renaissance' of gynaecology we examined in the previous chapter obviously was notable precisely because, with the exception of the new midwifery texts, it excluded women. Here I wish to revisit the significance of Rösslin's *Rosegarden* within the larger context of women's medical literacy more generally. This broadened perspective shows that there was not one but two major developments in the ways women engaged with literate medicine in the sixteenth century. The first, the rise of midwifery texts, shows important continuities with the medieval period. The second, the appearance of what can be considered the first genre of women's medical writing, the recipe book, was an unprecedented and arguably far more radical development.

As we saw in Chapters 3 and 4, women's engagement with medical literature—not just gynaecology, but medical works of any sort—had not been extensive in the Middle Ages. Prior to Savonarola in the mid fifteenth century, midwives had not yet emerged as a specialized audience: aside from brief sections in works owned by clerics or surgeons that might be *read to* midwives, there were no texts focusing solely on childbirth and its management nor did any medical writer address his work to midwives. Such gynaecological texts as were addressed to female audiences were addressed to women in general, which in practice almost certainly meant upper-class or bourgeois women. Only among French aristocratic women is ownership of medical books regularly documented, and even here their medical interests mirror those of men of their class, being focused on basic regimen more than women's medicine specifically. We have only a handful of documented cases where women passed medical books directly to another woman or to a female institution.[42] Nor, with the exception of Costanza Calenda who sat in on medical lectures in Naples and was awarded a degree (there is no evidence

[40] Ellen E. Kittell and Kurt Gueller, ' "Whether Man or Woman": Gender Inclusivity in the Town Ordinances of Medieval Douai', *Journal of Medieval and Early Modern Studies* 30 (2000), 63–100; Judith M. Bennett, *Ale, Beer, and Brewsters in England: Women's Work in a Changing World, 1300–1600* (New York: Oxford University Press, 1996); Merry E. Wiesner, *Women and Gender in Early Modern Europe*, 2nd edn (Cambridge: Cambridge University Press, 2000).

[41] The essay has been reprinted many times. The most readily accessible version is in Joan Kelly, *Women, History, and Theory: The Essays of Joan Kelly* (Chicago: University of Chicago Press, 1984).

[42] Green, 'Possibilities'.

that she ever practised medicine), do we find any woman who read medicine in order to acquire an expertise in medical science equivalent to that of university-trained (and even some non-university-trained) male physicians and surgeons. While there was, therefore, some female engagement with medical literature, particularly in northern Europe, it did not usually penetrate down to the classes of women who might actually have to use their medical knowledge to make a living.

These trends continued into the sixteenth century: the number of texts addressed to women increased but these were written as often with the expectation that they would reinforce women's reliance on male physicians as encourage women's independence. Whereas Bernard Chaussade had been the only fifteenth-century writer to address a work on women's medicine to an individual female patron, several sixteenth-century writers recognized the potential of such a strategy and followed suit. Ludovico Bonaccioli directed his Latin *Enneas muliebris* to the humanistically educated Lucrezia Borgia in 1502/3, while in France Guillaume Chrestien (Willem Christiaan van der Boxe, d. *c*.1560) translated three learned texts on female physiology and generation for royal female patrons in the 1550s.[43] In Italy in 1563, Giovanni Marinelli composed an Italian treatise for women that included a surprising amount of detailed gynaecological information.[44] In not all cases, however, was female independence actively encouraged. In the 1580s, Jean Liebault, regent of the Faculty of Medicine in Paris, translated his own lengthy Latin text on the diseases of women into French; he advises his anticipated reader (whose gender he does not specify) that he or she should use the information contained therein only if they are already initiated into the 'mysteries and secrets' of medicine or if they are doing so under the supervision of 'a learned, wise, and well-informed physician'. In fact, he actually reduced the number of remedies in the text, and rendered some of what remained into Latin.[45] In the Low Countries, not only did the Dutch *Trotula* continue to circulate in manuscript (where, at last, we find our first certain evidence of female ownership),[46] but there was also published in Antwerp in 1550 (with four reprints up through 1600) a treatise with the simple title, *The Profit of Women* (*Das Profijt der Vrouwen*). This text covers pregnancy regimen and childbirth, gynaecological concerns and cosmetics, and such topics as how to restore sexual vigour in both men and women

---

[43] See Appendix 2, items 7, 30, 38, and 39. Diane de Poitier, dedicatee of one of these works, was also the dedicatee of Claude Valgelas's health regimen, *Commentaire de la conservation de santé, et prolongation de vie* (Lyons, 1559).

[44] See Appendix 2, item 44. I have consulted the revised edition of 1574.

[45] See Appendix 2, item 62. For a detailed analysis of Liebault's debts to Marinelli, see Valérie Worth-Stylianou, *Les Traités d'obstétrique en langue française au seuil de la modernité. Bibliographie critique des 'Divers Travaulx' d'Euchaire Rosslin (1536) à l' 'Apologie de Louyse Bourgeois sage-femme' (1627)* (Geneva: Droz, 2006), pp. 258–63. On Liebault's possible feminism, see Regine Reynolds-Cornell, 'Les Misères de la femme mariée: Another Look at Nicole Liébault and a Few Questions about the Woes of the Married Woman', *Bibliothèque d'Humanisme et Renaissance* 64, no. 1, 2002, 37–54.

[46] For 16th-century female owners of the Dutch *Trotula*, see Appendix 1, items 93 and 96.

'who served Venus excessively'.[47] In England, surprisingly, which had the longest tradition of directing texts on women's medicine to female audiences (starting, of course, with the Anglo-Norman texts of the thirteenth century), the coming of print brought a rupture: although it is clear that several of the fifteenth-century English gynaecological texts continued to be used in manuscript well into the sixteenth century (often by men), none made the transition into print nor were they replaced with any equivalent English work that combined obstetrics with gynaecology. Rather, in sixteenth-century England and elsewhere, the text that dwarfed all others was Eucharius Rösslin's *Rosegarden*.

The *Rosegarden* is generally described as a midwifery manual (as I myself did in the previous chapter), but in fact it served multiple purposes that show continuity with medieval uses of writings on 'women's secrets'.[48] First, it is clear that Rösslin's *Rosegarden* did at last give midwives their first professional handbook. An ordinance which probably dates from the sixteenth century for midwives in the countryside surrounding Nuremberg dictates that 'a midwife *should diligently read the books pertaining to her profession*, and in the summer she should attend the Wednesday lectures given by the instructor in Nuremberg'. An ordinance from Heilbronn says much the same thing.[49] In contrast, a description of the duties of the midwife coming from Württemberg around 1480, three decades before the appearance of Rösslin's work, says nothing that hinted at midwives' expected literacy; itself written in Latin, the injunction lays out practices and responsibilities that will be dictated *to* the midwife by a physician or Latinate overseer.[50] The municipal authorities of Nuremberg and Heilbronn thus seem to have been taking advantage of the novel opportunity afforded by the creation of the *Rosegarden* to transform midwifery into a literate medical profession with uniform standards of learning similar to those expected

---

[47] *The Profit of Women*, Appendix 2, item 29. My thanks to Orlanda S. H. Lie, of the University of Utrecht, for sharing with me a draft of her survey of late medieval and early modern Dutch texts on women's medicine.

[48] Besides the multiple reprints and translations of Rösslin's text, 16th-century midwifery texts included the 1541 *Libro del arte de las comadres o madrinas* by the Majorcan physician Damian Carbón, the 1554 *Ein shön lustig Trostbüchle von den Empfengknussen und Geburten der Menschen* by the Zurich city physician, Jakob Ruf (1500–58), and the 1595 *La commare o riccoglitrice* by the Venetian physician, Girolamo (or Scipione) Mercurio (*c*.1550–1615, not to be confused with the Pisan professor, Girolamo Mercuriale). See Appendix 2 for full details.

[49] Georg Burckhard, *Die deutschen Hebammenordnungen von ihren ersten Anfängen bis auf die Neuzeit* (Leipzig: W. Engelmann, 1912), pp. 109 and 124; regarding the dating of these documents, see Monica H. Green, 'The Sources of Eucharius Rösslin's *Rosegarden for Pregnant Women and Midwives* (1513)' (forthcoming). On the licensing of German midwives generally, see Sibylla Flügge, *Hebammen und heilkundige Frauen: Recht und Rechtswirklichkeit im 15. und 16. Jahrhundert*, 2nd edn (Frankfurt am Main: Stroenfeld, 2000).

[50] Walther Pfeilsticker, 'Eine württembergische Hebammenordnung von *c*.1480: Ein weiterer Beitrag zu Georg Burckhards *Hebammenordnungen*', *Archiv für Geschichte der Medizin* 20 (1928), 95–8. Unlike almost all oaths from the 15th or 16th century, this *ordinatio* is extremely specific on therapeutic matters (including Caesarean section). It begins by stating that midwives will take an oath four or at least two times a year promising correct care of the parturient.

of physicians, apothecaries, and even some surgeons and barbers for the past two to three centuries.

While there is thus no question that the *Rosegarden* and its progeny helped to elevate midwifery to a true profession for women (at least in Germany), it was perhaps less epochal than has often been claimed for four principal reasons. First, precisely by focusing primarily on birth and care of the child, the *Rosegarden* reinforced the separation of gynaecology from obstetrics. It was a manual for the still female-dominated birthing room and nursery, not a guidebook for general gynaecological care. Second, although Rösslin included more information on medicines and pathological conditions than had Savonarola in his own vernacular book for the women of Ferrara,[51] both writers shared a similar, central concern: they wished to manage the whole culture of reproduction, from conception to the rearing of the child. The midwife was therefore just one of the players involved; instructing her alone was never the goal. Rösslin's full title, after all, was *The Rosegarden for Pregnant Women and Midwives*. It was meant to inform pregnant women (or women hoping to become pregnant) how to manage themselves reproductively and how to assess any midwife who might attend them. In Germany, the *Rosegarden* was also used by *Ehrbare Frauen*, the upright matrons who supervised the midwives.[52] Thus, although Rösslin does more to place the midwife at the centre of the birth event than had the female-addressed medieval gynaecological texts, precisely because she must share her 'professional book' with her clients this newly literate midwife did not enjoy the same esoteric knowledge that distinguished most learned male practitioners from their patients.

Third, Rösslin's *Rosegarden* came to serve an additional function, one not in the least surprising given the medieval heritage of other texts on women's medicine: it was used to instruct lay people in the 'science' of generation. In England, where the pseudo-Albertan text had never had much influence, the *Rosegarden* stepped into the double role that the medieval English gynaecological texts had earlier played. When Richard Jonas published the first English translation in 1540, he dedicated the text to Henry VIII's most recent wife, Katherine Howard, but made clear that he really intended the work for 'the utility and wealth of all women'.[53] Midwives were only a subsidiary category of that larger group. In 1545, Thomas Raynalde incorporated into his revised English translation some new anatomical material, explaining to his female readers that it would aid them

---

[51] There was a hidden irony in Rösslin's having chosen as his source Savonarola's Latin compendium, which was written for his fellow male practitioners. Savonarola's Italian text for women had not been nearly so detailed about medicines etc., to be used.

[52] Caroline Gisela March-Long, 'Early Modern German Obstetrical Manuals: *Das Frauenbüchlein* (*c.*1495) and *Der Rosengarten* (1513)', MA thesis, Duke University, 1993; Merry E. Wiesner, 'The Midwives of Southern Germany and the Private/Public Dichotomy', in *The Art of Midwifery*, ed. Hilard Marland (London: Routledge, 1993), pp. 77–94.

[53] Richard Jonas, (trans), *The Byrth of Mankynde, Newly Translated out of Laten into Englysshe* (London: T[homas] R[aynald], 1540), f. AB i verso.

in discussing their conditions with (male) physicians,[54] as well as some cosmetics. Like Jonas, he hardly mentioned midwives as readers; indeed, he suggested his work could serve in their place.[55] Both Jonas and Raynalde, moreover, like the authors of the *Knowing of Woman's Kind* and the *Sickness of Women* before them, also recognized that men would be among their readers, with the inherent possibilities for misuse. Jonas warned men to use the book 'only to the profit of their neighbors',[56] while Raynalde developed a more elaborate rhetoric that shamed any man who might misuse the text while still allowing for sympathetic male readers. As if trying to exorcise the ghost of Jankyn, he asserted 'it shall be no displeasure to any honest and loving woman that her husband should read such things'.[57] Yet he also notes that midwives already complained that 'every boy and knave [has access to] these books, reading them as openly as the tales as Robin Hood'. Similar uses of both midwifery texts and the older genre of 'women's secrets' as instructional manuals for male heads of house are amply documented in Germany. Indeed, already within a decade and a half of its initial publication, the German *Rosegarden* was joined by Rösslin's own son with the pseudo-Albertan text and several other texts into a compendium on 'Marriage Medicine'.[58] And throughout Europe the rhetorical warnings against 'misuse' of these writings continued.[59] Thus, whether making knowledge of midwifery the common property of all women (and thus diminishing the midwife's claim to her own esoteric knowledge that would have distinguished her as a professional) or turning texts on women's medicine into compendia of 'women's secrets', the

---

[54] Thomas Raynalde, (ed. and trans), *The Byrth of Mankynde, Otherwyse Named the Womans Booke. Newly set furth, corrected and augmented* (London: Thomas Raynalde, 1545), f. B iiii recto.

[55] Raynalde, *Byrth,*, f. C viii recto-verso: 'to them whiche diligently wyll aduert, and geue hede to thenstructions [*sic*] of this lytell booke, it may supply the roome and place of a goud mydwyfe: and aduise them many tymes of sundry cases, chaunses, and remedies, wherin peraduenture right wise wemen and goud mydwifes shalbe full ignorant'.

[56] Jonas, *Byrth*, f. AB i verso.   [57] Raynalde, *Byrth*, f. C vii recto.

[58] See Appendix 2, item 14. Margaret R. Schleissner, 'A Fifteenth-Century Physician's Attitude Toward Sexuality: Dr. Johann Hartlieb's *Secreta mulierum* Translation', in Joyce A. Salisbury (ed.), *Sex in the Middle Ages* (New York: Garland, 1991), pp. 110–25, argues that the incorporation of 'secrets of women' texts into 16th- and 17th-century 'housefather' books suggests that women were being addressed in order to teach them attitudes about their bodies that supported the goals of patriarchy. Similarly, Kathleen Crowther-Heyck, 'Wonderful Secrets of Nature: Natural Knowledge and Religious Piety in Reformation Germany', *Isis* 94 (2003), 253–3, cites one German author claiming that 'many honorable people have read this German text on the secrets of nature with reverence . . . They read this book of secrets alone and with their wives, in private [*in geheim*] and away from their children and maids' (p. 273). It should not surprise us, therefore, that by the end of the century it would be assumed that women regularly read the *Secreta mulierum* themselves: in 1594, the German writer Johann Fischart advised his female readers to bind his book with their daily prayerbooks or with the work of Albertus Magnus, no doubt the *Secreta mulierum*. See Margaret R. Schleissner, 'Pseudo-Albertus Magnus: *Secreta mulierum cum commento*, Deutsch: Critical text and commentary', PhD dissertation, Princeton University, 1987, p. 34.

[59] For example, Jean Liébault, *Trois Livres appartenant aux infirmitez et maladies des femmes, pris du Latin de M. Jean Liebaut, Docteur Médecin à Paris, et facts François* (Paris: Jacques de Puys, 1585), f. iiii: 'lesquels à la verité pour l'honneur, excellence et grauité de l'art de medecine ne doibuent estre prophanez ny diuulguez au populaire'.

midwifery texts of the sixteenth century did not function all that differently from the gynaecological texts of the late Middle Ages. What differed was the sheer scale on which such books could now circulate in men's as well as women's hands.

A fourth and final feature of Rösslin's *Rosegarden* is that it solidified the rhetoric of midwives' ignorance that the Dominican preacher Thomas of Cantimpré had first introduced 300 years earlier. Thomas, of course, had not been the first to question midwives' intelligence. Muscio, writing in late Antiquity, had bemoaned midwives' fading command of Greek in his day and deliberately 'dumbed down' his Latin translation of Soranus out of consideration for women's 'weaker minds'.[60] Yet he never blamed midwives for the loss of maternal or foetal life that presumably was just as high in his own day as it was 1000 years later. Thomas's concern for the religious implications of foetal death was supported, from the medical side, by casual statements like Avicenna's who listed 'the fault of the midwife' as one of several different reasons that birth could go badly.[61] But it is only in the fifteenth and sixteenth centuries that birth attendants move from being seen as occasionally incompetent (something that even the author of the Salernitan *Treatments for Women* acknowledged) to being seen as generally ignorant and even dangerous. Rösslin's opening poem deploring the ignorance of midwives was perhaps the most extreme example of this though, as we have seen above, his sentiments were echoed by many others.[62] True, neither Thomas nor Rösslin had universally condemned *all* midwives nor had they made any universal claims about women's intelligence. Yet neither did they give any thought to how the gendered structures of society contributed to the inherent problems of accumulating obstetrical knowledge.

From our modern perspective, the problems seem obvious. Although uncomplicated births do not differ that much from one another, complicated births can differ in myriad ways. Certain foetal malpresentations, such as shoulder dystocia, occur on average only once in every 100 births (some even more rarely than that), meaning that the chances are small that anyone other than the most specialized midwife will encounter such a situation more than a few times.[63] Justine Siegemund, the seventeenth-century midwife, delivered 6,199

---

[60] See Chapter 1 above.

[61] Avicenna, *Liber canonis* (Venice, 1507; repr. Hildesheim: Georg Olms, 1964), Bk III, fen XXI, cap. xxi, f. 369rb.

[62] Savonarola, in his Italian text, asserts that 'all midwives and attendants [need] to be taught the rules they must observe in birth, for it is clear that through their ignorance many babies and mothers either die or suffer harm'; Giovanni Michele Savonarola, *Il trattato ginecologico-pediatrico in volgare 'Ad mulieres ferrarienses de regimine pregnantium et noviter natorum usque ad septennium'*, ed. Luigi Belloni (Milan: Società Italiana di ostetricia e ginecologia, 1952), p. 116. In contrast, in his Latin text, he merely follows Avicenna in listing 'the fault of the midwife' as one of eight possible causes of difficulty; *Practica maior*, tract. VI, cap. xxi, rubr. 32, f. 267v.

[63] The current estimate of US incidence for children of normal birthweight of shoulder dystocia (when the foetus's shoulder becomes lodged on the symphysis pubis after its head has already entered

babies over the course of her career; a local neighbour woman might only assist at a few hundred or even just a few dozen.[64] For the latter, the opportunity to learn anything from one abnormality and then be able to apply it the next time is slim. To be sure, there may well have been oral traditions among midwives that preserved this very specialized information, but at the moment we have no evidence of any such lore, certainly nothing comparable to the written information on malpresentations that accompanied the series of foetal images from Muscio (Figs. 3.5 and 3.6 above) which, of course, we have never been able to document in the hands of midwives prior to the publication of the *Rosegarden* in the sixteenth century.

How sixteenth-century midwives responded to Rösslin's *Rosegarden* or the other midwifery manuals we still don't know. Midwives, unlike most other medical practitioners, did not regulate themselves through their own guilds or confraternities or medical colleges. Although we can find some intriguing evidence for 'collective action' among midwives (for example, municipal midwives in Basel petitioning in the early sixteenth century for an improvement in their salary, midwives in seventeenth-century London doing the same thing),[65] they were regulated from above and thus did not enjoy any particular autonomy. Male physicians had authority to approve German midwives in the late fifteenth century[66] and a midwife's possession of a single handbook no more changed that power imbalance than Perretta's book of remedies had made her the equal of male surgeons in the fifteenth century. The regulation of midwives continued apace in the sixteenth century, spurred on in some cases by Protestant efforts to redefine religious practices surrounding birth,[67] and an argument could be made that that increased scrutiny diminished midwives' autonomy even more. Nevertheless, midwifery did finally emerge as a field in which women not only practised but could claim authority. In the seventeenth century we finally witness the publication of the first female-authored texts on women's medicine since

the birth canal) is 0.6 to 1.4%. Estimates of rates in historical populations are, of course, inherently difficult not simply from lack of terminologically commensurable data but because obstetrical complications are affected by such historically variable factors as nutrition, co-morbidity (such as tubercular infection), and the kinds of obstetrical interventions that are made.

[64] Siegemund, *Court Midwife*. Adrian Wilson, 'A Memorial of Eleanor Willughby, a Seventeenth-Century Midwife', in *Women, Science and Medicine, 1500–1700: Mothers and Sisters of the Royal Society*, ed. Lynette Hunter and Sarah Hutton (Phoenix Mill: Sutton, 1997), 138–77, provides an excellent analysis of just this point about the slim chances that the *average* midwife would gain *expertise* in dealing with complicated births.

[65] Gordon P. Elmeer, 'The Regulation of Germany Midwifery in the 14th, 15th and 16th Centuries', MD thesis, Yale University School of Medicine, 1964; Doreen A. Evenden, *The Midwives of Seventeenth-Century London* (Cambridge: Cambridge University Press, 2000).

[66] Thomas G. Benedek, 'The Changing Relationship Between Midwives and Physicians During the Renaissance', *Bulletin of the History of Medicine* 51 (1977), 550–64.

[67] For England, see James Hitchcock, 'A Sixteenth Century Midwife's License', *Bulletin of the History of Medicine* 41 (1967), 75–76; and Mary E. Fissell, 'The Politics of Reproduction in the English Reformation', *Representations* no. 87 (Summer 2004), 43–81. On regulation in Germany, see Flügge, *Hebammen*.

Trota's day: Louise Bourgeois's and Marguerite Du Tertre de La Marche's works in France (published between 1609 and 1626, and in 1677, respectively), Jane Sharp's in England (1671), and Justine Siegemund's in Germany (1690).[68] While La Marche and Siegemund stayed closely to the midwife's defined territory (Siegemund focusing solely on management of difficult births), Bourgeois and Sharp attempted to redefine the midwife's province more broadly, including aspects of the physician's territory of gynaecological disease and infertility. Yet even here, women's entry into medical literacy does not reveal an 'underground world' of women's gynaecological or obstetrical traditions that rivalled the body of knowledge created and circulating among men: both Bourgeois and Sharp relied on the writings of male authors for much of their material (Bourgeois most heavily on the male obstetrical pioneer, Ambroise Paré) and even Siegemund credits her reading of earlier obstetrical texts (which probably included but was not limited to the German translation of Bourgeois) as the basis of her knowledge. Thus, as original as they may be in many respects, none of these four writers presents us with evidence for a 'parallel universe' where women created their own medical traditions completely separate from men's.

Something approaching a distinct women's tradition of literate medicine can be found, but not in midwifery. As I argued at the beginning of this book, the traditional equation of midwifery with 'women's medicine' in its entirety has caused historians to overlook other aspects of women's health and engagements with medicine. One of these areas is the female tradition of exchanging medical recipes which, far from existing outside of time, very much demands to be historicized. Given women's minimal engagements with medical literacy overall, it is not surprising to find little evidence for recipe exchanges in the Middle Ages. Beginning, however, in the fifteenth century, recipe exchanges began to pass from the oral realm into writing when women more regularly corresponded with one another. These shared recipes, in turn, eventually grew into whole collections of medical (and culinary and cosmetic) recipes made by women themselves.[69] This was a domestic medicine, one firmly inscribed within women's roles as managers of households, posing little threat to the authority of male medical professionals. It represents, however, a major shift in the role that literacy played within domestic medical traditions since the male dominance of the household book we witnessed earlier now gave way to a new feminine model.[70] By the end of the sixteenth century, we find the first printed, female-authored recipe collection, a cookbook more than a medical

---

[68] Lianne McTavish, *Childbirth and the Display of Authority in Early Modern France* (Aldershot: Ashgate, 2005), p. 44, also identifies an unpublished summary of obstetrical practices written in 1671 by a Mademoiselle Baudoin, who had trained at the Hôtel Dieu in Paris. The first female-authored midwifery text in Italy did not appear until 1787 (Teresa Ployant's *Breve compendio dell'arte ostetricia*), and even then its author was a Frenchwoman, not a native Italian.

[69] Green, 'Possibilities', pp. 42–8.   [70] See Chapter 4 above.

treatise, but one that recognized women's needs for obstetrical care.[71] And we are only beginning to assess the numbers of such collections that remained in manuscript.

The literary scholar Rebecca Krug has recently proposed a radical re-interpretation of the meaning of women's writing in the late Middle Ages.[72] Women like the English family of the Pastons, she argues, engaged in writing because they were fulfilling feminine duties in the context of patriarchy. Maintenance of their bourgeois households while their men were away at court or on business demanded that they emulate men in employing their literate skills to write correspondence, keep books, etc. Writing, for them, was not a defiant act. I would argue that women's first large-scale engagement with medical literacy—not the writing of midwifery texts but the collection of recipes—needs to be viewed from this same perspective. Just as the midwife re-emerged as a specialist out of the fluidity of women's roles as mothers, so women's roles as household managers seem to have led to a new sense among women that they were also responsible for collecting the best remedies available to them in order to maintain the health and good order of their households (a category that might, in the case of noble women, expand metaphorically to their entire realm). This new-found literacy could, in turn, create real confidence. Dorothea Susanna von der Pfalz, Duchess of Saxony-Weimar (1544–92), for example, not only compiled a recipe collection and engaged in medical correspondence with other women, but is also distinctive as the first German woman whom we can prove owned a copy of the *Trotula*, in this case Johannes Hartlieb's paired translations of the pseudo-Albertan *Secrets of Women* and *Das Buch Trotula*, wherein 'Trotula' is referred to not simply as an important medical authority but a queen.[73] Was Dorothea Susanna a prelude to the German countess, Aemilie Juliane of Schwarzburg-Rudolstadt, who in the 1680s not only had her own handwritten apothecary manual, but was intimately involved in supervising the provision of obstetrical care in her territory, composing for women her own handbook of spiritual advice for all the eventualities of childbearing?[74] However we eventually answer that question, it is clear even now that in the sixteenth and seventeenth centuries, at the same time middle-class women's professional roles

---

[71] Anna Weckerin, *Ein Köstlich new Kochbuch von allerhand Speisen . . . fürnehmlich vor Krancke in allerlay Krankheiten und Gebrästen; auch Schwangere Weiber, Kindbetterinnen und alte schwache Leute* (Amberg, 1598; repr. Munich, 1977).

[72] Rebecca Krug, *Reading Families: Women's Literate Practice in Late Medieval England* (Ithaca, NY: Cornell University Press, 2002).

[73] Breslau (or Wrocław, in current-day Poland), Dombibliothek, MS C 120, an. 1570–3. For information on Dorothea Susanna's medical collection and correspondence, I am grateful to Alisha Rankin. For a general survey of this phenomenon, see Alisha Michelle Rankin, 'Medicine for the Uncommon Woman: Experience, Experiment, and Exchange in Early Modern Germany', PhD dissertation, Harvard University, 2005.

[74] Judith P. Aikin, 'The Welfare of Pregnant and Birthing Women as a Concern for Male and Female Rulers: A Case Study', *Sixteenth Century Journal* 35.1 (2004): 9–41.

in medicine were contracting, upper-class women ironically turned into what we might call 'professional amateurs'. And they used their medical literacy to do it.

'THE HIGHEST ATTAINABLE STANDARD OF HEALTH'

Sometime before the middle of the fifteenth century, a woman in London, having been told by various physicians that the abnormal swelling and collection of fluids in her uterus was incurable, decided to take matters into her own hands. The woman, 'through her own wit', prepared for herself a special diet of herbal drinks and bread made of beans, salves to use after phlebotomy, and special baths and plasters.[75] The narrator of this account did not indicate the outcome of these self-ministrations, though presumably he could not have reported them in such detail had they not worked and saved her life. There are several ways we can interpret this woman's self-cure. We could say that it proves how generally inefficacious pre-modern medicine was, though that is hardly a helpful (or even necessarily true) observation. After all, she was as 'pre-modern' as her doctors. Or we could say that it proves how worthless the medicine of learned *men* was when it came to gynaecological conditions and that the woman was right to trust 'her own wit' in seeking a cure. But the fact that she initially sought help from the physicians proves she had faith in their skill.

The lessons I would prefer to take from this story are these: first, that new medical knowledge was probably always being created, sometimes by trial and error and sometimes by a reasoned belief that certain kinds of knowledge (about anatomy, bodily processes, the effective qualities of medicines) would yield certain results. And second, that medieval women, by and large, could not participate in the intellectual technologies that many men enjoyed (reading, writing, and the techniques of analysis learned in formal education) to share in the reproduction and refinement of that knowledge. Yes, this woman 'through her own wit' could create an apparently effective treatment for uterine dropsy, but unless she was literate she had no way to communicate this knowledge to other women beyond the circle of her own acquaintances. Unless she was literate, she had no way to refine her treatment by comparison with the opinions of others distant from her in time or space. It took a literate male to record, preserve, and disseminate her learning to a broader 'textual community', which now, of course, includes us.

As twenty-first-century biomedicine attempts to carve out a field of 'women's medicine' and an understanding of the ways in which biological sex and social gender interact to produce health or illness in women's bodies, it does so in the context of debates about health disparities and whether access to healthcare

---

[75] Anonymous, *Sickness of Women*, ed. Green and Mooney, chap. 6, p. 520, lines 938–62.

is a human right. I have argued above that the Middle Ages was no 'golden age' in terms of women's ability to practise medicine on a level fully equal with men. Here I wish to turn to the question of the female patient. Was she in any way disadvantaged by the structure of medieval medicine? Assessing medieval medicine's 'clinical efficacy', whether practised by men or women, is a fruitless task, I believe, not because medieval medical treatments were inherently worthless but because any comparison with the complex and expensive technologies of modern biomedicine is impossible given the incommensurability of their epistemological paradigms and technological resources with ours. Does the 'dropsy' from which the London woman suffered correspond precisely to anything we would now find in a medical textbook? If we cannot even be sure what condition she suffered from, how can we know (again according to our own epistemological standards) whether or not her cure was spontaneous, having nothing to do with her novel therapy? We could, to be sure, attempt to assess whether the masculine birth of gynaecology correlated with any larger trends in mortality or morbidity or demographic growth, but at the moment there seems to be little correlation between the timing of the great demographic changes in medieval and early modern Europe and the work of a handful of medical practitioners.[76]

Nor do I think we can use any universal standard to assess the quality of medieval medicine on the belief that we know 'what women want'. Studies by medical historians and anthropologists confirm that women universally do not share the same concept of health or expect the same things from their healthcare. While many women in the modern United States, for example, may seek out pain relief as a desired goal of medical intervention in birth, many women in southern India ask for drugs to *induce* more intense labour pains, on the belief that pain is necessary for successful childbirth and the stronger the pain, the quicker the birth.[77] When we find no evidence of contraceptives either in

[76] There is as yet an insufficient body of archeological or demographic information differentiated by sex to assess any impact that changes in medical practice may have had. Clearly, both the rise of literate medicine in the 12th century and the new composition of fertility treatises in the 14th came long after the well-documented rise of European population beginning before 1100. For the later medieval period, Klapisch-Zuber's data on female mortality from early 15th-century Florence (which shows approximately 20% mortality rates for women during their childbearing years) come from a period when there was already considerable involvement of male physicians in women's medicine; see Christiane Klapisch-Zuber, 'Le dernier enfant: fécondité et vieillissement chez les Florentines XIVᵉ–XVᵉ siècles', in *Mesurer et comprendre: Mélanges offerts à Jacques Dupaquier,* ed. Jean-Pierre Barder, François Lebrun, and René Le Mée (Paris: Presses Universitaires de France, 1993), pp. 277–90. Rather than having any discernible *effect* on overall demographic trends, I rather think the shifts in masculine involvement in women's medicine are more likely a *response* to the catastrophic mortality of the plague and other, more personal anxieties about succession. For a brief overview of paleopathological work on medieval women, see Green, 'Bodies'. On intellectual *interests* in population growth, see Peter Biller, *The Measure of Multitude: Population in Medieval Thought* (Oxford: Oxford University Press, 2000).

[77] Cecilia Van Hollen, 'Invoking *Vali*: Painful Technologies of Modern Birth in South India', *Medical Anthropology Quarterly,* n.s. 17, no. 1 (March 2003), 49–77.

Trota's own work or even in the translations made for female audiences of *Conditions of Women* (which in its original form had included both a justification for the use of contraceptives and several amuletic methods), should we assume that this absence reflects a censoring by later scribes who wished to condemn contraceptives, or a self-censoring by women themselves who preferred not to put such controversial material in writing? Or might the absence reflect something completely different: women's own sense that the medical control they wished to have over their fertility was to enhance it, not to suppress it, knowing how much their social worth depended on reproductive success?[78] To judge from most medical writings, the medieval definition of a healthy woman was that she be regularly menstruating, heterosexually active, and reproductively successful (especially by producing sons). Celibate religious women, as we have seen, were inherently unhealthy, menstruating too little or too much, and needing medical intervention to help them cope with the side effects of sexual continence. The medieval definition of women's health is not, therefore, terribly unlike those underlying the structures of medical systems in ancient Greece or China or in certain societies today.[79] Moreover, women did not necessarily grant authority to other women or always see that they had 'common cause' with them. As modern theorists have noted, women often engage in 'bargains with patriarchy' in order to shore up their own personal advantage at the expense of other women.[80] Women across Europe accepted the ministrations of male physicians, everyone from the Lombard princess Sichelgaita in the eleventh century to the above-mentioned woman in fifteenth-century London, and for the moment we have no reason to believe that they did not believe that the medicine to be had from learned men was, in fact, the best available. But to acknowledge that women accommodate to the patriarchal structures they live in is hardly a revelation.

There is, however, a different perspective we can adopt to assess what difference it made that men and women were unequally involved in the formulation and provision of women's healthcare between the twelfth and the sixteenth centuries. And that is simply the question whether women, as much as men, could achieve

---

[78] My thinking on this matter was enormously expanded upon discovery of Marcia Inhorn's anthropological work on infertility on modern Egypt: Marcia C. Inhorn, *Quest for Conception: Gender, Infertility, and Egyptian Medical Traditions* (Philadelphia: University of Pennsylvania Press, 1994), and *Infertility and Patriarchy: The Cultural Politics of Gender and Family Life in Egypt* (Philadelphia: University of Pennsylvania Press, 1996). For work rethinking the modern western assumption that all use of emmenagogues (substances to induce menstruation) are intended as contraceptives or abortifacients, see Etienne van de Walle and Elisha P. Renne, eds., *Regulating Menstruation: Beliefs, Practices, Interpretations* (Chicago: University of Chicago Press, 2001).

[79] See Helen King, *Hippocrates' Woman: Reading the Female Body in Ancient Greece* (London and New York: Routledge, 1998); Charlotte Furth, *A Flourishing Yin: Gender in China's Medical History, 960–1665* (University of California Press, 1999).

[80] Deniz Kandiyoti, 'Bargaining with Patriarchy', *Gender and Society* 2, no. 3 (September 1988), 274–90.

'the highest attainable standard of health' then available, the goal of medicine that is now being articulated by advocates of health as a human right.[81]

In terms of its effects on the medical care that women actually received, the masculine birth of gynaecology can be reduced to two main elements. First, if we can take medical texts as an indicator, there is no question that in the later medieval centuries there was an increasing level of *interest* in women's health and even, I would argue, in the actual level of care offerred to women. Interest in generation as an abstract question began in the thirteenth century, while specific concerns to address infertility, which had already been a concern for the Salernitans, took on new import in the fourteenth century. Interventions in childbirth, in turn, show a marked upsurge in the fifteenth century. Not simply is this a matter of more manuscripts being copied or more specialized texts being composed. Rather, there is clearly a change in the level in *intellectual investment* that was made. Comparing Copho's perfunctory gynaecological remedies in the twelfth century with, say, Giovanni Matteo Ferrari da Grado's (d. 1472) extraordinarily detailed *consilia* 300 years later for a German countess suffering from dysuria during her pregnancies or a noblewoman who laboured with difficult breathing as well as menstrual retention,[82] there can be no question that gynaecological conditions (at least in women of the upper classes) grew enormously in importance during the later medieval centuries.

Secondly, the masculine birth of gynaecology is characterized by an increased dissemination of formal medical knowledge on women's conditions and, apparently, a greater standardization of such knowledge within the textual community of literate medical practitioners across Europe. As the first Latin surgical writers of the late twelfth and thirteenth centuries recognized, the transition from strictly oral dissemination of knowledge to a written medium created a broadened community of masters and students, a community from which, fundamentally, women remained excluded or dependent upon men for their admittance. To be sure, the textual medium itself had a conservative effect: whereas some early medieval gynaecological texts might have had several dozen different disease

---

[81] The definition of women's health offered in the platform statement of the Fourth World Conference on Women in Beijing in 1995 is perhaps the most capacious: 'Health is a state of complete physical, mental and social well-being and not merely the absence of disease or infirmity. Women's health involves their emotional, social and physical well-being and is determined by the social, political and economic context of their lives, as well as by biology. . . . A major barrier for women to the achievement of the highest attainable standard of health is inequality, both between men and women and among women in different geographical regions, social classes and indigenous and ethnic groups'; Fourth World Conference on Women (Beijing, September 1995), Platform for Action, Section C, paragraph 89.

[82] Giovanni Matteo Ferrari da Grado, *Perutilia consilia ad diversas aegritudines* (Pavia: J. de Zerbo, 1482), *Consilium* lxxiii: Consilium pro quadam magnifica domina Germana omni anno fecundante partu naturali cum difficultate vrinandi cum mictu sanguineo et interdum sanioso (ff. 57va–59ra); *Consilium* lxxix: Pro vxore domini zenonis de hugino de difficultate anhelitus cum subtractione menstruorum (f. 62rb).

categories,[83] after the influx of learned Arabic medicine the gynaecological and obstetrical nosological canon remained remarkably limited and stable. The same minimalist classification of female reproductive conditions found in Ibn al-Jazzār's *Zād al-musāfir* served as the foundation for the 'women's section' in virtually every medical encyclopedia written between the twelfth and fifteenth centuries, from *Conditions of Women* on.[84] New textual sources might on occasion expand this nosological model: the ancient disease category of the uterine mole, for example, which no Salernitan author had addressed (or at least not under that name), was added back into the litany of women's diseases in the thirteenth century with the influence of Avicenna's *Canon*. And there was even latitude for new empirical observation: the gynaecological disease of 'white flowers' (some kind of vaginal discharge) first appears in medical writings around the turn of the fifteenth century.[85] The gynaecological canon was also open enough to allow the incorporation of therapeutic developments, including such novelties as the medicated pillow on which a fifteenth-century London practitioner has women sit as a treatment for menstrual retention and his rather extraordinary concern to offer interventions to expel a foetus that has died *in utero*.[86] As we have seen, from time to time this openness could also allow for the incorporation of women's empiricism.

But the male approach to gynaecology had two major failings, both of which had to do with the inadequate recognition of the problem of sexuality, of the practitioners as well as the patients, as an inevitable component of reproductive medicine. First, as we have seen over and over again, whether men realized it or not, the same gender system that privileged them educationally also mitigated against their treatment of the intimate conditions of their female patients. Whether, like the author of *Conditions of Women* and many of his translators, we locate this problem of shame in women themselves or rather see men's own anxieties about sexual access to 'other men's women' as the cause, there was a real limit to how far the educated physician or surgeon could apply the knowledge he obtained from books or, for that matter, increase it through empirical observation of women's diseases as they manifested themselves in women's bodies. Since women were not available as educated caretakers to take up the slack (William of Saliceto, for example, believed that the midwives who assisted him even had to be taught the anatomy of the vagina),[87] this left a gaping hole in the care a woman could expect to receive.

---

[83] For example, a work edited under the title *De diversis causis mulierum* has ninety-one chapters, reflecting nearly as many different disease categories.

[84] See Table 1.1 above.

[85] The uterine mole first reappears as a regular gynaecological category in William of Saliceto's work. The disease of 'white flowers' is found in the anonymous French text, *On the Diseases Which Can Occur in the Generative Organs of Women*; in a variety of works by Italian authors; and even in some random recipes in English.

[86] On this anonymous Middle English text, *Sickness of Women 2*, see Chapter 4 above.

[87] Helen Lemay, 'William of Saliceto on Human Sexuality', *Viator* 12 (1981), 167–81.

Consider, for a moment, the parallel conditions of inguinal hernia and uterine prolapse, the former far more common in men, the latter (by definition) unique to women.[88] In modern medical understanding both are considered 'mechanical' defects, caused by structural weaknesses and particular stresses on the ligaments and muscles that support the lower abdominal wall, in the one case, or the pelvic floor, in the other. Since these conditions are not due to infection, we can suppose, for the sake of argument, that they occurred at more or less the same rates in historical populations as they do today.[89] Inguinal hernia seems to have been a perennial concern for surgeons, though the pace of innovation in treatment increased noticeably in the late thirteenth century. Taking inspiration from Arabic descriptions of hernial operations, surgeons refined their techniques to such an extent that hernias became the first area of surgical specialization in fourteenth-century Europe.[90] As we have seen, uterine prolapse was also almost always mentioned, at least perfunctorily, in gynaecological writings and general medical textbooks from the Salernitans on. But whereas inguinal hernia saw increasing theorization by surgical writers and increasing innovation in practical techniques, uterine prolapse remained decidedly untheorized well into the fifteenth century. Did it also remain untreated? As we saw in Chapter 2, Trota's strikingly original recommendations for treating prolapse and preventing reoccurrence of vaginal fistulae in later births were never incorporated into the work of any male medical or surgical writer in the thirteenth century save for Gilbertus Anglicus; later, the southern Italian writer, Francesco da Piedemonte, would incorporate them into his work, though he too erased Trota's existence, attributing her procedures to 'the counsels from an expert'.[91] In other words, even when the hands-on learning of a female practitioner was available to men, they did not exploit it. Instead, the kinds of treatments male practitioners recommended continued to stay on the level of potions, abdominal massages, and other hands-off treatments that characterized men's gynaecological practice in general. The first known vaginal hysterectomy, performed on a woman with a prolapsed uterus by Berengario da Carpi's father in the late fifteenth century,

---

[88] Inguinal hernia, the protrusion of any part of the intestines or abdominal fluid through an extended portion of the peritoneum called the processus vaginalis (which in males is usually obliterated after the testicles descend during foetal development), occurs about twelve times more often in males than in females. Medieval surgical writers seem to have conceived of it exclusively as a male condition since they defined it as the extrusion of the intestines into the scrotal sac.

[89] Because modern societies that make extensive use of Caesarean section have probably skewed 'natural' rates of prolapse, I looked for incidence rates for populations in Southeast Asia and Africa in the 'Older Women Annotated Bibliography' gathered by *Reproductive Health Outlook* <http://www.rho.org/html/older-b–01.htm#alqutob01> accessed 23 April 2005. Here, incidence rates of genital prolapse ranged from 19–70% with the higher figures common for older populations.

[90] Michael R. McVaugh, 'Treatment of Hernia in the Later Middle Ages: Surgical Correction and Social Construction', in Roger French, *et al.*, *Medicine from the Black Death to the French Disease* (Aldershot: Ashgate, 1998), pp. 131–55; and 'Cataracts and Hernias: Aspects of Surgical Practice in the Fourteenth Century', *Medical History* 45 (2001), 319–40.

[91] See Chapter 2 above.

seems to come directly out of male surgical traditions, not female empiricism.[92] Female practitioners attempting to treat prolapse would have been handicapped by the gender system, too, since they did not have their own literate traditions to preserve empirical learning such as Trota's. Perhaps in southern Italy the traditions of apprenticeship-based oral instruction were strong enough among women to maintain a direct line between, say, the illiterate fourteenth-century surgeon Raymunda de Taberna and her forebear, the Salernitan Trota, that could ensure transmission of techniques for repairing a vaginal fistula, restoring a prolapsed uterus, and even for distinguishing, as did Trota, between an intestinal complaint and a uterine one. But how many other women in Europe would have been able to benefit from this knowledge? Thus, where the ancients, according to Caelius Aurelianus, had instituted the tradition of writing on women's conditions precisely so that women could benefit from learned female healers and avoid the problem of sexual shame,[93] no one in the Middle Ages seems to have thought of that possibility. From the perspective of the female patient, the gender gap in the accumulation and transfer of medical knowledge had very real consequences.

A second, more pernicious effect of the gendered structure of later medieval women's medicine—more pernicious precisely because it was deliberate—is the way in which men came to use gynaecological literature against women. As we have seen, misogynous views of women were embedded in the training that boys received in grammar school, which in turn laid a foundation both for prurience among 'boys whether in age or in morals' and for a suspicious need among adult men to establish control over women and their 'secrets'. Male interest in generation need not necessarily be misogynous, of course. Under a patriarchal system, especially one that restricted men to monogamy for the production of legal heirs, men could have as much concern about progeny as women. Yet precisely because medieval society was patriarchal, information about anatomy, reproductive physiology, the signs of pregnancy, and the ways in which reproductive outcomes could be manipulated was powerful knowledge. It was also inherently problematic knowledge, since it involved deliberate discourse on matters of sex. Ever since Antiquity, it was assumed that it was *women* who did not wish to discuss the diseases of their genitalia, though as we have seen it was equally problematic for men to engage in any practices that involved access to the genitalia of 'other men's' women. If gynaecological conditions are seen simply as 'women's matters' (the literal meaning of the Greek *gynaikeia*), then the problem of women's exclusion from literate medical discourses revolved around how to transfer knowledge from men (who owned, read, and wrote the books)

---

[92] Though the stories of Flore Nicole and Dulceta of Marseille (see Chapter 2 above) suggest that women themselves or their kin might conceive of surgical intervention as an obvious course of relief.

[93] See Chapter 1 above.

to women. If, however, the reproductive capacities of the female body are seen as 'women's secrets'—'secrets' hidden from men that they wish to uncover—then women's exclusion from the production and dissemination of medical/scientific views on women becomes part of the structures of patriarchy, a means by which men like the English gentleman Humphrey Newton establish control over their 'patrimony' or, like the fictitious Jankyn, try (sometimes unsuccessfully) to browbeat and humiliate women. To be sure, the contestation over uses of gynaecological knowledge had some surprising results: the author of the English *Knowing of Woman's Kind* turned concern about slander into a novel distillation of written lore on women's diseases and childbirth for a female audience. In Germany, the same environment that produced and sustained an extraordinary level of engagement with the pseudo-Albertan *Secrets of Women* would also produce the first printed texts for midwives. But neither English laywomen nor German midwives truly 'owned' this new literature. Concerns about men's prurient or manipulative reading of gynaecological literature continued and the midwifery manuals of the sixteenth century came to serve as default guides to sex education.[94] Hence the need of vernacular translators and authors to attempt to convince their female audiences that these works were meant for women's benefit, not their harm. The gap in communication between women and men, and between women and other women, was costly in more ways than one.

Thus, we are left in the rather heretical position of concluding that by the end of the Middle Ages, the women who received the best medical care according to the standards of the time were the upper-class women of northern Italy. By breaching, at least partially, the taboo against male inspection of the female genitalia, north Italian male practitioners were actually able to bring to women something approaching the same quality of care they gave their male patients. Although the discourse of 'women's secrets' existed there as well, as yet no trace has been found of a female protest against disparaging male uses of gynaecological knowledge that writers in northern Europe had to warn against.[95] Savonarola is full of cordial respect for the upper-class women who made up his valued clientele, the *noblesse oblige* of someone very secure in the distance that separates him from

---

[94] Fear that his gynaecological text might be misused appears in the work of the Majorcan author, Damián Carbón, *Libro del arte de las comadres o madrinas, y del regimiento de las preñadas y paridas y de los niños* ([Majorca City: Hernando de Cansoles,] 1541). For similar concerns in various versions of Eucharius Rösslin's *Rosegarden*, see Monica H. Green, 'Gender and the Vernacularization of Women's Medicine in Late Medieval and Early Modern Europe' (forthcoming).

[95] One of the two known Italian translations of the *Trotula* was called *Segrete cose delle donne*. Not only did it trim down the text to a focus on fertility, but it also circulated in similar codicological contexts as the Italian translation of the pseudo-Albertus Magnus, which was called *Segreti delle femmine*; see Green, 'Gender and the Vernacularization of Women's Medicine'. As Katharine Park shows, patrician women readily consulted male physicians, even to the point of requesting that the latter autopsy them after death; *Secrets of Women: Gender, Generation, and the Origins of Human Dissection* (New York: Zone Books, 2006), chapter 3.

the people dependent on him. The hierarchies of gender and learning were so securely established in northern Italy that there was no need either for laws to drive women out of medical practice or even polemics against female practice beyond the most subtle reminder, 'this is not the work of women'.

This same confidence among male practitioners that they were providing women the best that learned medicine could offer, unaccompanied by any awareness of why there were no female practitioners of comparable learning beside them, would characterize gynaecology up through the twentieth century. The intellectuals preoccupied with the *Querelle des femmes* ('Debate about Women') in the fifteenth through seventeenth centuries did not raise questions about the presence of women in medicine, but perhaps we can. What if the upper-class women of northern Italy had had a *choice* between a Savonarola and an equally learned woman healer? What if Trota really had held a professorial chair in medicine at Salerno, had had the same command of Latin and dialectical argument as the male medical masters, had engaged in anatomical work alongside Copho, and had established a tradition of training other such women? What if such women existed to offer the patrician women of Florence or Bologna or Ferrara, whose sexual chastity was considered their chief virtue, or even better, what if they existed to offer all women of whatever class, the *option* of being taken into a female practitioner's home 'so that secretly she could determine the cause of [their] illness'?

Even this exercise in counterfactual speculation carries a whiff of Whiggism, of course, the assumption that the past can be judged by how well or poorly it accords with our own notions of what is 'best'. Yet we have already had ample evidence that people in the Middle Ages were accustomed to having a relatively open medical marketplace, an array of choices that ranged from learned medicine to the passing empiric to the saint's shrine down the road. The trials of Jacoba Felicie and Perretta Petone show that satisfied patients were willing to protest when their options were curtailed. It may be relevant, therefore, to bring in one more element of modern medical discourse for comparison.

A characteristic of new arguments about health as a human right is that those most affected by any science or technology must be parties to its creation, both so that they can guide the enterprise according to their own wants or needs and so that they can be vigilant against the abuse of knowledge against them.[96] The Office of Women's Health Research at the United States National Institutes of Health was founded in 1990 with the mandate both to advance research on women and to promote the careers of female researchers and clinicians. The politicians, health practitioners, and political activists who worked to have the

---

[96] On the general concept of health as a human right, see Sofia Gruskin and Daniel Tarantola, 'Health and Human Rights', in *Oxford Textbook of Public Health*, 4th edn, ed. Roger Detels, James McEwen, Robert Beaglehole and Heizo Tanaka (Oxford: Oxford University Press, 2004), pp. 311–36.

Office established, many of whom had participated with the nascent women's health movement of the 1960s and 1970s, recognized that the two objectives had to work hand in hand: too many aspects of women's health had been ignored, they argued, because too few women existed at the decision-making levels of medical research and education. Similar efforts to improve women's health by increasing the representation of women in the healthcare fields have been pursued in other nations, as well as at the international level by the Office of Women's Health at the World Health Organization (WHO).[97] The very existence of these organizations is an argument that the quality of women's healthcare is affected, perhaps even determined, by the gendered structures of women's health education, research, and policy. However much modern biomedicine has helped women live longer lives less compromised by disability and disease, precisely because it has such power women must be centrally involved as the producers and transmitters of its knowledge.

In the present day, major health disparities occur in access to expensive medical technologies and life-saving vaccines and drugs.[98] Medieval Europe had no such powerful technologies and I have found no particular disparities between the genders in terms of therapies employed.[99] Rather, in the Middle Ages the most valuable commodity traded in the medical marketplace was learning, particularly the disciplined learning that came from reading, studying, and in a few but important cases, composing books. Female patients were never totally denied the benefits of learned medicine: as we have seen, most male physicians did not hesitate to diagnose and treat women. But the structures of the medieval gender system set real limits to how far the male physician could go, both in his verbal interrogations and his visual and manual inspections and treatments. That same gender system set equally real limits to how far a female practitioner might go in gaining the same expanded knowledge that the male practitioner got from his books and from the reasoned discourse they made possible. Whether we judge that book learning worthwhile or not, women's inability to attain it meant their gradual exclusion from any authoritative stature in the medical marketplace. The inequalities of gender can perhaps be best summarized by this simple fact: whereas the first professional handbooks of surgery written by surgeons appear within

[97] For an overview of the development of 'women's medicine' from the 1970s through 2002, see Monica H. Green, 'Defining Women's Health: An Interdisciplinary Dialogue—Background', posted 15 April 2002 on <http://www.fas.harvard.edu/womenstudy/events/proposal.htm>.

[98] And not even necessarily expensive ones. See Institute of Medicine, *Unequal Treatment: Confronting Racial and Ethnic Disparities in Health Care* (Washington, DC: National Academies Press, 2003).

[99] In terms of gender, I have not yet found for the Middle Ages anything comparable to Heinrich von Staden's discovery, in 'Women and Dirt', *Helios* 19, no. 1–2 (1992), 7–29, of a pronounced use of dung in Hippocratic gynaecological remedies in contrast to other areas of medicine where it was never used. The biggest disparities in healthcare (and almost certainly also in health) were between rich and poor, urban and rural, and not between men and women generically. On rich vs. poor, see Chapter 1 above. As Savonarola himself admitted, with rather shocking candour, 'the physician does not busy himself very much with the poor' (*Practica major*, f. 268ra).

decades of the field's re-emergence as a specialization in the twelfth century, 400 years were to pass between the re-emergence of professional midwives in the thirteenth century and the appearance of the first textbook actually composed by a midwife, Louise Bourgeois's *Diverse Observations* in 1609. A 400-year gap can, I think, by any measure be called a disparity. And that, in the end, is what gender is about: the unequal distribution of power, access, and authority between men and women.

TROTA, 'TROTULA', AND THE USES OF HISTORY

I began this book with the assertion that the 'Trotula Question', traditionally defined around the historicity of a single female practitioner, was wrong-headed or at the very least inadequate. We needed to look at how gender structured the whole field of women's medicine and not simply focus on one iconic individual. But there remains the question, relevant not so much to the Middle Ages as to our own times: why *did* 'Trotula' become an icon, a placeholder on the monumental plinth of women's medical history, a figurehead whose specific historical details, if we follow the thinking of the nineteenth-century physician Marie Zakrzewska, really didn't matter?

This book has chronicled how both Trota and 'Trotula's' status as an authoritative female figure gradually eroded over the later medieval centuries. In her own day, Trota clearly had considerable authority. Even if her male Salernitan peers were largely oblivious to her written work, she had enough effect on some part of her community to generate a reputation that spread all the way to Normandy and England. That esteem itself seems to have led to the creation of *Treatments for Women* and it continued at least into the thirteenth century if we can judge from the Anglo-Norman cosmetic writer who readily proclaims his fidelity to the teachings of 'madame Trote de Salerne'. Yet there is precious little evidence after the thirteenth century that medieval women found Trota/'Trotula' to be an estimable figure, assuming they had heard of her at all. Aside from the women who may have read the English *Book of Rota* and the Dutch *Liber Trotula*, the only two vernacular translations of the *Trotula* that presented 'Rota' or 'Trotula' as the author of a text clearly intended for female readers, and aside from Dorothea Susanna who owned a copy of Johannes Hartlieb's German *Buch Trotula* (where Trotula' was praised as a queen), I have found no evidence that any women knew about Trota/'Trotula' again until the eighteenth century. None of the seventeenth-century female midwife authors—Louise Bourgeois, Jane Sharp, Elizabeth Cellier, and Justine Siegemund—knew about any medieval forebears.[100] For them, the history of their profession was limited to references to

---

[100] Cellier, a London midwife (fl. 1668–88), did not write a midwifery manual, though she does employ historical arguments in one of her two polemical tracts supporting female midwifery.

midwives in the Bible or legends from Antiquity. Moreover, when early modern learned women—authors such as Lucrezia Marinella (1571–1653), a physician's daughter like Christine de Pizan two centuries before her, or Sor Juana Inés de la Cruz (1648–95), a Mexican nun—began compiling their own histories of accomplished women, they made no mention of any female medical authorities at all.[101] Despite the engagement of early modern women in recipe-collecting and charitable healing, I have found no evidence that they imagined that women had ever held positions of medical authority in the past outside the field of midwifery.

That the legend of 'Trotula' survived at all was due, ironically, to certain narrow learned traditions that kept alive enough remnants of her story for later ages to weave new narratives. A year before Georg Kraut turned his sharp-edged humanist pen on the *Trotula* to recreate it as an exemplar of ancient medicine in 1544, another humanist scholar, the French lawyer André Tiraqueau, addressed the question whether the practice of medicine was ennobling to those who practised it. He answered in the affirmative, and said this was true even of women; he then provided a list of some notable female practitioners, among whom he included 'Trota, or Trotula the Salernitan, who wrote on the diseases of women and their treatment'.[102] Similarly, in 1620, an Italian bishop, Francesco Agostino della Chiesa, referred to 'Tertulia [*sic*], or Trota Salernitana' in his *Theater of Learned Women*, an alphabetical listing of several dozen different names.[103] Most influential of all in terms of defining the modern 'Trotula' legend was Antonio Mazza who, in 1681, for the first time referred explicitly to 'Trotula' (and several other women) as holding professorial chairs at the university of Salerno. An Italian natural philosopher, Giuseppa Eleonora Barbapiccola, in turn recycled Mazza's list of famous Salernitan female practitioners—Abella, Mercuriade, Rebecca, Trotta, Sentia Guarna, and Costanza Calenda—in the introduction to her translation of Descartes' *Principles of Philosophy* in 1722.[104]

---

[101] Marinella and de la Cruz's works listing female authorities were, respectively, *The Nobility and Excellence of Women and the Defects and Vices of Men* (1600), and *Response to Sor Filotea de la Cruz* (1691). Marinella's father was Giovanni Marinelli, author of the Italian *Medicine Pertaining to the Diseases of Women* discussed above. Her brother and husband were physicians, too.

[102] This post-medieval fate of 'Trotula's' fame is recounted in Monica H. Green, 'In Search of an "Authentic" Women's Medicine: The Strange Fates of Trota of Salerno and Hildegard of Bingen', *Dynamis: Acta Hispanica ad Medicinae Scientiarumque Historiam Illustrandam* 19 (1999), 25–54.

[103] Francesco Agostino della Chiesa, *Theatro delle donne letterate, con vn breue discorso della preminenza, e perfettione del sesso donnesco* (Mondovi: Gislandus and Rossus, 1620), where 'Tertulia, ò sia Trota Salernitana' is described as having 'dar fuori al giuditio vniuersale vn bel volume di salutiferi rimedi alle infirmità donnesche'. Della Chiesa had studied law and may, therefore, have been familiar with Tiraqueau's work.

[104] On Mazza, see Green, 'In Search'. My thanks to Paula Findlen of Stanford University for bringing the citation from Barbapiccola's work to my attention. A friend of the historian Giovanni Battista Vico's daughter and probably a resident of Naples, Barbapiccola no doubt encountered Mazza's book in her native Salerno.

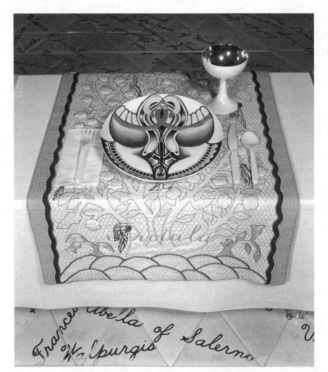

FIG. C.I place setting for 'Trotula' at Judy Chicago's *The Dinner Party* (1979).

These two rhetorical strands—the 'learned women/feminist' and the 'Salernitan/patriotic'—would coexist or even intertwine for the next 250 years. The most important Salernitan medical historian of the nineteenth century, Salvatore De Renzi, revived Mazza's opinion that women held positions of instructional authority at Salerno (he called them *maestre*, rather than *professoresse*),[105] while the feminist physicians, Melina Lipinska, a Polish emigré to Paris, and Kate Campbell Hurd-Mead, the American obstetrician, eagerly adopted 'Trotula' and her embellished story from De Renzi, setting her up as one of the great monuments of the history of women's medicine. Little wonder, then, that when 'second wave' feminism and the new women's health movement were developing in the 1960s and 1970s, the ready-made heroine 'Trotula' should be adopted as one of the great lost women from the past: she was one of only six medieval women and one of only two physicians invited to sit at the table of Judy Chicago's feminist art masterpiece, *The Dinner Party*, in 1979 (Fig. C.1). Scholarly scepticism over 'Trotula's' existence persisted into the twentieth century, with a new theory coming along every few years, some more ridiculous or misogynistic

---

[105] De Renzi, apparently something of a feminist himself, used these *maestre* to chide his fellow academics about their objections to contemporary efforts to admit women to medical study.

than others, each claiming to be the last nail in her coffin. The most recent stage of scholarship, of course, argues for the need to distinguish between the broadly skilled and highly original (if marginally literate and definitely untenured) historic practitioner, Trota, from the metasticized textual persona 'Trotula'. Perhaps it is not surprising, however, that these painstaking philological arguments, quite obscure to the non-medievalist, have had no effect in dislodging the popular myth of 'Trotula', 'the first female professor of medicine', from the western psyche. As Marie Zakrewska presciently recognized in 1881, there was—and apparently still is—greater need for a *symbolic* 'first woman physician' (or first female medical professor) than for a specific historically documentable woman.[106]

In musing upon the idea of a statue to 'the first woman physician', Zakrzewska was thinking in contemporary terms: she wanted some commemoration of the women of her own age who had wedged their feet in the doors of Europe's and North America's medical schools, opening the way for others who followed. Zakrzewska had no thought of turning to the Middle Ages for inspiration, though her keen insights on the uses of history help explain why the medieval period has since come to function as a sort of 'golden age' for women's medicine, when women allegedly had control over their own bodies without any male involvement. This book has shown that the only constant of the twelfth through sixteenth centuries is that women had uncontested control over birth or, to put it another way, that only the management of normal childbirth was gendered unambiguously as feminine. And as the Faculty of Medicine at Paris would declare in 1423 in the case of the male practitioner Jean Domrémi, what women did in the process of assisting each other in birth was not considered medicine. Clearly, this book has not shared the Parisian Faculty's opinion in defining the work of Trota and countless other medieval women out of existence in the history of medicine. When looking at the achievements of Trota in Salerno, therefore, and the handful of other women we have found who actively engaged with the *literate* aspects of medical knowledge and practice, the question should not be 'How did she do it?' but rather 'Why weren't there dozens or even hundreds more like her?' Aside from Trota's contemporary, Hildegard of Bingen, it would not be until the sixteenth and seventeenth centuries that other women would appear as full-fledged medical authors, and it would not be until the feminist movements of the nineteenth and twentieth centuries reconfigured women's place within the medical hierarchy that women would gain an equal footing in the formal systems of medical education that first took root in twelfth-century Salerno.

---

[106] In that same letter of 28 May 1881, Zakrzewska wrote 'You all know how little appreciation I have for Fame; but whenever I go to places like [Westminster] Abbey, Fame presents to me another aspect. It is entirely impersonal—names are of no consequence, *but the reasons why these landmarks of civilization are placed there for the beholder are of intense interest*'. As cited in Vietor, *Woman's Quest*, p. 404, my emphasis.

When looking for monuments in women's medical history, therefore, we can certainly turn to Trota or Perretta Petone or their countless female peers who practised medicine in medieval Europe. We can celebrate their achievements or bemoan the ways the gendered structures of medieval society kept them from achieving more. Either way, we should remember to ask why we want or need monuments at all. Marie Zakrzewska felt that 'the fact that a woman can work and make an impression upon civilization needs to be known to be remembered'. In the nineteenth century when she was writing, women's ability to 'make an impression upon civilization' as fully trained independent medical practitioners was neither known nor, obviously, could it be remembered. In the early twenty-first century, that fact is now embodied in the hundreds of thousands of women throughout the world who are making their own impressions upon civilization through their medical work. Although one cannot yet claim that women have an equal role in the formulation of the science of gynaecology and its delivery as clinical medicine (the percentage of women practising OB/GYN in the United States, for example, continues to rise yet men still overwhelmingly hold the authoritative positions in academic OB/GYN departments), the fields of medical history and medical sociology have grown attentive enough to gender analysis to ensure that these modern women's stories are known.

Perhaps the kinds of monuments we need now are different. Two thousand years ago, a Greek woman named Antiochis, daughter of Diadotos, was noted 'for her experience in the medical art'.[107] She could have looked around her and seen that medical practice by women, although subordinate within what was as fundamentally a patriarchal society as medieval Europe, was nevertheless normative. No abstract narrative of women's general accomplishments was needed. Antiochis erected a statue that Dr Zakrzewska probably could not have conceived as possible in her own day but which, I believe, she would have ultimately admired. Antiochis erected a statue . . . to herself.

---

[107] Rebecca Flemming, *Medicine and the Making of Roman Women: Gender, Nature, and Authority from Celsus to Galen* (Oxford: Oxford University Press, 2001), p. 391.

APPENDIX 1

Medieval and Renaissance Owners of *Trotula* Manuscripts

PART 1 OWNERS OF LATIN MANUSCRIPTS

Owner (and means of acquisition, if known)	*Manuscript*[1] or *Witness* (if lost or unidentified)
England	
[1] Walter of St George (fl. 1286), a monk at St Augustine's, Canterbury,[2] was very likely a medical practitioner, as thirteen of the fifteen books he donated to St Augustine's contained medical texts; among them were two copies of the *Trotula*	Late 15th-century catalogue of St Augustine's Abbey in Canterbury lists one copy of *Trocula maior* and one of *Cure trocule* (item nos. 1235h and 1255f)[3]
[2] William of Chichester (late 13th century?), perhaps a medical practitioner given his ownership of nine medical volumes, had a text identified by the 15th-century cataloguer as *De infirmitatibus mulierum et earum curis*, which, given its context amid Constantinian texts, may have been a copy of the *Trotula*[4]	*Ibid.* (item 1249e)
[3] John of London (fl. 1310–30), also a monk at St Augustine's and an	*Ibid.* two copies of *Trotula maior de curis mulierum*, one of *Trotula*

---

[1] Full bibliographical and biographical references for most of the extant manuscripts can be found in my essays, Green, 'Handlist I' and 'Handlist II'. The notes here are limited to information that supplements or corrects that earlier work.

[2] A. B. Emden, *Donors of Books to S. Augustine's Abbey, Canterbury*, Oxford Bibliographical Society, Occasional Publication, 4 (Oxford, 1969), p. 16.

[3] See Montague Rhodes James, *The Ancient Libraries of Canterbury and Dover: The Catalogues of the Libraries of Christ Church Priory and St Augustine's Abbey at Canterbury and of St Martin's Priory at Dover* (Cambridge: Cambridge University Press, 1903), catalogue of St Augustine's, pp. 341 and 345. The corrected orthography is from Bruce Barker-Benfield (personal communication, 21 June and 28 June 2002), who is re-editing the St Augustine's catalogue.

[4] This title is found with several extant copies of the transitional *Trotula* ensemble.

astronomer, gave a massive donation of eighty-three volumes to the monastery, of which a quarter were medical; he owned three copies of the *Trotula*; he also owned a copy of a text called, by a later 15th-century cataloguer, *Practica de Genescie de secretis mulierum*, which may, given its context amid Salernitan texts, have been the *Trotula*

maior et minor (items 1187j, 1219j and 1599f [= CTC, MS R.14.30 (903), s. xiii ex., France]); *Practica Genescie de secretis mulierum* (item 1262a)[5]

[4]   Michael of Northgate (fl. 1340), monk, translator, and author of works in Middle English,[6] copied with his own hand selections from *Women's Cosmetics*; at his death he donated the volume to St Augustine's, together with twenty-three other volumes on theology, devotional works, natural science, medicine, arboriculture, and alchemy

Ibid., here called *Depilatoria* (item 1170k [= Oxford, Corpus Christi College, MS 221, s. xiv[1] (England)])

[5]   John of Chesterford (before 1349?)[7]donated one copy to St Augustine's

Ibid., *Trotula minor* (item 1225b)

[6]   Simon Bredon, a fellow of Merton College, canon of Chichester, and sometime physician to Elizabeth de Burgh (d. 1360), seems to have owned a copy of the standardized ensemble; he willed it, together with a massive collection of more than two dozen medical and other scientific books, to Merton College

Oxford, Merton College, MS 230, s. xiv in. (England, probably Oxford)

---

[5] James, *Ancient Libraries*. On John of London, see Wilbur R. Knorr, 'Two Medieval Monks and their Astronomy Books', *Bodleian Library Record* 14 (1991–4), 269–84; and Richard Sharpe, *A Handlist of the Latin Writers of Great Britain and Ireland before 1540* (Turnhout: Brepols, 1997), pp. 277–8. Since, according to my findings, 'secreta mulierum' was still not commonly used as a title in the early 14th century, I think it unlikely that John of London's manuscript had it as the original title. The St Augustine's cataloguer was responsible for assigning the title 'de secretis mulierum' to the text by 'Ascarus' in item 1599 (which is actually the *Genecia Cleopatre* with a unique, fictitious prologue, now CTC, MS R.14.30 [903]), and so may have added a similar title to this text owned by John of London. See Chapter 5.

[6] Also known as Dan Michael, he translated into the Kentish dialect the French confessor's manual *Somme le Roi* under the title *Ayenbite of Inwit*.

[7] Emden was unable to locate any biographical information on J. de Chesterford. He speculates, however, that most of the donors with names in the form of 'de' before a territorial title probably date from before the mid 14th century (*Donors*, p. 24).

[7]	Merton College received a copy in 1368 from Simon Bredon (see above); the copy has remained there up to the present day	(as above)
[8]	William Rede, Bishop of Chichester (1369–85) and a noted astronomer, bequeathed a copy of the proto-ensemble to New College, Oxford	Oxford, New College, MS 171, s. xiii[1] (S. France or Italy)
[9]	New College, Oxford, received in 1385 Rede's manuscript (as above), where it remains to the present day	(as above)
[10]	Henry Whitfield, who held degrees in arts, medicine, and theology, was an ordained priest and fellow of Queen's College, Oxford; in 1383 or 1387 he gave to Stapledon Hall (later Exeter College) a manuscript containing the transitional ensemble and *Women's Cosmetics* 3	Oxford, Exeter College, MS 35, s. xiv[1] (England)
[11]	Stapledon Hall (later Exeter College), Oxford, received in 1383 or 1387 Whitfield's manuscript	(as above)
[12]	John Erghome (d. *c.*1385), prior of the convent of Augustinian friars at York and apparently a man of remarkable learning, owned among some 300 books (twenty-two of which were medical) one copy of 'trotula maior de secretis mulierum'	Catalogue of the convent library made in 1372[8]
[13]	Convent of Augustinian friars at York received Erghome's copy of 'trotula maior de secretis mulierum'[9]	(as above)
[14]	Benedictine priory at Dover owned two copies of *Conditions of Women* or	Catalogue of 1389[10]

---

[8] K. W. Humphreys (ed.), *The Friars' Libraries*, Corpus of British Medieval Library Catalogues (London: British Library in association with the British Academy, 1990), p. 136. Erghome's books may have been listed in 1372, or they may have been added later. Erghome also owned a copy of Muscio's *Gynaecia* in a volume containing *inter alia* Hildegard of Bingen's *Physica* (*ibid.*, p. 110). On Erghome's library in general, see Aubrey Gwynn, *The English Austin Friars in the Time of Wyclif* (London: Humphrey Milford, Oxford University Press, 1940), pp. 130–4.

[9] Of Erghome's 300 books, twenty-two were primarily medical in content. The convent library seems to have had only one medical book that was not Erghome's.

[10] William P. Stoneman, *Dover Priory*, Corpus of British Medieval Library Catalogues, 5 (London: British Library, 1999), pp. 141 and 143. Both copies are identified as the *Trotula maior* and have the normal incipit of *Conditions of Women*, 'Cum auctor uniuersitatis'.

perhaps the whole ensemble by 1389;
the names of the donors are not known

[15]	Abbey of Premonstratensian Canons at Titchfield owned one copy by 1400; the name of the donor is not known	Catalogue of 1400 lists volume comprising twenty-eight medical works, including a 'Summa tractule [*sic*] de cura sue sexus'[11]
[16]	Richard Stapleton, Master of Balliol College (*c.*1430), copied and annotated with his own hand a copy of the proto-ensemble; he later left it to his college's library	OBL, MS Digby 29 (SC 1630), s. xv in. (England)
[17]	John Stnetesham (or Stetesham, d. 1448), chancellor of Exeter, donated a copy of the proto-ensemble to Exeter Cathedral	OBL, MS Wood empt. 15 (SC 8603), s. xv[1] (England)
[18]	Edmund Lacy, bishop of Exeter (d. 1455), passed on a manuscript with a fragment of the proto-ensemble to Exeter Cathedral upon his death	OBL, MS Bodley 786 (SC 2626), s. xiii med. (England)
[19]	Exeter Cathedral owned at least two copies of the *Trotula* by 1455	(see entries above)
[20]	Gilbert Kymer, chancellor of Oxford (1431–34, 1446–53), dean of Salisbury (1449–63), and personal physician to Humphrey, Duke of Gloucester, had the professional scribe Hermannus Zurke of Greifswald copy for him an unusual assemblage of the three independent *Trotula* texts	OBL, MS Bodley 361 (2462), an. 1453–9 (Salisbury)
[21]	Robartus Glaspullus, owned a copy of the *Women's Cosmetics* 1 in 1451	Edinburgh, Edinburgh University Library, MS 167, s. xiii[1] (England)
[22]	John Harryson (or Herryson, fl. 1443–73), a cleric and MD who early in his career served as chaplain to the nuns of St Radegund's Priory in Cambridge, owned a copy of the proto-ensemble (Erfurt Group)	BLL, MS Royal 12.E.VII, s. xv[1] (England)
[23]	Roger Marchall (*c.*1417–77), physician and fellow of Peterhouse, Cambridge, owned a copy of the	Cambridge, Gonville & Caius College, MS 117/186, s. xiii med. (England) and BLL, MS

---

[11] R. M. Wilson, 'The Medieval Library of Titchfield Abbey', *Proceedings of the Leeds Philosophical and Literary Society. Literary and Historical Section* 5/3 (February 1940), 150–177 and 5/4 (June 1941), 252–76: MS. K. IX. (pp. 174–5); David N. Bell (ed.), *The Libraries of the Cistercians, Gilbertines and Premonstratensians*, Corpus of British Medieval Library Catalogues 3 (London: British Library, in association with the British Academy, 1992), p. 213.

	revised ensemble and, in another codex, some selections from *Women's Cosmetics* 1; he seems to have donated the ensemble copy to Gonville Hall in Cambridge	Sloane 420, s. xiv in. (England)
[24]	Gonville Hall (now Gonville & Caius College), Cambridge, has retained Marchall's copy to the present day	(as above)
[25]	King Edward IV (r. 1461–83) obtained what is now the earliest extant copy of the proto-ensemble before his accession; this would later pass into Henry VIII's library[12]	BLL, MS Royal 12.E.XV, s. xii ex. (E. France)
[26]	Benedictine Abbey of St Augustine's, Canterbury: in addition to the six copies donated by Walter of St George, John of London, Michael of Northgate, and John of Chesterford (see above), by the late 15th century the collection also included a copy of the transitional ensemble plus two copies of what was probably the Salernitan *Women's Cosmetics* (here attributed to 'Cleopatra')[13] given by unspecified donors	late s. xv catalogue, item no. 1274 = New York, New York Academy of Medicine, MS SAFE, s. xiii med. (France);[14] and items 1137.23 and 1195.10

[12] James P. Carley (ed.), *The Libraries of King Henry VIII*, Corpus of British Medieval Library Catalogues, 7 (London: The British Library in association with the British Academy, 2000), p. 160. Since Henry's cataloguer failed to note the presence of any of the medical texts in the codex (the manuscript was identified only as containing the *Secreta secretorum* ascribed to Aristotle), it is unlikely that Henry, at least, had any interest in the *Trotula*.

[13] I believe that these two copies of 'Cleopatra's' cosmetic text do not reflect an otherwise un-attested Latin translation of 'her' Greek *Cosmetics* (which were probably themselves apocryphal), but instead are copies of the Salernitan cosmetic text. My reasons stem from item 1274 in the St Augustine's catalogue, now extant as New York Academy of Medicine, MS SAFE, s. xiii med., which may have been compiled for Richard de Fournival. (See Green, 'Handlist I', item 64.) Here, there is a fragment of the Salernitan *Women's Cosmetics* right after the *Gynaecology of Cleopatra*. (*Women's Cosmetics* is left incomplete apparently because the scribe realized that he had already copied the text within the *Trotula* ensemble, which appears earlier in the manuscript). I have found no other extant manuscripts where *Women's Cosmetics* similarly follows the *Gynaecology of Cleopatra*, but I can imag-ine that the St Augustine's cataloguer assumed that *Women's Cosmetics* was, like the preceding text, by 'Cleopatra'; then, when he found two other copies of the same text in other manuscripts, he attributed these, too, to 'Cleopatra'. I would point out that all three instances of a text *de ornatu mulierum* in the St Augustine's catalogue are ascribed to specific authors (items 1137, 1195, and 1236). Since, with one exception, the Salernitan *Women's Cosmetics* is in extant manuscripts (some thirty altogether) always anonymous, it might have been ripe for such an appealing ascription in the eyes of this cataloguer. My thanks to Dr Richard Sharpe for a query that helped me clarify my thinking on this attribution.

[14] James, *Ancient Libraries*, p. 347. The 'liber de ornatu faciei' in item 1277 (now Oxford, Corpus Christi College 125) is not *Trotula*. The nearby cathedral priory of Christ Church (whose

[27]	Augustinian Abbey of Leicester owned a copy of 'Trocula maior de secretis mulierum' by the end of the 15th century at the latest; the *Trotula* appears here amid a massive collection of mostly astronomical and astrological texts	late s. xv catalogue, item no. A20.1160v[15]
[28]	John Argentine (*c.*1443–1508), doctor of medicine, churchman, and later provost of King's College, Cambridge, was possibly the owner of a copy of the intermediate ensemble[16]	Cambridge, Gonville & Caius College, MS 84/166, *c.*1215–35 (England)
[29]	Friar W[illiam?] Ffrothyngham made an index of the contents of a later 15th-century manuscript that included excerpts from *Treatments for Women* 2; whether he himself owned the manuscript or whether it was owned by a house to which he belonged is unclear	LWL, MS 550, s. xv² (England)
[30]	'Iohannes eccam', 'Iohn Han(?)', 'Iohn wallton', 'Hughe drapere merchaunt', 'Iohn Bosgrove' owned a copy of the cosmetic section of the intermediate ensemble in late s. xv and s. xvi	San Marino, California, Huntington Library, HM 64, s. xv ex. (England)
[31]	A certain Henricus de Sutton adds his own remedy for paralysis at the end of a copy of the standardized ensemble; he can perhaps be identified with Henry Sutton (d. 1501), a cleric and MD in Salisbury[17]	Glasgow, Glasgow University Library, MS Hunter 341 (U.8.9.), s. xiii ex./xiv in. (N. France)

early 14th-century catalogue is also edited by James, *Ancient Libraries*) also possessed several gynaecological and cosmetic texts, though not apparently the *Trotula*. The 'Practica domine Trote ad prouocanda menstrua' at Christ Church (cat. no. 475) is the genuine work of Trota.

[15] T. Webber and A. G. Watson, eds., *The Libraries of the Augustinian Canons*, Corpus of British Medieval Library Catalogues, 6 (London: British Library, 1998), p. 320. My thanks to Tessa Webber for sharing with me portions of her edition of the Leicester catalogue prior to publication.

[16] On Argentine, see L. D. Riehl, 'John Argentein and Learning in Medieval Cambridge', *Humanistica Lovaniensia* 33 (1984), 71–85; J. D. North, *Horoscopes and History* (London: The Warburg Institute, University of London, 1986), pp. 141–2.

[17] C. H. Talbot and E. A. Hammond, *The Medical Practitioners in Medieval England: A Biographical Register* (London: Wellcome Historical Medical Library, 1965), pp. 84–85; Sharpe, *Handlist of the Latin Writers*, p. 175.

[32] Thomas Grovis, abbot (1524–35) of Augustinian Abbey of Darley (Derbyshire), possibly owned a copy of the intermediate ensemble that may have previously been owned by John Argentine

Cambridge, Gonville & Caius College, MS 84/166

[33] John Dee (1527–1608), mathematician and astrologer, owned the manuscripts that John of London and Michael of Northgate, respectively, had donated to St Augustine's, Canterbury, in the early 14th century; he also owned the copy that Richard Stapleton had left to Balliol College

CTC, MS R.14.30 (903), s. xiii ex. (France) and Oxford, Corpus Christi College, MS 221, s. xiv[1] (England); OBL, Digby 29 (SC 1630), s. xv in. (England)

[34] John Edward de Chyrke, knight (s. xvi), marked his name and a Welsh motto on a volume which may at that time have included the transitional ensemble[18]

Dublin, Trinity College, MS 367, s. xiii[2] (France)

France

[35] Richard de Fournival (d. before 1260), poet, physician, and high church official at Amiens, commissioned a large volume of surgical and gynaecological texts, including a copy of the transitional *Trotula* ensemble

His *Biblionomia* describes a manuscript containing 'the gynaecology of Lady Trotula, the Salernitan healer'[19]

[36] An unidentified male surgeon (*cyrurgicus*) owned a copy of the standardized ensemble in Laon in the early 14th century; from him, it passed to the Cathedral of Laon

Laon, Bibliothèque Municipale, MS 417, s. xiv in. (Italy)

[37] Cathedral of Laon, which supervised the Hospital of Notre-Dame, owned a copy of the standardized ensemble in the 14th century; the several hands

(as above)

---

[18] It is not clear when the three manuscripts that make up Dublin MS 367 were brought together. De Chyrke's ownership mark is at the beginning of the first ms, *Trotula* is in the second.

[19] Léopold Delisle, *Le cabinet des manuscrits de la Bibliothèque Nationale*, 3 vols. (Paris: Imprimerie Nationale, 1874), 2: 535: *Domne Trotule sanatricis salernitane liber geneciarum de eisdem* [sc. *causis mulierum*]. Fournival's description is of a manuscript he apparently commissioned but which was never completed. It was found in the late 15th century at the Benedictine abbey of St Augustine's, Canterbury (item 1274, see above) and is now in New York Academy of Medicine, MS SAFE. See Green, 'Handlist I'.

	annotating the text may be those of canons who practised medicine[20]	
[38]	Cathedral of Reims may have owned a copy of the intermediate ensemble perhaps as early as the 14th century; it has numerous annotations listing remedies prepared for canons of the cathedral; it is not clear when the cathedral acquired its second *Trotula*, a copy of the standardized ensemble	Reims, Bibliothèque Municipale, MS 1002, s. xiii med. (N. France) and MS 1004, s. xiii² (France)[21]
[39]	Library of the Sorbonne, Paris: between 1321 and the late 1320s, the *magna libraria* (i.e., the reference collection of chained books) contained a volume with the *Practica domine Trote de secretis mulierum*, which was a copy of the *Conditions of Women* or perhaps the whole ensemble—see also the following three items	Inventory of chained collection and analytical catalogue compiled by late 1320s[22]
	At an unknown later date, the Sorbonne also acquired a copy of *Women's Cosmetics* 3	BNF, MS lat. 16089, s. xiii ex. (France?)
[40]	Gérard of Utrecht (d. betw. 1326 and 1338), a theologian, owned a copy of the standardized ensemble; he left it to the Sorbonne at his death	BNF, MS lat. 16222, s. xiv in. (N. France)

[20] The date of acquisition is uncertain, but Alain Saint-Denis observes that Laon ms 417 presents that same characteristic annotations as other medical manuscripts owned by the cathedral. See Alain Saint-Denis, *L'Hôtel-Dieu de Laon, 1150–1300: Institution hospitalière et société aux XIIe et XIIIe siècles* (Nancy: Presses Universitaires de Nancy, 1983), pp. 111–13.

[21] Although the late 15th-century catalogue of Reims cathedral lists only four medical books, these are only the books that were *chained* in the library. Colette Jeudy speculates that the cathedral library may well have had many more medical books in its collection; see her 'Traductions françaises d'oeuvres latines et traductions médicales à la bibliothèque cathédrale de Reims d'après l'inventaire de 1456/1479', *Scriptorium* 47 (1993), 173–85.

[22] The presence of at least the *Conditions of Women* is certain because the catalogue provides the incipit 'Cum auctor'. See Delisle, *Cabinet* 3:91; this codex (labelled Z.d. in the library's inventory), also included *Tractatus compendiosus de animalibus* and *Sompnia Danielis* (*ibid.*, pp. 83 and 109). The text in the chained collection identified by the cataloguer Master Adalbertus Ranconis in the mid 14th century as *Trotula de secretis mulierum* is not *Trotula* but modified selections from Muscio's *Gynaecia*. See the description of BNF, MS lat. 15081 in Green, 'Handlist II', at p. 103; and *eadem*, 'From "Diseases of Women" to "Secrets of Women": The Transformation of Gynecological Literature in the Later Middle Ages', *Journal of Medieval and Early Modern Studies* 30 (2000), 5–39, at p. 22.

[41]	Jacques de Padua, master of arts, medicine, and doctor of theology at Paris (fl. 1342–53), likewise bequeathed his copy of the standardized ensemble to the Sorbonne	BNF, MS lat. 16191, s. xiv in. (France)
[42]	King Charles V (r. 1364–80) owned at least two copies in his library of some 900 volumes: one (a French translation) he gave away to a surgeon, Master Pierre, sometime before 1380 (see below under vernacular translations); the second copy, in Latin, probably a version of the ensemble, was still in the library in 1424 when the booksellers of the University of Paris assessed the value of all the books remaining in the royal library at the death of his successor, Charles VI (r. 1380–1422)	One copy of 'le petit et le grant Trotole' was listed in an inventory of 1373 and noted as missing in 1380; a copy of 'Medicina Trotula, domina mulierum' was listed in inventories from 1373 to 1424; this latter copy was valued at 6 sous in 1424[23]
[43]	Bertrand Cormerii (fl. 1435), a student of medicine at Paris, sold a volume containing the standardized ensemble and *Women's Cosmetics* 2 for five gold sous [*quinque scutorum auri*] to Jean Caillau	BNF, MS lat. 6964, an. 1305 (Montpellier)
[44]	Jean Caillau (d. after 1472), physician to the duke of Orléans, who was called on at least one occasion to attend the lying-in of the Duchess of Blois, purchased Bertrand Cormerii's copy; Jean in turn gave it to his patron, the Duke of Orléans	(as above)
[45]	Duke Charles d'Orléans (1391–1465) received the same volume as a gift from Jean Caillau	(as above)

---

[23] BNF, MS fr. 2700, ff. 5r and 24r. Cf. Léopold Delisle, *Recherches sur la librairie de Charles V, roi de France, 1337–1380*, 2 vols. (Paris, 1907; repr. Amsterdam: van Heusden, 1967), 2:135* (item 828) and 136* (item 838); and Louis Douët-d'Arcq (ed.), *Inventaire de la Bibliothèque du Roi Charles VI fait au Louvre en 1423 par ordre du Régent Duc de Bedford* (Paris: Société des Bibliophiles, 1867), p. 115. On my reasons for identifying the first copy as a French translation, see Green, 'Traittié', p. 174, n. 46. The second folio incipit of the Latin volume, *parcium postea*, refers to a phrase in ¶19 of the *Trotula* ensemble; this particular reading is not found in the independent *Conditions of Women*.

[46]	Johannes de Bursalia (fl. 1433–55), a physician trained at Paris and Montpellier, copied out sections of the *Trotula* into a miscellaneous collection	Seville, Biblioteca Capitolar y Colombina, MS 5-1-45, an. 1452–53 (France)[24]
[47]	Ant[onius] Payxius (15th century) noted receipt of collateral for a loan in a copy of excerpts from the standardized ensemble	Carpentras, Bibliothèque Municipale, MS 320, s. xv (France?)
[48]	A certain count Robert, master of arts and medicine (otherwise unidentifiable), owned a late 13th- or early 14th-century copy of the revised ensemble in the 15th century	Montpellier, Faculté de Médecine, MS 317, *c.*1300 (S. France)
[49]	Guichard Bessonat, who describes himself as 'natif de Lion, demourant a Paris, notaire et secretaire du Roy', purchased in 1512 a copy of the versified Latin *Trotula*	BNF, MS lat. 8161A, s. xiii med. (England)
[50]	Prior to *c.*1521, the Cistercian Abbey of Clairvaux acquired the copy of the revised ensemble that had been owned by count Robert, master of arts and medicine	(as above)

Germany

[51]	The hospital of Rothenburg ob der Tauber, founded in 1281, owned a copy of a *Tractatus de passionibus mulierum* by at least 1339; it contained *Conditions of Women* (and probably the whole ensemble), followed by Petrus Hispanus's *Thesaurus pauperum*	Catalogue of 1339[25]
[52]	Male Franciscans of St Jacob in Munich at some point owned a copy of the proto-ensemble	Munich, Bayerische Staatsbibliothek, Clm 8742, s. xiii ex./xiv in. (Germany)

[24] On Bursalia, see Danielle Jacquart (ed.), *Supplément* to Ernest Wickersheimer, *Dictionnaire biographique des médecins en France au Moyen Age* (Geneva: Librairie Droz, 1979), p. 149. The manuscript is described (though not identified as the *Trotula*) in José Francisco Saéz Guillén and Pilar Jiménez de Cisneros, *Catálogo de manuscritos de la Biblioteca Colombina de Sevilla* (Seville: Cabildo de la S. M. y P. I. de Sevilla—Institucion Colombina, 2002), pp. 80–3.

[25] Bayerische Akademie, *Mittelalterliche Bibliothekskataloge*, vol. 4, pt. 2, p. 931: 'Item libellus medicinalis continens primo quendam tractatum de passionibus mulierum. Deinde opusculum medicine, quod intitulatur: Thessaurus pauperum et incipitur: 'Cum actor universitatis', in parvo

[53]	Two monks, Heinrich and Friedrich, both of them rectors, jointly owned a copy of selections from the ensemble *c.*1400; they donated it to the Premonstratensian monastery of Mildenfurth in Thuringia	Jena, Thüringer Universität- sund Landesbibliothek, MS El. q. 17, s. xiv¹ (Germany)²⁶
[54]	Premonstratensian monastery of Mildenfurth retained this copy until the 16th century	(as above)
[55]	Johannes Medici alias Patzker (s. xv), master of arts from Paris, provost and canon of Sanctus Johannes Maior, and cantor of the church of the Holy Cross in Wrocław, had rebound a copy of the standardized ensemble; it later passed to the Dominican church of Wrocław	Wrocław (Breslau), Biblioteka Uniwersytecka, MS 2022, s. xiii² (Germany)
[56]	Amplonius Ratinck (or Ratingen) of Rheinberg (1363/64–1435), doctor of medicine and master of liberal arts, owned four, perhaps five copies of the *Trotula* texts. Listed in a 1412 inventory of Ratinck's private library of 635 volumes, three of the copies are still extant: a copy of the proto-ensemble (Erfurt Group), a copy of the transitional ensemble, and a copy of the *meretrices* version of the proto-ensemble; lost are a compendium of natural philosophical and philosophical *dicta* with the *Liber Trotule de passionibus mulierum* and an anonymous *Liber de ornatu mulierum*, which may have been a copy of *Women's Cosmetics 3*	Ratinck's inventory of 1412:²⁷ extant are Erfurt, Wissenschaftliche Bibliothek, MS Amplonian Q 15, *c.*1352–4 (Cremona and Erfurt); Pommersfelden, Bibliothek der Grafen von Schönborn, HS 178, s. xiii ex./xiv in. (Italy); and HS 197, s. xiv² (Germany)

volumine in asseribus obductis albo corio'. My thanks to Florence Eliza Glaze for bringing this reference to my attention.

²⁶ My thanks to Dr Bernhard Tönnies of the Stadt- und Universitätsbibliothek, Frankfurt am Main, for graciously providing me with his description of this manuscript from his forthcoming catalogue of the Jena manuscripts.

²⁷ Wilhelm Schum, *Beschreibendes Verzeichniss der amplonianischen Handschriften-Sammlung zu Erfurt . . .* (Berlin: Weidmann, 1887): pp. 801–2 (MS Math. 29: *Liber de ornatu mulierum*); p. 814 (MS Phil. nat. 46: *Liber Trotule de passionibus mulierum*); p. 815–16 (MS Phil. nat. 49 [= ms 22]: *Liber Trotule de passionibus mulierum*); p. 825 (MS Med. 28 [= ms 94]: *Trotula de passionibus mulierum*); p. 829 (MS Med. 75 [= ms 95]: *Trotula maior et minor de morbis mulierum*). In Amplonius's lost MS math. 29, the *Liber de ornatu mulierum* immediately followed Pietro d'Abano's tract on physiognomy.

[57]	Collegium Amplonianum in Erfurt, founded by Amplonius Ratinck in 1412, receives all his books	(as above)
[58]	Martin von Geismar (d. 1450), who received his master of arts degree from Erfurt and a licentiate in canon law from Heidelberg and served as head of the chapter of St Peter's in Fritzlar (diocese of Mainz) and later a canon in Worms, owned a copy of the revised ensemble amidst his private library of some fifty-seven volumes; on the opening flyleaf, there is a 'disease woman' figure	Kassel, Stadt- und Landesbibliothek, 2° Ms. med. 7, *c*.1435 (Germany)
[59]	Cathedral of St Peter's in Fritzlar inherited Geismar's copy in 1457, along with many of his other books	(as above)
[60]	Johannes Spenlin (d. 1458) of Rothenburg, a doctor of both medicine and theology who studied for a time at Paris, owned a copy of the standardized ensemble, bound together with Muscio's *Gynaecology*); perhaps in 1455, he gave the codex to Kurfürst Friedrich I[28]	BAV, MS Pal. lat. 1304, s. xiii² (Italy)
[61]	Kurfürst Friedrich I received Johannes Spenlin's copy *c*.1455 (see above); it was then deposited in the Palatine Library in Heidelberg	(as above)
[62]	Martin Rentz, Ordinarius of Medicine at the University of Heidelberg from 1480 to 1503, bound together (and may have owned) a collection of seven fascicles of natural philosophical and medical content, one of which included a copy of the proto-ensemble (*Conditions of Women* only); the volume became part of the Palatine collection	BAV, MS Pal. lat. 1382, s. xiv² (SW Germany)

---

[28] On Spenlin's career in Paris, where he studied and taught from *c*.1401 through at least 1414, and later in Heidelberg, see Jeanne Vieillard and Marie-Henriette Jullien de Pommerol, eds., *Le Registre de prêt de la Bibliothèque de Collège de Sorbonne (1402–1536)* (Paris: CNRS, 2000), pp. 258–59; and Ernest Wickersheimer, *Dictionnaire biographique des médecins en France au Moyen Âge*, 2 vols. (1936; repr. Geneva: Librairie Droz, 1979), 2: 486.

[63] Palatine Library in Heidelberg had, as of the early 16th century, received at least two copies of the *Trotula*

(see two previous items)

[64] Dr Hermann Schedel of Nuremberg (1410–85), a humanist and MD who had studied in Leipzig and Padua and served as physician to Elector Frederick III of Brandenburg and the leading families of Nuremberg, owned three manuscripts: a copy of selections from the proto-ensemble, a copy of *Women's Cosmetics 3*, and a copy of the revised ensemble, to which he or another hand added the heading from the *meretrices* version

Munich, Bayerische Staatsbibliothek, Clm 381, s. xiii med. (Germany); Clm 444, s. xiv ex. (S. Germany); and Clm 660, s. xv¹ (Germany)

[65] Erhard Manseer de Salina (near Salzburg, d. after 1495), a cleric and later bishop of Seeon, wrote a portion of a copy of the standardized ensemble while he was studying in Leipzig; it was probably he who took the volume back to Salzburg

Salzburg, Erzabtei St Peter, MS b V 22, *c*.1456 (Leipzig)

[66] At the end of the 15th century, the Charterhouse of Salvatorberg in Erfurt owned a *Rapularius medicine* (a collection of medical excerpts) that included 'The medical disputations of Trotula on all the parts of the body made to the envy of the masters'

s. xv ex. catalogue²⁹

[67] Hartmann Schedel (1440–1516) inherited his older cousin Hermann's three copies and acquired for himself yet another copy with *Conditions of Women 3* and *Women's Cosmetics 2*

As above in item 64, plus Clm 570, s. xiv¹ (Germany)

²⁹ Bayerische Akademie, *Mittelalterliche Bibliothekskataloge*, vol. 2, p. 439: *Excepciones trocule artis phisice facte ad invidiam magistrorum de omnibus partibus corporis*. I have been able to trace only one of Salvatorberg's several *Rapularii*: Liverpool, University Library, MS F.2.12, which is a theological collection. Since the medical *Rapularius* no longer seems to be extant, it must remain undetermined whether it was a copy of the *Trotula* (in which case we might expect a title more like *Excepciones . . . de omnibus partibus corporis mulierum*) or, on the contrary, a copy of Trota's *Practica*, which might better fit this description.

[68]	Siegmund Gotzkircher (*c.*1410–75), a court physician at Munich, personal physician to Margarethe, Marchioness of Brandenburg (for whom he may have written a fertility regimen),[30] and friend of Johannes Hartlieb (d. 1468, author of one of the German translations of the *Trotula*), owned a copy of the revised ensemble	Wolfenbüttel, Herzog-August-Bibliothek, MS 784 Helmst., s. xv med. (Germany)
[69]	Johannes Rudolt, a physician of Klattau (Bohemia), made his own copy of the standardized ensemble, rearranging the chapters to suit his own tastes	Munich, Bayerische Staatbibliothek, Clm 3875, an. 1478–9
[70]	Count Arnold II (1546–1614) von Manderscheid-Blankenheim (in the diocese of Trier) purchased a copy of the revised ensemble; this, together with his five other medical books, were incorporated into the large library of Latin and German books assembled by his brother, Count Hermann (1543–1604)[31]	Darmstadt, Hessische Landes- und Hochschulbibliothek, MS 463, after an. 1493
[71]	Henricus Scholer (no biographical information found) owned a copy of the standardized ensemble in 1598	LWL, MS 548, s. xv med. (Germany or Flanders)

Italy

| [72] | A certain Sinibaldus was the scribe and probable owner of a copy of the intermediate ensemble; he was possibly a surgeon and a member of the ancient Florentine Sinibaldi family | Florence, Biblioteca Laurenziana, Plut. 73, cod. 37, s. xiii[2] (Florence) |
| [73] | Marianus Jonathan de Anglono (otherwise unknown) owned a copy of the intermediate ensemble | Naples, Biblioteca Nazionale, MS VIII D. 59, s. xiii ex. (Italy) |

---

[30] Karl Sudhoff, 'Ein Fruchtbarkeitsregimen für Margaretha, Markgräfin von Brandenburg', *Sudhoffs Archiv* 9 (1915–16), 356–9.

[31] For the history of this library, see Alan R. Deighton, 'Die Bibliothek der Grafen von Manderscheid-Blankenheim', *Archiv für Geschichte des Buchwesens* 26 (1986), 259–83.

The Netherlands

[74] Johannes Alphensis 'and friends' owned in the 15th century a copy of excerpts from the proto-ensemble amid a collection of alchemical, magical, and natural philosophical texts in Latin and Dutch; it seems to have been later owned by Jan Meesten

LWL, MS 517, s. xv (Flanders)

Spain

[75] Bernat Serra (d. June 1338), surgeon to Jaume II and Alfons III, kings of the Crown of Aragón

An inventory of his estate describes over twenty technical books on surgery and general medicine, among which was a copy of *Trotula*[32]

[76] Fernand Columbus (1488–1539), son of Christopher Columbus and a noted bibliophile, acquired one copy on 10 April 1531 in Padua of excerpts from the intermediate ensemble; he acquired a second manuscript with excerpts from *Conditions of Women* in Lyons in 1535

Seville, Biblioteca Capitular y Colombina, MS 7-4-25, s. xv[1] (probably Italy); and MS 5-1-45, an. 1452–53

Switzerland

[77] Carthusian house of Basel owned in the 15th century a copy of *Women's Cosmetics* (as extracted from the intermediate ensemble) amid a collection of Aristotelian texts and medical writings

Basel, Öffentliche Universitätsbibliothek, MS F II 19, s. xiii/xiv

---

[32] Josep Hernando, *Llibres i lectors a la Barcelona del s. XIV*, 2 vols., Textos i Documents, 30 (Barcelona: Fundació Noguera, 1995), pp. 136: 'Item, quendam alium librum, vocatum *Trotula*, scriptum in papiro'. For Bernat's biography, see Michael R. McVaugh, 'Royal Surgeons and the Value of Medical Learning: The Crown of Aragon, 1300–1350', in *Practical Medicine from Salerno to the Black Death*, ed. Luis García-Ballester, Roger French, Jon Arrizabalaga, and Andrew Cunningham (Cambridge: Cambridge University Press, 1994), pp. 221–36, at 231–2.

OWNERS OF VERNACULAR TRANSLATIONS

Owner (and means of acquisition, if known)	*Manuscript Number*
	England
[78]	Robert de Barry, rector of Begelly, Pembrokeshire, may have been the original owner of an early 14th-century Anglo-Norman verse version of the *Trotula, Si com Aristocele nous dit*	CTC, MS O.2.5 (1109), s. xiv[1] (England)[33]
[79]	A mid 15th-century copy of *Knowing of Woman's Kind*, the earliest Middle English translation, bears the inscription of 'Jhon Barcke' *c*.1500; the volume was probably owned in the later 16th century by John Twynne of Canterbury (d. 1581)	OBL, MS Bodley 483 (SC 2062), s. xv med. (England)
[80]	Richard Nix, Bishop of Norwich from 1501 to 1535, owned a copy of one of the earlier French translations, the *Quant Dex nostre Seignor*	Formerly Thomas Phillipps collection, MS 1109, s. xiv ex. (England)[34]
[81]	Humphrey Newton (1466–1536), a Cheshire country gentleman and amateur poet, bound the Middle English translation entitled *Secrets of Women* and several texts on urines into a miscellany alongside legal and notarial notes, the fables of Aesop, and his own poems	OBL, MS Lat. misc. c. 66, s. xv ex. (England)
[82]	Robert Green of Welby copied out *The Book of Rota* along with Latin surgical texts for his own use in 1544	Glasgow, Glasgow University Library, MS Hunter 403 (V.3.1), an. 1544 (England)

[33] Robert de Barry is attested in a deed, bound into the codex, dated 1270. If he did own this manuscript, it must have been very late in his life.

[34] This manuscript was sold at Sotheby's, London, on 30 November 1965. I have not been able to trace its current whereabouts.

France

[83]   In addition to his Latin copy (see above), King Charles V owned a French translation; he gave it away to a surgeon, Master Pierre, sometime before 1380 (see below)

One copy of 'le petit et le grant Trotole' listed in inventory of 1373 and noted as missing in 1380 (see item 42 above)

[84]   Master Pierre, 'le cirurgien', is said to have come to Paris from Montpellier with a physician named Jean; sometime before 1380, King Charles V gave him a volume containing a French translation of the *Trotula* together with surgical and pharmaceutical texts[35]

(as above)

[85]   The inscription 'Williamus Pauli' in a 15th-century hand is found in a copy of *Quant Dex nostre Seignor*, an early French prose translation of *Conditions of Women 1*

BLL, MS Sloane 3525, s. xiv in. (France?)

[86]   The name Saudon (?) is written on the verso of the first fly-leaf in an early 15th-century hand in another copy of the same text; on the verso of the second fly-leaf in a 16th- or 17th-century hand is written: 'Ce present liure appartient a Berthellemy le Roy demeurant paris en la Rue de la riviere au dit lieu au lougis de monsieur de Vignaulx'

LWL, MS 546, s. xiv med. (France?)

[87]   A copy of a modified redaction of *Quant Dex nostre Seignor* was later owned by Bauduin Cauwet, an inhabitant of Lille

Lille, Bibliothèque Municipale, MS 863, s. xv med.

Germany

[88]   The physician Hermann Bach (fl. mid 15th century) owned a German rendition of the proto-ensemble among a large collection of German and Latin medical tracts

Los Angeles, University of California at Los Angeles Library, MS Benjamin 11, *c.*1444 (central Germany)

---

[35] Another book (item 800) was also given to Pierre, but unlike the *Trotole* volume it continues to appear in the inventories made up through 1424 and is assessed at 4 l. in that year. See Delisle, *Recherches*, 1:121–2 and 2:130.

[89]   The other German translation, that of
        Johannes Hartlieb (composed
        c.1460–65), was prepared expressly for
        the Duke of Bavaria-Munich,
        Siegmund, though none of the extant
        mss has been identified as the
        presentation copy. Its dedicatory
        preface was later altered for the
        Emperor Frederick III, but as the one
        extant ms of this latter version is
        incomplete it is unlikely to have been
        the presentation copy

[90]   Georg Palma (1543–91), a Nuremberg   Nuremberg, Stadtbibliothek,
        municipal physician, owned a copy of   MS Cent. VI,1, an. 1509[37]
        the cosmetic section of Johannes
        Hartlieb's German translation of the
        standardized ensemble[36]

[91]   Dorothea Susanna von der Pfalz,   Wrocław (Breslau)
        Duchess of Saxony-Weimar   Dombibliothek, MS C 120,
        (1544–92), had made for her own use   an. 1570–73
        a copy of Johannes Hartlieb's paired
        translations of the pseudo-Albertan
        Secrets of Women and *Das Buch Trotula*

The Netherlands

[92]   The Franciscan brothers of Utrecht   Utrecht,
        probably owned a copy of the earliest   Universiteitsbibliotheek, MS
        Dutch translation of the *Trotula, On*   1328, s. xiv in. (Utrecht)[38]
        the Secret Medicine of Women (*Van*
        heymeliken medicinen in
        vrouwen/Secreta mulierum)

---

[36] In Green, 'Handlist II', I identified this as an independent translation of the *Trotula* cosmetics. I have since realized that it is simply the cosmetic section of Johannes Hartlieb's translation; see Chapter 4. In fact, it is possible that this manuscript had originally had a complete copy of Hartlieb's *Secreta mulierum* and *Trotula* compendium.

[37] In her comprehensive study of the institutional owners of medieval manuscripts in Germany, *Handschriftenerbe des Deutschen Mittelalters*, 3 vols., *Mittelalterliche Bibliothekskataloge Deutschlands und der Schweiz*. Ergänzungsband I (Munich, Beck, 1989–90), Sigrid Krämer listed Nuremberg Cent. VI,1 as having been owned by the Dominican nuns of St Katharina's in Nuremberg. Dr Krämer has kindly informed me (personal communication, 18 January 2003) that she obtained that information from an earlier piece by W. Fries. Fries offers no citation in the medieval library catalogue to support his claim, and may have been assuming that Cent. VI,1 came from St Katharina's because the other surrounding manuscripts did. In any case, if it ever did belong to St Katharina's, it must have been after Palma owned it.

[38] For information on ownership, see W. F. Daems, *Boec van medicinen in Dietsche: Een middelnederlandse compilatie van medisch-farmaceutische Literatur, Janus* Suppléments 7 (Leiden: E. J. Brill, 1967), p. 69.

[93] The inscription 'Anna Sebastiaens' appears in a 16th-century manuscript containing this same Dutch version; this copy embeds the Dutch *Trotula* amid sundry gynaecological and obstetrical recipes and a treatise on embryological development; other contents include miscellaneous medical recipes, and short texts on plague, medicinal waters, and phlebotomy

Hattem, Gemeentearchief, MS 958, s. xvi[39]

[94] In the 16th century Godefridus Leonijs, a notary and apothecary in Mechelen, owned a volume of Dutch medical texts, including a long poem on generation that incorporated the *meretrices* version of the *Trotula* ensemble

Brussels, Bibliothèque Royale, MS 15624–41, an. 1351 (perhaps Brabant)

[95] In 1586, Max Schneider wrote his name in a copy of another one of the Dutch translations (this one addressed to women)

Copenhagen, Det Kongelige Bibliotek, MS GKS 1657, s. xv (perhaps Brabant)

[96] In the late 16th or early 17th century, Countess Maria Geborma of Berg and Sulenborth owned the last known copy of the early 14th century Dutch translation; this copy embeds the *Trotula* within a small handbook containing a plague treatise, a tract on horse medicine, and various medical, surgical, gynaecological, and cosmetic recipes

Amsterdam, Universiteitsbibliothek, MS II E 42, s. xvi[40]

Ireland

[no owners yet identified]

Italy

[no owners yet identified]

---

[39] The Hattem manuscript also has a recipe (f. 2r), added later, ascribed to the Countess Juliana, who was very likely the countess of that name whose dates are 1587–1643. Her father-in-law, Willem IV, count of Hessen, added his own inscription, 'HaEc willem lantgraue van hessen manu proprya', at the bottom of f. 1v. My thanks to Noor Versélewel de Witt Hamer and Marianne Elsakkers for providing information on this manuscript and the Amsterdam one cited below.

[40] On the front flyleaf is the inscription 'Det boeck beest myn vereert die Wolge boren frouw Maria Geborma Graefin zu dem Berg Grauin zu Sulenborth Anno 1608 den 17. Decembris'.

Spain

[97]	Joan Galceran, a tailor and surgeon in the Majorcan town of Sineu, owned a copy of a *Suma de Trotula* in 1544	Listed in the inventory of his estate along with three other books (none on medicine)[41]

---

[41] J. N. Hillgarth, *Readers and Books in Majorca, 1229–1550*, 2 vols. (Paris: Éditions du Centre National de la Recherche Scientifique, 1991), item 873 (p. 814). It is possible, of course, that this is not really the Salernitan *Trotula* but the Catalan cosmetic text by Joan Reimbamaco misleadingly entitled *Trotula*. See Chapter 4.

Printed Gynaecological and Obstetrical Texts, 1474–1600

Works that are later reprinted in one or more editions of the *Gynaeciorum libri* are marked with an asterisk (*). Works whose first appearance is within the *Gynaeciorum libri* are marked with a dagger (†).

#	DATE	TEXT	LANGUAGE
1	1474	Antonius Guainerius (d. 1440), *De propriis mulierum aegritudinibus seu De matricibus* (Padua or Venice: Albrecht von Stendal, 1474); repr. as part of his *Opera*, Pavia, 1481 and 1488; Venice, 1497 and 1500	Latin
2	1481	Niccolò Falcucci (d. 1411 or 1412), *Sermo sextus de membris generationis*, in *Sermones medicinales* (Pavia: Damianus de Confaloneriis de Binasco, for Johannes Antonius de Bassinis, 1481–84); repr. Venice, 1490–91, 1500, 1507, 1515, and 1533; repr. separately in Venice, *c*.1491 and *c*.1495	Latin
3	1490	Galen [attributed], *De passionibus mulierum*, in his *Opera omnia* (Venice: P. Pincius, 1490); although included in several reprints, this was rejected as spurious by 1541	Latin
4	1495	anonymous, *Frauenbüchlein* (Augsburg, *c*.1495; repr. 1525 [2x])	German
5	1495	Bernard de Gordon (*c*.1260–*c*.1318) [attributed], *Le secret des dames que peut entendre légèrement le gouvernement des fleurs des dames* (perhaps a tr. of excerpts from Gordon's *Lilium medicine*), printed Lyons, 1495, together with French trans. of the *Lilium*	French
6	1502	Gabriele Zerbi (1445–1505), *Anathomia matricis pregnantis et est sermo de anathomia et generatione embrionis*, follows *Liber anathomie* (Venice: Boneto Locatello, ed. Ottaviano	Latin

		Scoto, 1502; repr. Marburg: Eucharius Cervicornus, 1537)	
*7	1502	Ludovico Bonaccioli (d. *c*.1540), *Enneas muliebris* (Ferrara: Laurentius de Rubies?, *c*.1502–3)—dedicated to Lucrezia Borgia, at the time wife of Alfonso d'Este; portions were reprinted in 1536 and 1537; see also item 14 below	Latin
8	1504	*Tractatus de sterilitate tam ex parte viri quam ex parte mulieris continens duos tractatus*—an early 14th-century text variously attributed in manuscript to Arnau de Vilanova (d. 1311) and others; published in *Opera arnaldi* (Lyons 1504, Venice 1505, etc.)	Latin
9	1505	*Compilatio de conceptione*—an early 14th-century text attributed to Arnau de Vilanova; published in *Opera arnaldi* (Venice, 1505)	Latin
10	1513	Eucharius Rösslin (d. 1526), *Der Swangern frawen vnd hebammen roszgarten* (Hagenau: H. Gran, and Strasbourg: Martin Flach, 1513); repr. at least 16x up through 1541; see entries 14, 26, and 42 below for later revisions	German
11	1516	Eucharius Rösslin, *Den roseghaert vanden bevruchten vrouwen* (Brussels: Thomas van der Noot, 1516); see also the expanded 1528 edition below	Dutch
12	1525	Marco Fabio Calvi (d. 1527) (trans.), *Hippocratis Coi medicorum omnium longe principis, Octoginta volumina* (Rome: Franciscus Minitius, 1525)—includes *Diseases of Women 1, Diseases of Women 2, Diseases of Young Girls, Sterile Women*, and *On the Nature of the Child*	Latin
13	1526	Marco Fabio Calvi (trans.), *Hippocrates de foemina natura* (Paris: Claudius Chevallonius, 1526)—a reprinting in a cheap sextodecimo format of Calvi's 1525 translation of the Hippocratic gynaecological texts	Latin
14	1526	Eucharius Rösslin, Jr (ed.), *Ehstand Arzneybuch*, a compilation of his father's *Rosegarten*; (Erfurt: Wolfgang u. Gervasius Stürmer, 1526); repr. at least 14x thereafter—selections from a German translation of the pseudo-Albertus Magnus, *Secreta mulierum*; selections from a German translation of Ludovico Bonacciuoli's *Enneas*	German

		muliebris; Johannes Cuba's *Frauwen Artzney*; and Bartholomeus Metlinger's tract on pediatrics	
15	1527	Jason Pratensis (Iasonis a Pratis Zyricaei, Artium liberaliu[m] magistrii, ac medicinæ professoris, [= Jan Van de Velde], 1486–1558), *De pariente & partu, liber obstetricibus puerperis, nutricibusque utilissimus, in quo preter historiarum amœnitatem eruditio est non uulgaris* ([Cologne?]: [Hero Fuchs?], 1527; repr. at least 3x in 1657 in Amsterdam)	Latin
16	1528	Eucharius Rösslin, *Den roseghaert vanden bevruchten vrouwen. Ghecorrigeert ende vermeerdert uut die boecken van die alder expeertste scrivers, die van deser materien (te weten van die secreten, ontfanghinghe, baringhe, ende conste der vroevrouwen) int latijn ghescreven hebben, als Albertus Magnus, Aristoteles, Plinius, Avicenna, Marcus varro, ende meer andere. Ende oeck uut Jason a pratis, die een dat aldercotelijcste tractaet in latijn heeft bescreven van der vroevrouwen conste* (Antwerp: Simon Cock en Jacop van Liesveldt, 1528); repr. Reess, 1528; Antwerp, 1529; Antwerp, 1530; Antwerp, c.1540 (2x), etc.	Dutch
17	1532	Eucharius Rösslin, *De partu hominis, et quae circa ipsum accidunt*, (Frankfurt am Main: Christoph Egenolph, 1532); repr. Frankfurt 1534, 1544, 1551, 1554, 1556, and 1563; Paris 1532, 1535, and 1538; Venice, 1536 and 1537—a Latin translation of the *Rosegarden* by his son, Eucharius Rösslin, the younger	Latin
18	1532	Theodorus Priscianus, *Gynaecea, de mulierum accidentibus, et curis eorundem*, in his *Phaenomen euporiston* (Basel: Hieronymus Froben & Nicolaus Episcopius, 1532); repr. in *Rerum medicarum lib. quatuor* (Strasburg: Johann Schott, 1532)	Latin
19	1536	Constantine the African (d. before 1098/99) [attributed], *De mulierum morbis liber*, included in his *Opera* (Basel: Henricus Petrus, 1536)—this is the abbreviated Latin translation of the Greek Metrodora text, *De passionibus mulierum (Version A)*, which had	Latin

		been attributed to Galen in the 1490 edition of his work	
20	1536	Eucharius Rösslin, *Des diuers traualx et enfantements des femmes, et par quel moyen lon doit suruenir aux accidens qui peuuent escheoir deuant et apres iceulx trauaulx : Item quel lait et quelle nourrisse on doit eslire aux enfans ...* anon. trans. (Paris: Jehan Foucher, 1536); repr. 1539	French
21	1538	Eucharius Rösslin, *Libro nel qual si tratta del parto delhuomo e de tutte quelle cfose, che cerca esso parto accadeno, e delle infermita che po[sso]no accadere a i fanciulli, con tutti i suoi rimedii posti particolarmente* (Venice: Giovanni Andrea Vavassore, 1538)	Italian
22	1540	Eucharius Rösslin, *The byrth of mankynde: newly translated out of Laten into Englysshe*, tr. Richard Jonas (London: [Thomas Raynalde], 1540)	English
23	1541	Damián Carbón (d. 1554), a physician of Majorca, *Libro del arte de las comadres o madrinas, y del regimiento de las preñadas y paridas y de los niños* ([Majorca City: Hernando de Cansoles,] 1541)	Castillian
*24	1542	Nicolas de La Roche (fl. 1516–42), *De morbis mulierum curandis* (Paris: Joannes Foucherius, 1542); repr. in all three editions of the *Libri gynaeciorum* (1566, 1586–8, and 1597)	Latin
*25	1544	Georg Kraut (ed.), *Trotulae curandarum Aegritudinum Muliebrium, ante, in & post partum liber unicus, nusquam antea editus*, in *Experimentarius medicinae* (Strasburg: Joannes Schottus, 1544); reprinted (in different collections) in 1547, 1550, 1551, 1554, 1555, 1558, 1565, 1566, 1572, 1586, 1597, and 1778	Latin
26	1545	Walter Ryff (d. 1548), *Frawen Rosengarten. Von vilfaltigen sorglichen Zufällen und gebrechen der Mütter und Kinder, so jnen vor, in u. nach der Geburt begegnen mögenn* (Frankfurt am Main: Christian Egenolff, 1545); repr. 1561, 1569, 1572, and 1580—a plagiarized reworking of Rösslin's text	German
27	1545	Eucharius Rösslin, *The byrth of mankynde, otherwyse named the womans booke*, a revision of Richard Jonas's 1540 English translation	English

		by Thomas Raynalde (fl. 1540–51) (London, 1545); repr. 1552, 1560, 1565, 1598	
28	1549	Ambroise Paré (1510?–90), *Briefve collection de l'administration anatomique, avec la maniere de conjoindre les os: et d'extraire les enfans tant mors que vivans du ventre de la mere, lors que nature de soy ne peult venir a son effect* . . . (Paris: Guillaume Cavellat, 1549); repr. 1550	French
29	1550	*Tprofijt der vrouwen, in het welcke gheleert wordt de remedie teghen alle die ghebreken der Vrouwen, Weduwen, Meyskens, ende allen anderen persoonen* (Antwerp: Jan van Ghelen, 1550); repr. Antwerp, 1556, 1561, 1595, and *c.*1600	Dutch
30	1553	Hippocrates, *De la nature de l'enfant au ventre de la mère,* trans. Guillaume Chrestien [= Willem Christiaan van der Boxe] (Reims: N. Bacquenois, 1553)—with dedication to Duchesse de Buillon, the daughter-in-law of Diane de Poitiers	French
31	1554	Rufus of Ephesus & Soranus of Ephesus, *Rouphou Ephesiou Peri ton en kystei kai nephrois pathon. Peri ton pharmakon kathartikon. Peri theseos kai onomasias ton tou anthropou morion. Soranou peri metras kai gynaikeiou aidoiou. Ruffi Ephesii De vesicae renumque morbis. De purgantibus medicamentis. De partibus corporis humani. Sorani de vtero & muliebri pudendo* (Paris: Adr. Turnebum, 1554)	Greek & Latin
*32	1554	Giovanni Battista da Monte (1498–1551), *Opuscula de vterinis affectibus* (Venice: Balthassar Constantinus, 1554), repr. (Paris: Gilles Gourbin, 1556); repr. in Girolamo Donzellino (ed.), *Opuscula uaria et praeclara* (Basel: Widow of Michael Isengrin for Peter Ferma, 1558)	Latin
33	1554	Jakob Ruf (1500–58), *Ein shön lustig Trostbüchle von den Empfengknussen und Geburten der Menschen* (Zurich: Christoph Froschauer, 1554; repr. 1569)	German
*34	1554	Jakob Ruf, *De conceptu et generatione hominis: De matrice et eius partibus, nec non de conditione infantis in utero, et gravidarum cura et officio: . . . libri sex* . . . —a trans. of his German *Trostbüchle* by Wolfgang Haller with	Latin

		a new preface probably by Ruf himself (Zurich: C. Froschover, 1554); repr. with revisions, Frankfurt am Main, 1580 and 1587; also repr. in the 1586–8 and 1597 eds. of the *Gynaeciorum*	
*35	1555	Jacques Dubois (= Jacobus Sylvius, 1478–1555), *De mensibus mulierum et hominis generatione . . . commentarius* (Paris: Joannes Hulpeau, 1555); repr. Venice and Basel, 1556; Paris, 1561; Basel, 1566 in Wolff's *Gynaeciorum libri* and subsequent editions	Latin
36	1555	Mathias Cornax (d. 1564), *Historiae duae memorabiles: Prima, quomodo foemina Viennensis, quae foetum mortuum in utero ultra quadriennium gestauit, tandem ope medicorum, facta per uentrem incisione, euaserit & sanitati sit restituta. Secunda, quod eadem foemina denuo preter omnem rationem humanam concoeperit, & gestauerit foetum masculum, usq[ue] ad legittimum pariendi tempus* (Augsburg: per Iohannem Zimmerman, 1555), repr. Mathias Cornax, *Historia gestationis in utero foetus mortui*, in Rembert Dodoens (ed.), *Medicinalium obseruationum exempla rara* (Cologne: Maternus Cholinus, 1581)	Latin
37	1556	Soranus, *Ex Sorano De vulva et pudendo muliebri, Ioan. Baptista Rasario interprete* [published with Theophilus Protospatharius, *De corporis humani fabrica libri V, Iunio Paulo Crasso . . . interprete*] (Paris: Guil. Morelius, 1556)	Latin
38	1556	Galen, *De la formation des enfans au ventre de la mère*, trans. Guillaume Chrestien (Paris: Guillaume Cauellat, 1556)—dedicated to the French Queen Catherine de Medici	French
39	1559	Jacques Dubois (1478–1555), *Livre de la natvre et vtilité des moys des femmes, & de la curation des maladies qui en suruiennent*, trans. Guillaume Chrestien (d. 1560?) (Paris, Chez Guillaume Morel, 1559)—dedicated to Diane de Poitiers	French
40	1559	Boudewijn Ronsse (1525–97), *De hominis primordiis hystericisque affectibus centones* (Louvain: Antonius Maria Bergainge, 1559; repr. Lyons: Franciscus Raphelengium, 1594)	Latin
41	1561	Donato Antonio Altomare (1506–62), *Quod utero gerentibus pro praeservatione aborsus,*	Latin

		venae sectio non competat ex Hippocratis et Galeni sententia, in *Nonnulla opuscula* (Venice: Marco de Maria, 1561; repr. in his *Omnia . . . opera,* Lyons: Guillaume Rouillé, 1565)	
42	1562	Adam Lonitzer (1528–86, city physician of Frankfurt-am-Main) (ed.), *Hebammenbüchlin* (Frankfurt: Christian Egenolff, 1562), a re-edition of Rösslin's *Rosegarten;* repr. at least 6 times	German
43	1563	Eucharius Rösslin, *Des divers travavlx et enfantemens des femmes, par quel moyen lon doit suruenir aux accidens qui peuuent eschoir deuant et apres iceux trauaulx : item quel lait & quelle nourrisse on doit eslire aux enfans* . . . , tr. Paul Bienassis (Paris: Jean Foucher, 1563), repr. Paris, 1577 and 1586; Lyons, 1584	French
44	1563	Giovanni Marinelli (d. 1615), *Le medicine pertinenti allè infermità delle donne* (Venice: Francesco de Franceschi Senese, 1563); repr. 1574	Italian
45	1565	Taddeo Duno (1523–1613), *Muliebrium morborum omnis generis remedia, ex Dioscoride, Galeno, Plinio . . . collecta et disposita* (Strasboug: Iosias Rihelius, 1565)	Latin
*46	1566	[Moschionos peri gynakeion pathon]: *id est, Moschionis medici Graeci De morbis muliebribus liber vnus: cum Conradi Gesneri viri clariss. scholijs & emendationibus, nunc primùm editus opera ac studio Caspari Vuolphij Tigurini medici . . .* (Basel: Thomas Guarinus, 1566)	Greek[1]
47	1566	Caspar Wolf (also known as Hans Kaspar Wolf, 1532–1601) (ed.), *Gynaeciorum, hoc est de Mulierum tum aliis, tum gravidarum, parientium et puerperarum affectibus et morbis libri veterum ac recentiorem aliquot, partim nunc primum editi, partim multo quam ante castigatiores . . .* (Basel: Thomas Guarinus, 1566)—a collection of seven gynaecological texts, six of which are reprints (Albucasis's obstetrical chapters;	Latin & Greek

---

[1] This is a late medieval Greek translation of the fifth- or sixth-century Latin translation, by Muscio, of Soranus's second-century Greek *Gynaekeia*. Aside from the excerpts in item 37, Soranus's original Greek text was not to be rediscovered until the 19th century.

the *Trotula*, here for the first time attributed to
'Eros'; and works by La Roche, Bonacciuoli,
and Dubois; and the Greek Muscio).
New here is:

†48	1566	*Cleopatrae, Moschionis, Prisciani, et incerti cvivsdam Muliebrium libri, superfluis ac repetiis omnibus recisis, in vnam Harmoniam redacti, per Casp. VVolphivm, medicvm Tigvrinvm, nunc recens editi*	Latin
49	1566	Paracelsus (1493–1541), *Buch Meteororvm: Jtem: Liber qvartvs Paramiri de Matrice* (Cologne: Arnoldius Byrckmans Erben, 1566)	Latin
50	1567	Paracelsus, *Medici Libelli Physionomia morborum; De terebinthina & utroq. helleboro; Liber secundus de caduco matricis . . .* (Cologne: Arnoldus Birckmans Erben, 1567)	Latin
51	1573	Ambroise Paré (1510?–1590), *De la generation de l'homme, & maniere d'extraire les enfans hors du ventre de la mere, ensemble ce qu'il faut faire pour la faire mieux, & plus tost accoucher, avec la cure de plusieurs maladies qui luy peuvent survenir*, in *Deux livres de chirurgie* (Paris: André Wechel, 1573)	French
52	1574	Maurice de la Corde (fl. 1569–74), *Hippocrates Coi libellus Peri Parthenion, hoc est, De iis quae virginibus accidunt* (Paris: Bariel Buon, 1574)	Latin
53	1576	Giovanni Marinelli, *Vier Bücher von rechter, unverfälschter, eüsserlicher Zier der Weyber*, tr. Hieremiam Martium (Augsburg: Willers, 1576), repr. 1581	German
54	1576	Georg Pictorius (*c.*1500–69), *Frauwenzimmer: ein nützliches Büchlein, darausz die schwangeren Frawen mögen erlernen, wie sie sich vor, in, und nach der Geburt halten shollen, und wie sie alle weibliche Zufäl, besseren und ableinen mögen, mit anderen guten stücken die in ein Fraenzimmer gehörig sind. Sampt einem kurtzem angehenckten Tractat, wie in zufelligen kranckheiten den jungen Kindern zu helffen seye. Item, mit einem nothwendigen Bericht von den Spulwürmen . . . alles ausz Avicenna, Hippocrate, Galeno, Aegeneta, Aetio, Constantino, Plinio, und andern Gelehrten*	German

		(Frankfurt am Main: [Nicolaum Basse], 1576); repr. 1593	
*55	1577	Jean Le Bon (d. 1583), *Iohannis le Bon regis et cardinalis Gvisiani medici Therapia puerperarum* (Paris: DuBuys, 1577); repr. in 1586–8 and 1597 eds. of *Gynaeciorum libri*, and in Antoine Valet & Louis Paret, eds., *De morbis internis* (Frankfurt: Johann Wechel, 1589–91)	Latin
*56	1579	Luis Mercado (1520–1606), *De mulierum affectionibus: libri quatuor. Quorum primus de communibus mulierum passionibus disserit. Secundus virginum & viduarum morbos tractat. Tertius, sterilium & praegnantium. Quartus, puerperarum, & nutricum accidentia ad vnguem exequitur. Ad Philippvm secvndvm hispaniarvm indiarumque regem potentissimum* (Valladolid: D. Fernandez a Corduba, 1579); repr. Venice, 1587; Basel, in vol. 4 of 1586–8 ed. of *Gynaeciorum*; and Madrid, 1594	Latin
57	1580	Eucharius Rösslin, *Libro intitulado del parto humano, en el qual se contienen remedios muy utiles y usuales para el parto difficultoso de las mugeres, con otros muchos secretos a ello pertenescientes* (Alcalá: Juan Gracián, 1580), a Spanish version of the *Rosengarten* trans. by Francisco Nuñez de Oria (fl. 1560–*c*.1586)	Castillian
58	1580	Jakob Ruf, *Hebammen Buch* (Frankfurt: [for Sigmund Feyerabend], 1580, repr. 1588, 1600)—a revised version of his earlier *Trostbüchle*	German
59	1580	Jakob Ruf, *Thoeck van de vroet-wijfs, in 't welke men mach leeren alle heymeleyckheden van de vrouwen etc. na Jacob Ruff overgezet door Martyn Everaert* (Amsterdam, 1580), repr. 1591 (2x)—a Dutch translation of Ruf's 1554 German original	Dutch
60	1581	François Rousset (1535?–90?), *Traitté nouveau de Hysterotomotokie, ou enfantement caesarien. Qui est extraction de l'enfant par incision laterale du ventre, & matrice de la femme grosse ne pouvant autrement accoucher. Et ce sans prejudicier à la vie de l'un, ny de l'autre; ny empescher la foecondité maternelle par aprés* (Paris: D. Duval, 1581)	French
*61	1582	Jean d'Ailleboust (Joannes Albosius, fl. 1550–1600), *Portentosum lithopaedion, sive*	Latin

		embryon petrefactum urbis Senonensis. Adjecta . . . exercitatione . . . de hujus indurationis caussis naturalibus (Sens: J. Savine, 1582); repr. 1588	
62	1582	Jean Liebault, *Trois Livres appartenant aux infirmitez et maladies des femmes, pris du Latin de M. Jean Liebaut, Docteur Médecin à Paris, et facts François* (Paris: Jacques de Puys, 1582), repr. Paris 1585, 1587, 1597; Lyons 1598[2]	French
63	1582	Giovanni Battista Donati (1530–*c*.1591), *Commentarius in magni Hipocratis Coi librum de morbis virginum* (Lucca: J. Guidobonius, 1582); repr. Frankfurt, 1591	Latin
*64	1582	Ambroise Paré, *De hominis generatione*, a Latin translation of his earlier *De la generation de l'homme*, in *Opera Ambrosii Parei* . . . (Paris: Jacob Du-Puys, 1582); this would be reprinted in the 1586–8 edn of the *Gynaeciorum libri*	Latin
*65	1585	Albertino Bottonni (1528–96?), *De morbis muliebribus. Liber secundus* (Padua: Paolo Meietti, 1585), repr. Venice: Paolo Meietti, 1588	Latin
*66	1585	Maurice de la Corde, [commentary on] *Hippocratis Coi, Medicorum Principiis, liber prior de morbis mulierum* (Paris: Dionysius Duvallius, 1585); repr. in *Gynaeciorum*, 1586–88 and 1597	Latin
*67	1586	Vittore Trincavelli (1496–1568), *Consilia* (Venice, 1586)—three of his gynaecological *consilia* were reprinted in 1586–88 and 1597 editions of the *Gynaeciorum*	Latin
68	1586–88	*Gynaeciorum siue De mulierum affectibus commentarii Graecorum, Latinorum, Barbarorum iam olim & nunc recens editorum: in tres [i.e. quatuor] tomos digesti, et necessariis passim imaginibus illustrati* (Basel: Conradus Waldkirch, 1586–8), w/some material edited by Caspar Bauhin (1560–1624)?; vol. II bears title *Gynaeciorum physicus et chirurgicus:*	Latin & Greek

---

[2] In most of these later editions, it would bear the title *Thresor des remedes secrets pour les maladies des femmes*.

		continens inter caetera Hieron. Mercurialis antecessoris Patauini elegantissimi, Muliebrium libros IV. Franc. item Rousseti Hysterotomotokian e Gallico conuersam	
†69	1586–88	Felix Platter (1536–1614), *Felicis Plateri Medici Basiliensis de Mulierum partibus generationi dicatis Icones, vna cum explicationibus, ipsarum delineationem accurate ostendentes. Item Tabvlae, structuram vsumque methodice describentes. Quibus quoque, quo pacto ossa Mulieris a Viri ossibus hisce sedibus varient, breuiter adiecta fuerunt,* published in the 1586–8 of the *Gynaeciorum libri*—the images (there including one of the female skeleton) had originally appeared in a different format in Platter's *De corporis hvmani strvctvra et vsv . . . libri III* (Basel: Frobenius, 1583)	Latin
†70	1586–88	Girolamo Mercuriale (1530–1606), *Muliebrium libros IV,* published in the 1586–8 of the *Gynaeciorum libri*	Latin
71	1587	Girolamo Mercuriale, *De morbis muliebribus praelectiones ex ore Hieronymi Mercurialis,* ed. Michele Colombo (Venice: Felice Valgrisi, 1587)—the earlier edition of this text in the 1586 *Gynaeciorum* had been 'unauthorized', hence the *ex ore* here; repr. 1591 with excerpts from Caspar Bauhin (1560–1624)	Latin
72	1587	Gervais de la Tousche, *La tres-haute et tres-souveraine science de l'art et industrie naturelle d'enfanter. Contre la maudicte et perverse impericie des femmes que l'on appelle saiges femmes, ou belles meres, lesquelles par leur ignorance font journellement périr une infinité de femmes & d'enfans à l'enfantement . . .* (Paris: Didier Millot, 1587)	French
*73	1588	François Rousset, *Usterotomotókia . . . gallice primum edita, nunc vero Caspari Bauhini . . . opera latine reddita, multisque et variis historiis in appendice additis locupletata . . . Adiecta est Ioan. Albosii.. lithopaedii senonensis per annos XXIIX [sic] in utero contenti historia elegantissima* (Basel: Conr. Waldkirch, 1588)	Latin
74	1591	Séverin Pineau (d. 1619), *De integritatis et corruptionis virginum notis: graviditate item & partu naturali mulierum, opuscula*	Latin

		(Lugduni-Batavorum Apud Franciscum Hegerum., M D CXCI.; repr. Frankfurt, 1599)	
75	1591	[author?], *Schwangerer, kreistender, Wöchnerin vnnd seugender Regiment oder Vnterweisung, sampt einem Verzeichnus gesunder auch vngesunder Speisen vnd Tranck* (Hall in Sachsen: A. Lieskaw, in Verlegung J. Francken, 1591)	German
76	1594	Oswald Gabelkover (1539–1616), *Artzneybuch, darinnen . . . vast für alle, des menschlichen Leibs Anligen u. Gebrechen außerlesene unnd bewehrte Artzneyen . . . Theil 2: Kranckheiten des weiblichen Geschlechts und der jungen Kinder* (Tübingen: Gruppenbach, 1594)	German
77	1595	Girolamo (or Scipione) Mercurio (*c.*1550–1615), *La commare o riccoglitrice dell'ecc.mo s. Scipion Mercurii . . . divisa in tre libri* (Venice, 1595); a corrected edition was published in Venice: Gio. Bat. Ciotti, 1601	Italian
78	1595	Joannes Hiltprandus (1572–1601), *Ordnung und Nutzliche Vnderweysung fuer die Hebammen vnd Schwangeren Frawen* (Passau: M. Henninger, 1595)	German
79	1597	Israel Spach (1560–1610), ed. *Gynaeciorum sive de Mulierum tum communibus, tum gravidarum, parientium et puerperarum affectibus et morbis libri Graecorum, Arabum, Latinorum veterum et recentium quotquot extant, partim nunc primum editi, partim vero denuo recogniti, emendati* (Strasburg: Lazarus Zetzner, 1597)—the third and final edition of the great 16th-century collection. New here is:	Latin & Greek
†80	1597	Martin Akakia (identified here as *Galli*, presumably referring to Martin the younger, 1539–88), *De morbis muliebribus Libri II. nunc primum in lucem editi*	Latin
81	1597	Caspar Bauhin (1560–1624), *Anatomica corporis uirilis et muliebris historia* (Geneva: J. Jean Le Preux, 1597)	Latin
82	1597	Orazio Augenio (1527–1603), *De hominis partu libri ii*, in *Epistolarum &*	Latin

		consultationum medicinalium (Frankfurt: Claude de Marne & Johann Aubry, 1597)	
83	1598	Emilio Vezzosi (1565–1637), *Gynaecyeseos, sive de mulierum conceptu, gestatione, ac partu. Libri tres* (Venice: Gio. Ant. Rampazetti, 1598)	Latin
84	1598	Johannes Wittich (1537–98), *Tröstlicher Unterricht für schwangere und geberende Weiber. Item von Vorbereitunge zum Geberen damit ihnen ihre Geburt nicht zu schwer und sawer ankomme auch mit andern bösen Zufellen beydes schwangere Personen vnd die Frucht betreffende mit gutem Raht möge begegnet werde* ([Leipzig] In Vorlegung Bart. Voigts, 1598)	German
85	1599	Pieter van Foreest (1522–97), *Observationum et curationum medicinalium liber vigesimus-octavus de mulierum morbis* (Basel: Christophorus Raphelengius, 1599)	Latin
86	1600	Alessandro Massaria (1510–98), *Praelectiones de morbis mulierum, conceptus & partus* (Leipzig: Abraham Lamberg, 1600)	Latin
87	1600	Hieronymus Fabricius ab Aquapendente (*c.*1533–1619), *De formato foetu* (Venice: Lorenzo Pasquati for Francesco Bolzetta, 1600)	Latin

References

Abulafia, D. S. H., 'Joanna, Countess of Toulouse (1165–99)', *Oxford Dictionary of National Biography* (Oxford: Oxford University Press, 2004), online edition: <http://www.oxforddnb.com.library.lib.asu.edu:80/view/article/14818> accessed 15 May 2005.

Agrimi, Jole and Chiara Crisciani, 'The Science and Practice of Medicine in the Thirteenth Century according to Guglielmo da Saliceto, Italian Surgeon', in *Practical Medicine from Salerno to the Black Death*, ed. Luis García-Ballester, Roger French, Jon Arrizabalaga, and Andrew Cunningham (Cambridge: Cambridge University Press, 1994), pp. 60–87.

_____ and _____ *Les 'consilia' medicaux*, trans. Caroline Viola, *Typologie des sources du moyen âge occidental*, fasc. 69 (Brepols: Turnhout, 1994).

Aikin, Judith P., 'The Welfare of Pregnant and Birthing Women as a Concern for Male and Female Rulers: A Case Study', *Sixteenth Century Journal* 35 (2004): 9–41.

Albucasis, *Albucasis on Surgery and Instruments. A Definitive Edition of the Arabic Text with English Translation and Commentary*, ed. and trans. M. S. Spink and G. L. Lewis (London: The Wellcome Institute of the History of Medicine, 1973).

Archer, Janice Marie, 'Working Women in Thirteenth-Century Paris', PhD dissertation, University of Arizona, 1995.

Archimatheus Salernitanus, *Practica Archimathaei*, in De Renzi, *Collectio Salernitana*, 5:350–76.

_____ *Erklärungen zur hippokratischen Schrift Prognostikon. Nach der Handschrift Trier Bischöfliches Priesterseminar 76*, ed. Hermann Grensemann (Hamburg 2002/rev. 2004), at <http://www.uke.uni-hamburg.de/institute/geschichte-medizin/index_18229> accessed 7 October 2006.

_____ *Glossae in Isagogas Johannitii: Ein Kursus in mittelalterlicher Physiologie nach dem Codex Trier Bischöfliches Priesterseminar 76A und dem Codex Toletanus Archivo y Biblioteca Capitulares 97–14*, ed. Hermann Grensemann (Hamburg 2004), electronic publication: <http://www.uke.uni-hamburg.de/institute/geschichte-medizin/index_18229.php> accessed 6 June 2005.

Arderne, John, *Treatises of Fistula in ano*, in *Treatises of Fistula in Ano, Haemorrhoids and Clysters by John Arderne*, ed. D'Arcy Power, Early English Text Society o.s. 139 (London: Oxford University Press, 1910; repr. 1968),

Avicenna, *Liber canonis* (Venice, 1507; repr. Hildesheim: Georg Olms, 1964).

Bailbon, W. P., *Records of the Honorable Society of Lincoln's Inn: The Black Books*, 5 vols. (London: Lincoln's Inn, 1897–1968).

Barkaï, Ron, 'A Medieval Hebrew Treatise on Obstetrics', *Medical History* 33 (1989), 96–119.

_____ *Les Infortunes de Dinah: le livre de la génération. La gynécologie juive au Moyen-Age*, trans. Jacqueline Barnavi and Michel Garel (Paris: Cerf, 1991).

_____ *A History of Jewish Gynaecological Texts in the Middle Ages* (Leiden: Brill, 1998).

Barratt, Alexandra (ed.), *The Knowing of Woman's Kind in Childing: A Middle English Version of Material Derived from the 'Trotula' and Other Sources*, Medieval Women: Texts and Contexts, 4 (Turnhout: Brepols, 2001).

Bäuml, Franz, 'Varieties and Consequences of Medieval Literacy and Illiteracy', *Speculum* 55 (1980), 237–65.

Bayerische Akademie der Wissenschaften, *Mittelalterliche Bibliothekskataloge Deutschlands und der Schweiz*, 4 vols., repr. (Munich: Beck, 1969–83).

Bazin-Tacchella, Sylvie, 'Adaptations françaises de la *Chirurgia Magna* de Guy de Chauliac et codification du savoir chirurgical au XVᵉ siècle', in *Bien dire et bien aprandre: Actes du colloque du Centre d'Études Médiévales et Dialectales de Lille III. 'Traduction, transposition, adaptation au Moyen Age'*, Lille, 22–24 septembre 1994, t. 14 (1996), pp. 169–88.

Beccaria, Augusto, *I codici di medicina del periodo presalernitano (secoli IX, X e XI)* (Rome: Storia e Letteratura, 1956).

Behrmann, Thomas, 'The Development of Pragmatic Literacy in the Lombard City Communes', in Britnell (ed.), *Pragmatic Literacy*, pp. 25–42.

Bell, David N. (ed.), *The Libraries of the Cistercians, Gilbertines and Premonstratensians*, Corpus of British Medieval Library Catalogues 3 (London: British Library, in association with the British Academy, 1992).

Benedek, Thomas G., 'The Changing Relationship Between Midwives and Physicians During the Renaissance', *Bulletin of the History of Medicine* 51 (1977), 550–64.

Benedetti, Alessandro, *De omnium a uertice ad plantam morborum signis, causis, differentijs, indicationibus et remedijs tam simplicibus quam compositis*, in *Alexandri Benedicti veronensis, Medici ac Philosophi multis nominibus clarissimi, de re medica* (Basel: Henricus Petrus, 1549).

Bennett, Judith M., 'Misogyny, Popular Culture, and Women's Work', *History Workshop* issue 31 (Spring 1991), 166–88.

——*Ale, Beer, and Brewsters in England: Women's Work in a Changing World, 1300–1600* (New York: Oxford University Press, 1996).

Benton, John F., 'Trotula, Women's Problems, and the Professionalization of Medicine in the Middle Ages', *Bulletin of the History of Medicine* 59, no. 1 (Spring 1985), 30–53.

Berengario da Carpi, Jacopo, *Commentaria cum amplissimis additionibus super anatomia Mundini* (Bologna: Girolamo Benedetti, 1521).

Bernard de Gordon, *Lilium medicine* (Naples: Franciscus de Tuppo, 1480).

Biller, Peter, *The Measure of Multitude: Population in Medieval Thought* (Oxford: Oxford University Press, 2000).

—— 'Medicine and Heresy', in Peter Biller and Joseph Ziegler, eds., *Religion and Medicine in the Middle Ages*, York Studies in Medieval Theology, 3 (York: York Medieval Press, 2001), pp. 155–74.

Bird, Jessalynn, 'Medicine for Body and Soul: Jacques de Vitry's Sermons to Hospitallers and their Charges', in Peter Biller and Joseph Ziegler, eds., *Religion and Medicine in the Middle Ages*, York Studies in Medieval Theology, 3 (York: York Medieval Press, 2001), pp. 91–108.

—— 'Texts on Hospitals: Translation of Jacques de Vitry, *Historia Occidentalis* 29, and Edition of Jacques de Vitry's Sermons on Hospitallers', in Peter Biller and Joseph Ziegler, eds., *Religion and Medicine in the Middle Ages*, York Studies in Medieval Theology, 3 (York: York Medieval Press, 2001), pp. 109–34.

Blamires, Alcuin (ed.), *Woman Defamed and Woman Defended: An Anthology of Medieval Texts* (Oxford: Clarendon, 1992).

Blonquist, Lawrence B. (trans.), *L'Art d'amours (The Art of Love)* (New York: Garland, 1987).

Blumenfeld-Kosinski, Renate, *Not of Woman Born: Representations of Caesarean Birth in Medieval and Renaissance Culture* (Ithaca, NY: Cornell University Press, 1990).

Boccaccio, Giovanni, *The Decameron*, terza giornata, novella nona, ed. V. Branca (1992), available online at <http://www.brown.edu/Departments/Italian_Studies/dweb/> accessed 9 October 2004.

——— *The Decameron*, trans. G. H. McWilliam, 2nd edn (New York: Penguin, 1995).

Bodarwé, Katrinette, 'Pflege und Medizin in mittelalterlichen Frauenkonventen', *Medizinhistorisches Journal* 37 (2002), 231–63.

pseudo-Boethius, *De disciplina scolarium*, ed. Olga Weijers, Studien und Texte zur Geistesgeschichte des Mittelalters, 12 (Leiden: Brill, 1976).

Boffey, Julia, 'Bodleian Library, MS Arch. Selden.B.24 and Definitions of the "Household Book"', in *The English Medieval Book: Studies in Memory of Jeremy Griffiths*, ed. A. S. G. Edwards, Vincent Gillespie, and Ralph Hanna (London: The British Library, 2000), pp. 125–34.

Bonaccioli, Ludovico, *Enneas muliebris* (Ferrara: Laurentius de Rubies?, *c.* 1502–3?).

Bosselmann-Cyran, Kristian, 'Ein weiterer Textzeuge von Johann Hartliebs '*Secreta mulierum*'-und '*Buch Trotula*'-Bearbeitung: Der Mailänder Kodex AE.IX.34 aus der Privatbibliothek des Arztes und Literaten Albrecht von Haller', *Würzburger medizinhistorische Mitteilungen* 13 (1995), 209–15.

——— (ed.), '*Secreta mulierum*' *mit Glosse in der deutschen Bearbeitung von Johann Hartlieb*, Würzburger medizinhistorische Forschungen, 36 (Pattensen/Hannover: Horst Wellm, 1985).

Braddy, Haldeen, 'The French Influence on Chaucer', in *Companion to Chaucer Studies*, ed. Beryl Rowland, rev. edn (New York and Oxford: Oxford University Press, 1979), pp. 143–59.

Braekman, Willy, 'Johannes Conincks Instructies voor Vroedvrouwen uit de zestiende eeuw', in *Volkskunde* 88 (1987), 120–30.

Bresc, Henri, *Livre et société en Sicile (1299–1499)* (Palermo: Centro di Studi Filologici e Linguisitici Siciliani, 1971).

Briggs, Charles F., 'Literacy, Reading, and Writing in the Medieval West', *Journal of Medieval History* 26 (2001), 397–420.

Britnell, Richard, 'Pragmatic Literacy in Latin Christendom', in *idem*, *Pragmatic Literacy, East and West: 1200–1330* (Woodbridge, Suffolk: Boydell, 1997), pp. 3–24.

——— (ed.), *Pragmatic Literacy, East and West: 1200–1330* (Woodbridge, Suffolk: Boydell, 1997).

Broomhall, Susan, *Women's Medical Work in Early Modern France* (Manchester: University of Manchester Press, 2004).

Brundage, James A., *Law, Sex, and Christian Society in Medieval Europe* (Chicago: University of Chicago Press, 1987).

Bruzelius, Caroline A., 'Hearing is Believing: Clarissan Architecture, *c.*1213–1340', *Gesta* 31, no. 2 (1992), 83–91.

Bryce, Judith, 'Les Livres des Florentines: Reconsidering Women's Literacy in Quattro-cento Florence', in *At the Margins: Minority Groups in Premodern Italy*, ed. Stephen J. Milner (Minneapolis: University of Minnesota Press, 2005), pp. 133–61.

Buck, R. A., 'Women and Language in the Anglo-Saxon Leechbooks', *Women and Language* 23, 2 (Fall 2000), 41–50.

Burckhard, Georg, *Die deutschen Hebammenordnungen von ihren ersten Anfängen bis auf die Neuzeit* (Leipzig: W. Engelmann, 1912).

Burghetti, P. Benv[enuto], 'De regimine Clarissarum durante saec. XIV', *Archivum Franciscanum Historicum* 13 (1920), 89–135.

Burnett, Charles S. F., 'Physics before the *Physics*: Early Translations from Arabic of Texts Concerning Nature in MSS British Library, Additional 22719 and Cotton Galba E IV', *Medioevo: Rivista di Storia della Filosofia Medievale* 27 (2002), pp. 53–109.

Butler, Judith, *Gender Trouble: Feminism and the Subversion of Identity* (New York: Routledge, 1990).

Bylebyl, Jerome, 'The Medical Meaning of *Physica*', *Osiris*, 2nd ser., 6 (1990) 16–41.

Caballero Navas, Carmen, 'Algunos "secretos de mujeres" revelados: El *Še'ar yašub* y la recepción y transmisión del *Trotula* en hebreo [Some "secrets of women" revealed: The *She'ar yašub* and the reception and transmission of the *Trotula* in Hebrew]', *Miscelánea de Estudios Árabes y Hebraicos, sección Hebreo* 55 (2006), 381–425.

—— 'Secrets of Women: Naming Female Sexual Difference in Medieval Hebrew Medical Literature', *Nashim: A Journal of Jewish Women's Studies and Gender* 12 (2006), 39–56.

Cabré i Pairet, Montserrat, 'Kate Campbell Hurd-Mead (1867–1941) and the Medical Women's Struggle for History', *Collections. The Newsletter of the Archives and Special Collections on Women in Medicine. The Medical College of Pennsylvania*, Philadelphia, PA, issue 26 (February 1993), pp. 1–4, 8.

—— 'From a Master to a Laywoman: A Feminine Manual of Self-Help', *Dynamis: Acta Hispanica ad Medicinae Scientiarumque Historiam Illustrandam* 20 (2000), 371–93.

—— 'Nacer en relation', in *De dos en dos: Las practicas de creación y recreación de la vida y de la convivencia*, ed. Marta Beltran i Tarres (Madrid: Hora y Hora, 2000), pp. 15–32.

—— (trans.), 'Public Record of the Labour of Isabel de la Cavalleria. January 10, 1490, Zaragoza', *The Online Reference Book for Medieval Studies* <http://orb.rhodes.edu/birthrecord.html>. accessed 13 October 2003.

—— and Fernando Salmón Muñiz, 'Poder académico *versus* autoridad femenina: La Facultad de Medicina de París contra Jacoba Félicié (1322)', *Dynamis* 19 (1999), 55–78.

Cadden, Joan, *Meanings of Sex Difference in the Middle Ages: Medicine, Science and Culture* (Cambridge: Cambridge University Press, 1993).

Caelius Aurelianus, *Caelius Aurelianus, Gynaecia: Fragments of a Latin Version of Soranus' Gynaecia from a Thirteenth Century Manuscript*, ed. Miriam and Israel Drabkin (Baltimore: Johns Hopkins University Press, 1951).

Calvanico, Raffaele, *Fonti per la storia della medicina e della chirurgia per il regno di Napoli nel periodo angioino (a. 1273–1410)* (Naples: L'Arte Tipografica, 1962).

Cambell, Jacques, *Vies occitanes de Saint Auzias et de Sainte Dauphine, avec traduction française, introduction et notes* (Rome: [Pontificium Athenaeum antonianum], 1963).

362   *References*

Camille, Michael, 'Seeing and Reading: Some Visual Implications of Medieval Literacy and Illiteracy', *Art History* 8 (1985), 26–49.

_____ *Image on the Edge: The Margins of Medieval Art* (Cambridge, MA: Harvard University Press, 1992).

Camus, Jules, 'La Seconde Traduction de la Chirurgie de Mondeville (Turin, Bibl. nat. L.IV.17)', *Bulletin de la Société des Anciens textes français* 28 (1902), 100–19.

Cantimpré, Thomas de, *Liber de natura rerum*, ed. H. Boese, vol. 1 (Berlin/New York: Walter de Gruyter, 1973).

Carbón, Damián, *Libro del arte de las comadres o madrinas, y del regimiento de las preñadas y paridas y de los niños* ([Majorca City: Hernando de Cansoles,] 1541).

Carley, James P. (ed.), *The Libraries of King Henry VIII*, Corpus of British Medieval Library Catalogues, 7 (London: The British Library in association with the British Academy, 2000).

Carlino, Andrea, *Paper Bodies: A Catalogue of Anatomical Fugitive Sheets*, trans. Noga Arika. Medical History, Supplement No. 19 (London: Wellcome Institute for the History of Medicine, 1999).

Carruthers, Mary, *The Book of Memory* (Cambridge: Cambridge University Press, 1990).

Chaucer, Geoffrey, *Canterbury Tales*, in *The Riverside Chaucer*, ed. Larry Benson, 3rd edn (Boston: Houghton Mifflin, 1987).

Chiarelli, Leonard C., 'A Preliminary Study on the Origins of Medical Licensing in the Medieval Mediterranean', *Al-Masaq: Islam and the Medieval Mediterranean* 10 (1998), 1–11.

Christ, Karl, 'Mittelalterliche Bibliotheksordnungen für Frauenklöster', *Zentralblatt für Bibliothekswesen* 59, nos. 1/2 (Jan./Feb. 1942), 1–29.

Cifuentes, Lluís, 'La Promoció intellectual i social dels barbers-cirurgians a la Barcelona medieval: L'obrador, la biblioteca i els béns de Joan Vicenç (*fl.* 1421–64)', *Arxiu de Textos Catalans Antics* 19 (2000), 429–79.

Cifuentes i Comamala, Lluís, *La ciencia en catala a l'edat mitjana* (Barcelona: Universitat de Barcelona, 2001).

Clanchy, Michael T., *From Memory to Written Record: England 1066–1307*, 2nd rev. edn (Oxford: Blackwell, 1993).

_____ 'England in the Thirteenth Century: Power and Knowledge', in *England in the Thirteenth Century: Proceedings of the 1984 Harlaxton Symposium*, ed. W. M. Ormrod (Woodbridge, Suffolk: Boydell Press, 1986), pp. 1–14.

Clare of Assisi: Early Documents, ed. and trans. Regis J. Armstrong, rev. edn (Saint Bonaventure, NY: Franciscan Institute Publications, Saint Bonaventure University, 1993).

Coleman, Joyce, *Public Reading and the Reading Public in Late Medieval England and France* (Cambridge: Cambridge University Press, 1996).

Colker, Marvin L. (ed.), *Analecta Dublinensia: Three Medieval Latin Texts in the Library of Trinity College Dublin* (Cambridge, MA: Medieval Academy of America, 1975).

Conde Parrado, Pedro, Enrique Montero Cartelle, and M.ª Cruz Herrero Ingelmo (eds.), *Tractatus de conceptu; Tractatus de sterilitate mulierum*, Lingüística y filología, 37 (Valladolid: Universidad de Valladolid, 1999).

Congourdeau, Hélène, ' "Métrodôra" et son oeuvre', in *Maladie et société à Byzance*, ed. Evelyne Patlagean (Spoleto: Centro Italiano di Studi sull'Alto Medioevo, 1993), pp. 57–96.

Corner, George Washington, *Anatomical Texts of the Earlier Middle Ages* (Washington, DC: Carnegie Institution of Washington, 1927).

Crowther-Heyck, Kathleen, 'Wonderful Secrets of Nature: Natural Knowledge and Religious Piety in Reformation Germany', *Isis* 94 (2003), 253–73.

Curion, Johannes and Jacob Crell (eds.), *De conservanda bona valetudine opusculum scholae Salernitanae, ad regem Angliae, versibus conscriptum* (Frankfurt: Christian Egenolph, 1551).

Daems, W. F., *Boec van medicinen in Dietsche: Een middelnederlandse compilatie van medisch-farmaceutische Literatur, Janus* Suppléments 7 (Leiden: E. J. Brill, 1967).

Daremberg, Charles (ed.), *Liber de secretis mulierum*, in *Collectio Salernitana ossia documenti inediti, e trattati di medicina appartenenti alla scuola medica salernitana*, ed. Salvatore De Renzi, 5 vols. (Naples: Filiatre-Sebezio, 1852–59; repr. Bologna: Forni, 1967), 4:1–38.

d'Argellata, Pietro, *Chirurgia* (Venice: Benedictus Senuensis, 1480).

Dean, Trevor, 'Gender and Insult in an Italian City: Bologna in the Later Middle Ages', *Social History* 29 (2004), 217–31.

Deighton, Alan R., 'Die Bibliothek der Grafen von Manderscheid-Blankenheim', *Archiv für Geschichte des Buchwesens* 26 (1986), 259–83.

Delisle, Léopold, *Le cabinet des manuscrits de la Bibliothèque Nationale*, 3 vols. (Paris: Imprimerie Nationale, 1874).

——*Recherches sur la librairie de Charles V, roi de France, 1337–1380*, 2 vols. (Paris, 1907; repr. Amsterdam: van Heusden, 1967).

della Chiesa, Francesco Agostino, *Theatro delle donne letterate, con vn breue discorso della preminenza, e perfettione del sesso donnesco* (Mondovi: Gislandus and Rossus, 1620).

Delva, Anna (ed.), *Vrouwengeneeskunde in Vlaanderen tijdens de late middeleeuwen*, Vlaamse Historische Studies 2 (Brugge: Genootschap voor Geschiedenis, 1983).

Denecke, Ludwig, 'Die Bibliothek des Fritzlarer Stiftsherrn Martin von Geismar († 1450)', *Hessisches Jahrbuch für Landesgeschichte* 28 (1978), 80–109.

Denifle, Henri (ed.), *Chartularium universitatis Parisiensis*, 4 vols. (Paris, 1891–99; repr. Brussels: Culture et Civilisation, 1964).

De Renzi, Salvatore (ed.), *Collectio Salernitana ossia documenti inediti, e trattati di medicina appartenenti alla scuola medica salernitana*, 5 vols. (Naples: Filiatre-Sebezio, 1852–59; repr. Bologna: Forni, 1967).

Deutsches Wörterbuch von Jacob und Wilhelm Grimm, <http://www.dwb.uni-trier.de/index.html> accessed 9 October 2004.

Dhonnchadha, Aoibheann Nic, 'Medical Writing in Irish, 1400–1700', in *Two Thousand Years of Irish Medicine*, ed. J. B. Lyons (Dublin, 1999); repr. *Irish Medical Journal of Medical Science* 169, no. 3 (July–Sept. 2000), 217–20; available at <http://www.celt.dias.ie/gaeilge/staff/rcsi1.html> accessed 13 July 2004.

Dickson, J. H., and W. W. Gauld, 'Mark Jameson's Physic Plants: A Sixteenth Century Garden for Gynaecology in Glasgow?', *Scottish Medical Journal* 32 (1987), 60–2.

Dolea, Carmen, and Carla AbouZahr, 'Global Burden of Obstructed Labour in the Year 2000', <http://www.who.int/healthinfo/statistics/bod_obstructedlabour.pdf> accessed 4 October 2006.

Douët-d'Arcq, Louis (ed.), *Inventaire de la Bibliothèque du Roi Charles VI fait au Louvre en 1423 par ordre du Régent Duc de Bedford* (Paris: Société des Bibliophiles, 1867).

Doviak, Ronald, 'The University of Naples and the Study and Practice of Medicine in the Thirteenth and Fourteenth Centuries', PhD dissertation, City University of New York, 1974.

Drancourt, Michel, *et al.*, '*Yersinia pestis Orientalis* in Remains of Ancient Plague Patients', *Emerging Infectious Diseases*, 2007, Feb. <http://www.cdc.gov/EID/content/13/2/332.htm> accessed 10 February 2007.

Dubois, Pierre, *De recuperatione Terre Sante. Traité de politique générale*, ed. Ch.-V. Langlois (Paris: Alphonse Picard, 1891).

Dubreuil-Chambardel, Louis, *Les médecins dans l'ouest de la France aux XIe et XIIe siécles* (Paris: Secrétaire général de la Société française d'histoire de la médecine, 1914).

Dumas, Geneviève, 'Les femmes et les pratiques de la santé dans le "Registre des plaidoiries du Parlement de Paris, 1364–1427"', *Canadian Bulletin of Medical History/Bulletin canadien d'histoire de la médecine* 13 (1996), 3–27.

—— and Faith Wallis, 'Theory and Practice in the Trial of Jean Domrémi, 1423–1427', *Journal of the History of Medicine and Allied Sciences*, 54, no. 1 (Jan. 1999), 55–87.

Elmeer, Gordon P., 'The Regulation of Germany Midwifery in the 14th, 15th, and 16th Centuries', MD thesis, Yale University School of Medicine, 1964.

Emden, A. B., *Donors of Books to S. Augustine's Abbey, Canterbury*, Oxford Bibliographical Society, Occasional Publication, 4 (Oxford: Oxford Bibliographical Society, 1969).

Encarnación, Karen Rosoff, 'The Proper Uses of Desire: Sex and Procreation in Reformation Anatomical Fugitive Sheets', in *The Material Culture of Sex, Procreation, and Marriage in Premodern Europe*, ed. Anne L. McClanan and Karen Rosoff Encarnación (New York: Palgrave, 2002), pp. 221–49.

Erler, Mary C., *Women, Reading, and Piety in Late Medieval England* (Cambridge: Cambridge University Press, 2002).

Evenden, Doreen A., 'Gender Differences in the Licensing and Practice of Female and Male Surgeons in Early Modern England', *Medical History* 42 (1998), 194–216.

—— *The Midwives of Seventeenth-Century London* (Cambridge: Cambridge University Press, 2000).

Everett, Nicholas, *Literacy in Lombard Italy, c.568–774* (Cambridge: Cambridge University Press, 2003),

Falcucci, Niccolò, *Sermonum liber scientie medicine* (Venice: [B. Locatellus for Heirs of O. Scotus], 1507).

Farmer, Sharon, 'The Leper in the Master Bedroom: Thinking Through a Thirteenth-Century Exemplum', in *Framing the Family: Narrative and Representation in the Medieval and Early Modern Periods*, ed. Rosalynn Voaden and Diane Wolfthal (Tempe, AZ: Arizona Center for Medieval and Renaissance Studies, 2005), 79–100.

Fausto-Sterling, Anne, *Sexing the Body: Gender Politics and the Construction of Sexuality* (New York: Basic Books, 2000).

Ferrari da Grado, Giovanni Matteo, *Perutilia consilia ad diversas aegritudines* (Pavia: J. de Zerbo, 1482).

Ferzoco, George, 'The Massa Marittima Mural', *Toscana Studies* 1 (2004), 71–105.

Fidelis, Fortunatus, *Bissus, seu medicinae patrocinium quatuor libris distinctum* (Palermo, 1598).

Fissell, Mary E., 'The Politics of Reproduction in the English Reformation', *Representations*, no. 87 (Summer 2004), 43–81.

Flahaut, Jean, 'L'exercise de la pharmacie par les veuves d'apothicaires du XVe au XVIIIe siècles. 1ere partie: Aspects réglementaires', *Revue d'histoire de la pharmacie* 50, no. 335 (2002), 367–78.

_____ 'L'exercise de la pharmacie par les veuves d'apothicaires du XVe au XVIIIe siècles: 2e partie: Aspects humains', *Revue d'Histoire de la Pharmacie* 40, no. 336 (2002), 543–54.

Flemming, Rebecca, *Medicine and the Making of Roman Women: Gender, Nature, and Authority from Celsus to Galen* (Oxford: Oxford University Press, 2001).

Flügge, Sibylla, *Hebammen und heilkundige Frauen: Recht und Rechtswirklichkeit im 15. und 16. Jahrhundert*, 2nd edn (Frankfurt am Main: Stroenfeld, 2000).

Fourth World Conference on Women (Beijing, September 1995), Platform for Action.

Franciscus de Pedemontium, *Supplementum in secundum librum secretorum remediorum Ioannis Mesuae, quae vocant De appropriatis*, in *Supplementum in secundum librum Compendii secretorum medicinae Ioannis Mesues medici celeberrimi tum Petri Apponi Patavini, tum Francisci de Pedemontium medicorum illustrium* (Venice: Iunta, 1589).

French, Katherine. ' "To Free Them from Binding": Women in the Late Medieval English Parish', *Journal of Interdisciplinary History* 27, no. 3 (1997), 387–412.

Friedman, John Block, 'The Cipher Alphabet of John de Foxton's *Liber Cosmographiae*', *Scriptorium* 36 (1982), 219–35.

_____ (ed.), *John de Foxton's 'Liber cosmographiae' (1408)* (Leiden: E. J. Brill, 1988).

Fürbeth, Frank, 'Die spätmittelalterliche Adelsbibliothek des Anton von Annenberg: ihr Signaturensystem als Rekonstruktionshilfe', in *Sources for the History of Medieval Books and Libraries*, ed. Rita Schlusemann, Jos. M. M. Hermans, and Margriet Hoogvliet (Groningen: Egbert Forstern, 1999), pp. 61–78.

Furth, Charlotte, *A Flourishing Yin: Gender in China's Medical History, 960–1665* (University of California Press, 1999).

Gadd, I., 'Raynald, Thomas (fl. 1539–1552?)', *Oxford Dictionary of National Biography* (Oxford: Oxford University Press, 2004), online edition, <http://www.oxforddnb.com.library.lib.asu.edu:80/view/article/23209> accessed 24 December 2004.

Gairdner, J. (ed.), *The Historical Collections of a Citizen of London in the Fifteenth Century*, Camden Society, n.s. 17 (London, 1876; repr. New York: Johnson Reprint Corp., 1965).

Galante, Maria, 'Il notaio e il documento notarile a Salerno in epoca longobarda', in *Per una storia del notariato meridionale*, ed. Mario Amelotti, Studi storici sul notariato italiano, VI (Rome: Consiglio Nazionale del Notariato, 1982), 71–94.

García-Ballester, Luís, 'Tres bibliotecas médicas en la Valencia del siglo XV', *Asclepio* 18–19 (1966–67), 383–405.

_____ Michael R. McVaugh, and Agustín Rubio-Vela, *Medical Licensing and Learning in Fourteenth-Century Valencia, Transactions of the American Philosophical Society* 79, pt. 6 (Philadelphia: American Philosophical Society, 1989).

Garrigues, Laurent, 'Les Professions médicales à Paris au début du XVe siècle: Praticiens en procès au parlement', *Bibliothèque de l'École des Chartes* 156 (1998), 317–67.

Garufi, Carlo Alberto, *Necrologio del Liber confratrum di S. Matteo di Salerno*, Fonti per la Storia d'Italia, 56 (Rome: Tipographico del Senato, 1922).

Gauvard, Claude, Mary and Richard Rouse, and Alfred Soman, 'Le Châtelet de Paris au début du XVe siecle d'après les fragments d'un registre d'écrous de 1412', *Bibliothèque de l'École des Chartes* 157 (1999), 565–606.

Gentilcore, David, *Healers and Healing in Early Modern Italy*, Social and Cultural Values in Early Modern Europe (Manchester: Manchester University Press, 1998).

Getz, Faye Marie, 'Charity, Translation, and Language of Medical Learning in Medieval England', *Bulletin of the History of Medicine* 64 (1990), 1–17.

―――― *Healing and Society in Medieval England: A Middle English Translation of the Pharmaceutical Writings of Gilbertus Anglicus* (Madison, Wisconsin: University of Wisconsin Press, 1991).

Giacosa, Piero, *Magistri Salernitani nondum editi* (Turin: Fratelli Bocca, 1901).

Gill, Katherine, 'Women and the Production of Religious Literature in the Vernacular, 1300–1500', in *Creative Women in Medieval and Early Modern Italy*, ed. E. Ann Matter and John Coakley (Philadelphia: University of Pennsylvania Press, 1994), pp. 64–104.

Giovanni da Vigo, *Practica in chirurgia* (Lyons: Jacob Myr, 1516).

Giraudet, Christophe, 'Le milieu médical à Decize à la fin du Moyen Âge', *Annales de Bourgogne* 72 (2000), 237–64.

Glaze, Florence Eliza, 'Medical Writer: "Behold the Human Creature"', in *Voice of the Living Light: Hildegard of Bingen and her World*, ed. Barbara Newman (Berkeley: University of California Press, 1998), pp. 125–48.

Glaze, Florence Eliza, 'The Perforated Wall: The Ownership and Circulation of Medical Books in Medieval Europe, *c*.800–1200'. PhD dissertation, Duke University, 2000.

Green, Monica H., 'The Transmission of Ancient Theories of Female Physiology and Disease Through the Early Middle Ages', PhD dissertation, Princeton University, 1985.

―――― 'The *De genecia* Attributed to Constantine the African', *Speculum* 62 (1987), 299–323; repr. in Green, *Women's Healthcare*, Essay III.

―――― 'Women's Medical Practice and Health Care in Medieval Europe', *Signs: Journal of Women in Culture and Society* 14 (1989–90), 434–73; repr. in *Sisters and Workers in the Middle Ages*, ed. J. Bennett, E. Clark, J. O'Barr, B. Vilen, and S. Westphal-Wihl (Chicago: University of Chicago Press, 1989), pp. 39–78; and in Green, *Women's Healthcare*, Essay I.

―――― 'Gynäkologische und geburtshilfliche Illustrationen in mittelalterlichen Manuskripten: Sprechende Bilder halfen den Frauen', *Die Waage* 30, no. 4 (1991), 161–7.

―――― 'Obstetrical and Gynecological Texts in Middle English', *Studies in the Age of Chaucer* 14 (1992), 53–88; repr. in Green, *Women's Healthcare*, Essay IV.

―――― 'Documenting Medieval Women's Medical Practice', in *Practical Medicine from Salerno to the Black Death*, ed. Luis García-Ballester, Roger French, Jon Arrizabalaga, and Andrew Cunningham (Cambridge: Cambridge University Press, 1994), pp. 322–52; repr. in Green, *Women's Healthcare*, Essay II.

―――― 'The Re-Creation of *Pantegni, Practica*, Book VIII', in *Constantine the African and 'Alī ibn al-'Abbās al-Mağūsī: The 'Pantegni' and Related Texts*, ed. Charles Burnett and Danielle Jacquart (Leiden: E. J. Brill, 1994), pp. 121–60.

―――― 'The Development of the *Trotula*', *Revue d'Histoire des Textes* 26 (1996), 119–203; repr. in Green, *Women's Healthcare*, Essay V.

_____ 'A Handlist of the Latin and Vernacular Manuscripts of the So-Called *Trotula* Texts. Part I: The Latin Manuscripts', *Scriptorium* 50 (1996), 137–75.

_____ 'A Handlist of the Latin and Vernacular Manuscripts of the So-Called *Trotula* Texts. Part II: The Vernacular Texts and Latin Re-Writings', *Scriptorium* 51 (1997), 80–104.

_____ ' "Traittié tout de mençonges": The *Secrés des dames*, "Trotula", and Attitudes Towards Women's Medicine in Fourteenth- and Early Fifteenth-Century France', in *Christine de Pizan and the Categories of Difference*, ed. Marilynn Desmond (Minneapolis: University of Minnesota Press, 1998), pp. 146–78; repr. in Green, *Women's Healthcare*, Essay VI.

_____ 'In Search of an "Authentic" Women's Medicine: The Strange Fates of Trota of Salerno and Hildegard of Bingen', *Dynamis: Acta Hispanica ad Medicinae Scientiarumque Historiam Illustrandam* 19 (1999), 25–54.

_____ 'Books as a Source of Medical Education for Women in the Middle Ages', *Dynamis: Acta Hispanica ad Medicinae Scientiarumque Historiam Illustrandam* 20 (2000), 331–69.

_____ 'From "Diseases of Women" to "Secrets of Women": The Transformation of Gynecological Literature in the Later Middle Ages', *Journal of Medieval and Early Modern Studies* 30 (2000), 5–39.

_____ 'Medieval Gynecological Texts: A Handlist', in *Women's Healthcare*, Appendix, pp. 1–36.

_____ 'The Possibilities of Literacy and the Limits of Reading: Women and the Gendering of Medical Literacy', in Green, *Women's Healthcare*, Essay VII.

_____ *Women's Healthcare in the Medieval West: Texts and Contexts*, Variorum Collected Studies Series, CS680 (Aldershot: Ashgate, 2000).

_____ (ed. and trans.), *The 'Trotula': A Medieval Compendium of Women's Medicine* (Philadelphia: University of Pennsylvania Press, 2001).

_____ 'Defining Women's Health: An Interdisciplinary Dialogue—Background', posted 15 April 2002 on <http://www.fas.harvard.edu/womenstudy/events/proposal.htm>

_____ 'Gendering the Audiences of Medieval Scientific Texts: The Case for Chiromancy' (presented at the 38th International Medieval Congress, Kalamazoo, Michigan, May 2003).

_____ 'Masses in Remembrance of "Seynt Susanne": A Fifteenth-Century Spiritual Regimen', *Notes and Queries* n. s. 50, no. 4 (December 2003), 380–4.

_____ 'Bodies, Gender, Health, Disease: Recent Work on Medieval Women's Medicine', *Studies in Medieval and Renaissance History* 3rd ser. 2 (2005), 1–49.

_____ 'Flowers, Poisons, and Men: Menstruation in Medieval Western Europe', in *Menstruation: A Cultural History*, ed. Andrew Shail and Gillian Howie (New York: Palgrave, 2005), pp. 51–64.

_____ 'Reconstructing the *Oeuvre* of Trota of Salerno', in *La Scuola medica Salernitana: Gli autori e i testi*, ed. Danielle Jacquart and Agostino Paravicini Bagliani, Edizione Nazionale 'La Scuola Medica Salernitana', 1 (Florence: SISMEL/Edizioni del Galluzzo, 2007), pp. 183–233.

_____ 'Gender and the Vernacularization of Women's Medicine in Late Medieval and Early Modern Europe' (forthcoming).

_____ 'Slander and the Secrets of Women: The *Meretrices* Version of the *Trotula* Ensemble' (forthcoming).

Green, Monica H., 'The Sources of Eucharius Rösslin's *Rosegarden for Pregnant Women and Midwives* (1513)' (forthcoming).

_____ and Linne R. Mooney, 'The *Sickness of Women*', in *Sex, Aging, and Death in a Medieval Medical Compendium: Trinity College Cambridge MS R.14.52, Its Texts, Language, and Scribe*, ed. M. Teresa Tavormina, Medieval and Renaissance Texts and Studies, 292, 2 vols. (Tempe, AZ: Arizona Center for Medieval and Renaissance Studies, 2006), vol. 2, pp. 455–568.

_____ and Daniel Lord Smail, 'The Trial of Floreta d'Ays (1403): Jews, Christians, and Obstetrics in Later Medieval Marseille', *Journal of Medieval History* (forthcoming).

Grensemann, Hermann, 'Die Schrift *De adventu medici ad aegrotum* nach dem Salernitaner Arzt Archimatheus', *Würzburger medizinhistorische Mitteilungen* 14 (1996) 233–51.

Grubmüller, Klaus, 'Hartlieb, Johannes', in *Die deutsche Literatur des Mittelalters: Verfasserlexikon*, rev. edn., ed. Kurt Ruh *et al.*, 10 vols. (Berlin: De Gruyter, 1978–99), Bd. 3, coll. 480–96.

Grundmann, Herbert, 'Litteratus-illiteratus: Der Wandel einer Bildungnorm vom Altertum zum Mittelalter', in Grundmann, *Ausgewählte Aufsätze, 3: Bildung und Sprache*, Monumenta Germaniae Historica Schriften 25:3 (Stuttgart: Hiersemann, 1978), pp. 1–66.

Gruskin, Sofia, and Daniel Tarantola, 'Health and Human Rights', in *Oxford Textbook of Public Health*, 4th edn, ed. Roger Detels, James McEwen, Robert Beaglehole, and Heizo Tanaka (Oxford: Oxford University Press, 2004), pp. 311–36.

Guardiola, Ginger Lee, 'Within and Without: The Social and Medical Worlds of the Medieval Midwife, 1000–1500', PhD dissertation, University of Colorado at Boulder, 2002.

Guillén, José Francisco Saéz and Pilar Jiménez de Cisneros, *Catálogo de manuscritos de la Biblioteca Colombina de Sevilla* (Seville: Cabildo de la S. M. y P. I. de Sevilla—Institucion Colombina, 2002).

Guy de Chauliac, *Inventarium sive Chirurgia magna*, ed. Michael R. McVaugh, with Margaret S. Ogden, Studies in Ancient Medicine, vol. 14, I and II (Leiden: Brill, 1997).

Gwynn, Aubrey, *The English Austin Friars in the Time of Wyclif* (London: Humphrey Milford, Oxford University Press, 1940).

Hall, Susan P., *The 'Cyrurgia magna' of Brunus Longoburgensis: A Critical Edition*, DPhil thesis, Oxford University, 1957.

Hamilton, George L., 'Trotula', *Modern Philology* 4 (1906), 377–80.

Hanna, Ralph, III, '*Compilatio* and the Wife of Bath: Latin Backgrounds, Ricardian Texts', in *Latin and Vernacular: Studies in Late-Medieval Texts and Manuscripts*, ed. Alistair Minnis (Woodbridge: D. S. Brewer, 1989), pp. 1–11.

_____ and Traugott Lawler (eds.), *Jankyn's Book of Wikked Wyves* (using materials collected by Karl Young and Robert A. Pratt) (Athens: University of Georgia Press, 1997).

_____ 'Humphrey Newton and Bodleian Library, MS Lat. misc. c. 66', *Medium Aevum* 69 (2000), 279–91.

Hanson, Ann Ellis, 'Hippocrates: *Diseases of Women* 1', *Signs: Journal of Women in Culture and Society* 1, no. 2 (Winter 1975), 567–84.

_____ 'A Division of Labor: Roles for Men in Greek and Roman Births', *Thamyris* 1 (1994), 157–202.

_____ 'The Correspondence between Soranus, Antonius and Cleopatra' (forthcoming).

_____ and Monica H. Green, 'Soranus of Ephesus: *Methodicorum princeps*', in Wolfgang Haase and Hildegard Temporini, eds., *Aufstieg und Niedergang der römischen Welt*, Teilband II, Band 37.2 (Berlin and New York: Walter de Gruyter, 1994), pp. 968–1075.

Harkness, Deborah E., 'Managing an Experimental Household: The Dees of Mortlake and the Practice of Natural Philosophy', *Isis* 88 (1997), 247–62.

Harvey, L. P., 'In Granada Under the Catholic Monarchs: A Call from a Doctor and Another from a *Curandera*', in *The Age of the Catholic Monarchs, 1474–1516: Literary Studies in Memory of Keith Whinnom*, ed. Alan Deyermond and Ian Macpherson (Liverpool: Liverpool University Press, 1989), pp. 71–5.

Heinrich von dem Türlin, *The Crown: A Tale of Sir Gawein and King Arthur's Court*, trans. J. W. Thomas (Lincoln, Neb. and London: University of Nebraska Press, 1989).

Heldris of Cornwall, *Silence: A Thirteenth-Century French Romance*, trans. Sarah Roche-Mahdi (East Lansing: Michigan State University Press, 1992).

Hernando, Josep, *Llibres i lectors a la Barcelona del s. XIV*, 2 vols., Textos i Documents, 30 (Barcelona: Fundaciò Noguera, 1995).

Hewson, M. Anthony, *Giles of Rome and the Medieval Theory of Conception: A Study of the 'De formatione corporis humani in utero'*, University of London Historical Studies, 38 (London: Athelone Press, University of London, 1975).

Hiersemann, Conrad, *Die Abschnitte aus der Practica des Trottus in der Salernitanischen Sammelschrift 'De Aegritudinum Curatione'. Breslau Codex Salern. 1160–1170*, inaugural dissertation, Leipzig 1921.

Hillgarth, J. N., *Readers and Books in Majorca, 1229–1550*, 2 vols. (Paris: Éditions du Centre National de la Recherche Scientifique, 1991).

Hitchcock, James, 'A Sixteenth Century Midwife's License', *Bulletin of the History of Medicine* 41 (1967), 75–6.

Hobby, Elaine, 'Gender, Science and Midwifery: Jane Sharp, *The Midwives Book* (1671)', in *The Arts of Seventeenth Century Science: Representations of the Natural World in European and North American Culture*, ed. Claire Jowitt and Diane Watt (Aldershot: Ashgate, 2002), pp. 146–59.

Humphreys, K. W., 'The Medical Books of the Medieval Friars', *Libri: International Library Review* 3 (1954), 95–103.

_____ (ed.), *The Friars' Libraries*, Corpus of British Medieval Library Catalogues (London: British Library in association with the British Academy, 1990).

Hünemörder, Christian, and Kurt Ruh, 'Thomas von Cantimpré OP', in *Die deutsche Literatur des Mittelalters: Verfasserlexikon*, rev. edn, ed. Kurt Ruh *et al.*, 10 vols. (Berlin: De Gruyter, 1978–99), vol. 9 (1995), coll. 838–51.

Hunt, R. W., 'The Medieval Library', in *New College Oxford, 1379–1979*, ed. John Buxton and Penry Williams (Oxford: Wardens and Fellows of New College, 1979), pp. 317–45.

Hunt, Tony, *The Medieval Surgery* (Woodbridge, Suffolk: Boydell Press, 1992).

_____ *Anglo-Norman Medicine*, 2 vols. (Cambridge: D. S. Brewer, 1994–7).

Hurd-Mead, Kate Campbell, 'Trotula', *Isis* 14 (1930), 349–67.

Huws, Daniel, 'MS Porkington 10 and its Scribes', in Jennifer Fellows, *et al.*, eds., *Romance Reading on the Book: Essays on Medieval Narrative presented to Maldwyn Mills* (Cardiff, 1996), pp. 208–20.

Hyginus, *Fabulae*, ed. Peter K. Marshall (Stuttgart: Teubner, 1993).

Inhorn, Marcia C., *Quest for Conception: Gender, Infertility, and Egyptian Medical Traditions* (Philadelphia: University of Pennsylvania Press, 1994).

——— *Infertility and Patriarchy: The Cultural Politics of Gender and Family Life in Egypt* (Philadelphia: University of Pennsylvania Press, 1996).

Innocent IV, Pope, 'The Form of Life of Pope Innocent IV (1247)', in *Clare of Assisi: Early Documents*, ed. and trans. Regis J. Armstrong, rev. edn (Saint Bonaventure, NY: Franciscan Institute Publications, Saint Bonaventure University, 1993), pp. 118–19.

Institute of Medicine, *Unequal Treatment: Confronting Racial and Ethnic Disparities in Health Care* (Washington, DC: National Academies Press, 2003).

Irblich, Eva (ed.), *Abū'l Qāsim Halaf Ibn 'Abbas al-Zahrāuī, Chirurgia. Faksimile und Kommentar* (Graz: Akademische Druck- und Verlagsanstalt, 1979).

Jacquart, Danielle, *Le milieu médical en France du XIIe au XVe siècle: En annexe 2e supplément au 'Dictionnaire' d'Ernest Wickersheimer* (Geneva: Librairie Droz, 1981).

——— 'Aristotelian Thought in Salerno', in *A History of Twelfth-Century Philosophy*, ed P. Dronke (Cambridge: Cambridge University Press, 1988), pp. 407–28.

——— (ed.), *Supplément* to Ernest Wickersheimer, *Dictionnaire biographique des médecins en France au Moyen Age* (Geneva: Librairie Droz, 1979).

——— and Françoise Micheau, *La médecine arabe et l'occident médiéval* (Paris: Maisonneuve et Larose, 1990).

——— and Claude Thomasset, 'Albert le Grand et les problèmes de la sexualité', *History and Philosophy of the Life Sciences* 3 (1981), 73–93.

——— and ——— *Sexuality and Medicine in the Middle Ages*, trans. Matthew Adamson (Cambridge: Polity Press; Princeton: Princeton University Press, 1988).

James, Montague Rhodes, *The Ancient Libraries of Canterbury and Dover: The Catalogues of the Libraries of Christ Church Priory and St Augustine's Abbey at Canterbury and of St Martin's Priory at Dover* (Cambridge: Cambridge University Press, 1903).

Jeudy, Colette, 'Traductions françaises d'oeuvres latines et traductions médicales à la bibliothèque cathédrale de Reims d'après l'inventaire de 1456/1479', *Scriptorium* 47 (1993), 173–85.

John of Gaddesden, *Rosa anglica practica medicine a capite ad pedes noviter impressa et perquam diligentissime emendata* (Venice: Bonetus Locatellus for Octavianus Scotus, 1502).

Johnson, Michael, 'Science and Discipline: The Ethos of Sex Education in a Fourteenth-Century Classroom', in *Homo Carnalis: The Carnal Aspect of Medieval Human Life*, ed. Helen Rodnite Lemay, Acta XIV, Center for Medieval and Early Renaissance Studies (Binghampton: SUNY Center for Medieval and Renaissance Studies, 1990), pp. 157–172.

Johnson, Penelope D., *Equal in Monastic Profession: Religious Women in Medieval France* (Chicago: University of Chicago Press, 1991).

Jonas, Richard (trans.), *The Byrth of mankynde, Newly Translated out of Laten into Englysshe* (London: T[homas] R[aynald], 1540).

Jones, Peter Murray, *Medieval Medicine in Illuminated Manuscripts*, rev. edn (London: British Library [by] arrangement with Centro Tibaldi, 1998).

Jordan, Mark D., 'Medicine as Science in the Early Commentaries on 'Johannitius'', *Traditio* 43 (1987): 121–45.

Jordan, Mark D., 'The Construction of a Philosophical Medicine: Exegesis and Argument in Salernitan Teaching on the Soul', *Osiris*, 2nd ser., 6 (1990): 42–61.

Jordan, William Chester, *The Great Famine: Northern Europe in the Early Fourteenth Century* (Princeton, NJ: Princeton University Press, 1996).

Junius, Hadrianus, *Animadversionum libri sex, omnigenae lectionis thesaurus, in quibus infiniti penè autorum loci corriguntur et declarantur, nunc primùm et nati, et in lucem aediti* (Basel: Isengrinus, 1556).

Kaeppeli, Thomas, and E. Panella, *Scriptores Ordinis Praedicatoris Medii Aevi*, Bd. 4 (Rome: S. Sabina, 1993).

Kandiyoti, Deniz, 'Bargaining with Patriarchy', *Gender and Society* 2, no. 3 (September 1988), 274–90.

Karras, Ruth Mazo, *From Boys to Men: Formations of Masculinity in Late Medieval Europe* (Philadelphia: University of Pennsylvania Press, 2003).

Kealey, Edward J., *Medieval Medicus: A Social History of Anglo-Norman Medicine* (Baltimore and London: Johns Hopkins University Press, 1981).

Keil, Gundolf, 'Ludwig V', in *Die deutsche Literatur des Mittelalters: Verfasserlexikon*, rev. edn., ed. Kurt Ruh *et al.*, 10 vols. (Berlin: De Gruyter, 1978–99), vol. 5, coll. 1016–30.

—— 'Die Frau als Ärtzin und Patientin in der medizinischen Fachprosa des deutschen Mittelalters', in *Frau und spätmittelalterlicher Alltag: Internationalaler Kongress, Krems an der Donau, 2. bis 5. Oktober 1984* (Vienna: Österreichischen Akademie der Wissenschaften, 1986), pp. 157–211.

—— 'Der Hausvater als Arzt', in *Haushalt und Familie in Mittelalter und früher Neuzeit*, ed. Trude Ehlert *et al.* (Sigmaringen: Jan Thorbecke, 1991), pp. 219–43.

Kelly, Joan, *Women, History, and Theory: The Essays of Joan Kelly* (Chicago: University of Chicago Press, 1984).

King, Helen, 'Agnodike and the Profession of Medicine', *Proceedings of the Cambridge Philological Society* 32 (1986), 53–77.

—— *Hippocrates' Woman: Reading the Female Body in Ancient Greece* (London and New York: Routledge, 1998).

—— *The Disease of Virgins: Green Sickness, Chlorosis, and the Problems of Puberty* (New York: Routledge, 2003).

—— 'The Mathematics of Sex: One to Two, or Two to One?', *Studies in Medieval and Renaissance History* 3rd ser. 2 (2005), 47–56.

Kinzelbach, Annemarie, ' "wahnsinnige Weyber betriegen die unverstendigen Poeffel": Anerkennung und Diffamierung heilkundiger Frauen und Männer, 1450 bis 1700', *Medizinhistorisches Journal* 32 (1997), 29–56.

Kittell, Ellen E. and Kurt Gueller, ' "Whether Man or Woman": Gender Inclusivity in the Town Ordinances of Medieval Douai', *Journal of Medieval and Early Modern Studies* 30 (2000), 63–100.

Klapisch-Zuber, Christiane, 'Le dernier enfant: fécondité et vieillissement chez les Florentines XIVᵉ–XVᵉ siècles', in *Mesurer et comprendre: Mélanges offerts à Jacques Dupaquier*, ed. Jean-Pierre Barder, François Lebrun, and René Le Mée (Paris: Presses Universitaires de France, 1993), pp. 277–90.

Knorr, Wilbur R., 'Two Medieval Monks and their Astronomy Books', *Bodleian Library Record* 14 (1991–4), 269–84.

Kooper, Erik (ed.), *Medieval Dutch Literature in its European Context* (Cambridge: Cambridge University Press, 1994).

Kowaleski, Maryanne, 'Women's Work in a Market Town: Exeter in the Late Fourteenth Century', in *Women and Work in Preindustrial Europe*, ed. Barbara A. Hanawalt (Bloomington: University of Indiana Press, 1986), pp. 145–64.

Krämer, Sigrid, *Handschriftenerbe des Deutschen Mittelalters*, 3 vols., *Mittelalterliche Bibliothekskataloge Deutschlands und der Schweiz*. Ergänzungsband I (Munich, Beck, 1989–90).

Kristeller, Paul Oskar, 'Fonti per la medicina Salernitana del Sec. XII', *Salerno—Civitas Hippocratica* 1, no. 1–2 (1967), 19–26.

——— 'Learned Women of Early Modern Italy: Humanists and University Scholars', in *Beyond Their Sex: Learned Women of the European Past*, ed. Patricia H. Labalme (New York: New York University Press, 1984), pp. 91–116.

Krochalis, Jeanne, 'The Benedictine Rule for Nuns: Library of Congress, MS 4', *Manuscripta* 30 (1986), 21–34.

Krug, Rebecca, *Reading Families: Women's Literate Practice in Late Medieval England* (Ithaca, NY: Cornell University Press, 2002).

Krüger, Paul (ed.), *Corpus iuris civilis*, vol. II: *Codex Iustinianus* (Berlin: Weidmann, 1954).

Kruse, Britta-Juliane, 'Neufund einer handschriften Vorstufe von Eucharius Rößlins Hebammenlehrbuch *Der schwangeren Frauen und Hebammen Rosengarten* und des *Frauenbüchleins* Ps.-Ortolfs', *Sudhoffs Archiv* 78 (1994), 220–36.

——— *Verborgene Heilkünste: Geschichte der Frauenmedizin im Spätmittelalter*, Quellen und Forschungen zur Literatur- und Kulturgeschichte, 5 (Berlin: Walter de Gruyter, 1996).

Kurvinen, Auvo, 'MS Porkington 10: Description with Extracts', *Neuphilologische Mitteilungen* 54 (1953), 33–67 (repr. Modern Language Society, Helsinki. Amsterdam: Swets and Zeitlinger, 1968).

Kusche, Brigitte, 'Laatmiddelnederlandse Fragmenten uit de *Chirurgie* van Albucasis', *Verslagen en mededelingen*, Koninklijke Academie voor Nederlandse Taal- en Letterkunde (Gent, 1980), pp. 370–420.

——— *Frauenaufklärung im Spätmittelalter: Eine philologisch-medizinhistorische Untersuchung und Edition des gynäkologisch-obstetrischen GKS 1657 Kopenhagen*, Acta Universitatis Umensis (Stockholm: Almqvist and Wiksell International, 1990).

Lanfranc of Milan, *Cyrurgia magna*, in *Cyrurgia Guidonis de Cauliaco. et Cyrurgia Bruni, Teodorici, Rolandi, Lanfranci, Rogerii, Bertapalie* (Venice, 1519), ff. 166va–210vb.

Lang, S. J., 'John Bradmore and His Book *Philomena*', *Social History of Medicine* 5 (1992), 121–30.

——— 'The *Philomena* of John Bradmore and its Middle English Derivative: A perspective on Surgery in Late Medieval England', PhD dissertation, University of St Andrews, 1998.

Lansing, Carol, 'Concubines, Lovers, Prostitutes: Infamy and Female Identity in Medieval Bologna', in *Beyond Florence: The Contours of Medieval and Early Modern Italy* (Stanford, CA: Stanford University Press, 2003), pp. 85–100 and 256–8.

Lawler, Traugott, 'The Chaucer Library: 'Jankyn's Book of Wikked Wyves'', *The Chaucer Newsletter* 7 (1985), 1 and 3–4.

Lawn, Brian, *The Prose Salernitan Questions* (London: British Academy/Oxford University Press, 1979).

Lemay, Helen, 'William of Saliceto on Human Sexuality', *Viator* 12 (1981), 167–81.

_____ (trans.), *Women's Secrets: A Translation of Pseudo-Albertus Magnus' 'De secretis mulierum' with Commentaries* (Albany: State University of New York Press, 1992).

L'Estrange, Elizabeth, *Holy Motherhood: Gender, Dynasty, and Visual Culture in the Later Middle Ages* (Manchester: Manchester University Press, 2008).

Lewis, Katherine J., 'Model Girls? Virgin-Martyrs and the Training of Young Women in Late Medieval England', in *Young Medieval Women*, ed. Katherine J. Lewis, Noël James Menuge, and Kim M. Phillips (Phoenix Mill: Sutton, 1999), pp. 25–46.

Liébault, Jean, *Trois Livres appartenant aux infirmitez et maladies des femmes, pris du Latin de M. Jean Liebaut, Docteur Médecin à Paris, et facts François* (Paris: Jacques de Puys, 1585).

Liliencron, Rochus von, *et al.* (eds.), *Allgemeine Deutsche Biographie*, 56 vols. (Leipzig: Duncker and Humblot, 1875–1912).

Lonie, I. M., 'Literacy and the Development of Hippocratic Medicine', in François Lasserre and Philippe Mudry, eds., *Formes de pensée dans la collection Hippocratique* (Geneva: Droz, 1983), pp. 145–61.

McCracken, Peggy, *The Curse of Eve, the Wound of the Hero: Blood, Gender, and Medieval Literature* (Philadelphia: University of Pennsylvania Press, 2003).

McKitterick, Rosamond, *The Carolingians and the Written Word* (Cambridge: Cambridge University Press, 1989).

_____ (ed.), *The Uses of Literacy in Early Mediaeval Europe* (Cambridge: Cambridge University Press, 1990).

McTavish, Lianne, *Childbirth and the Display of Authority in Early Modern France* (Aldershot: Ashgate, 2005).

_____ 'Blame and Vindication in the Early Modern Birthing Chamber', *Medical History* 50 (2006), 447–64.

McVaugh, Michael R., *Medicine Before the Plague: Practitioners and Their Patients in the Crown of Aragon, 1285–1345* (Cambridge: Cambridge University Press, 1993).

_____ 'Royal Surgeons and the Value of Medical Learning: The Crown of Aragon, 1300–1350', in *Practical Medicine from Salerno to the Black Death*, ed. Luis García-Ballester, Roger French, Jon Arrizabalaga, and Andrew Cunningham (Cambridge: Cambridge University Press, 1994), pp. 221–36.

_____ 'Treatment of Hernia in the Later Middle Ages: Surgical Correction and Social Construction', in Roger French, *et al.*, *Medicine from the Black Death to the French Disease* (Aldershot: Ashgate, 1998), pp. 131–55.

_____ 'Surgical Education in the Middle Ages', *Dynamis: Acta Hispanica ad Medicinae Scientiarumque Historiam Illustrandam* 20 (2000), 283–304.

_____ 'Cataracts and Hernias: Aspects of Surgical Practice in the Fourteenth Century', *Medical History* 45 (2001), 319–40.

Manly, John M., and Edith Rickert (eds.), *The Text of the Canterbury Tales, Studied on the Basis of All Known Manuscripts*, 8 vols. (Chicago: University of Chicago Press, 1940).

March-Long, Caroline Gisela, 'Early Modern German Obstetrical Manuals: *Das Frauenbüchlein* (*c.*1495) and *Der Rosengarten* (1513)', MA thesis, Duke University, 1993.

Marie de France, *The Lais of Marie de France*, trans. Glyn S. Burgess and Keith Busby (Harmondsworth/New York: Penguin, 1986).

Marland, Hilary (ed.), *The Art of Midwifery: Early Modern Midwives in Europe* (London: Routledge, 1993).

Marquis de Pastoret, M. le (ed.), *Ordonnances des rois de France de la troisième race, recueillies par ordre chronologique*. Vol. 19 (Paris: Imprimerie Royale, 1835; repr. Farnborough: Gregg, 1968).

Marsh, Deborah [*see also* Youngs, Deborah], ' "I see by sizt of evidence": Information Gathering in Late Medieval Cheshire', in *Courts, Counties and the Capital in the Late Middle Ages*, ed. Diana E. S. Dunn (New York: St Martin's, 1996), pp. 71–92.

Matheson, Lister, 'Constantinus Africanus: *Liber de coitu (Liber creatoris)*', in *Sex, Aging, and Death in a Medieval Medical Compendium: Trinity College Cambridge MS R.14.52, Its Texts, Language, and Scribe*, ed. M. Teresa Tavormina, Medieval and Renaissance Texts and Studies, 292, 2 vols. (Tempe, AZ: Arizona Center for Medieval and Renaissance Studies, 2006), vol. 1, pp. 287–326.

Meale, Carole M., and Julia Boffey, 'Gentlewomen's Reading', in *The Cambridge History of the Book in Britain, vol. III: 1400–1557*, ed. Lotte Helinga and J. B. Trapp (Cambridge: Cambridge University Press, 1999), pp. 526–40.

Menestò, Ernesto (ed.), *Il Processo di canonizzazione di Chiara da Montefalco* (Regione dell 'Umbria: La Nuova Italia, 1984).

Mews, Constant J., 'Orality, Literacy, and Authority in the Twelfth Century Schools', *Exemplaria* 2, no. 2 (Fall 1990), 475–500.

—— 'Introduction', in *Listen, Daughter: The 'Speculum virginum' and the Formation of Religious Women in the Middle Ages*, ed. Constant J. Mews (New York: Palgrave, 2001), pp. 1–14.

Miller, Gordon, 'Literacy and the Hippocratic Art: Reading, Writing, and Epistemology in Ancient Greek Medicine', *Journal of the History of Medicine and Allied Sciences* 45 (1990), 11–40.

Millett, Bella, and Jocelyn Wogan-Browne (eds. and trans.), *Medieval English Prose for Women: From the Katherine Group and 'Ancrene Wisse'*, rev. edn (Oxford, Clarendon, 1992).

Mondeville, Henri de, *Die Chirurgie des Heinrich von Mondeville (Hermondaville): nach Berliner, Erfurter und Pariser codices*, ed. Julius Leopold Pagel (Berlin: August Hirschwald, 1892).

Montero Cartelle, Enrique, *Tractatus de sterilitate: Anónimo de Montpellier (s. XIV). Attribuido a A. de Vilanova, R. de Moleris y J. de Turre*, Lingüística y Filología, no. 16 (Valladolid: Universidad de Valladolid and Caja Salamanca y Soria, 1993).

—— and María Cruz Herrero Ingelmo, 'Las *Interrogaciones in cura sterilitatis* en el marco de la literatura médica medieval', *Faventia* 25, no. 2 (2003), 85–97.

Montford, Angela, 'Dangers and Disorders: The Decline of the Dominican *Frater Medicus*', *Social History of Medicine* 16, no. 2 (2003), 169–91.

Mooney, Catherine M., 'The Authorial Role of Brother A. in the Composition of Angela of Foligno's Revelations', in E. Ann Matter and John Coakely, eds., *Creative Women in Medieval and Early Modern Italy: A Religious and Artistic Renaissance* (Philadephia: University of Pennsylvania Press, 1994), pp. 34–63.

Mooney, Linne R., 'The Scribe', in *Sex, Aging, and Death in a Medieval Medical Compendium: Trinity College Cambridge MS R.14.52, Its Texts, Language, and Scribe*, ed. M. Teresa Tavormina, Medieval and Renaissance Texts and Studies, 292, 2 vols. (Tempe, AZ: Arizona Center for Medieval and Renaissance Studies, 2006), vol. 1, pp. 55–64.

Morantz-Sanchez, Regina Markell, *Sympathy and Science: Women Physicians in American Medicine* (New York: Oxford University Press, 1985).

Moulinier, Laurence (ed.), *Beate Hildegardis Cause et cure*, Rarissima mediaevalia, 1 (Berlin: Akademie Verlag, 2003).

Mowbray, Donald, 'A Community of Sufferers and the Authority of Masters: The Development of the Idea of Limbo by Masters of Theology at the University of Paris (*c*.1230–1300)', in *Authority and Community in the Middle Ages*, ed. Ian P Wei, Donald Mowbray, and Rhiannon Purdie (Stroud: Sutton, 1999), pp. 43–68.

Musacchio, Jacqueline Marie, *The Art and Ritual of Childbirth in Renaissance Italy* (New Haven and London: Yale University Press, 1999).

[Muscio], *Sorani Gynaeciorum vetus translatio latina*, ed. Valentin Rose (Leipzig: Teubner, 1882).

Narbona-Cárceles, Maria, 'Woman at Court: A Prosopographic Study of the Court of Carlos III of Navarre (1387–1425)', *Medieval Prosopography* 22 (2001), 31–64.

Naylor, Eric W., ' "Nunca le digas trotera" (*Libro de buen amor*, 926c)', in *Homenaje al Profesor Antonio Vilanova*, ed. Adolfo Sotelo Vázquez and Marta Cristina Carbonell (Barcelona: Universidad de Barcelona, 1989), pp. 461–74.

Newman, Barbara, 'Authority, Authenticity, and the Repression of Heloise', *Journal of Medieval and Renaissance Studies* 22, no. 2 (Spring 1992), 121–57.

——— (ed.), *Voice of the Living Light: Hildegard of Bingen and Her World* (Berkeley: University of California Press, 1998).

Nicaise, Edouard, *Chirurgie de Maitre Henri de Mondeville: chirurgien de Philippe le Bel, roi de France, composée de 1306 à 1320* (Paris: Félix Alcan, 1893).

North, J. D., *Horoscopes and History* (London: The Warburg Institute, University of London, 1986).

Nutton, Vivian, 'The Rise of Medical Humanism: Ferrara, 1464–1555', *Renaissance Studies* 11 (1997), 2–19.

——— ' "A Diet for Barbarians": Introducing Renaissance Medicine to Tudor England', in *Natural Particulars: Nature and the Disciplines in Renaissance Europe*, ed. A. Grafton, N. G. Siraisi (Cambridge, MA: MIT Press, 2000), 275–94.

——— and Christine Nutton, 'The Archer of Meudon: A Curious Absence of Continuity in the History of Medicine', *Journal of the History of Medicine and Allied Sciences* 58, no. 4 (October 2003), 401–27.

O'Boyle, Cornelius, 'Surgical Texts and Social Contexts: Physicians and Surgeons in Paris, *c*.1270 to 1430', in *Practical Medicine from Salerno to the Black Death*, ed. Luis García-Ballester, Roger French, Jon Arrizabalaga, and Andrew Cunningham (Cambridge: Cambridge University Press, 1994), pp. 156–85.

Oliver, Judith, *Gothic Manuscript Illumination in the Diocese of Liege (c.1250–c.1330)*, 2 vols. (Leuven: Uitgeverij Peeters, 1988–90).

Ong, Walter, 'Latin Language Study as a Renaissance Puberty Rite', *Studies in Philology* 56 (1959), 103–24.

Ordericus Vitalis, *The Ecclesiastical History*, ed. Marjorie Chibnall, 6 vols. (Oxford: Clarendon, 1969–80).

Ovid, *L'Art d'amours: Traduction et commentaire de l'Ars amatoria d'Ovide*, ed. Bruno Roy (Leiden: E. J. Brill, 1974).

Pächt, O., and J. J. G. Alexander, *Illuminated Manuscripts in the Bodleian Library*, Oxford, vol. III British School (Oxford: Clarendon, 1973).

Palmer, Richard, 'Pharmacy in the Republic of Venice in the Sixteenth Century', in *The Medical Renaissance of the Sixteenth Century*, ed. A. Wear, R. K. French, and I. M. Lonie (Cambridge: Cambridge University Press, 1985), 100–17.

Paré, Ambroise, *Briefve collection de l'administration anatomique, avec la maniere de conjoindre les os: et d'extraire les enfans tant mors que vivans du ventre de la mere, lors que nature de soy ne peult venir a son effect . . .* (Paris: Guillaume Cavellat, 1550).

Park, Katharine, *Doctors and Medicine in Early Renaissance Florence* (Princeton: Princeton University Press, 1985).

―――― 'The Rediscovery of the Clitoris: French Medicine and the *Tribade*, 1570–1620', in David Hillman and Carla Mazzio, eds., *The Body in Parts: Fantasies of Corporeality in Early Modern Europe* (New York: Routledge, 1997), pp. 171–93.

―――― 'Medicine and Magic: The Healing Arts', in *Gender and Society in Renaissance Italy*, ed. Judith C. Brown and Robert C. Davis (London: Longman, 1998), pp. 129–49.

―――― *Secrets of Women: Gender, Generation, and the Origins of Human Dissection* (New York: Zone Books, 2006).

Parkes, M. B., 'The Literacy of the Laity', in *Literature and Western Civilization*, vol. II: *The Mediaeval World*, ed. David Daiches and Anthony Thorlby (London: Aldus, 1973), pp. 555–77; repr. in M. B. Parkes, *Scribes, Scripts and Readers: Studies in the Communication, Presentation and Dissemination of Medieval Texts* (London/Rio Grande, Ohio: The Hambledon Press, 1991), pp. 275–298.

Pasca, Maria (ed.), *La Scuola medica salernitana: storia, immagini, manoscritti dall'XI al XIII secolo* (Naples: Electa Napoli, 1988).

Paviot, Jacques, 'Les livres de Jeanne de Chalon, comtesse de Tonnerre (v. 1388–v. 1450)', in P. Henriet and A.-M. Legras, eds., *Au cloître et dans le monde. Femmes, hommes et société (IXe–XVe siècle). Mélanges en l'honneur de Paulette L'Hermite-Leclercq*, Cultures et civilisations médiévales, 23 (Paris: Presses de l'Université de Paris-Sorbonne, 2000), pp. 247–56.

Payer, Pierre J., *The Bridling of Desire: Ideas of Sex in the Later Middle Ages* (Toronto: University of Toronto Press, 1993).

Pedersen, Else Marie Wiberg, 'The In-carnation of Beatrice of Nazareth's Theology', in *New Trends in Feminine Spirituality: The Holy Women of Liège and their Impact*, ed. Juliette Dor, Lesley Johnson, and Jocelyn Wogan-Browne, Medieval Women: Texts and Contexts, 2 (Turnhout: Brepols, 1999), pp. 61–79.

Pelling, Margaret, 'The Women of the Family? Speculations around Early Modern British Physicians', *Social History of Medicine* 8, no. 3 (Dec. 1995), 383–401.

―――― with Frances White, *Medical Conflicts in Early Modern London: Patronage, Physicians, and Irregular Practitioners, 1550–1640* (Oxford: Clarendon Press; New York: Oxford University Press, 2003).

Penketh, Sandra, 'Women and Books of Hours', in Jane H. M. Taylor and Lesley Smith, eds., *Women and the Book: Assessing the Visual Evidence* (London: British Library, 1997), pp. 266–80.

Pesenti, Tiziana, 'Le *Divisiones librorum Ypocratis* nei commenti all'*Articella*', *Medicina nei secoli* 14 (2002), 417–37.

Pesenti Marangon, Tiziana, 'Michele Savonarola a Padova: L'ambiente, le opere, la cultura medica', *Quaderni per la Storia dell'Università di Padova* 9–10 (1976–7), 45–102, plus genealogical tables.

Pfeilsticker, Walther, 'Eine württembergische Hebammenordnung von *c.*1480: Ein weiterer Beitrag zu Georg Burckhards *Hebammenordnungen*', *Archiv für Geschichte der Medizin* 20 (1928), 95–8.

Pierro, Francesco, 'Nuovi contributi alla conoscenza delle medichesse nel regno di Napoli negli ultimi tre secoli del medioevo', *Archivio Storico Pugliese* 17, fasc. 1–4 (1964), 231–41.

Pizan, Christine de, *The Book of the City of Ladies*, trans. Earl Jeffrey Richards (New York: Persea, 1982).

Pomata, Gianna, *Contracting a Cure: Patients, Healers, and the Law in Early Modern Bologna*, translated by the author, with the assistance of Rosemarie Foy and Anna Taraboletti-Segre (Baltimore: Johns Hopkins University Press, 1998).

Powell, Morgan, 'The Mirror and the Woman: Instruction for Religious Women and the Emergence of Vernacular Poetics, 1120–1250', PhD dissertation, Princeton University, 1997.

—— 'The *Speculum virginum* and the Audio-Visual Poetics of Women's Religious Instruction', in *Listen Daughter: The 'Speculum virginum' and the Formation of Religious Women in the Middle Ages*, ed. Constant J. Mews (New York: Palgrave, 2001), pp. 111–36.

Power, Eileen, 'Some Women Practitioners of Medicine in the Middle Ages', *Proceedings of the Royal Society of Medicine* 15, no. 6 (April 1922), 20–3.

Pratt, Robert A., 'Jankyn's Book of Wikked Wyves: Medieval Antimatrimonial Propaganda in the Universities', *Annuale mediaevale* 3 (1962), 5–27.

Processus Canonizationis et legendae variae Sancti Ludovici O.F.M., Episcopi Tolosani, Analecta Franciscana, vol. 7 (Quaracchi/Florence: Fratri Collegii S. Bonaventurae, 1951).

Rankin, Alisha Michelle, 'Medicine for the Uncommon Woman: Experience, Experiment, and Exchange in Early Modern Germany', PhD dissertation, Harvard University, 2005.

Rasmussen, Ann Marie, *Mothers and Daughters in Medieval German Literature* (Syracuse: Syracuse University Press, 1997).

Rawcliffe, Carole, *Medicine and Society in Later Medieval England* (Phoenix Mill: Alan Sutton, 1995).

Raynalde, Thomas (ed. and trans.), *The Byrth of Mankynde, Otherwyse Named the Womans Booke. Newly set furth, corrected and augmented* (London: Thomas Raynalde, 1545).

Reynaert, Joris, '*Der vrouwen heimelijcheit* als secundaire bron in de Zuid-Nederlandse bewerking van de *Chirurgia Magna* van Lanfranc van Milaan', in *Verslagen en Mededelingen van de Koninklijke academie voor Nederlandse Taal- en Letterkunde* 111, no. 1 (2001), pp. 165–88.

Reynolds-Cornell, Regine, 'Les Misères de la femme mariée: Another Look at Nicole Liébault and a Few Questions about the Woes of the Married Woman', *Bibliothèque d'Humanisme et Renaissance* 64, no. 1, 2002, 37–54.

Riehl, L. D., 'John Argentein and Learning in Medieval Cambridge', *Humanistica Lovaniensia* 33 (1984), 71–85.

Ritzinger, E. and H. C. Scheeben, 'Beitrage zur Geschichte der Teutonia in der zweiten Hälfte des 13. Jahrhunderts', *Archiv der deutschen Dominikaner* 3 (1941), 11–95.

Robbins, Rossell Hope, 'The Poems of Humfrey Newton, Esquire, 1466–1536', *Publications of the Modern Languages Association of America* 65 (1950), 249–81.

Roberts, Julian, and Andrew G. Watson (eds.), *John Dee's Library Catalogue* (London: Bibliographical Society, 1990).

Rollo-Koster, Joëlle, 'The Women of Papal Avignon. A New Source: The *Liber divisionis* of 1371', *Journal of Women's History* 8 (1996), 36–59.

Rosenthal, Carl Oskar, 'Zur geburtshilflich-gynaekologischen Betätigung des Mannes bis zum Ausgange des 16. Jahrhunderts', *Janus* 27 (1923), 117–48 and 192–212.

Rosenthal, Joel, 'Mediaeval Longevity and the Secular Peerage, 1350–1400', *Population Studies* 27 (1973), 287–93.

Rösslin, Eucharius, *Der Swangern Frauwen und hebammen Rosegarten*, facsimile reproduction of the 1513 Strasburg edition, ed. Huldrych M. Koelbing (Zürich: Verlag Bibliophile Drucke von J. Stocker, 1976).

Rothwell, W., 'Anglo-French and Middle English Vocabulary in *Femina nova*', *Medium Aevum* 69 (2000), 34–58.

Rouse, Mary A., and Richard H. Rouse, 'The Book Trade at the University of Paris, *c.*1250–*c.*1350', in Rouse and Rouse, *Authentic Witnesses: Approaches to Medieval Texts and Manuscripts* (Notre Dame, Indiana: University of Notre Dame Press, 1991), pp. 259–338.

Rouse, Richard H., and Mary A. Rouse, *Manuscripts and their Makers: Commercial Book Producers in Medieval Paris, 1200–1500*, 2 vols. (Turnhout: Harvey Miller, 2000).

Rubin, Miri, 'The Person in the Form: Medieval Challenges to Bodily "Order"', in *Framing Medieval Bodies*, ed. Sarah Kay and Miri Rubin (Manchester: Manchester University Press, 1994), pp. 100–22.

Saenger, Paul, *Space between Words: The Origins of Silent Reading* (Stanford, CA: Stanford University Press, 1997).

Saint-Denis, Alain, *L'Hôtel-Dieu de Laon, 1150–1300: Institution hospitalière et société aux XIIe et XIIIe siècles* (Nancy: Presses Universitaires de Nancy, 1983).

Salvat, Michel, 'L'Accouchement dans la littérature scientifique médiévale', *Senefiance* 9 (1980), 87–106.

Saunier, Annie, 'Le visiteur, les femmes et les "obstetrices" des paroisses de l'archidiaconé de Josas de 1458 à 1470', in *Santé, médecine et assistance au moyen âge, Actes du 110ᵉ Congrès National des Sociétés Savantes, Montpellier, 1985,* Section d'histoire médiévale et de philologie, 2 vols. (Paris: Editions du C.T.H.S., 1987), 1:43–62.

Savonarola, Michele, *Practica maior* (Venice: Vincentius Valgrisium, 1561).

——*Il trattato ginecologico-pediatrico in volgare 'Ad mulieres ferrarienses de regimine pregnantium et noviter natorum usque ad septennium'*, ed. Luigi Belloni (Milan: Società Italiana di ostetricia e ginecologia, 1952).

Schalick, Walton O, III, 'The Face Behind the Mask: 13th- and 14th-Century European Medical Cosmetology and Physiognomy', in *Medicine and the History of the Body: Proceedings of the 20th, 21st and 22nd International Symposium on the Comparative History of Medicine, East and West*, ed. Yasuo Otsuka, Shizu Sakai, and Shigehisa Kuriyama (Tokyo: Ishiyaku EuroAmerica, 1999), pp. 295–312.

Schenck, Johannes, *Elenchus auctorum in re medica cluentium, qui gynaecia scriptis clararunt et illustrarunt*, published in Joannes Andernacus Guinterius (1487–1574), *Gynaeciorum commentarius, de gravidarum, parturientium puerperarum et infantium, cura. Nunc primum a Schenkiana bibliotheca in lucem emissus.* (Strasburg: Lazar Zetzner, 1609), pp. 37–56.

Schenck, Johannes Georg, *[PINAX] auctorum in re medica, graecorum, latinorum priscorum, Arabum, Latinobarbarum, Latinorum recentiorum, tum et peregrinis linguis cluentium, Exstantium, MS. promissorum vel desideratorum: qui gynaecia, sive muliebria pleno argumento sive ex instituto scriptis excoluerunt et illustrarent* (Strasburg: Lazar Zetzner, 1606).

Schleissner, Margaret R., 'Pseudo-Albertus Magnus: *Secreta mulierum cum commento*, Deutsch: Critical text and commentary', PhD dissertation, Princeton University, 1987.

——— 'A Fifteenth-Century Physician's Attitude Toward Sexuality: Dr. Johann Hartlieb's *Secreta mulierum* Translation', in *Sex in the Middle Ages*, ed. Joyce A. Salisbury (New York: Garland, 1991), pp. 110–25.

Schmidt, Erich W. G., *Die Bedeutung Wilhems von Brescia als Verfasser von Konsilien. Untersuchung über einen medizinischen Schriftsteller des XIII.–XIV. Jarhhunderts*, inaugural-dissertation (Leipzig: Emil Lehmann, 1922).

Schnell, Bernhard, 'Die volkssprachliche Medizinliteratur des Mittelalters—Wissen für wen?', in *Laienlektüre und Buchmarkt im späten Mittelalter*, ed. Thomas Kock and Rita Schlusemann (Frankfurt am Main: Peter Lang, 1997), pp. 129–45.

Schum, Wilhelm, *Beschreibendes Verzeichniss der amplonianischen Handschriften-Sammlung zu Erfurt . . .* (Berlin: Weidmann, 1887).

Scott, Kathleen L., *Later Gothic Manuscripts 1390–1490*, 2 vols., *A Survey of Manuscripts Illuminated in the British Isles*, general ed., J. J. G. Alexander, VI (London: Harvey Miller, 1998).

Seebohm, Almuth, *Apokalypse, Ars moriendi, Medizinische Traktate, Tugend- und Lasterlehren: Die erbaulich-didaktische Sammelhandschrift, London, Wellcome Institute for the History of Medicine, Ms. 49* (Munich: H. Lengenfelder, 1995).

Sharpe, Richard, *A Handlist of the Latin Writers of Great Britain and Ireland before 1540* (Turnhout: Brepols, 1997).

Shatzmiller, Joseph, *Médecine et justice en Provence médiévale: Documents de Manosque, 1262–1348* (Aix-en-Provence: Publications de l'Université de Provence, 1989).

——— and Rodrigue Lavoie, 'Médecine et gynécologie au moyen-âge: un exemple provençal', *Razo: Cahiers du Centre d'Études Médiévales de Nice*, no. 4 (Nice: Faculté des Lettres et Sciences Humaines, Université de Nice, 1984), 133–43.

Sheridan, Bridgette Ann Majella, 'Childbirth, Midwifery, and Science: The Life and Work of the French Royal Midwife Louise Bourgeois (1563–1636)', PhD dissertation, Boston College, 2002.

Sherman, Claire Richter, 'The Queen in Charles V's "Coronation Book": Jeanne de Bourbon and the "Ordo ad reginam benedicendam" ', *Viator* 8 (1977), 255–99 and plates.

Siegemund, Justine, *The Court Midwife*, ed. and trans. Lynne Tatlock (University of Chicago Press, 2005).

Sigal, Pierre André, 'La grossesse, l'accouchement et l'attitude envers l'enfant mort-né à la fin du moyen âge d'après les récits de miracles', in *Santé, médecine et assistance au moyen âge, Actes du 110ᵉ Congrès National des Sociétés Savantes, Montpellier, 1985* (Paris: Editions du CTHS, 1987), pp. 23–41.

Sigerist, Henry E., 'Johannes Hartlieb's Gynaecological Collection and the Johns Hopkins Manuscript 3 (38066)', in *Science, Medicine and History: Essays on the Evolution of*

Scientific Thought and Medical Practice in Honor of Charles Singer, ed. E. A. Underwood, 2 vols. (London and New York: Oxford University Press, 1953), 1:231–46.

Signori, Gabriela, 'Defensivgemeinschten: Kreißende, Hebammen und "Mitweiber" im Spiegel spätmittelalterlicher Geburtswunder', *Das Mittelalter* 1 (1996), 113–34.

Simons, Walter, *Cities of Ladies: Beguine Communities in the Medieval Low Countries, 1200–1565* (Philadelphia: University of Pennsylvania Press, 2001).

Singer, Charles, and Dorothea Singer, 'The Origin of the Medical School of Salerno, the First University: An Attempted Reconstruction', in *Essays on the History of Medicine Presented to Karl Sudhoff on the Occasion of His Seventieth Birthday November 26th 1923*, ed. Charles Singer and Henry E. Sigerist (London: Oxford University Press, 1924; repr. Freeport, NY: Books for Libraries Press, 1968), pp. 121–38.

Siraisi, Nancy G., *Taddeo Alderotti and His Pupils: Two Generations of Italian Medical Learning* (Princeton: Princeton University Press, 1981).

_____ 'How to Write a Latin Book on Surgery: Organizing Principles and Authorial Devices in Guglielmo da Saliceto and Dino del Garbo', in *Practical Medicine from Salerno to the Black Death*, ed. Luis García-Ballester, Roger French, Jon Arrizabalaga, and Andrew Cunningham (Cambridge: Cambridge University Press, 1994), pp. 88–109.

Skinner, Patricia, 'Women, Literacy and Invisibility in Southern Italy, 900–1200', in Lesley Smith and Jane H. M. Taylor, eds., *Women, the Book and the Worldly: Selected Proceedings of the St Hilda's Conference, 1993*, vol. 2 (Cambridge: D. S. Brewer, 1995), pp. 1–11.

Solterer, Helen, *The Master and Minerva: Disputing Women in French Medieval Culture* (Berkeley: University of California Press, 1995).

Soranus of Ephesus, *Soranus' Gynecology*, trans. Owsei Temkin (Baltimore: Johns Hopkins University Press, 1956; repr. 1991).

Spach, Israel, *Nomenclator scriptorum medicorum. Hoc est: Elenchus eorum, qui artem medicam suis scriptis illustrarunt, secundum locos communes ipsius Medicinae; cum duplici Indice et rerum et authorum* (Frankfurt: Nicolaus Bassaeus and Lazarus Zetznerus, 1591).

_____ (ed.), *Gynaeciorum sive de Mulierum tum communibus, tum gravidarum, parientium et puerperarum affectibus et morbis libri Graecorum, Arabum, Latinorum veterum et recentium quotquot extant, partim nunc primum editi, partim vero denuo recogniti, emendati* (Strasburg: Lazarus Zetzner, 1597).

Stabile, G., 'Bonaccioli, Ludovico', *Dizionario biografico degli Italiani*, vol. 11 (1969), pp. 456–58.

Staden, Heinrich von, *Herophilus: The Art of Medicine in Early Alexandria* (Cambridge: Cambridge University Press, 1989).

_____ 'Women and Dirt', *Helios* 19, no. 1–2 (1992), 7–29.

Stock, Brian. *The Implications of Literacy: Written Language and Models of Interpretation in the Eleventh and Twelfth Centuries* (Princeton: Princeton University Press, 1983).

Stolberg, Michael, 'A Woman Down to Her Bones: The Anatomy of Sexual Difference in Early Modern Europe', *Isis* 94 (2003), 274–99.

Stoneman, William P., *Dover Priory*, Corpus of British Medieval Library Catalogues, 5 (London: British Library, 1999).

Strocchia, Sharon, 'Gender and the Rites of Honour in Italian Renaissance Cities', in *Gender and Society in Renaissance Italy*, ed. Judith C. Brown and Robert C. Davis, Women and Men in History Series (London and New York: Longman, 1998), pp. 39–60.

Strohm, Paul, *Social Chaucer* (Cambridge, MA: Harvard University Press, 1989).

Stoudt, Debra L., 'The Production and Preservation of Letters by Fourteenth-Century Dominican Nuns', *Mediaeval Studies* 53 (1991), 309–26.

——— 'Medieval German Women and the Power of Healing', in *Women Healers and Physicians: Climbing a Long Hill*, ed. Lilian R. Furst (Lexington: University of Kentucky Press, 1997), pp. 13–42.

Sudhoff, Karl, 'Ein Fruchtbarkeitsregimen für Margaretha, Markgräfin von Brandenburg', *Sudhoffs Archiv* 9 (1915–16), 356–9.

Summit, Jennifer, *Lost Property: The Woman Writer and English Literary History, 1380–1589* (Chicago: University of Chicago Press, 2000).

Taglia, Kathryn, 'Delivering a Christian Identity: Midwives in Northern French Synodal Legislation, *c.*1200–1500', in Peter Biller and Joseph Ziegler, eds., *Religion and Medicine in the Middle Ages*, York Studies in Medieval Theology, 3 (York: York Medieval Press, 2001), pp. 77–90.

Talbot, C. H., and E. A. Hammond, *The Medical Practitioners in Medieval England: A Biographical Register* (London: Wellcome Historical Medical Library, 1965).

Thomas de Cantimpré, *Liber de natura rerum: Editio princeps secundum codices manuscriptos*, vol. I: *Text*, ed. Helmut Boese (New York and Berlin: De Gruyter, 1973).

Thomasset, Claude (ed.), *Placides et Timéo ou Li secrés as philosophes: Edition critique avec introduction et notes* (Geneva and Paris: Droz, 1980).

——— *Une vision du monde à la fin du XIIIe siècle: Commentaire du Dialogue de 'Placides et Timéo'* (Geneva: Droz, 1982).

Thompson, Guy Llewelyn, *Paris and its People Under English Rule: The Anglo-Burgundian Regime 1420–1436*, Oxford Historical Monographs (Oxford: Clarendon, 1991).

Thorndike, Lynn, 'Further Consideration of the *Experimenta, Speculum astronomiae*, and *De secretis mulierum* Ascribed to Albertus Magnus', *Speculum* 30 (1955), 413–43.

Tovar, Claude de, 'Les versions françaises de la *Chirurgia parva* de Lanfranc de Milan. Étude de la tradition manuscrite', *Revue d'Histoire des Textes* 12–13 (1982–83), 195–262.

Traister, Barbara, ' "Matrix and the Pain Thereof": A Sixteenth-Century Gynaecological Essay', *Medical History* 35 (1991), 436–51.

Tuchman, Arleen Marcia, 'Situating Gender: Marie E. Zakrzewska and the Place of Science in Women's Medical Education', *Isis* 95 (2004), 34–57.

Turner, D. H., 'The Eric Millar Bequest to the Department of Manuscripts. I. The Medieval and Renaissance Manuscripts', *British Museum Quarterly* 33 (1968–9), 16–37 and pl. 8.

Uebel, Michael, 'Pornography', in *Dictionary of the Middle Ages. Supplement I*, William C. Jordan, editor-in-chief (New York: Charles Scribner's Sons, 2004), pp. 490–3.

Ussery, Huling E., *Chaucer's Physician: Medicine and Literature in Fourteenth-Century England*, Tulane Studies in English 19 (New Orleans: Tulane University, Department of English, 1971).

Valesco de Taranta, *Philonium* (Lyons: Scipio de Gabiano, 1535).

Valgelas, Claude, *Commentaire de la conservation de santé, et prolongation de vie* (Lyons, 1559).

Valls, Helen, 'Studies on Roger Frugardi's *Chirurgia*', PhD dissertation, University of Toronto, 1995.

van de Walle, Etienne, and Elisha P. Renne (eds.), *Regulating Menstruation: Beliefs, Practices, Interpretations* (Chicago: University of Chicago Press, 2001).

Van Hollen, Cecilia, 'Invoking *Vali*: Painful Technologies of Modern Birth in South India', *Medical Anthropology Quarterly*, n.s. 17, no. 1 (March 2003), 49–77.

van Houts, Elisabeth, 'Gender and Authority of Oral Witnesses in Europe (800–1300)', *Transactions of the Royal Historical Society*, Sixth Series 9 (1999), 201–20.

Veit, Raphaela. 'Quellenkundliches zu Leben und Werk von Constantinus Africanus', *Deutsches Archiv für Erforschung des Mittelalters* 59 (2003), 121–52.

Vielliard, Jeanne, and Marie-Henriette Jullien de Pommerol (eds.), *Le Registre de prêt de la Bibliothèque de Collège de Sorbonne (1402–1536)* (Paris: CNRS, 2000).

Vietor, Agnes C. (ed.), *A Woman's Quest: The Life of Marie E. Zakrzewska, MD* (New York: D. Appleton and Co., 1924; repr. New York: Arno Press, 1972).

Viganò, Anna, Patrizia Tomba, and Luciano Merlini, 'A Manuscript Worth a Villa: Vittorio Putti's Acquisition of the Guy de Chauliac Manuscript', *Acta orthopaedica Scandinavica* 70, no. 6 (December 1999), 531–5.

Voigts, Linda Ehrsam, 'Multitudes of Middle English Medical Manuscripts, or the Englishing of Science and Medicine', in *Manuscript Sources of Medieval Medicine: A Book of Essays*, ed. Margaret R. Schleissner, Garland Medieval Casebooks, 8 (New York: Garland,1995), pp. 183–95.

—— 'What's the Word? Bilingualism in Late-Medieval England', *Speculum* 1:4 (1996), 813–26.

—— and Patricia Deery Kurtz, (eds.), *Scientific and Medical Writings in Old and Middle English: An Electronic Reference*, The Society for Early English and Norse Electronic Texts, CD-ROM (Ann Arbor: University of Michigan Press, 2000).

Wack, Mary F., 'The Measure of Pleasure: Peter of Spain on Men, Women, and Lovesickness', *Viator* 17 (1986), 173–96.

—— *Lovesickness in the Middle Ages: The 'Viaticum' and its Commentaries* (Philadelphia: University of Pennsylvania Press, 1990).

Webber,T., and A. G. Watson, *The Libraries of the Augustinian Canons*, Corpus of British Medieval Library Catalogues, 6 (London: British Library, 1998).

Weckerin, Anna, *Ein Köstlich new Kochbuch von allerhand Speisen . . . fürnehmlich vor Krancke in allerlay Krankheiten und Gebrästen; auch Schwangere Weiber, Kindbetterinnen und alte schwache Leute* (Amberg, 1598; repr. Munich, 1977).

Weisheipl, James A. (ed.), *Albertus Magnus and the Sciences: Commemorative Essays, 1980*, Studies and Texts 49 (Toronto: Pontifical Institute of Mediaeval Studies, 1980).

Wells, Susan, *Out of the Dead House: Nineteenth-Century Women Physicians and the Writing of Medicine* (Madison: University of Wisconsin Press, 2001).

Wheeler, Bonnie (ed.), *Listening to Heloise: The Voice of a Twelfth-Century Woman* (New York: St Martin's, 2000).

Wickersheimer, Ernest, 'Les secrets et conseils de maître Guillaume Boucher et de ses confrères: Contribution à l'histoire de la médecine à Paris vers 1400', *Bulletin de la Société Française d'Histoire de la Médecine* 8 (1909), 199–305.

Wickersheimer, Ernest, 'La descente de matrice d'une bourgeoise de Paris et la monstre bicéphale d'Aubervilliers. Deux observations du XV siècle', *Progrès Médical* no. 47 (Nov. 17, 1931), p. 2099.

_____ *Dictionnaire biographique des médecins en France au Moyen Age*, 2 vols. (1936; repr. Geneva: Librairie Droz, 1979).

Wiesner, Merry E., 'The Midwives of Southern Germany and the Private/Public Dichotomy', in *The Art of Midwifery*, ed. Hilard Marland (London: Routledge, 1993), pp. 77–94.

_____ *Women and Gender in Early Modern Europe*, 2nd edn. (Cambridge: Cambridge University Press, 2000).

Wiethaus, Ulrike, 'Street Mysticism: An Introduction to *The Life and Revelations* of Agnes Blannbekin', in *Women Writing Latin from Roman Antiquity to Early Modern Europe*, vol. 2: *Medieval Women Writing Latin*, ed. Laurie J. Churchill, Phyllis R. Brown, and Jane E. Jeffrey (New York: Routledge, 2002), pp. 281–307.

William of Saliceto, *Summa conseruationis; Chirurgia* (Piacenza: Johannes Petrus de Ferriatis, 1476).

Wilson, Adrian, 'William Hunter and the Varieties of Man-Midwifery', in W. F. Bynum and Roy Porter (eds.), *William Hunter and the Eighteenth-Century Medical World* (Cambridge: Cambridge University Press, 1985), pp. 343–69.

_____ *The Making of Man-Midwifery: Childbirth in England, 1660–1770* (Cambridge, MA: Harvard University Press, 1995).

_____ 'A Memorial of Eleanor Willughby, a Seventeenth-Century Midwife', in *Women, Science and Medicine, 1500–1700: Mothers and Sisters of the Royal Society*, ed. Lynette Hunter and Sarah Hutton (Phoenix Mill: Sutton, 1997), 138–77.

Wilson, R. M., 'The Medieval Library of Titchfield Abbey', *Proceedings of the Leeds Philosophical and Literary Society. Literary and Historical Section* 5/3 (February 1940), 150–77 and 5/4 (June 1941), 252–76.

Witt, Ronald G., '*In the Footsteps of the Ancients': The Origins of Humanism from Lovato to Bruni*, Studies in Medieval and Reformation Thought, 74 (Brill: Leiden, 2000).

Wogan-Browne, Jocelyn, ' "Reading is Good Prayer": Recent Research on Female Reading Communities', *New Medieval Literatures* 5 (2002), 229–97.

_____ Nicholas Watson, Andrew Taylor, and Ruth Evans (eds.), *The Idea of the Vernacular: An Anthology of Middle English Literary Theory, 1280–1520* (University Park, PA: Pennsylvania State University Press, 1999).

Wolf, Caspar (ed.), *Gynaeciorum, hoc est de Mulierum tum aliis, tum gravidarum, parientium et puerperarum affectibus et morbis libri veterum ac recentiorem aliquot, partim nunc primum editi, partim multo quam ante castigatiores* . . . (Basel: Thomas Guarinus, 1566).

Wölfel, Hans, *Das Arzneidrogenbuch 'Circa instans' in einer Fassung des XIII. Jahrhunderts aus der Universitätsbibliothek Erlangen. Text und Kommentar als Beitrag zur Pflanzen- und Drogenkunde des Mittelalters* (Berlin: A. Preilipper, 1939).

Woods, Marjorie Currie, 'Rape and the Pedagogical Rhetoric of Sexual Violence', in *Criticism and Dissent in the Middle Ages*, ed. Rita Copeland (Cambridge: Cambridge University Press, 1996), pp. 56–86.

_____ 'Shared Books, Primers, Psalters, and the Adult Acquisition of Literacy among Devout Laywomen and Women in Orders in Late Medieval England', in *New Trends in Feminine Spirituality: The Holy Women of Liège and Their Impact*, ed. Juliette Dor, Lesley Johnson, and Jocelyn Wogan-Browne, Medieval Women: Texts and Contexts, 2 (Turnhout: Brepols, 1999), pp. 177–93.

Worth-Stylianou, Valérie, *Les Traités d'obstétrique en langue française au seuil de la modernité. Bibliographie critique des 'Divers Travaulx' d'Euchaire Rosslin (1536) à l' 'Apologie de Louyse Bourgeois sage-femme' (1627)* (Geneva: Droz, 2006).

Yearl, Mary K. K. H., 'The Time of Bloodletting', PhD dissertation, Yale University, 2005.

York, William Henry, 'Experience and Theory in Medical Practice during the Later Middle Ages: Valesco de Tarenta (fl. 1382–1426) at the Court of Foix (France)', PhD dissertation, The Johns Hopkins University, 2003.

Youngs, Deborah [*see also* Marsh, Deborah], 'Servants and Labourers on a Late Medieval Demesne: The Case of Newton, Cheshire, 1498–1520', *Agricultural History Review* 47 (2000), 145–60.

Ziegler, Joseph, 'Practitioners and Saints: Medical Men in Canonization Processes in the Thirteenth to Fifteenth Centuries', *Social History of Medicine* 12 (1999), 191–225.

Zieman, Katherine, 'Reading, Singing and Understanding: Constructions of the Literacy of Women Religious in Late Medieval England', in *Learning and Literacy in Medieval England and Abroad*, ed. Sarah Rees Jones (Turnhout: Brepols, 2003), 97–120.

Zimmermann, Karin, 'Ein unbekannter Textzeuge der *Secreta mulierum* und *Trotula*-Übersetzung des Johannes Hartlieb in Cod. Pal. germ. 280', *Zeitschrift für deutsches Altertum* 131 (2002), 343–5.

General Index

Medieval figures up through ca. 1300 are indexed under the personal name. Anonymous texts are indexed under their title. Bold numbers denote reference to illustrations.

Index of Manuscripts Cited

Bold numbers denote reference to illustrations.